Short Review of TUMOUR

Third Edition

Rachna Chaurasia MD (Radiodiagnosis)
Lecturer
MLB Medical College, Jhansi, Uttar Pradesh, India
(Ex-Registrar, Indraprastha Apollo Hospital, New Delhi)

Anshul Jain MD (Anaesthesia)
Lecturer
MLB Medical College, Jhansi, Uttar Pradesh, India
(Ex-Senior Resident, Anaesthesiology
All India Institute of Medical Sciences, New Delhi)

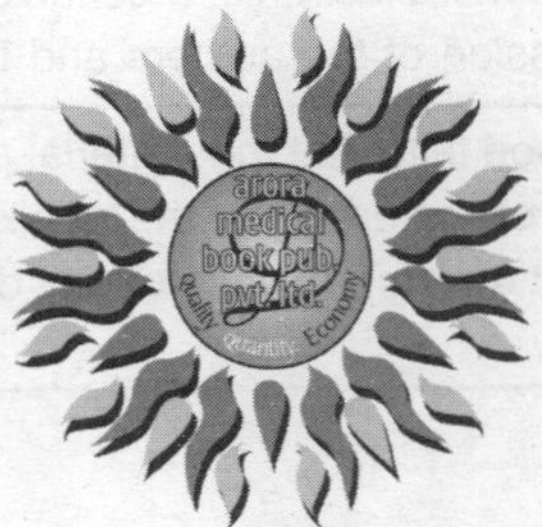

the arora medical book publishers pvt. ltd.
A Group of Jaypee Brothers Medical Publishers (P) Ltd.

Published by

Jitendar P Vij

Jaypee Brothers Medical Publishers (P) Ltd

Corporate Office

4838/24 Ansari Road, Daryaganj, **New Delhi** - 110002, India, Phone: +91-11-43574357
Fax: +91-11-43574314

Registered Office

B-3 EMCA House, 23/23B Ansari Road, Daryaganj, **New Delhi** - 110 002, India
Phones: +91-11-23272143, +91-11-23272703, +91-11-23282021
+91-11-23245672, Rel: +91-11-32558559, Fax: +91-11-23276490, +91-11-23245683
e-mail: jaypee@jaypeebrothers.com, Website: www.jaypeebrothers.com

Offices in India

- **Ahmedabad**, Phone: Rel: +91-79-32988717, e-mail: ahmedabad@jaypeebrothers.com
- **Bengaluru**, Phone: Rel: +91-80-32714073, e-mail: bangalore@jaypeebrothers.com
- **Chennai**, Phone: Rel: +91-44-32972089, e-mail: chennai@jaypeebrothers.com
- **Hyderabad**, Phone: Rel:+91-40-32940929, e-mail: hyderabad@jaypeebrothers.com
- **Kochi**, Phone: +91-484-2395740, e-mail: kochi@jaypeebrothers.com
- **Kolkata**, Phone: +91-33-22276415, e-mail: kolkata@jaypeebrothers.com
- **Lucknow**, Phone: +91-522-3040554, e-mail: lucknow@jaypeebrothers.com
- **Mumbai**, Phone: Rel: +91-22-32926896, e-mail: mumbai@jaypeebrothers.com
- **Nagpur**, Phone: Rel: +91-712-3245220, e-mail: nagpur@jaypeebrothers.com

Overseas Offices

- **North America Office, USA,** Ph: 001-636-6279734,
  e-mail: jaypee@jaypeebrothers.com, anjulav@jaypeebrothers.com
- **Central America Office, Panama City, Panama,** Ph: 001-507-317-0160
  e-mail: cservice@jphmedical.com Website: www.jphmedical.com
- **Europe Office, UK,** Ph: +44 (0) 2031708910
  e-mail: info@jpmedpub.com

Short Review of TUMOUR

Third Edition: **2010**

ISBN 978-93-5025-132-4

Typeset at JPBMP typesetting unit

Printed at Rajkamal Electric Press, Plot No. 2, Phase-IV, Kundli, Haryana.

Dedication

Dedicated

to

Our family members, teachers

and above all God

who created us

Contributors

We are extremely grateful to our teachers and seniors for contributing their knowledge, sharing their experiences and devoting their precious time for making our book errorfree and excellent.

Ganesh Kumar MD, MICR
Professor and Head, Department of Radiodiagnosis
MLB Medical College, Jhansi, Uttar Pradesh, India
Radiological Diagnosis

Sachin Mahour MD
Associate Professor and Head, Department of Radiotherapy
MLB Medical College, Jhansi, Uttar Pradesh, India
Cancer Radiotherapy

VC Pandit MCh
Consultant Neurosurgeon
Head and Neck Tumour

H Ramesh Gupte MCh
Consultant Paediatric Surgeon
Paediatric Tumour

Kamni Malhotra MS
Consultant Gynaecologist
Gynaecological Tumour

Ashok Sharma MD
Consultant Pathologist
Haematological Tumour

HK Bist MS
Consultant Ophthalmologist
Ophthalmic Tumour

Santosh Karnatak MS
Consultant, Orthopaedic Surgeon
Bone Tumour

Vikas Chaurasia MS
Consultant, ENT Surgeon
Oropharyngeal Tumour

Preface

"Schedule a daily time for relaxing, reflecting, planning and brainstorming"

Postgraduate Medical Entrance Examination (PGMEE) is a battlefield in which everyone fights for success but only few succeed because only few knew the correct use of weapon of "knowledge, hardwork and guidance".

So, guys learn the golden words:

Winners do things
What looser do not do

Similarities among various tumour provoked us to create a text which includes all tumour under one cover.

In every PGMEE, there are 10 to 15% questions of tumour and most of them are new. This book enables you to solve one of the most difficult aspect of examination.

Why this book is different?

- This book provides systemic approach to the tumour of whole body.
- Each chapter consists of theory followed by its questions, so theory portion helps in solving new questions.
- This pattern of book allows you to revise all tumour very quickly and efficiently.

How to use this book?

- Read the theory first then do questions. You realize that this way of learning makes topic easy to understand and easy to grasp for long-term memory.
- Try to complete each topic in one sitting.
- In the last, we would like to say 'All the Best' for your PGMEE preparation and hope you will work hard with positive attitude in your mind.

Always keep one thing in your mind:

"There's one thing, we cannot recycle and that's wasted time"

Acknowledgements

"To Bhagwan Mahavir and Ganesha whose blessing made our goal possible"

We will extremely grateful and obliged to our teachers

Dr Ganesh Kumar (Principal, MLB Medical College, Jhansi)
Dr Chandralekha (Prof and Head of Department, Anaesthesia, AIIMS, New Delhi)
Dr AK Gupta (Prof and Head of Department, Radiodiagnosis, SN Medical College, Agra)
Dr Dinesh Kapoor (Senior Consultant, Radiology, Indraprastha Apollo Hospital, New Delhi)
Dr Chhavi (Asstt Prof, Anaesthesia, JPN Trauma Centre, AIIMS, New Delhi)
Dr Babita (Asstt Prof, Anaesthesia, JPN Trauma Centre, AIIMS, New Delhi)
Dr Veena Gupta (Prof, Anaesthesia, MLB Medical College, Jhansi)
Dr Sachin Mahour (Lecturer Radiotherapy, MLB Medical College, Jhansi)

We would always remain obliged to our lifelong teachers Dr B C Tiwari, Dr Atish Sharma, Mr Amod Yadav
We would be extremely thankful to Dr Vikas Chaurasia, Dr Gaurav Tiwari whose inspiration makes the task possible.
We are higly grateful to our contributors for reviewing and updating the text.
We would like to thank the following students for their suggestion:

Dr Ashwin (Bengaluru)
Dr Priyadarshni (Chennai)
Dr Kiran Rao (Hyderabad)
Dr Manjeet Kaur (Amritsar)
Dr Akhlesh Yadav (Patna)
Dr Santosh (Mumbai)

We extend our sincere thanks and gratitude to our beloved family members for their encouragement and useful suggestions:

Father : Dr PC Chaurasia
Mother : Mrs Shakuntla Chaurasia
Uncle and Aunty : Mr Subhash Chandra Chaurasia and Mrs Rashmi Chaurasia
Brother and Bhabhi : Dr Vikas Chaurasia and Dr Mrs Anahita Chaurasia, Mr Vishal Chaurasia and Mrs Kavita Chaurasia
Nephew and Niece : Priyanshu, Aashi and Paras

– Rachna Chaurasia

Father : Dr DB Jain
Mother : Mrs Saroj Jain
Sisters : Ayusha Jain and Ankita Jain
Brother : Mr Kapil Jain

– Anshul Jain

And above all to our little baby Riya whose innocence empower us in every moment.

We offer cordial thanks to our colleagues for their support:

Dr Apoorva Abhinandan Mittal, MD Anaesthesia (STD), BRDMC, Gorakhpur
Dr Ankur, Senior Resident, Orthopaediac, AIIMS, New Delhi
Dr Deepak Singhal, Senior Resident, Anaesthesia, JPN Trauma Centre, AIIMS, New Delhi
Dr Hazari M Shukla, Senior Resident, ESI Hospital, Delhi
Dr Kapil Soni, Senior Resident, Anaesthesia, JPN Trauma Centre, AIIMS, New Delhi
Dr Keshav, DM, Neuroanaesthesia (STD), AIIMS, New Delhi
Dr Manish Singhal, Senior Resident, General Surgery, AIIMS, New Delhi
Dr Naveen SR, Neuroanaesthesia, AIIMS, New Delhi
Dr Manoj Sharma, Registrar Radiodiagnosis, Apollo, New Delhi
Dr Sameer, DNB Radiodiagnosis (STD) Apollo, New Delhi
Dr Sachin Maheshwari, Senior Resident, Anaesthesia, GTB Hospital, New Delhi
Dr Saurabh Jain, DLO (STD), Safdarjung Hospital, New Delhi
Dr Tumul, DM Neuroanaesthesia (STD), AIIMS, New Delhi
Dr RK Singh, Dr Dushyant Agarwal, Dr Monika Agarwal, Dr Nidhi Singh, Dr Neha, Dr Anil Kumar Suryavanshi

We would like to acknowledge Mr Bhupesh Arora for his all time support.

We cannot forget to acknowledge:

Mr Bishan Lal (Librarian, MLB Medical College, Jhansi) and All Staff.
Mr CP Lavania (Librarian, SN Medical College, Agra) and All Staff.

We would also like to acknowledge: Mr Sandeep Tiwari, Mr Adeep Tiwari, Mr CP Lamba
Our gratitudes are due to Shri Jitendar P Vij (Chairman and Managing Director), Mr Tarun Duneja (Director-Publishing) and all staff members of our publisher M/s Jaypee Brothers Medical Publishers (P) Ltd who took keen interest in this project and for speedy completion of this mega task.

Last but not least, most important we gratefully acknowledge all readers, who will act as a guide to improve and upgrading the content of this book.

Contents

SECTION—D: MISCELLANEOUS ONCOLOGY

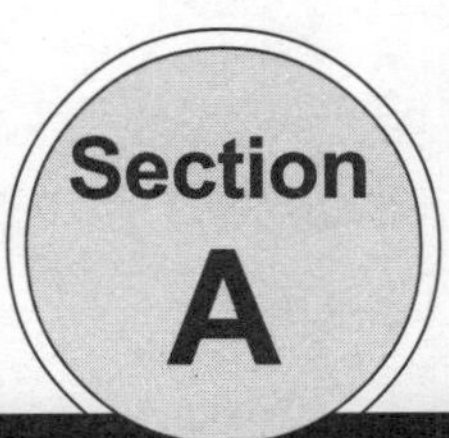

General Oncology

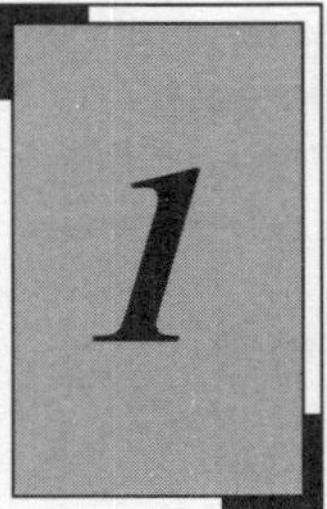

Cancer Cell Genetics and Biology

What's Important ?

- Names of Oncogenes and Tumour suppressor genes
- Rb and p53 genes, Telomerase
- Radiation carcinogenesis
- Tumour markers

Neoplasia is an *abnormal* mass of tissues, the growth of which exceeds and is uncoordinated than that of the normal tissues and persist in the same excessive manner even after cessation of the stimuli. *All neoplasm ultimately depend on the host for their nutrition and vascular supply.*

All tumours have two basic components	
Parenchyma	***Supportive stroma***
– Consist of proliferating neoplastic cells – Determine the *nature of tumour* – Form the basis of nomenclature	– Consist of connective tissue and blood vessels – Determine growth and evolution of tumour – If it is scanty, tumour is soft and fleshy while if it is abundant than it is called as ***desmoplasia***

DEFINITIONS

Benign Tumour : They are designated by attaching the suffix **-oma** to the cell of origin e.g. *fibroma; chondroma.*

Malignant Tumour :

- If arise from ***mesenchymal tissue*** then malignant tumour are called as Sarcoma.
- If arise from ***epithelial cell*** than called as Carcinoma.

Mixed Tumour : Arise by divergent differentiation of single line of parenchymal cells, usually they are *composed of cells representative of single germ layers* e.g. pleomorphic adenoma of salivary gland.

Teratoma : It consist of variety of parenchymal cells containing elements of *more than one germ layer,* usually all three. They arise from ***totipotential cells*** and so are principally encountered in the gonads, although rarely they occur in sequestered primitive cell nest elsewhere.

Choristoma : It is ***ectopic rest*** of normal tissue i.e. *normal tissue at abnormal place.*

Hamartoma : Mass of aberrantly differentiated but ***mature specialized cells*** / tissue indigenous to the particular site i.e. *abnormal tissue at normal place.* It is totally benign.

Differentiation and Anaplasia : Differentiation refers to the ***extent to which parenchymal cells resemble comparable normal cells*** both morphologically and functionally while anaplasia is lack of differentiation which includes *pleomorphism; hyperchromatism; atypical bizarre mitotic figures; tumour or division giant cell; loss of normal polarity.*

Remember : Anaplasia is considered a hallmark of malignant transformation.

Dysplasia

- It is disordered growth seen usually in the epithelium as a ***loss in the uniformity*** of individual cells as well as loss in their ***architectural orientation.***
- Dysplastic cells are hyperchromatic, pleomorphic, with abundant mitotic figures in abnormal locations but normal pattern.
- It is partially reversible and doesn't necessarily progress to cancer. When dysplastic changes are marked and involve the entire thickness of epithelium, the lesion is considered preinvasive precancerous, neoplasia known as carcinoma in situ.
- ***Carcinoma in situ*** displays the cytologic features of malignancy without invasion of the basement membrane or *with no tumour in sub epithelial stroma.*

Remember :
- Usually benign tumours are encapsulated except hemangioma.
- Usually malignant tumours metastasize except glioma (malignant neoplasm of glial cells in the CNS) and basal cell carcinoma. They are locally invasive.
- Metastasis is most reliable feature that differentiates malignant from benign tumours, Invasiveness is next reliable feature.
- *Most common* pathway for initial dissemination of carcinoma is lymphatic while that of sarcoma is hematogenous route.

MOLECULAR BASIS OF CANCER

Cancer genes : Genes which are related to human carcinogenesis

Growth promoting Oncogenes	***Growth inhibiting tumour suppressor gene***	***Genes that regulate programmed cell death***	***Genes involved in DNA repair***
(*Derived from proto Oncogenes*). They are dominant gene	They are recessive with few exceptions.	(*apoptosis*) They are dominant or recessive	

Characteristics of cancer genes :

i. Genetic damage or *mutation* should be *nonlethal.*

ii. Mutation cause clonal expansion of single precursor cell forming tumour so *"Tumors are monoclonal".*

Most commonly *used method to determine tumour clonality involves the analysis of methylation patterns adjacent to highly polymorphic locus of human androgen receptor gene (HUMARA).*

Remember :
- Loss of functions of tumour suppressor gene caused by damage of single allele is called ***haploinsufficiency.***
- DNA repair genes affect cell proliferation or survival indirectly by influencing the ability of organism to repair nonlethal damage. So defect in DNA repair genes can predispose to mutation in genome and hence to neoplastic transformation. Such propensity to mutation is called ***"Mutator phenotype."*** They are usually recessive.
- Carcinogenesis is multistep process at both phenotypic and genetic levels.

ESSENTIAL ALTERATIONS FOR MALIGNANT TRANSFORMATION

There are seven fundamental changes in cell physiology that together determine malignant phenotype.

Oncogenes are created by mutations in protooncogenes and are characterized by the ability to promote cell growth in the absence of normal growth promoting signals. Product of oncogenes (oncoproteins) resemble the normal product of protooncogenes except that oncoproteins are devoid of important internal regulatory elements.

1. Protooncogene involved in human cancer

Category of Oncoproteins	Protooncogene	Associated human tumour
Growth factors		
PDGF β chain	SIS	Astrocytoma, Osteosarcoma
Fibroblast growth factors	HST-1	Stomach cancer
	INT-2	Bladder cancer, Breast cancer, Melanoma
TGFα	TGFα	Astrocytomas, Hepatocellular carcinomas
HGF	HGF	Thyroid cancer
Growth Factor Receptors		
EGF-receptor family	ERB-B1 (EGFR)	Squamous cell carcinomas of lung, gliomas
	ERB-B2 (HER-2/Neu)	Breast and ovarian cancers
CSF-1receptor	FMS	Myeloid leukemia
Receptor for neurotrophic factors	RET	Multiple endocrine neoplasia 2A and B, familial medullary thyroid carcinomas, adrenal and parathyroid tumour
PDGF receptor	PDGF-R	Gliomas
Receptor for stem cell *(steel)* factor	KIT	Gastrointestinal stromal tumours and other soft tissue tumours
Proteins Involved in Signal Transduction		
GTP binding	K-RAS	Colon, lung, and pancreatic tumours
	H-RAS	Bladder and kidney tumours
	N-RAS	Melanomas, hematologic malignancies
Nonreceptor tyrosine kinase	ABL	Chronic myeloid leukemia (not CLL) Acute lymphoblastic leukemia, AML
RAS signal transduction	BRAF	Melanomas
WNT signal transduction	β-catenin	Hepatoblastomas, hepatocellular carcinoma

Nuclear Regulatory Proteins		
Transcriptional activators	C-MYC	Burkitt lymphoma; Mantle cell; follicular lymphoma ,T cell ALL
	N-MYC	Neuroblastoma, small cell carcinoma of lung
	L-MYC	Small cell carcinoma of lung
Cell-Cycle Regulators		
Cyclins	CYCLIN D	Mantle cell lymphoma, Breast and esophageal cancers,
	CYCLIN E	Breast cancer
Cyclin-dependent kinase	CDK4	Glioblastoma, melanoma, sarcoma
Others		
	FES, FOS, MLL, EWS, JUN, SRC gene	

Remember :
- In sporadic papillary thyroid carcinoma, cMET (growth factor receptor) is overexpressed in almost every case.
- Monoclonal antibodies can be directed against growth factors. This therapy is called ***Targeted therapy.*** Used in ***ERB-B2 or HER-2*** / Neu gene of breast and ovarian cancer; CKIT gene in stromal tumour of gastrointestinal tract.

Mechanism of some important oncoproteins

- ***GTP binding protein (G proteins) :*** RAS is signal transducing protein. It receives signals from outside the cell and transmit it to nucleus.
- Most common abnormality of dominant oncogene in human tumours is *point mutation of RAS family oncogene.*

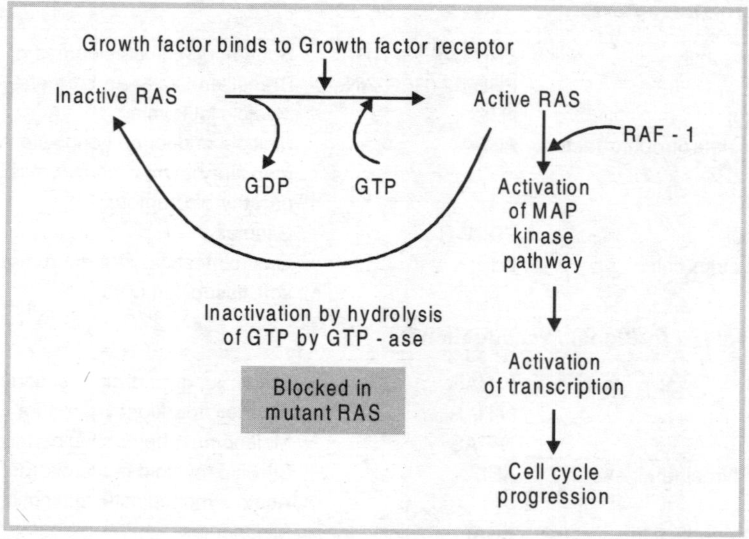

Inactive RAS is GDP bound. Active RAS is GTP bound with intrinsic GTP ase activity and GTP ase activating protein (GAP).

GAP function as brakes by converting GTP to GDP. So it prevents uncontrolled RAS activity which is lost in mutant RAS. Mutant RAS proteins bind GAP, but their GTP-ase activity fails to be augmented, so ras protein is entrapped in excited GTP bound form. This causes uncontrolled proliferation.

Remember :
- *Most common* gene involved in category of nuclear regulatory proteins is ***'Myc'.***
- *Protoncogene with role in apoptosis :* ***myc, abl.***

... Robbin's 6/e, p 282

2. **Insensitivity to growth inhibitory signals of tumour suppressor gene**

   To understand carcinogenesis by tumour suppressor recessive gene **Knudson** proposed ***"two hit"*** hypothesis of oncogenesis i.e. cancer associated with these recessive cancer genes occur only when cell becomes homozygous for mutant allele or cell loses heterozygosity for normal gene **(know as LOH).**

Tumour suppressor genes involved in Human neoplasms

Subcellular Location	Gene	Function	Tumors Associated
Cell surface	TGF-β receptor	Growth inhibition, Cell adhesion	Colon and gastric Ca
Inner aspect of plasma membrane	NF-1	Inhibition of RAS signal transduction and of p21 cell cycle inhibitor	Neuroblastomas, Neurofibromatosis type 1and sarcomas
Cytoskeleton	NF-2	Cytoskeletal stability	Schwannomas & meningiomas, Neurofibromatosis type 2
Cystosol	APC/β-catenin	Inhibition of signal transduction	Carcinomas of stomach colon, pancreas; melanoma Familial adenomatous polyposis coli colon cancer
	PTEN	PI-3 kinase signal transduction	Endometrial and prostate cancers
	SMAD2 and SMAD4	TGF-β signal transduction	Colon, pancreas tumours
Nucleus	RB 1	Regulation of cell cycle	Retinoblastoma; osteosarcoma, Glioblastoma, carcinomas of breast, colon, lung, bladder
	p53	Cell-cycle arrest and apoptosis in response to DNA damage	*Most human cancers,* ***Li-Fraumeni syndrome;*** multiple carcinomas and sarcomas
	WT-1	Nuclear transcription	Wilms tumour
	p16 (INK4a)	Regulation of cell cycle by inhibition of cyclin dependent kinases	Pancreatic, breast, esophageal cancers, Malignant melanoma
	BRCA-1 and BRCA-2	DNA repair	Carcinomas of female breast and ovary; prostate colon; carcinomas of male breast, melanoma
	KLF6	Transcription factor	Prostate

Mechanism of important tumour suppressor gene

RB Gene : It is *first tumour suppressor* gene discovered. It is located on chromosome 13 q 14.

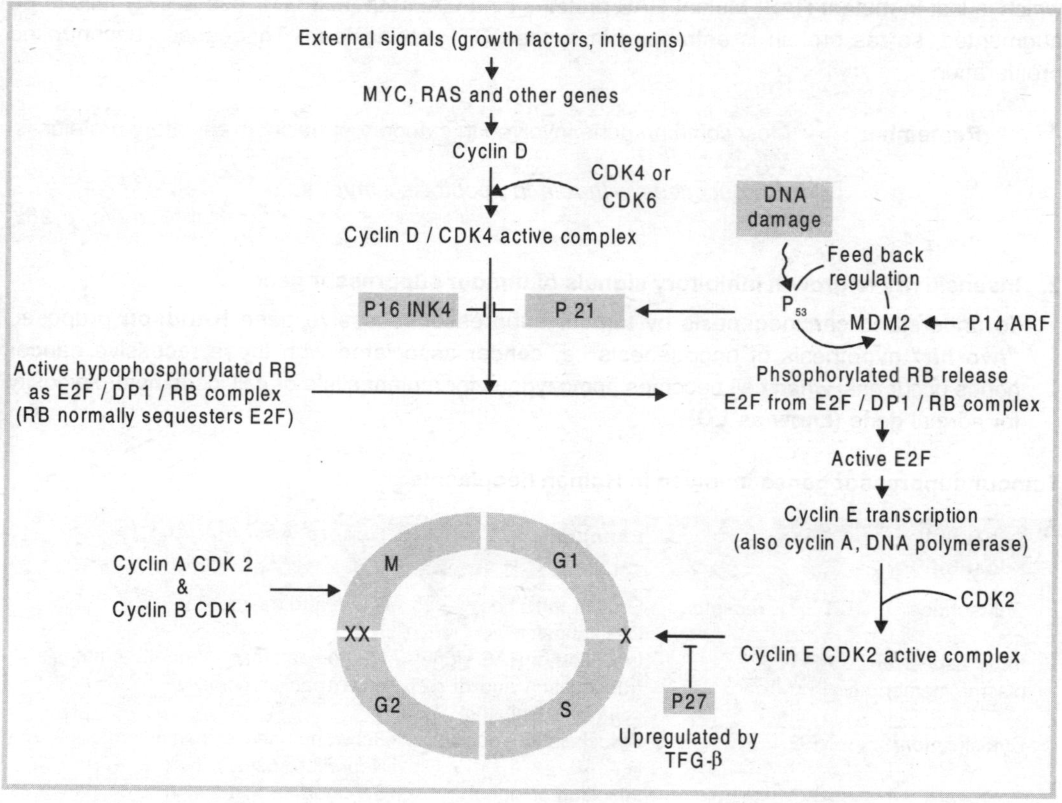

X : Denotes G_1 / S checkpoint which is mostly mediated by p53.

XX : Denotes G_2 / M checkpoint which involves both p53 dependent and independent mechanism.

Remember :
- Phosphorylation of RB is molecular ***ON-OFF switch*** for cell cycle.
- ***P_{53}*** act as ***G_1/S checkpoint*** allows cell for repair of DNA damage and prevent replication of cells with defective DNA. If damage is not repairable, apoptic pathways are activated.
- The ***main mediator*** that propels the cell beyond prophase is ***cyclin B- CDKI complex.***
- CDKs are expressed constitutively while cyclins are synthesized during specific phase of cell cycle.
- Cells damaged by ***ionizing*** radiation activate ***G_2/ M*** checkpoint and arrest in G_2 phase.

Main Cell-Cycle Components and their Inhibitors

Cell-Cycle Component	Main Function
Cyclin-Dependent Kinases	
• CDK4	Forms a complex with cyclin D. The complex phosphorylates or inactivate RB, allowing the cell to progress through the G_1 restriction point.
• CDK2	Forms a complex with cyclin E in late G_1, which is involved in the G/S transition. Forms a complex with cyclin A at the S phase that facilitates the G_2/M transition.
• CDK1	Forms a complex with cyclin B, which acts on the G_2/M transition.
Inhibitors	
• p21, p27	Block the cell cycle by binding to cyclin-CDK complexes. p21 is induced by the tumour suppressor p53. p27 responds to growth suppressors such as transforming growth factor -β.
• 1NK4/ARF family	p161NK4a binds to cyclin D-CDK4 and promotes the inhibitory effects of p16INK4A; p14ARF RB. p14ARF increases p53 levels by inhibiting MDM2 activity.
Checkpoint Components	
• p53	Tumour suppressor altered in the majority of cancers; causes cell-cycle arrest and apoptosis. Acts mainly through p21 to cause cell-cycle arrest. Causes apoptosis by inducing the transcription of pro-apoptotic genes such as BAX. Levels of p53 are negatively regulated by MDM2 through a feedback loop. p53 is required mainly for the G_1/S checkpoint.
• Ataxia-telangiectasia mutated (ATM)	Activated by mechanisms that sense double stranded DNA breaks. Transmits signals to arrest the cell cycle after DNA damage. Acts through p53 in the G_1/S checkpoint. At the G_2/M checkpoint, it acts both through p53 dependent mechanisms and independent mechanism which link DNA damage with cell-cycle arrest and apoptosis.

Remember : Simian virus 40, polyomavirus large T antigens, adenoviruses E - 7 protein and HPV E-7 protein binds to RB pocket so E2F is freed and proliferation is enhanced.

P53 gene :

- Also called as ***guardian of genome / Molecular policeman*** located on chromosome **17p13.1**
- It is the most common target for genetic alteration in human tumours.
- Most of the mutation are sporadic except of **Li-Fraumeni** syndrome (***inherited mutation in one p53 allele***) in which multiple primary tumours (Most common sarcomas, breast cancer, leukemia, brain tumours and carcinoma of adrenal cortex) occur at younger age.
- Major *functional activities of p 53* protein are *cell cycle arrest and initiation of apoptosis.*

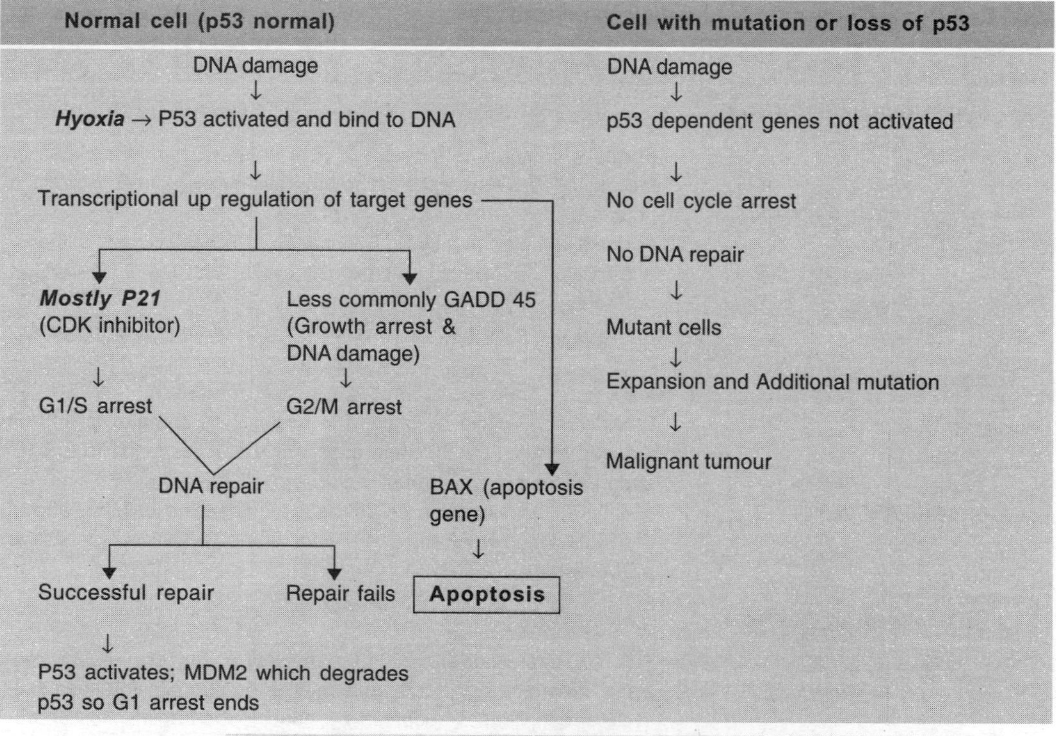

Remember :
- **E_6 protein of HPV also degrades P53**
- **P73** gene (***big brother of P53***) located on *1p36*
- ***Newest*** member of this family ***P63***
- VHL and Patched (PTCH) is also tumour suppressor gene.

3. **Evasion of Apoptosis :**
   Tumour forms if antiapoptic gene increased (bcl-2, bcl-xL,) or proapoptic gene decreased (bax, bad, bcl-xs, BID).
   Other genes associated with apoptosis :
   - **p53** : It increase transcription of pro-apoptoic gene bax, BID.
   - ***MYC*** : Triggers proliferation when growth factor is available while induces p53 when growth factor is not available.
4. **Defects in DNA repair genes**
   DNA repair genes themselves are *not oncogenic* but their abnormalities allow mutation in other genes. So, Person who born with mutation in DNA repair protein are at increased risk of developing cancer. This is known as ***genomic instability syndromes.*** DNA repair defects involve three systems :
   i. **Mismatch repair (MMR) genes**
   MMR gene act as ***spell checkers.*** With defective MMR, contraction and expansion of defective repeats occur creating alleles not found in normal cells. This is known as *Microsatellite instability eg HNPCC* (Hereditary nonpolyposis cancer syndrome).
   ii. **Nucleotide excision repair (NER)**
   This is defective in xeroderma pigmentosum.
   iii. **Defects in DNA repair by Homologous recombination**
   Occur in :
   - *Ataxia telangiectasia*
   - *Blooms syndrome*
   - *Fanconi anemia*
   - *BRCA-1 and BRCA-2 gene*

5. **Limitless replicative potential :** *Activation of telomerase* which maintain telomere length (essential for maintenance of replication in cancer cells) provide limitless replication. Telomere shortening is tumour suppressive mechanism.
   - Most normal human cells have a capacity of 60-70 doublings. This is due to progressive shortening of telomers. Activation of telomerase can make cell immortal.

6. **Development of sustained angiogenesis**
   - Tumors *cannot enlarge* beyond *1 to 2 mm* in diameter or thickness unless they are vascularized.
   - Neovascularization is requisite not only for continued tumour growth but also for metastases.
   - Tumour blood vessels differ from normal vasculature by being tortuous, irregularly shaped, disorganized, leaky (due to VEGF) and grow continuously.
   - Two most important tumour associated angiogenic factors are VEGF and basic fibroblast growth factor (bFGF).
   - ***p53 inhibits angiogenesis*** by increasing antiangiogenic factors thrombospondin 1 and decreasing angiogenic factors.

   Remember : Angiostatin, endostatin and tumstatin are other antiangiogenic factors.

7. **Invasion and Metastasis**
   - Both are biologic hallmarks of malignant tumours.
   - They are the **major cause** of *cancer-related morbidity and mortality.*
     - Metastases occur due to rare variant clones which develop in primary tumour as well as due to metastatic gene signature.
     - Metastatic gene signature depends on tumour cells, stroma, infiltrating immune cells and angiogenesis.
   - Metastatic cascade divide into two phases :

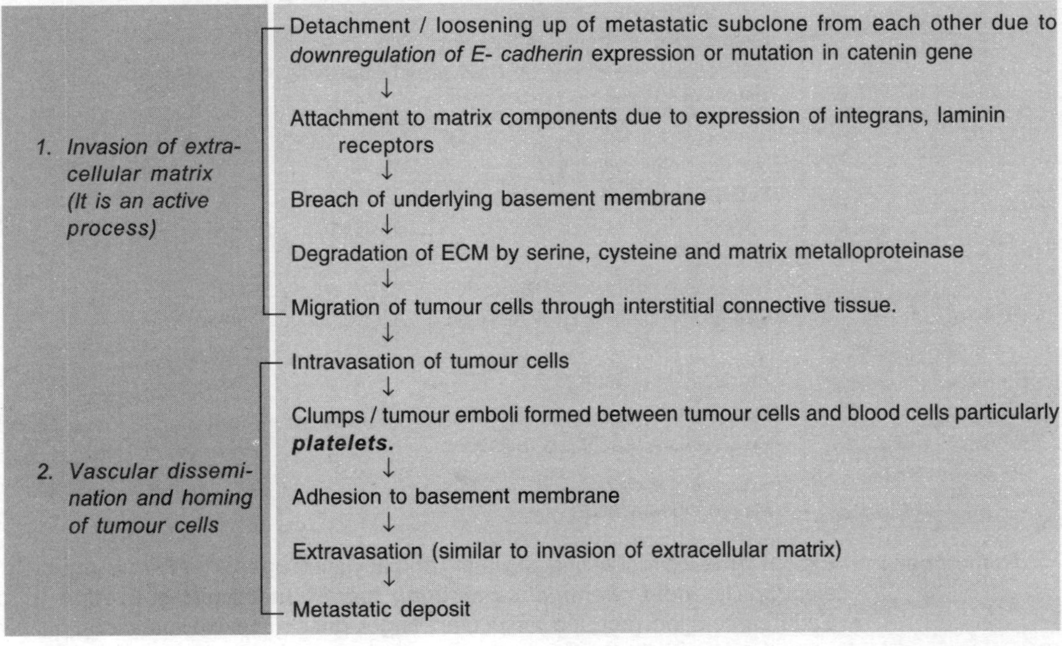

Remember : **CD-44** is adhesion molecule that expressed on normal T lymphocytes which is used by tumour cells to migrate to selective sites in lymphoid tissue.

MOLECULAR BASIS OF MULTISTEP CARCINOGENESIS

- Most human cancers occur due to ***multiple genetic alterations*** involving activation of several oncogenes and loss of two or more tumour suppressor gene.
- **Gate keeper genes : Directly** regulate entry of cell into tumorigenic path Eg. oncogenes and tumour suppressor genes.
- **Caretaker genes :** They do **not directly** control tumour growth but affect genomic instabilities Eg DNA repair genes.
- **Carcinogenesis is of three types :** – Chemical
  – Radiation
  – Microbial

1. Chemical Carcinogenesis

- ***Most potent*** chemical carcinogen : ***Polycyclic aromatic hydrocarbons.***
- Carcinogenicity of **most aromatic amines and azo** dyes is exerted mainly in *liver* except β naphthylamine which cause *bladder cancer.*
- Promoters of chemical carcinogenesis - phenol esters, hormones (estrogen), phenols, drugs, (Diethylstilbestrol phenobarbital) cigarette smoke, viral infections, bile salts, fat (bile acids), alcohol.
- Majority of initiating chemicals are mutagenic.
- ***Mutagenic potential*** are investigated most commonly by **Ames test.**

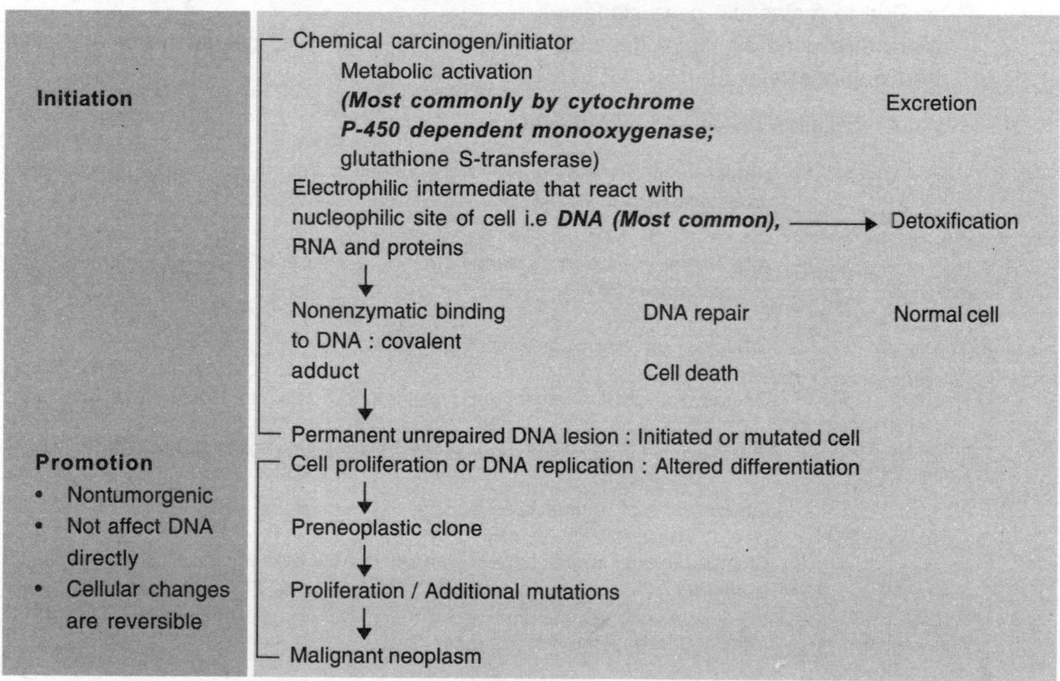

Remember :
- Except for few direct acting alkylating and acylating agents that are intrinsically electrophilic ***most chemical carcinogen require metabolic activation.***
- Each carcinogen produce molecular "finger print" (specific mutation).

2. Radiation Carcinogenesis :

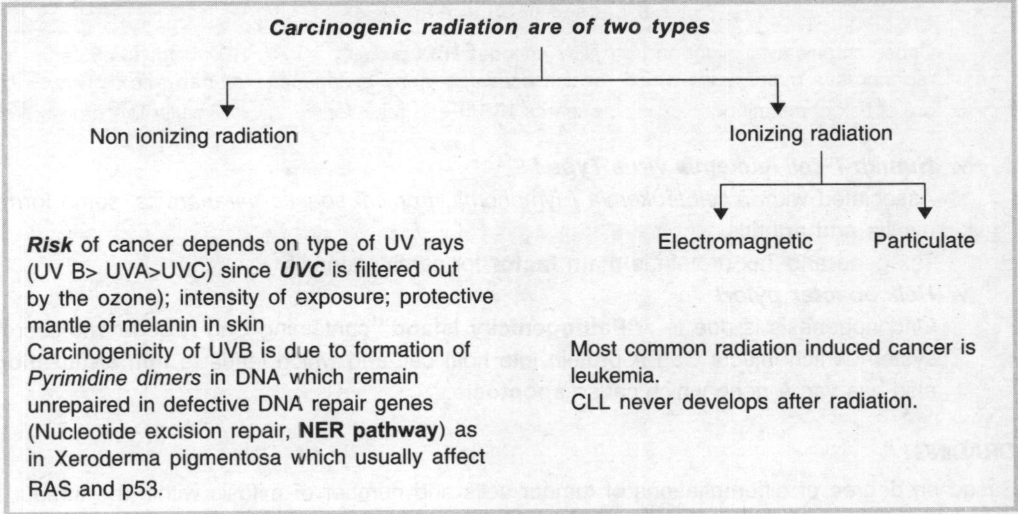

3. Microbial carcinogenesis

i. Human papillomavirus :

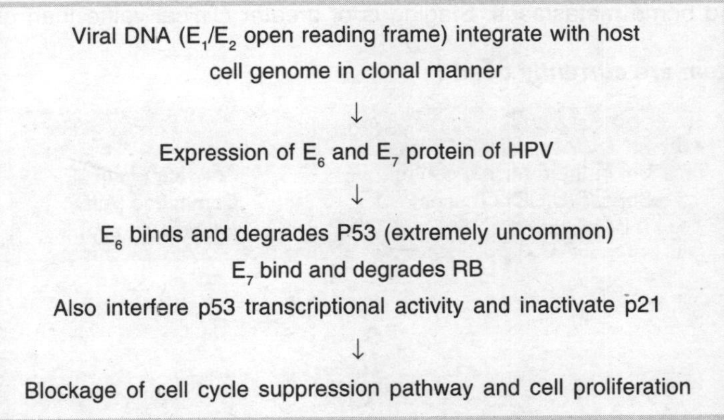

Remember : HPV infection act as initiating agent and additional somatic mutation are essential for malignant transformation.

ii. Epstein barr virus :

- It infects epithelial cells of oropharynx and B lymphocytes.
- It gains **entry into B cells** through CD21 molecule which is expressed on all B cells.
- ***Latent membrane protein* - 1** (LMP-1) of virus activate CD-40 receptor of B cells (NF-KB and JAK/STAT signaling pathway) and promotes B cell survival **(immortalization of B cells).**

iii. ***Hepatitis B virus -***

It causes carcinogenesis as :		
Cause chronic liver injury and regenerative hyperplasia which are at risk of mutation	HBV encodes **HBX** protein which *activates* many oncogenes such as **IGF II** and receptors	**HBX** binds to **p53** and interfere, its activity for insulin like growth factor I

iv. ***Human T cell leukemia virus Type I :***

Associated with *T cell leukemia / lymphoma, tropical spastic paraparesis,* some forms of uveitis and arthritis.

Tax gene and Tax protein is **main factor** for carcinogenesis.

v. ***Helicobacter pylori***

Onconogenesis is due to : **"Pathogenicity island"** containing Cag A gene and secretory system which injects Cag A protein into host cell and which leads to **immortalization**. It also has vac A gene which cause **apoptosis**.

GRADING :

Based on degree of differentiations of tumour cells and number of mitosis within the tumour and correlates of the neoplasm aggressiveness.

STAGING :

Based on size of primary lesion, its extent of spread to regional lymph nodes and presence or absence of blood borne metastases. Staging is of greater clinical value than grading.

Two major system are currently used :

Staging	
Union International centre Cancer (UICC) - It uses TNM system	American joint Committee (AJC) (stages 0 to IV)

QUESTIONS

1. All of the following cell types contain the enzyme telomerase which protect the length of telomers at the end of chromosomes except : [AI 06]
a. Germinal
b. Somatic
c. Haemopoetic
d. Tumour

2. The normal cellular counter parts of oncogenes are important for the following functions except : [AI 06]
a. Promotion of cell cycle progression
b. Inhibition of apoptosis
c. Promotion of DNA repair
d. Promotion of nuclear transcription

3. An example of a tumour suppressor gene is : [AI 05]
a. Myc.
b. Fos
c. Ras
d. Rb

4. The following is not a feature of malignant transformation by cultured cells : [AI 05]
a. Increased cell density
b. Increased requirement for growth factors
c. Alterations of cytoskeletal structures
d. Loss of anchorage

5. A simple bacterial test for mutagenic carcinogens is : [AI 05]
a. Ames test
b. Redox test
c. Bacteriophage
d. Gene splicing

6. In which of the following disease, the overall survival is increased by screening procedure : [AI 05]
a. Prostate cancer
b. Lung cancer
c. Colon cancer
d. Ovarian cancer

7. Which of the following is an antiapoptic gene ? [PGI 10]
a. C-myc
b. P_{53}
c. Bcl-2
d. Bax

8. AFP increased in [PGI 09, 08]
a. HCC
b. Cirrhosis with Activity
c. Hepatoblastoma
d. Endodermal sinus tumor

9. Which is not a tumor suppressor gene? [AIIMS 08]
a. WT-1
b. Rb
c. p53
d. RAS

10. Which of the following oncogenes is a growth factor? [AI 08]
a. fos
b. myc
c. jun
d. sis

11. Which of the following statements is not correct regarding p53 gene? [AI 08]
a. Located on chromosome 17
b. Arrests cell cycle at G1 phase
c. Is a 53 kD protein
d. Wild type is associated with tumours

12. True about tumour marker is: [PGI 08]
a. PSA is used for Ca prostate
b. Tumour marker is used to diagnose residual/recurrence of disease
c. Can be used for diagnosis of cancer
d. Ca-19 is used for colon cancer

13. Cytokeratin positioning is seen in: [AIIMS 10]
a. Adenoma
b. Melanoma

c. Carcinoma
d. Sarcoma

14. Antibody against tumour cells: [PGI 08]
a. MHC-I
b. MHC-II
c. Anti viral
d. Differentiated antigen

15. Which of the following statements about carcinogenesis is false : [AIIMS 06]
a. Asbestosis exposure increases the incidence of lung cancer
b. Papilloma viruses produce tumours in animals but not in humans
c. Exaposure to aniline dyes predisposes to cancer of the urinary bladder
d. Hepatitis B virus has been implicated in hepatocellular carcinoma

16. An undifferentiated malignant tumor on immunohistochemical stain shows cryptoplasmic positivity of most of the tumor cells for cytokeratin. The most probable diagnosis of the tumor is :
a. Sarcoma [AIIMS 06]
b. Lymphoma
c. Carcinoma
d. Malignant melanoma

17. For which one of the following tumors Gastrin is a biochemical marker :
a. Medullary carcinoma of thyroid
b. Pancreatic neuroendocrine tumor
c. Pheochromocytoma [AIIMS 05]
d. Gastrointestinal stromal tumor

18. Which of the following is known as the "guardian of the genome" ? [AIIMS 05]
a. p53
b. Mdm2
c. p14
d. ATM

19. The most common cancer, affecting both males and females of the world is :
a. Cancer of the pancreas
b. Buccal mucosa [AIIMS 05]
c. Lung cancer
d. Colo-rectal cancer

20. Which of the following has a normal level of alpha fetoprotein value in serum ?
a. Ovarian dysgerminoma
b. Hepatoblastoma [AIIMS 05]
c. Embryonal carcinoma
d. Yolk sac tumor

21. V7-Which of the following is the most common inherited malignancy :
a. Infant leukemia [AIIMS 05]
b. Retinoblastoma
c. Wilms tumour
d. Neuroblastoma

22. In which of the following tumors alpha fetoprotein is elevated ? [AIIMS 05]
a. Choriocarcinoma
b. Neuroblastoma
c. Hepatocellular carcinoma
d. Seminoma

23. The tumor suppressor gene P53 induces cell cycle arrest at : [AIIMS 05]
a. G_2M phase
b. S-G_2 phase
c. G1-S phase
d. Go phase

24. Xeroderma pigmentosum is caused due to a group of closely related abnormalities in : [AIIMS 05]
a. Mismatch repair
b. Base excision repair
c. Nucleotide excision repair [NER]
d. SOS repair

25. The following disease have defect in DNA repair mechanism except for : [AIIMS 05]
a. Xeroderma pigmentosa
b. Fanconi syndrome
c. Huntington's dise2stric carcinoma

27. Rise in AFP is seen in all except: [AI 10]
a. Pure choriocarcinoma
b. Yolk sac tumor
c. Hepatoma
d. Pure embryonal carcinoma

28. DNA repair defect is seen in: [AIIMS 09]
a. Xeroderma pigmentosum
b. Icthyosis
c. Marfan's syndrome
d. Mosaicism

ANSWERS, REFERENCES, EXPLANATIONS WITH INFORMATIVE ILLUSTRATIONS

1. **Ans. is b i.e. Somatic** *Ref. Harrison 17/e, p 500*

Telomere

- Each human chromosome contains two specialized structures: a centromere and two telomers.
- Centromere or primary constriction, divides the chromosome into short (p) and long (q) arms.
- Telomere is ***short repeated sequences of DNA*** present at linear ends of chromosome.
- Some portion of this sequence is lost during each cell division known as telomere shortening.
- Telomere shortening cause growth arrest called as *replicative senescence.*
- Telomerase is enzyme that adds TTAGGG (= telomere) repeat on 3 end of chromosome and RNA component that provides template for telomere extension.
- Thus the cell with telomerase are able to divide continuously.
- Most normal somatic cells do not express telomerase except stem cells of hematopoietic tissues, gut and skin epithelium and germ cells.
- More than 90% of human cancer express high levels of telomerase.
- Therapeutic agents which inhibit telomerase can leads to tumor cells apoptosis (or acts as anticancer agents).

2. **Ans. is c i.e. Promotion of DNA repair**

Ref. Robbin's 8/e, p 279-280; Chandrasoma Taylor 3/e, p 279 - 280

- **Oncogenes** are genes *that promote autonomous cell growth in cancer.*
- The are derived from their ***normal cellular counter parts*** called as protooncogene which are physiologic regulators of cell proliferation and differentiation.
- Oncogenies promote cell growth in the absence of normal mitogenic signals.
- Products of oncogene are called as oncoproteins which *resemble normal product of protooncogene **except that :***
  a. Oncoproteins are devoid of normal regulatory elements.
  b. Their production in the transformed cells does not depend on growth factors or other external signals.
- If oncogenes are transferred to animals using retroviruses as vectors, they transform normal animal cells in vitro to cancer cells.
- **Functions of oncogenes are :**
  - Act as growth factor eg SIS, int, hst
  - Act as growth factor receptor eg erb-B, erb-B_2 (Her 2/neu)
  - Act as signal transduction/relay factors e.g. ret
  - Act as transcription factors eg myc
  - Cell cycle controller eg bcl-1 (PRAD1), mdm-2 (P53 antagonist)
  - Apoptosis blocker eg bcl-2.

Remember : Tumor suppressor gene have role in cell cycle brakes, Mismatch DNA repair, induction of apoptosis.

3. **Ans. is d i.e. Rb** *Ref. Robbin's 8/e, p 287*

Tumor suppressor gene regulate the cell growth. Protein product of these gene apply brakes to cell proliferation. They are *recessive* cancer gene. So, cancer develop only when cell become homozygous for mutant allele or both normal allele are inactivated ***(Knudson's two hit theory of oncogenesis).***

Remember :
- Rb gene is located an chromosome 13q 14.
- Tumor associated with Rb gene mutation - Retinoblastoma; Osteosarcoma; Glioblastoma; Carcinoma breast, colon, lung, bladder. **myc, fos, and ras are oncogene (dominant cancer gene).**

4. **Ans. is b i.e. Increased requirement for growth factors** *Ref. Harper 26/e, p 654*

Changes shown by cultured cells which suggest the malignant transformation are :

- *Alterations of morphology :* Transformed cells often have a much rounder shape than control cells.
- *Increased cell density (loss of contact inhibition of growth) :* Transformed cells often form multilayers, while control cells usually form a monolayer.
- *Loss of anchorage dependence :* Transformed cells can grow without attachment to the surface of the culture dish and will often grow in agar.
- *Loss of contact inhibition of movement :* Transformed cell grow over one another, while normal cells stop moving when they come into contact with each other.
- A *variety of biochemical changes,* including an increased rate of glycolysis, alterations of the cell surface (eg, changes in the composition of glycoproteins or glycosphingolipids), and secretion of certain proteases.
- *Alterations of cytoskeletal structures,* such as actin filaments.
- ***Diminished requirement for growth factors*** and, often, increased secretion of certain growth factors into the surrounding medium.

5. **Ans. is a i.e. Ames test** *Ref. Robbin's 7/e, p 320; Harper 26/e, p 650*

"Ames assay has proved useful in screening for potential carcinogen."

- Majority of initiating chemicals are mutagenic so their mutagenic potential has to be determined before introducing commercially.
- Mutagenic potential has been determined most commonly by using **Ames test.**

AMES Test :

- ***Ames test uses the ability of chemical to induce mutation in bacterium*** *'Salmonella typhimurium'.*
- If chemicals are mutagenic than it convert His$^-$ salmonella to Hist$^+$ salmonella so it can synthesize histidine and can grow in medium lacking histidine.
- *Ames test identifies approximately 90% of known carcinogen.*
- Compounds giving positive reaction should undergo further testing, including assessment of carcinogenicity in animals.
- ***Advantage of Ames test -*** more rapid and less expensive than detecting tumors in animals.

- ***Limitation -*** *It can't detect carcinogenicity of chemicals* which require activation, as monooxygenase is absent in bacteria.

  However, this is overcome by incubating chemical to be tested in a post mitochondrial supernatant of rat liver (contain fragment of endoplasmic reticulum).

6. **Ans. is c i.e Colon cancer** *Ref. Sabiston 17/e, p 1465; Devita 8/e, p 664*

"Colorectal cancer is an ideal candidate for screening strategies."

Because, – it is common
– has precursor lesion
– it is slow growing
– testing is available.

So, its detection by screening well increase survival.

Screening methods for colorectal carcinoma
- Fecal occult blood testing
- Stool DNA testing
- Endoscopy
- Imaging CT colonography (Virtual colonoscopy)
- Capsule endoscopy

Tumour in which screening is done are :

Cancer	Screening technique
Ovarian cancer	Ca-125, Transvaginal sonography
Cervical cancer	Pap smear
Breast cancer	Mammography
Prostate cancer	Digital rectal examination, prostate specific antigen
Lung	Chest X-ray, sputum cytology

7. **Ans. is c i.e. Bcl-2** *Ref. Robbin's 8/e, p 295-296*

Cell survival is affected by gene that promote (proapoptotic gene) or inhibit apoptosis (antiapoptotic gene).

Proapoptotic gene (decrease tumor growth) :	– Bax, Bad – BID	– Bcl-xS – BAK
Antiapoptotic gene (increased cell proliferation) :	– Bcl-2 – MCL-1	– Bcl-XL

Remember : – Most common translocation in lymphoid malignancies is t(14:18) translocation, causes activation of Bcl-2 gene.
– P53 has proapoptotic action (by upregulation of bax gene) and c-myc is apoptotic in the absence of growth factors.

8. **Ans. is a, b, c and d i.e. All options are correct**

Ref. Harrison 17/e, p 582; Robbin's 8/e, p 327

AFP is
Glycoprotein synthesized normally early in fetal life by yolk sac, fetal liver and fetal GIT

Causes of rise in AFP is	
Neoplastic causes	***Nonneoplastic causes***
• Primary carcinoma of liver (HCC) • Hepatoblastoma • Non seminomatous germ cell tumor of testis (not in seminoma) • Ovarian germ cell tumor • Carcinoma of colon, Lung, Pancreas, Breast, Renal and Gastric	• Toxic liver injury • Hepatitis • Pregnancy (especially with fetal distress or death) • Cirrhosis

"AFP levels > 500 μg/L are found in about 70-80% of patients with HCC. Lower levels may be found in patients with large metastases from gastric or colonic tumors and in some patients with acute or chronic hepatiis. High levels of serum AFP (>500-1000 μg/L) in adult without liver disease and without an obvious GIT tumor strongly suggest HCC."

9. **Ans. is d i.e. RAS** *Ref. Robbin's 8/e, p 287*

Tumor suppressor genes	
Location	Gene
Cell surface	TGF β receptor, E-cadherin
Plasma membrane	NF-1
Cytoskeleton	NF-2
Cytosol	APC/β, PTEN, SMAD-2, SMAD-4
Nucleus	RB-1, p53, WT-1, p16/INK4a, BRCA, KLF6

10. **Ans. is d i.e. sis** *Ref. Robbin's 8/e, p 281*

Growth factor oncogenes
- SIS
- HST-1
- INT2
- TGFA
- HGF

11. **Ans. is d i.e. Wild type is associated with tumors**

Ref. Devita 6/e, p 19; Robbins 8/e, p 292

P53 gene :
- Also called as guardian of genome/ Molecular policeman, located on chromosome 17p13.1

- Derives its name from its protein product which is a 53 KD protein
- It is the most common target for genetic alteration in human tumors
- Most of the mutation are sporadic except of Li-Fraumeni syndrome (inherited mutation in one p53 allele) in which multiple primary tumors (Most common sarcomas, breast cancer, leukemia brain tumours and carcinoma of adrenal cortex) occur at younger age.
- Major functional activities of p53 protein are cell cycle arrest for DNA repair and initiation of apoptosis.
- P53 mediated cell cycle arrest occurs in late G1 phase and is caused mainly by transcription of CDK inhibitor (DKNIA (p21))

Remember : Mdm 2 is negative feedback regulator of p53;p-14 is inhibitor of Mdm2, while ATM senses double stranded DNA breaks and have role in G_1/S as well as G_2/M checkpoint.

12. Ans. is a, b, c, d i.e. All options are correct *Ref. Robbin's 8/e, p 326*

Selected tumor marker

Markers	Associated cancers
Hormones	
Beta human chorionic gonadotropin (B-HCG)	Trophoblastic tumors, nonseminomatous / seminomatous testicular tumors
Calcitonin	Medullary carcinoma of thyroid
Catecholamine and metabolites	Pheochromocytoma and related tumors
Oncofetal antigens	
α-Fetoprotein	**Tetraembryonal** carcinoma, ovarian GCT, Liver cell cancer nonseminomatous germ cell tumors of testis
Carcinoembryonic antigen	Carcinomas of the colon; pancreas, lung, stomach, & heart, breast ovary
Isoenzymes	
LDH	Lymphoma, **Ewings**, ovarian; Seminoma/ Nonseminoma testicular tumor
Prostatic and phosphatase (PAP)	Prostate cancer
Neuron-specific enolase	Small cell cancer of lung, neuroblastoma
Specific proteins	
Abnormal immunoglobulins (paraproteins), β2 microglobulins	Multiple myeloma and other gammopathies, macroglobulinemia
Prostate specific antigen and prostate specific membrane antigen	Prostate cancer
Thyroglobulin	Thyroid cancer (papillary and follicular) cervix, fallopian tube, pancreas, breast, lung, colon
Mucins and other Glycoproteins	
CA-125	Epithelial ovarian cancer, Endometrial cancer, stomach cancer, uterine sarcoma

CA-19-9	Colon cancer, pancreatic cancer, cholangio Ca, GB cancer, ovarian tumor
CA-15-3, CA 27-29	Breast cancer
CD-30	Hodgkin's anaplastic large cell lymphoma
New molecular markers	
p53, APC, RAS mutations in stool and serum	Colon cancer
p53 and RAS mutations in sputum and serum	Pancreatic cancer
p53 mutations in urine	Lung cancer
p53 mutations in urine	Bladder cancer
CD 25	Hairy cell leukemia, Adult T cell leukemia lymphoma
Urinary steroids	Adrenal carcinoma, paraneoplastic cushing's syndrome
5 Hydroxyindole acetic acid	Carcinoid syndrome
Placental alk phosphatase (PLAP)	Germ cell tumor (type of pancreatic neuroendocrine tumor)
Gastrin	Gastrinoma or zolinger - ellison syndrome, MEN-I
VIP	VIP-oma/WDHA syndrome / verner morrison syndrome
HIAA	Carcinoid syndrome

Applications of Tumor markers :

Detection	Screening in asymptomatic persons
Diagnosis	Differentiating malignant from benign conditions
Monitoring	Predicting effect of therapy and detecting recurrent cancer
Classification	Choosing therapy and predicting tumor behavior (prognosis)
Staging	Defining extent of disease
Localization	Nuclear scanning of injected radioactive antibodies
Therapy	Cytotoxic agents directed to marker containing cells

13. Ans. is c i.e Carcinoma

Ref. Harrison 16/e, p 563; Chandrasoma Taylor 3/e, p 307; Robbin's 8/e, p 324

'Cytokeratin filament are found in epithelial tumors (carcinoma)"

Evaluation	Primary site / Neoplasm
Immunohistology	
Leukocyte common antigen (LCA,CD 45)	Lymphoid neoplasm
Leu-MI	Hodgkin's disease
Epithelial membrane antigen	Carcinoma
Cytokeratin	Carcinoma
HMB-45	Melanoma
Desmin, Vimentin	Sarcoma
Myoglobin	Rhabdomyosarcoma
PSA/prostatic acid phosphatase	Prostate
S-100 protein	Neuroendocrine tumor, melanoma
Gross cystic fluid protein	Breast

Contd...

Contd...

Factor VIII	Kaposi's sarcoma, angiosarcoma
Thyroid transcription factor-1 (TTF-1)	Lung adenocarcinoma, thyroid
Ultrastructure	
Actin-myosin filament	Rhabdomyosarcoma
Secretory granules	Neuroendocrine tumors
Desmosomes	Carcinoma
Premelanosomes	Melanoma
Neurofilaments	Neural tumors
Viamentin	Non specific : mesenchymal tumors, some carcinoma
Glial Fibrillary acid protein	Glial tumors
Chromagranin and neuron specific enolase	Neuroendocrine tumor, some lung cancers
PNCA, K-67	Assessement of tumor growth rate

A. **MHC-I** *Ref. Robbins 7/e, p 328-330*

Both cell mediated and humoral immunity have been demonstrated against tumor, ***the principal mechanism of tumor immunity is killing of tumor cells by CD8+ Cytotoxic T-lymphocytec.*** CTLs recognize peptide derived from cytoplasmic proteins that are displayed bound to class I MHC molecules

- The immune response against the tumor cells is mediated through
  - Cytotoxic T lymphocytes (CTL)
  - Natural killer cells
  - Macrophage
  - Antibodies: Kill tumor cells by complement activation or antibody depend cell-mediated cytotoxicity

Tumour antigen are formed by:

i. Products of oncogene and tumor suppressor genes
ii. Products of other mutated genes
iii. Overexpressed or aberrantly expressed cellular proteins
iv. Tumour antigens produced by oncogenic virus
v. Oncofetal antigens
vi. Altered cell-surface glycolipids and glycoproteins, e.g. G_{M2}, G_{D2} G_{D3}
vii. Cell type-specific differentiation antigens, e.g. CD10, CALLA

14. Ans. is a i.e. MHC-1 *Ref. Robbins 17/e, p 328-330*

- Both cell mediated and humoral immunity have been demonstrated against tumor, ***the principal mechanism of tumor immunity is killing of tumor cells by CD8+ Cytotoxic T-lymphocyte.*** CTLs recognize peptide derived from cytoplasmic proteins that are displayed bound to Class I MHC molecules.
- The immune response against the tumor cells is mediated through
  - Cytotoxic T lymphocytes (CTL)
  - Natural killer cells
  - Macrophage
  - **Antibodies:** Kill tumor cells by complement activation or antibody dependent cell-mediated cytotoxicity.
- **Tumor antigen are formed by:**

  i. Products of oncogene and tumor suppressor genes
  ii. Products of other mutated genes

iii. Overexpressed or aberrantly expressed cellular proteins
iv. Tumor antigens produced by oncogenic virus
v. Oncofetal antigens
vi. Altered cell-surface glycolipids and glycoproteins, e.g. G_{M2},G_{D2} G_{D3}
vii. Cell type-specific differentiation antigens, e.g. CD10, CALLA

15. **Ans. is b ie. Papilloma viruses produce tumours in animals but not in humans**

Ref. Harrison 17/e, p 689, 487

Papilloma virus is the most common causative factor for cervical cancer.

Oncogenic microbes and parasites

Organism	Neoplasm
Human papilloma virus (papovaviridae)	Cervical, vulvar, penile cancers, squamous cell carcinoma, oropharyngeal carcinoma
HSV type 2	Cervical carcinoma
Hepatitis B virus (Hepadnaviridae)	Hepatocellular carcinoma
Hepatitis C virus (Flaviviridae)	Hepatocellular carcinoma, Lymphoplasmacytic lymphoma
HTLV – I (Retroviridae)	Adult T cell leukemia/lymphoma
HTLV – II (Retroviridae)	T cell variant of hairy cell leukemia
HTLV – III (Retroviridae)	AIDS related malignancies, NHL, Kaposi sarcoma, SCC (esp of UG tract), Diffuse large B cell lymphoma, Burkitt's lymphoma
Epstein barr virus (Herpesviridae)	Mixed cellularity Hodgkin's, Nasopharyngeal carcinoma (anaplastic), African Burkitt's lymphoma, Post organ transplant lymphoma, Primary CNS diffuse large B cell lymphoma, Extranodal NK/T cell lymphoma (nasal type)
H. Pylori	Gastric malt lymphoma, Gastric cancer
Human Herpes virus B	Primary effusion lymphoma, Multicentric Castleman's disease
Schistosoma hematobium	Bladder cancer (squamous cell)
Clonorchis	Cholangio carcinoma
Opisthorchis	Cholangio carcinoma

Important chemical carcinogens

Chemical agent	Neoplasm
• Alkylating agents	AML; Bladder Ca.
• Aromatic amines (dyes)	Bladder Ca.
• Arsenic	Lung Ca
• Asbestos	Lung Ca, Pleural Ca, Peritoneal Ca
• Benzene	AML
• Chromium	Lung Ca
• Nickel dust	Ca of paranasal sinus; lung Ca
• Polycyclic hydrocarbons	Ca of skin; Lung Ca
• Vinyl chloride	Liver Ca

16. Ans. is c i.e. Carcinoma *Ref. Robbin's 8/e, p 324*

Keratin filaments are characteristic of epithelial cells, so would be suggestive of carcinoma.

Filament	Cell	Malignancy
Cytokeratin	Epithelial	Carcinoma
Desmin	Muscle cell	Sarcoma
Vimentin	Connective tissue	Sarcoma
Glial filament	Astrocyte	Glioma

17. Ans. is b i.e. Pancreatic neuroendocrine tumor *Ref. Robbin's 8/e, p 326*

Already explained

18. Ans. is a i.e. p53 *Ref. Robbin's 8/e, p 292*

Remember :

- Most common target for genetic alteration in human tumors is p53 (A little over 50% of human tumors contain mutation in this gene).
- Most common target for genetic alteration among protooncogene is ras.
- Most common target for genetic alteration among nuclear regulatory proteins is myc.
- Most common target for genetic alteration among cell cycle regulators is CDK-4.

19. Ans. is c i.e. Lung Cancer *Ref. Park 19/e, 318; Park 18/e, p 302*

"In terms of incidence the most common cancer worldwide are lung cancer >breast cancer >colorectal cancer."

- Most common cancer in India (male) Mouth/oropharynx, oesophagus, stomach, lower respiratory tract
- Most common cancer in India (female) cervix, Breast;Mouth,oropharynx and oesophagus
- In Delhi/Mumbai, most common cancer in women is breast

- ***In developing world :*** – *Males* : Lung > Prostate > Colorectum > Stomach > Bladder
  – *Females* : Cervix > breast > Stomach > Lung > Mouth / Oropharynx
- ***In developed world :*** – *Males* : Lung > Prostate > Colorectum > Stomach > Bladder
  – *Females* : Breast > Colorectum > Lungs > Stomach > Cervix
- ***Most common cancer causing death*** : – *Males* : Lung>stomach> liver> colorectum >oesophagus
  – *Females* : Breast>Stomach> Colorectal>Cervix>Ovary

20. Ans. is a i.e. Ovarian dysgerminoma *Ref. CGDT 10/e, p 875*

Tumor markers that may be elevated in the presence of germ cell neoplasms.

Neoplasm	AFP	hCG
Dysgerminoma	–	+/-
Endodermal sinus tumor (Yolk sac tumour)	+	–
Immature teratoma	+/-	–
Mixed germ cell tumor	+/-	+/-
Choriocarcinoma	–	+
Embryonal carcinoma	+/-	+

Other tumor markers of Ovarian cancer :

• CA-125	– Malignant epithelial cell cancer
• LDH	– Germ cell and epithelial cell tumor
• Placental alkaline Phosphatase	– Germ cell ovarian tumor
• CEA	– Ovarian tumor

Remember : Cells of endodermal sinus/yolk sac tumor are rich in alpha 1 antitrypsin

21. Ans. is b i.e. Retinoblastoma *Ref. Robbin's 7/e, p 287*

Learn it.

22. Ans. is c i.e. Hepatocellular carcinoma *Robbin's 8/e, p 327*

Already explained, kindly see answer no. 10

23. Ans. is c i.e. G1-S phase *Ref. Devita 8/e, p 86; Robbin's 8/e, p 286*

P53 is required for G_1S check point and is a component of the G_2M checkpoint.

- ***The primary mechanism underlying the G_2 DNA damage (G_2M) checkpoint is p53 independent.***

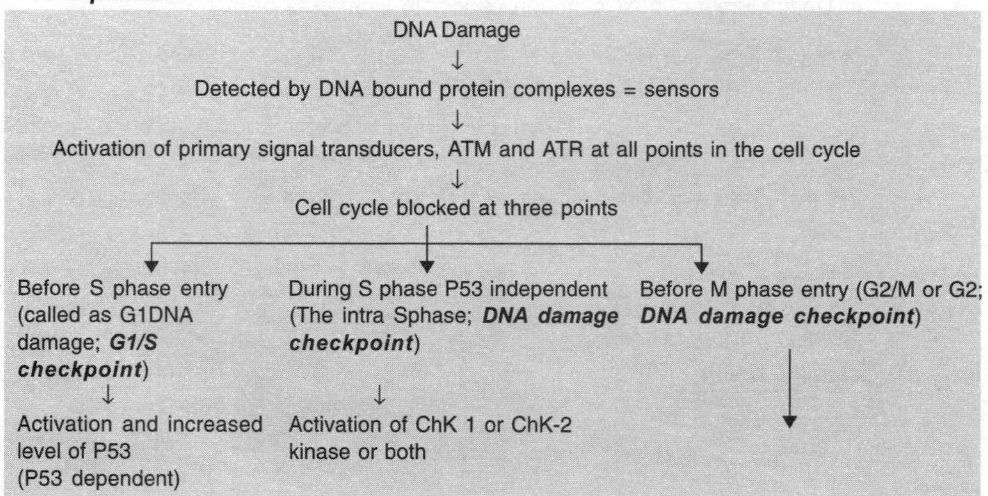

Contd...

Contd...

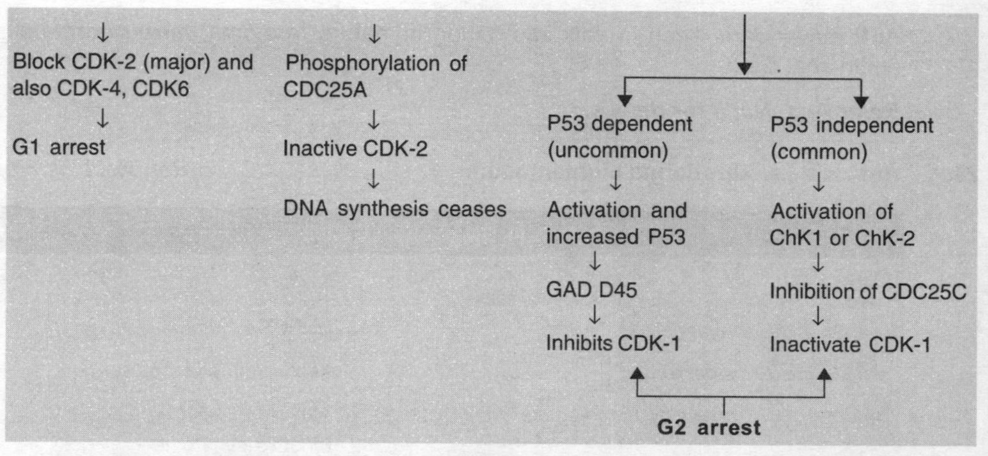

Cell cycle phase	Cycline/CDKs	CDK Inhibitors
G_1 – S transition by phosphorylating Rb	Cyclin D/CDK4 Cyclin D/CDK-6 Cyclin E/CDK-2	INK inhibitors (p 15, 16,18,19)
S phase	Cyclin A/CDK2 Cyclin A/CDK1	
G2-M transition	Cyclin B/CDK1	

Remember : p21,p27,p57 can inhibit all CDKs.

24. Ans. is c i.e. Nucleotide excision repair (NER) *Ref. Robbin's 8/e, p 302*

Types of defect in DNA repair gene	Disease / Gene
i. Defect in Mismatch repair(MMR) gene	– Hereditary nonpolyposis cancer syndrome (HNPCC)(MSH2,MLH1,PMS,PMS2 gene) – Pancreatic cancer (PRSS1)
ii. Defect in nucleotide excision repair (NER)	– Xeroderma pigmentosa
iii. Defect in DNA repair by Homologous recombination	– Ataxia Telangiectasia (ATM gene) – Bloom syndrome – Fanconi anemia – BRCA-1 and BRCA-2 gene

25. Ans. is c i.e. Huntington's disease *Ref. Robbin's 8/e, p 302*

Already explained, kindly see answer no. 24

26. Ans. is a, b and d i.e. Adenocarcinoma of colon; Pancreatic ca; and Ovarian ca

Ref. Harrison 16/e, p 439

Remember : CEA is increased in :

Heart	**B**reast	**O**vary	**L**ung
Colon	**G**astric	**P**ancreas	

Mnemonic – **H**ungry **B**oys **O**ften **L**ook **C**ute **G**irls **P**leasently

27. Ans. is a i.e. Pure choriocarcinoma *Ref. COGDT 13/e, p 875*

AFP elevation is seen in yolk sac tumor, immature teratoma, mixed germ cell tumor, embryonal Ca.

Refer Ans. No. 8 for details.

28. Ans. is a i.e. Xeroderma pigmentosum *Ref. Robbins 8/e, p 302*

Defect in DNA repair Genes	
Subclass	**Disease**
Mismatch repair genes	HNPCC syndrome
Nucleotide excision repair	Xeroderma pigmentosum
Defect in DNA repair by homologous recombination	Ataxia telangiectasia Bloom's syndrome Fanconi anemia

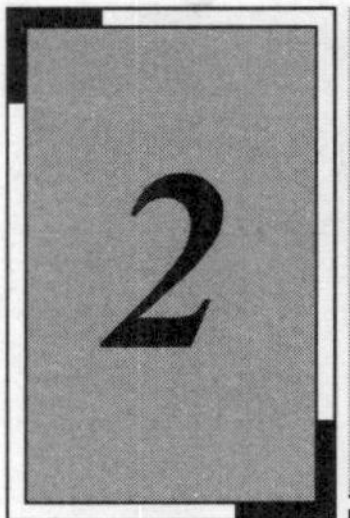

Cancer Radiotherapy

What's Important ?

- **Mechanism of Radiotherapy?**
- **Radiosensitive tumours**
- **Radioisotopes used**

The goal of cancer treatment is to *eradicate* the cancer. If this is *not accomplished; goal shifts to palliation,* amelioration of symptoms and preservation of quality of life.

Cancer treatments are divided into Four main types :

a. Surgery

- Surgery is most effective method of treating cancer (both for eradication and palliation).
- Aim of cancer surgery is to excise the tumor completely with an adequate margin of normal tissue touching the tumor to prevent vascular and lymphatic spread.

Remember :

- ***Neoadjuvant therapy :*** Initial chemotherapy and radiotherapy (to reduced the size of tumor) followed by surgery to remove residual mass. Used in bulky testicular cancer, stage III breast cancer.
- ***Abscopal effect :*** *Splenectomy* **in some cases of lymphoma (especially CLL, prolymphocytic leukemia) may cause regression of tumour.**

  Surgery may be curative in some patients with metastatic disease also e.g. in patient with colon cancer who have liver metastasis restricted to one lobe, hepatic lobectomy may produce long term survival.

b. Radiation therapy (*including photodynamic therapy*)

- For *certain tumor complete surgical removal is not possible* or disabling, under these circumstances ionized radiation are used in treatment of cancer.

c. Chemotherapy (including conventional chemotherapy and molecularly targeted therapy)

d. Biological therapy (including immunotherapy and gene therapy)

RADIOTHERAPY

It is the therapeutic use of high energy ionizing radiation in the treatment / management of malignant disease.

Ionizing radiation					
Electromagnetic (They posses no mass)		***Particulate*** (They have definite mass)			
X-ray	*Gamma rays*	*Electron*	*Proton*	*Neutron*	*α Particle*
	Uncharged	–ve Charge	+ve Charge	Uncharged	+ve Charged

X-rays

They are ***produced as a result of abrupt mechanical decceleration of electrons striking a heavy target*** such as tungsten.

- *X-rays cause ionization in three major ways :*
  a. **Photoelectric effect** seen in ***low energy*** X-rays, useful in diagnostic radiology.
  b. **Compton effect** seen in ***high energy*** X-rays, useful in therapeutic radiology.
  c. **Pair production** seen with ***very high energy*** X-rays, no role in medical field.

γ - rays : Produced by ***nuclear disintegration of radioisotopes*** such as cobalt, radium.

β Particles (Electrons) : Small ***negatively charged particles*** penetrate only to a limited depth. So used to treat superficial problems only.

Protons : ***Positively charged*** and have a mass about 2000 times of that of electron. Due to heavy mass they stop abruptly and give their energy to cause ionization. This region of enhanced ionization is called Bragg peak.

Neutrons : ***Uncharged particle*** produced by colliding charged particle in to a suitable target. Neutron beams are more effective in treating salivary gland tumors.

α Particle : ***Helium nuclei*** consisting of two proton and two neutron ($^{4}_{2}He$). Due to its high mass they are *not able to penetrate even a piece of paper.*

Radiation used to treat cancer

- **X-rays and γ rays are *most common* form of radiation used to treat cancer.**
- **X-rays and γ rays are** *sparsely ionizing* **radiation**

- **Electron beams (β rays)** : For intraoperative radiation, skin tumor like mycosis fungoides
- **Neutron beams** : For salivary gland tumor
- **α-rays** : Because of low penetrability they are not used for treating cancer.

Infrared rays are non ionizing radiation and are not used in cancer treatment.

Relative biologic effect : The equal doses of different radiation do not produce equal biologic effect. The biologic effects can be quantified in terms of relative biologic effects (RBE), ***higher the RBE, higher will be the biologic effects*** of given radiation.

RBE (in decreasing order) : Neutron > a particle > X rays > g rays > electrons.

LET (Linear energy transfer)

- It is the *amount of ionization occurring per unit length* of radiation track.
- ***Low LET*** radiation must produce multiple hits on DNA *to destroy a cell;* hypoxic cells are resistant to low LET radiation. X-rays produce DNA damage by low LET.
- **High LET** radiation produce only a *single hit on DNA* to *kill a cell,* oxygenated and hypoxic cells responds similarly to high LET irradiation. Protons and nutrons produce DNA damage by high LET.

Penetrability : Penetrability of various radiation (in decreasing order) is γ rays > **X** ray > β rays > α particle.

BIOLOGIC EFFECTS OF RADIATION

Molecular effect

- Ionizing radiation causes base damage, single stranded breaks, double stranded breaks sugar damage as well as DNA-DNA, and DNA-protein cross links.
- Radiation must produce **double strand break** in DNA to kill a cell *(as single strand break can be repaired).*
- Radiation interacts with water to generate free radical. ***Most X-ray induced cell damage*** is due to formation of hydroxyl ($OH^{\bullet}$) radical.
- Radiation induced ***chromosomal aberration*** typically occurs in cell irradiated in G1 *phase of cell cycle.*
- The frequency of *chromosomal aberration in peripheral circulating lymphocyte* can be used to correlate the total body dose received.

Cellular effect

- Cells are most sensitive to radiation at **G2 / M** interface followed by **M** phase > **G1** phase and **most resistant** towards *ends of 'S' phase.*
- Process that follow radiation exposure are : **[4R]** i.e.
  - ***Repair***
  - ***Reoxygenation***
  - ***Repopulation***
  - ***Redistribution***
- *Hypoxic cells are more resistant* to radiations than oxygenated cells.
- **Sulphydryl compound** interfere with free radical generation and thus act as ***radiation protectors.***

Factors that effect the response of tumors to radiation

1. DNA repair
2. **Split Dose repair:** If the given dose of radiation is administered in two fractions, the effect is decreased on tumor cells.
3. **Dose rate effect:** For sparsely ionizing radiation dose rate plays critical factor in cell killing. Lowering the dose rate thereby increasing exposure time, reduces the effectiveness of killing by X-rays.
4. **Check point pathways:** The major events in the cell cycle are DNA synthesis, which occurs in S-phase, and cell divison which occurs in mitosis. **The S-phase is most resistant, while G_2-M is most sensitive.**

Measurement of Ionizing Radiation

Roentgen (R)	Radiation adsorbed dose (RAD)
– Unit of *exposure* – It measure ionization produced per unit volume of air by X-rays and gamma rays and cannot be used for photon energies above 3MeV – **SI** unit of exposure is Coulomb per Kilogram i.e. C/Kg – ***Conversion is:*** 1R = *2.58 x10⁴ C/Kg air* *1cGy = 1 rad*	– Measure biologically significant effects – *Absorbed dose* = De/dm, De is the mean anergy imparted by ionizing radiation to material of mass dm – SI unit of absorbed dose is *Gray (Gy)* which defined as 1Gy = 1J/kg. Old unit is rad. – ***Conversion is:*** *1 rad = 100 erg/g* *1Gy = 100 rad*

Rem (Roentigen equivalent in man) : Unit that reflects biologic response. It is used to compare various types of radiation.

Methods of Delivery of Radiotherapy

External beam irradiation	Brachytherapy	Internal or systemic radiotherapy
– Source is at distance of 80-100 cm usually	It used sealed or closed container radioactive sources	– It use non-sealed radioactive sources either enterally, intracavitarly or intravenously
Types :	***Types :***	***Types :***
a. 60 Co Teletherapy b. X-ray such as linear accelerators	a. Intracavitary used in Ca cervix, Ca rectum b. Interstitial used in prostatic, GIT cancer. It is of two types temporary and permanent c. Surface molds or Plaques used in skin, eye cancer, radium or radon, ***Cs^{137}, Ir^{192}, Au^{198}, I^{125}*** d. Intraluminal used in lung Ca e. Intravascular	a. Iodine ***(I^{131})*** b. Phosphorus ***(P^{32})*** c. Samarium ***(Sm^{153})*** d. Strontium ***(Sr^{89})*** e. Rhenium ***(Re)*** **Used in :** – Ca thyroid – Bone tumours – Thyrotoxicosis

Indications of Radiotherapy

Curative Radiotherapy		Adjuvant RT (Surg+RT+/-CT)
Stage I and II :		
Head and neck cancers		Head and neck cancer (locally advanced)
Oesophagus cancer		Brain tumours
Skin	– Basal cell and squamous cell ca	Breast cancer
Lymphatic	– Hodgkin's lymphoma	Rectal cancer
Bladder	– Transitional cell ca	Soft tissue sarcoma
Prostate	– Adenocarcinoma	Bone sarcoma
Anal canal	– Carcinoma	Endometrial Ca, Cervical Ca
Lung	– Non-small cell cancer	*Paediatric solid tumours* (Wilms', rhabdomyosarcoma neuroblastoma)

Remember :

Combination of radiotherapy (RT) with chemotherapy (CT)		
Neoadjuvant Chemotherapy	*Adjuvant chemotherapy*	*Concurrent Chemotherapy*
↓	↓	↓
1-3 courses of CT before definite RT	CT given after completion of RT	CT given during course of RT

NEWER TECHNIQUES IN RADIOTHERAPY

i. **3D-Conformal Radiotherapy** ***(3-Dimensional treatment planning and conformal dose delivery i.e 3 DCRT).***

Features :
- Patient immobilization
- Image guided treatment planning
- Volumetric computer controlled treatment delivery.

Advantages : – Radiation dose is given accurately to cancer cell avoiding normal cells so dose of radiation can be increased if necessary without increasing toxicity to normal tissues.

ii. **IMRT (Intensity Modulated Radiation therapy)**

- It is advanced form of 3D CRT.
- It is the most advanced modality among the external beam radiation therapy.
- ***Feature :*** It use radiations broken into thousand tiny pencil-thin beams.
- ***Advantages :***
  - Same as 3D CRT
  - *Retreat* the cancer which is previously irradiated
  - Treat the ***tumours*** that lie close to delicate organs like eye, spinal cord or rectum.
- ***Indication :***
  - Prostate cancer, Pancreatic tumors, Lung cancer
  - Metastatic brain tumours, Primary brain tumours (glioblastomas, gliomas etc)
  - Liver tumours (metastases, hepatocellular carcinoma)
  - Head and neck cancer (larynx, tongue, sinus, base of skull, mouth etc)
  - Radiosurgery (single fraction) and stereotactic radiation therapy (Fractionated).

iii. **SRS (Single fraction)/SRT (Multiple fraction) :** *(Stereotactic Radiosurgery and Radiotherapy)*

- ***Stereotactic radiosurgery is a single day procedure for treating small intracranial lesion.***

- ***Feature :***
  - High dose
  - Highly focused radiation (photon beams) for *small target lesion* (< 2-4cm)
  - Patient immobilization is essential
- ***Equipment :***
  - *Gamma knife* (multiple Co^{60} sources)
  - *X knife* (Modified linear accelerator).
- ***Use :***
  - *Intracranial neoplasm (meningiomas, acoustic neuromas, metastatic tumours)*
  - Ablation of *arteriovenous malformations*
  - Ocular melanomas.

Radiation tolerance of Various organs

Organ	Injury	TD5/5	TD50/5 (in rad)
Bone marrow	Aplasia, pancytopenia	250	450
		3000	4000
Liver	**Acute and chronic**	**2500**	**4000**
	hepatitis	**1500**	**2000**
Stomach	Perforation, ulcer,		
	hemorrhage	4500	5500
Intestine	Ulcer, perforation,	4500	5500
	hemorrhage	5000	6500
Brain	Infarction, necrosis	5000	6000
Spinal cord	Infarction, necrosis	45000	55000
Heart	Pericarditis, pancarditis	45000	5500
		7000	8000
Lung	Acute and chronic	3000	3500
	pneumonitis	1500	2500
Kidney	Acute and chronic	1500	2000
	nephrosclerosis	2000	2500
Fetus	**Death**	**200**	**400**

TD_5 : Dose when administered to a given patient population, resulting in severe complications in ≤ 5% of patients. Also called as minimal tolerance dose

$TD_{50/5}$: Dose that resulted in severe complications in ≥ 50%. Also called as maximal tolerance dose

Pregnancy : It is recomended that exposure should not exceed 0.05 rem in any month or 0.5 rem in whole pregnancy.

Radiation toxicity

Acute toxicities

- Mucositis
- Bone marrow toxicities
- Skin erythema (Ulceration in severe cases)
- Nausea and vomiting

Delayed Toxicity

Brain	Headache, Leukoencephalopathy, Neurocognitive defect, Seizures
Spine	Incontinence, L'hermitte syndrome
Lung	Cough, Chest pain, Dyspnea, Pulmonary fibrosis; Pneumonia
Skin	Scaliness, Edema, Pain, Ulceration
Heart	Angina pectoris, Pericarditis; CHF
Liver	Cirrhosis, Hepatitis
GIT	Enteritis, Nausea and Vomiting
Cell	Mutations in cells

QUESTIONS

1. **All of the following radioisotopes are used as systemic radionucleide, except:** **[AI 06]**
   a. Phosphorus 32
   b. Strontium 89
   c. Iridium 192
   d. Samarium 153

2. **Phosphorus 32 emits :** **[AI 06]**
   a. Beta particles
   b. Alpha particles
   c. Neutrons
   d. X-rays

3. **Which of one of the following has the maximum ionization potential :** **[AI 06]**
   a. Electron
   b. Proton
   c. Helium ion
   d. Gamma [γ] photon

4. **Which of the following malignant tumours is radioresistant :** **[AI 06; AIIMS 07]**
   a. Ewing's sarcoma
   b. Retino blastoma
   c. Osteosarcoma
   d. Neuroblastoma

5. **The most radiosensitive tumour among the following is :** **[AI 06]**
   a. Bronchogenic carcinoma
   b. Carcinoma parotid
   c. Dysgerminoma
   d. Osteogenic sarcoma

6. **Which of the following imaging techniques gives maximum radiation exposure to the patient :** **[AI 06]**
   a. Chest X-ray
   b. MRI
   c. CT Scan
   d. Bone scan

7. **The technique employed in radiotherapy to counteract the effect of tumor motion due to breathing is known as :** **[AI 05]**
   a. Arc technique
   b. Modulation
   c. Gating
   d. Shunting

8. **Which one of the following radioisotope is not used as permanent implant?** **[AI 05]**
   a. Iodine-125
   b. Pallodium-103
   c. Gold-198
   d. Caesium-137

9. **Which of the following elements is obsolete in radiotherapy :** **[AIIMS 09]**
   a. Cesium 137
   b. Cobalt 60
   c. Radium 226
   d. iridium 192

10. **Craniospinal irradiation is employed in the treatment of :** **[PGI 09]**
    a. Oligodendroglioma
    b. Pliocytic astrocytoma
    c. Mixed oligoastrocytoma
    d. Medulloblastoma
    e. Glioblastoma

11. **Which of the following is the most radiosensitive phase of the cell cycle?** **[AI 08]**
    a. G2M
    b. G2
    c. S
    d. G1

12. **Amifostine, protects all of the following except:** **[AI 09]**
    a. CNS
    b. Salivary glands
    c. Kidneys
    d. GIT

13. **Which of the following is the most radiosensitive tumor :** **[AIIMS 05]**
    a. Ewing's sarcoma
    b. Hodgkin's disease
    c. Carcinoma cervix
    d. Malignant fibrous histiocytoma

14. **For which malignancy, intensity modulated radiotherapy [IMRT] is indicated :** **[AIIMS 05]**
a. Lung
b. Prostate
c. Leukemias
d. Stomach

15. **Which of the following radioactive isotopes is not used in brachytherapy :** **[AIIMS 05]**
a. Iodine 125
b. Iodine 131
c. Cobalt 60
d. Iridium 192

16. **Which of the following is most radiosensitive phase of cellcycle : [PGI 08, 09]**
a. G1
b. S
c. G2M
d. M
e. G0

17. **High energy linear acclerators use :** **[PGI 06]**
a. X - Rays
b. γ-Rays
c. α - Rays
d. Infrared Rays
e. β-Rays

18. **Ionizing radiation cause maximum damage in :** **[PGI 05]**
a. Hypoxic cells
b. Cells in S phase
c. Cells in G_2M phase
d. Dividing cells
e. Neurons

ANSWERS, REFERENCES, EXPLANATIONS WITH INFORMATIVE ILLUSTRATIONS

1. **Ans. is c i.e. Iridium 192**

Ref. Priniciples of Radiation Oncology by Carlos & Luther 4/e, p 636 - 637

- **Systemic radionuclides** are non-sealed radio nuclides which are ***administered*** orally, intravenously or intracavitary.
- Before administering it, pregnancy should be ruled out.
- Discontinue breast feeding for 1 to 2 weeks.

Radioisotopes	T ½ (days)	Decay particles	Use
a. Sodium iodide (I^{131})	8	Gamma, beta	*Hyperthyroidism* (diffuse toxic goiter, toxic multinodular goiter, or solitary toxic thyroid nodule), thyroid carcinoma
b. Sodium phosphate (P^{32})	14.3	Beta	*Myeloproliferative* disorders (PCV and thrombo-cytosis)
Colloidal chromic phosphate			Intracavitary therapy of malignant ascites, malignant pleural effusion and brain cyst
c. Samarium 153 (Sm) chloride	1.9	Beta	*Painful bone metastases*
d. Strontium 89 (Sr) chloride	50.5	Beta	*Painful bone metastases*
e. Rhenium (Re)	3.8	Beta, Gamma	*Painful bone metastases*

2. **Ans. is a i.e. Beta praticles**

Ref. Priniciples of Radiation Oncology by Carlos & Luther 4/e, p 636

P-32 is produced by bombarding sulfur -32 with reactor produced neutrons. ^{32}P decays by pure b particle emission.

3. **Ans. is c i.e. Helium ion** *Ref. Harrison 16/e, p 484*

"Alpha particles (helium ion) and low energy neutrons are densely ionizing; x-rays and Gamma rays sparsely ionizing."

Ionizing radiation	
Particulate	***Electromagnetic***
Electron (β rays) Proton Neutron Alpha particle *(maximum ionization)*	X-ray Gamma ray *(maximum penetration)*

Radiation *(specially x-rays)* cause ionization in three major ways :

Photoelectric effect	At low energies (30-100 Kev), as in *diagnostic radiology*, the photoelectric effect predominates.
Compton effect	At higher energies, as used in *therapeutic radiology.*
Pair production	At very high energy (>102Mv), *usually accidental.*

Remember :

– **Penetrating power of various particles** (in *decreasing order*) γ rays (*high energy photons*) > X-rays > β rays (*high energy electron*) > a particles (*helium nuclei*). ***Or***

– **For same particle penetrability depend upon energy,** or 10 Mev photon will have higher penetrating power than 5 Mev photons.

4. **Ans. is c i.e. Osteosarcoma** *Ref. Essentials of Radiology by Bhaduri, p 502*

Radiosensitive Tumours	
Highly sensitive	**Highly Resistant**
1. Seminoma/Dysgerminoma 2. Lymphoma 3. Myeloma 4. Ewing's sarcoma 5. Wilms	– Melanoma – Osteosarcoma – Pancreatic carcinoma – Hepatoma

5. **Ans. is c i.e. Dysgerminoma** *Ref. Bailey & Love 24/e, p 221*

Seminoma or its female counter part dysgerminoma is most radiosensitive tumour.

Note : Though seminoma and dysgerminoma are most radiosensitive tumor the treatment of choice for these tumor is surgery.

6. **Ans. is c i.e. CT scan** *Ref. Bailey & Love 25/e, p 130*

Investigation	Effective radiation dose	Equivalent chest radiograph dose
Chest- X-ray	(MSV) 0.02	1
CT - head	2.3	115
CT - chest	8	400
CT abdomen or pelvis	10	500
Bone scan (^{99M}TC)	4	200
Renal scan (^{99M}TC)	1	50
Lung perfusion scan (^{99M}TC)	1	50
Thyroid scan	1	50

So, guys I think answer is clear.

Remember :
- **CT** is ***best imaging*** for *bone, hemorrhagic condition* and *other harder structure* such as renal calculi.
- **MRI** is ***best imaging*** for *soft tissue pathology, spine.*

7. **Ans. is c i.e. Gating**

Ref. Text book of Radiation Oncology by Leibe Phillips 2/e, p 192 - 194

Variation in treatment geometry for sites such as thorax and abdomen are significant due to breathing motion. Larger margin are required in these regions to define the planed target volume.

Currently, several techniques are being used to reduce the uncertainty due to respiratory motion.

These include :
- Respiratory gating (RG)
- Active breathing control (ABC)
- *Deep inspiration breath hold technique.*

Respiratory gating : *RG system permit breathing synchronized fluoroscopy on a treatment simulator.* System consist of charge coupled device (CCD). Video camera attached to an infrared illuminator that track a patients respiratory motion.

In simple words, *in this technique, source of radiation moves as tumour moves on respiration.*

Active breathing control : In this method patient *nose is clamped* and *he or she breathes through an ABC apparatus,* which simultaneously control radiation dose.

Deep Insipiration Breath Hold Technique (DIBH) : *This is a subjective in which patient is asked to hold his breath in deep inspiration, Technique has two advantages :*
- Breath hold minimize tumor motion
- It expand the lung to its maximum volume putting the healthy lung tissue out of the radiation field.

However, this technique is ***not useful for uncooperative patients.***

Other options

Modulation : *Method of sensitizing tumour cells* to radiotherapy Eg. oxygen is well known radiosensitizer. *... Principle & practice of radiation oncology 4/e, p 663*

Arc technique : It is a *type of electron beam therapy* used in *postmastectomy case for chest wall radiation.* It is more useful in women with barrel chest and bilateral disease.

... Principle & practice of radiation oncology 4/e, p 278

8. **Ans. is d i.e. Caesium 137** *Ref. Washington & Leaver Principles of Radiotherapy 2/e, p 326; Principles & Practice of Radiation Oncology by Carlos & Luther 4/e, p 508*

"I-125, P-103, Gold-198 are used as permanent implant."

In interstitial brachytherapy the radioactive sourcess are directly placed into or adjacent to the tumor or tumor bed.

Interstitial implants is of two types :

Permanent interstitial implants	Temporary interstitial implants
They are used when the tumor to be treated is inaccessible making the *removal of radioisotope impossible or impractical.* *These implants have usually short half lives* (Cesium 137 has half life of 30 years)	Temporary removable implants are used in anatomic areas where *there is no body cavity or orifice* to accept radioactive sources.
Isotope used : *Pallodium 103* *Iodine 125* *Gold – 198* ***Mnemonic :*** *PIG*	*Iridium – 192 (MC)* *Cesium – 137* ***Mnemonic :*** **ICT**= **I**ntra **C**ranial **T**ension
Use : Deep seated lesion in pelvis, abdomen, lung colorectum	***Use :*** Breast and Chest wall irradiation Anterior, lateral and posterior wall of vagina

Remember : Brachytherapy is of 5 types.

Brachytherapy				
External applicator or molds	**Interstitial brachytherapy**	**Intracavitary brachytherapy**	**Intraluminal brachytherapy**	**Intravascular brachytherapy**
	– GI T Cancer – Caprostate	– Ca Cervix – Ca rectum	Lung Ca	

9. **Ans. is c i.e. Radium 226**

Ref. Text book of Radiation Oncology Leibel Phillips 2/e, p 231

Isotope used in Brachytherapy			
Application	**Traditional**	**Current**	**Future**
Intracavitary implants	(not used now)		
Low dose rate	^{226}Ra	^{137}Cs	^{241}Am, Ir^{192I}, ^{169}Yb
High dose	^{60}Co	^{192}Ir	^{169}Yb, ^{192}Ir
Interstitial implants			
Nonafterloading	^{226}Ra	^{137}Cs	—
Afterloading	—	^{192}Ir	^{125}I, ^{103}Pd, ^{169}Yb
High dose rate	—	^{192}Ir	^{169}Yb, ^{192}Ir
Permanent implants			
Conventional dose rate	^{222}Rn	^{198}Au	^{198}Au, ^{131}Cs
Ultra-low dose rate	—	^{125}I, ^{103}Pd	^{125}I, ^{103}Ir
Intravascular brachytherapy			
Cardiac stents	—	^{32}P	—
Catheter-based cardiac	—	^{32}P, ^{90}Sr/Y^{90}, ^{192}Ir	^{169}Yb,
Catheter-based peripheral	—	^{192}Ir	^{125}I, ^{103}Pd, ^{169}Yb

- Co-60 is now only used in teletherapy.
- ***Radium 226 is not ued any more*** because of following reasons:
  - Longest half life among all isotopes
  - Emits alpha and gamma rays, which is the most dangerous combination.
  - Produces radon, a radiactive inert gas which is difficult to remove.

10. Ans. is d and e i.e. Medulloblastoma; Glioblastoma

... Ref. Devita 7/e, p 1844; Radiation Oncology by Leibel Phillips 2/e, p 489

Prophylactic craniospinal irradiation is recommended in primary tumour showing high propensity to metastasize to CSF and metastatic tumours of brain.

Prophylactic craniospinal irradiation	
Primary brain tumour	**Tumour with high risk of brain metastases**
• Medulloblastoma	• ALL
• Anaplastic ependymomas	• Non hodgkin lymphoma
• Glioblastoma	• Small cell Ca of lung
• Germcell tumors such as germinoma	*... Devita 7/e, p 1861*

Dose is ***30 Gy*** given in *10 daily fraction of 3 Gy each over 2 weeks.*

11. Ans. is a i.e. G_2 M phase

... Ref. Principles & Practice of Radiation Therapy by Washington lever 2/e, p 65

Susceptibilty of various phases of cell cycle to radiation.

- G_2 M > M > G1 > early S > late S phase.
- ***Most sensitive*** period is junction of G2-M phase.

Remember : Radiation causes cell damage by daming DNA; generating free radicals.

12. Ans. is a i.e. CNS ... *Ref. Devita 8/e, p 916, 316; Radiation oncology 8/e p 41*

"Amifostine offers no protection to the CNS as it does'nt cross blood brain barrier".

Mechanism of protection: Amifostine (Ethyol) scavenge free radicals produce by ionizing radiations.

Tissue protected : Gut lining; hematopoetic system, salivary glands

Note: Amifostine provide protection against hematologic and nonhematologic toxicity of cisplatin also.

Radiosensitizers	Radiation protectors
• Oxygen *(most effective radiosensitizer)*	• Amifostine
• Metronidazole*, misonidazole*, Tinadazole*	• IL-1
• Tirapazamine*	• GM-CSF
• 5-Fu *(non hypoxic cell sensitizer)*	
• Hydroxyurea *(non hypoxic sensitizer)*	
• BUDR and IUDR *(non hypoxic cell sensitizer)*	
• Cisaplatin; Paclitaxel; Gemcitabine; Mitomycin; Tropotecan; Vinorelbine	

* *Hypoxic cell sensitizer*

13. Ans. is a i.e. Ewing's sarcoma *Ref. Bailey & Love 24/e, p 221*

Radiosensitivity of various tumours	
Highly sensitive	**Moderately sensitive**
– Seminoma / Dysgerminoma – Lymphoma – Myeloma – Ewing's sarcoma – Wilms tumour	– Small cell lung carcinoma – Carcinoma Breast – Teratoma – Ovarian carcinoma – Basal cell carcinoma – Medulloblastoma – Dysgerminoma – Nasopharyngeal carcinoma
Relatively Resistant	**Highly Resistant**
– Squamous cell carcinoma lung – Hypernephroma (Renal cell carcinoma) – Rectal carcinoma/colon carcinoma – Bladder carcinoma – Soft tissue sarcoma (fibrosarcoma) – Carcinoma cervix	– Melanoma – Osteosarcoma – Pancreatic carcinoma – Hepatoma

14. Ans. is b i.e. Carcinoma prostate

Ref. Radiation Oncology by Leibel Phillips 2/e, p 315, 334

Intensity modulated radiotherapy (IMRT)

IMRT is a *specialized formed of radiotherapy* in which intensity of individual ray in each beam can be manipulated to increase control over the radiation fluency and enables optimum dose distribution.

In comparision to standard 3D conformal radiation therapy, ***dose distribution are far*** more conformal in IMRT.

Indication :

- Prostate cancer, Pancreatic tumors.
- Metastatic brain tumours, Primary brain tumours (glioblastomas, gliomas etc).
- Liver tumours (metastatses, hepatocellular carcinoma).
- Head and neck cancer (larynx, tongue, sinus, base of skull, mouth etc).

15. Ans. is c i.e. Cobalt 60 *Ref. Radiation Oncology Leibel Philips 2/e, p 231*

Cobalt 60 is used in teletherapy alone.

16. Ans. is c i.e. G_2

Already explained.

17. Ans. is a i.e. X-rays *Ref. Harrison 17/e, p 516*

X-rays and γ rays are the most common form of radiation used to treat cancer. X-rays are generated by linear accleration; gamma rays are generated from decay of atomic nuclei in radiosotopes such as cobalt and sodium.

Type of radiation	RBE
X-rays, gamma rays and electron	1
Neurons	3-20
Heavy particles (a particles)	1-20

18. Ans. is c and d i.e. Cells in G_2M phase; and Dividing cells *Ref. Harrison 17/e, p 516*

Factors ↑ radiosensitivity	Factors ↓ Radiosensitivity
Well oxygenation	Hypoxic environment
Rapid division	Slow or no division
G2M, M phase of cell cycle	S-phase of cell cycle
Radiation sensitizers	Radiation protectors (Amifostine)
(Nitroimidazoles, Alkylating agent)	

Note: The most important microenvironmental factor is molecular oxygen. This decreased killing by decreased oxygen can be expressed as oxygen enhancement ratio.

Oxygen enhancement ratio can be defined as ratio of doses required to kill same cell under hypoxic and normoxic conditions. This ratio is approx. 3

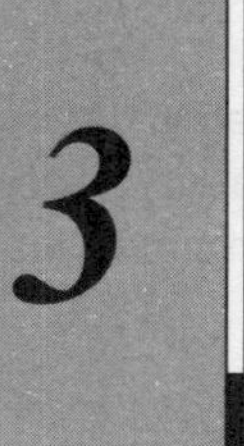

Cancer Chemotherapy and Complication

What's Important ?

- **Classification of Anti-cancer Drugs**
- **Mechanism of Action**

CLASSIFICATION

Anti Cancer drug are broadly classified into following classes :

– Alkylating agents	– Antimetabolites	– Antibiotics
– Topoisomerase poisons	– Mitotic spindle inhibitors	– Hormonal agents
– Miscellaneous drugs	– Molecularly targeted therapy	

- ***Anti metabolites*** and ***Mitotic spindle inhibitors*** are *cell cycle active, phase specific* i.e. *antimetabolites* ***kill cell in S phase*** while *mitotic spindle inhibitors* ***kills cell in M. phase.***
- ***Antibiotics and Alkylating agents*** are phase non specific, i.e. *they are active in all phases of cell cycle.*
- ***Cancer chemotherapeutic agents kills cancer cell by both necrosis and apoptosis*** .

..... Harrison 16/e, p 469

ALKYLATING AGENTS

Alkylating agents are electrophile molecules that react with *electron rich atom to form covalent bond.* It includes :

- **Nitrogen mustard :** Cyclophosphamide, Ifosfamide
- Mechlorethamine
- Melphalan
- Dacarbazine
- Thio TEPA
- Altretamine
- **Nitroso-ureas :** Carmustine, Lomustine.
- Chlorambucil
- Procarbazine
- Busulphan
- Temozolomide
- Cisplatin Carboplatin and Oxaliplatin (Not typical alkylating agents)

Mechlorethamine was the first alkylating agent used in human cancer management

... Devita 8/e p 407

Mode of Action

- On entering body these drugs changes in to reactive intermediates, that ***covalently*** *modify bases in DNA.* As a result DNA replication stops.

- In addition, they are potent activator of cell cycle check point and signaling pathway that can ***activate apoptosis.***
- The general mechanism of action involves intramolecular cyclization to form an ethyl carbonium ion that may directly or through formation of carbonium ion, transfer an alkyl group to DNA.
- *Major site of alkylation* within DNA is N7 portion of guanine. This results in cross linking; abnormal base pairing, and scission of DNA strand.

Pharmacologic effects

- Active alkylating agents can damage tissue at the site of injection as well as produce systemic toxicity.
- **Common Toxicities** of alkylating agents are : *Myelosuppresion, alopecia, gonadal dysfunction, pulmonary fibrosis, mucositis, second neoplasm (particularly leukemia).*

Drug resistance

Resistance to alkylating agents occur by :

- ***Decreased permeability*** of cell
- ↑ Capability ***of repair***
- ↑ production of ***glutathione*** which inactivates the drug.

Individual Drugs

Cyclophosphamide

- *Most useful* and *most frequently* used alkylating agent. It has prominent immunosuppressant property.
- Inactive as such metabolised in liver into alkylating species *"Aldophosphamide, Phosphoramide mustard"* as well as to *"acrolein". Acrolein cause chemical cystitis.* Chloramphenical retards the metabolism of cyclophosphamide.
- *Unique toxicity* of cyclophosphamide is characteristic ***hemorrhagic cystitis,*** acroline is responsible for it.
- To prevent cystitis excellent hydration should be maintained. If ***severe cystitis occur treat by Mesna (6 mercaptoethane sulphonate).***

Ifosphamide

- Also activated in liver but more slowly and require coadministration of Mesna, to prevent Cystitis.
- ***CNS*** effect includes somnolence, confusion and psychosis.

***Nitrosoureas* (Streptozocin; Carmustine; Lomustine)**

- Break down to carbamylating species that has DNA base pair toxicity and also modify proteins to cause cell death.
- Cause ***delayed Bone narrow toxicity.***
- *Streptozo tocin has glucose like structure*, and is specifically toxic to islet cells so ***used in endocrine pancreatic*** tumours.
- It is nephrotoxic also (cause *Fanconi syndrome and Renal tubular acidosis*).

Chlorambucil

- ***Slow acting*** alkylating agent.
- *Specially active* against ***lymphoid tissue;*** sparing myeloid tissue.

- First line drug for ***CLL.***
- Cause azoospermia and has pulmonary side effects in addition to common side effects of alkylators.

Melphalan

- Very effective drug in multiple myeloma.
- ***Bone marrow depression is most important toxicity.***
- ***Mucositis and pancreatitis*** are additional complication.

Procarbazine

- In addition to myelosuppression, it causes hypnotic and other effects.
- One of its ***metabolite is MAO Inhibitor,*** so produce *dangerous side effects when given with MAO inhibitors. It can cause disulfiram like syndrome on ingestion of ethanol.*
- It has leukemgenic properties, because of which its use is now restricted.

Dacarbazine

- Differs from other alkylating agents in having primary effect on RNA and protein synthesis (others mainly effects DNA).
- Major indication are melanoma and Hodgkins' disease.
- Cause severe nausea after use.

Busulphan

- It is ***highly specific for myeloid elements;*** granulocyte precursors being most sensitive. It is relatively lymphocytes sparing.
- Exerts cytotoxicity through alkylation of proteins ... *Devita 8/e 408*
- Cause ***severe myelosuppression. Pulmonary fibrosis*** is a specific side effect.
- Hyperuricemia is also common.
  Note : In *KDT 6/e, p 822* Busulphan is given as DOC for CML which is wrong. **Now DOC for CML is imatinib mesylate** a inhibitor of tyrosine kinase.

Temzolamide

- Newest alkylating agent
- Prodrug *that undergoes spontaneous actvation to produce MTIC a triazine derivative.*
- It can cross blood brain barrier, so is effective in the treatment of gliomas and melanomas.

ThioTEPA

- Highly toxic
- Now **use** is restricted to neoplastic meningitis in which it is administered intrathecally.

Cisplatin

- Inhibits DNA by forming platinum based cross links, RNA is spared. Effects are most pronounced during S phase.
- Very effective in metastatic testicular and ovarian carcinoma.
- Has very ***little effect on bonemarrow.***
- Nephrotoxic and intense emetogenic, so administered with diuretics and antiemetogenic agents.
- Other common toxicities include neurotoxicity with stocking and glove sensory motor neuropathy and hearing loss. Patient may develop AML after cisaplatin therapy.
- Hypomagnesemia and hypocalcema are also seen.

Carboplatin

- Less nephro and neurotoxic than cisplatin but cause more myelosuppresion.
- More effective than cisplatin in ovarian cancer, lung cancer

Oxaliplatin

- Used in refractory colon cancer
- *Neurotoxic*

ANTIMETABOLITES

- These are compounds ***structurally similar to purines / pyrimidines*** or that ***interfere with synthesis of purines and pyrimidines.*** So, they effect cell mainly in S-phase.
- **Common toxicities** include :
  - Stomatitis
  - Diarrhoea
  - Myelosupression
- Not associated with second malignancy.

Antimetabolites		
Purine antagonist	***Folic acid antagonist***	***Pyrimidine antagonist***
– Mercaptopurine – Thioguanines – Fludarabine – Cladarabine	– Methotrexate – Pemetrexed – Raltitrexed	– 5 FU – Cyatarbine = AraC – Gemcitabine – Capecitabine

I. Methotrexate

- It is ***folic acid antagonist.***
- *Binds to* dihydrofolate reductase, thus *blocks the conversion of dihydrofolic acid (DHFA) to tetrahydrofolic acid,* which acts as cofactor in synthesis of purines, thymidine, serine and methionine. There by interfering with the formation of DNA, RNA and protein.
- **Kill cells** in S phase.
- ***Toxicity***
  - Excreted primarily by kidney, so it is nephrotoxic.
  - Myelosupression, Hepatic fibrosis, arachnoiditis.
- *Toxicity of methotrexate* can be ***reversed*** by administration of leucovorin *(citrovorum factor – folinic acid).*
- **Used :**
  - Choriocarcinoma
  - Acute leukemia (for maintaining remission)
  - Rheumatoid arthritis
  - Psoriasis.
  - Osteosarcoma

Pemetrexed

- Noval folate directed antimetabolite, which inhibits the activity of ***multiple enzymes*** including *thymidylate synthetase, dihydrofolate reductase, and glycinamide ribonucleotide formyl transferase,* thereby affecting the synthesis of both purine and pyrimidine precursor.

II. Purine antagonist

A. Mercaptopurine and thioguanines

- They are *converted* in body to monoribonucleotides which *inhibits conversion of inosine monophosphate to adenine and guanine nucleotides.*
- Both are nephrotoxic, and cause myelosupression.
- **Used** mainly in childhood acute leukemia *(Thioguanine has synergistic action when used along with cytarabine).*
- 6 MP is metabolised by xanthine oxidase which is inhibited by allopurinol, so *dose of MP should be reduced if allopurinol is administered concurrently.*

B. Fludarabine and Cladribine

- Fludarabine is **prodrug** of F. adenine arabino-side (F – ara - A) which gets ***incorporated into DNA and cause cytotoxicity*** even in cells with low growth fraction.
- Primarily **used** in treatment of lymphoproliferative disease such as CLL and follicular B cell lymphoma.
- Main dose related **toxicity** is myelosupression and CNS dysfunction.
- **Cladribine** is similar drug which also incorporated in to DNA : ***Primarily used in treatment of hairy cell leukemia (DOC).***
- Both of these drugs are resistant to adenosine deaminase.

III. Pyrimidine antagonist :

These drugs have ***antineoplastic, antifungal and antipsoriatic*** properties

It includes :

A. Fluro uracil (5 FU) :

- *Converted* in body to **5FdUMP** which inhibits thymidylate synthetase, resulting in inhibition of DNA synthesis through *"thymine less death."* *... Katzung 8/e, p 934*
- In *addition it gets incorporated into RNA and cause single strand break,* thus effecting both DNA and RNA.
- Leucovarin augments the activity of 5 FU, by reducing folate, promoting formation of 5FU complexes. *... Harrison 16/e, p 476*
- **Used** in treatment of various adeno carcinoma (e.g. GIT).
- **Toxicity** include Mucositis and diarrhea (MC); myelosupression, hand foot syndrome, photosensitivity.

B. Cytarabine = Cytosine arabinoside = Arac

- S phase specific antimetabolite gets ***incorporated into DNA*** and its 5 trinucleotide 5 Ara (TP) ***inhibits DNA polymerase*** also.
- Can be given intrathecally.
- **Adverse effects** include nausea, diarrhoea, stomatitis, chemical conjunctivitis and cerebellar ataxia.
- **Used** is limited to AML.

C. Gemcitabine

- Similar to Ara C, it gets incorporated in DNA and make DNA susceptible to breakage.
- *In contrast to Ara C* it is ***effective in solid tumours*** (Mainly pancroatic ca, lung Ca, ovarian Ca).
- Main **toxicity** is myelosuppression, and *lacks other toxicities of AraC.*

ANTIBIOTICS

- They bind to DNA directly and generate free radical in close proximity to DNA leading to DNA damage in the form of single strand breaks and cross links. *... Harrison 17/e, p 524*
- All of the antitumour antibiotics are derived from various strains of soil microbe *Streptomyces*.
- Antibiotics anticancer drugs are :

– Anthracycline (Doxorubicin and Dauna rubicin)	– Bleomycin
– Dactinomycin	– Mithramycin
– Mitomycin	

Anthracyclines

- Doxorubicin is the most widely active and frequently used neoplastic drug.
- Anthracycline acts by **three modes :**

- Gets incorporated in to DNA and alter DNA structure, replication and topoisomerase.
- *Binds to membrane* to alter fluidity and ion transport.
- Generate free radicals and oxygen radical (responsible for their cardiotoxity) .

... Katzung 8/e, p 939

- Doxorubicin **used** in variety of tumours including Breast, endometrium, ovary, testicle. It is also useful in hematological cancer.
- *Daunorubicin is more effective than doxorubicin in acute leukemia.*
- **Doxorubicin** cause profound myelosupression and has specific cardiotoxicity in form of *ventricular and atrial dysrhythmias and irreversible cardiomyopathy.* **Other toxicities** include *stomatitis, alopecia and mucositis.*
- **Daunorubicin** have *similar toxicities* but cause less mucositis.
- Encapsulation of daunorubicin into liposome *attenuates its cardiotoxicity* and makes it effective in kaposi sarcoma and ovarian cancer. *... Harrison 17/e, p 525*

Bleomycin

- It is **mixture of glycopeptides** which form complex with Fe^{2+} and binds DNA. Oxidation of Fe^{++} *give rise to superoxide and hydroxide radical.*
- It leads to **accumulation** of cell in G_2 phase. (So cell cycle specific).
- It does **not** or cause very little myelosuppression.
- ***Most feared complication*** of bleomycin is pulmonary fibrosis.
- ***Earliest indication of pulmonary fibrosis is decline in*** *DLco.*
- Other ***common side effects*** include fever chills, facial flush, and Raynoud's syndrome.

Used in :
- Squamaus cell carcinoma, Testicular tumour.
- **Special use** is intracavitary therapy of malignant effusions in breast and ovarian cancer.

Dactinomycin (Actinomycin)

- **Binds** to *DNA* and *inhibit all forms of DNA dependent RNA synthesis. Ribosomal RNA synthesis being most affected.*
- **Cause** *severe myelosupression, nausea, alopecias, mucositis, defect in platelets, SIADH*
- **Used :** in treatment of Rhabdomyosarcoma, wilms tumour, chorio carcinoma.

Mithramycin

- **Binds to DNA** and interrupts DNA dependent RNA synthesis.
- **Cause :** *Myelosupression, nausea, vomiting and acute hemorrhagic syndrome.*
- Currently **use** is limited to hypercalcemia of malignancy.

Mitomycin C

- Undergoes reductive activation to **generate** alkylating agents which binds to DNA.
- ***Hypoxic tumour cells, solid tumours*** are *more sensitive.*
- It is the **best available drug** for use as an adjuvant to X-ray radiation to attack hypoxic tumour cell. *..... Katzung 8/e, p 439*
- In addition to nausea and vomiting its **toxicity** includes – *Delayed bronchospasm* (10-12 hour after dosing), chronic pulmonary fibrosis.
  - Myelosuppression
  - Cardiomyopathy
  - Hemolytic uraemic syndrome

Mitoxantrione

- *Synthetic analogue of doxorubicin with* ***lower cardiotoxicity,*** *though cardiomyopathy can occur.*

TOPOISOMERASE POISONS

- This include drugs that bind to ***topoisomerase*** *a enzyme that regulate the capacity of DNA to unwind, to allow normal replication and transcription.*
- DNA damage from these agents can occur in any phase of cell cycle, but tends to *arrest cell cycle in S-phase or G2.*
- They includes :
  - Etoposide
  - Tenioposide
  - Campothecins
  - Topotecan

Etoposide and Teniposide

- Etoposide was derived from plant product **podophyllotoxin.**
- **Binds** to topoisomerase II (two) and cause prominent G2 arrest.
- **Adverse effect** include – *Myelosuppression; Nausea; Transient hypotension, thrombocytopenia*
- Teniposide is its structural relative with **unique activity** in childhood ALL.
- When given in high does or very frequently these drugs ***may cause mucositis.***

Campothecin and Topotecan

- These **drugs binds** to Topoisomerase 1.
- Topotecan is approved for **use** in *ovarian carcinoma.*
- Toxicity of these drugs is limited to myelosupression and mucositis.
- **Irinotecan :**
  - Another campothecin derivative used in colon carcinoma.
  - In addition to myelosupression it cause **secretory diarrhea.**

MITOTIC SPINDLE INHIBITORS

- Mitotic spindles are made of microtubules along which various motile and secretory process occur during cell division. Thus inhibition leads block in M. phase.

  It includes :
  - Vinca alkaloids (Vinblastine and Vincristine)
  - Taxanes (Paclitaxel and Docetaxil)
  - Estramustine.

Vinblastine and Vincristine

- These drugs **binds** to tubulin dimer as a result micro tubules are disintegrated and cause **mitotic arrest** in **metaphase.**
- **Toxicity** of vinblastine includes *nausea, myelosuppression (Bone marrow supression) and alopecia.*
- Vincristine is not associated with myelosupression, but **causes** *neurotoxicity* in form of peripheral neuritis, *paralytic ileus, jaw pain and acute urinary retention* alopecia.
- Vincristine is **used** for inducing remission in *childhood acute leukemia.*

Paclitaxel and Docetaxil

- Taxanes are among the *most broadly active neoplastic agents.*
- In **contrast to vinca alkaloids,** these drugs *stabilize the tubules,* which are not able to undergo normal dynamic changes necessary for cell cycle completion.
- **Paclitaxel causes :** *Hypersenstivity reaction, myelosupression, neurotoxicity in form of* ***glove and stocking numbness*** *and paresthesia*
- **Docetaxil also has same toxicity,** but hypersensitivity reactions are less and in addition it causes fluid retention.

Estramustine :

- **Binds** to microtubule associated proteins, resulting in abnormal microtubule function.
- ***Specifically active in prostatic ca.***
- **CVS** *side effect* occur in form of worsened heart failure and thromboembolic phenomenon.

HORMONAL AGENTS

This include :

Class	Drug	Use
Antiestrogen	Tamoxifen	Breast ca
Antiandrogen	Flutamide	Prostate ca
GnRH agonist	Leuprolide, Goserelin	Prostate ca, Breast ca
Aromatase inhibitors	Aminoglutethimide Anastrozole, Letrozole	Metastatic breast ca
5a reductase inhibitros	Finasteride	Ca Prostate

MISCELLANEOUS DRUGS

Asparaginase

- Acts indirectly by ***inhibition of protein synthesis*** by depleting asparagine in neoplastic cells which requires external asparagine.

Hydroxyurea

- Analogue of urea, acts by inhibiting DNA synthesis by ***inhibiting ribonucleotide reductase.***
- **Used** in melanoma and CML.
- **Major toxicity** is bone marrow depression.

Retinoic acid derivative

- ***Trans retinoic acid*** – **Used** in cases of acute promyelocytic leukemia.
- ***Cis Retinoic acid*** – **Used** to prevent secondary tumours in patient with head and neck squamous cell carcinoma.

Amifostine (WH2721)

- Agent designed to **provide cytoprotection** to **normal cells** from *chemotherapy and radiotherapy.*
- Converted in normal tissue to its active thiolform WH 1065 which **binds free radicals** hence protect normal cells.

MOLECULARY TARGETED THERAPY

These agents are targeted against products of oncogenes, mediators of cellular immortality such as telomerase etc.

Important agents are :

Antitumour antibodies		
1. Monoclonal Antibodies	**Target**	**Use**
Rituximab	CD-20	Relapsed or Resistant lymphoma
Trastuzumab	HER-2/neu (C-erb-2) Coding for tyrosine Kinase	Metastatic breast ca
A lemtuzumab	CD-52	Resistant CLL
Cetuximab	EFGR	Resistant colorectal ca
Bevacizumab	VEGF	***First antiangiogenic agent approved*** Colorectal ca, RCC, Breast ca
2. Antibodies linked to radio isotopes		
Ibritumonab tiuxetal (Linked to yttrium 90)	CD-20	Lowgrade NHL Tositumemab (Linked to I^{131})

Tyrosine Kinase inhibitors

- Imatinib mesylate – **Blocks** active tyrosine kinase, **used** in CML.
- Gefitinib – **Block** the *intracellular component of epidermal growth factor receptor.*
- Netotinib – Similar to imitanib, but with increased potency and better tolerability.
- Dasatinib – Inhibitory to kinases of src-tyrosine protein kinase family
  – Effective in hematopoetic tumor and some solid tumors where src kinases are active
- Lapitinib – Combined EGF receptor and erb_2 tyrosine kinase antagonist with activity in breast cancer
- Erlotinib – EGF receptor tyrosine kinase antagonist, used in small cell lung cancer.

Other agents

Bortezonib : Proteosome inhibitor that has activity in multiple myeloma and certain lymphomas.
Vorinostat : Histone deacetylase inhibitor, that has activity in cutoneous T-cell lymphoma.
Soafenib : VEGF-R antagonist
Sunitinib : Anti VEGFR, as well as anti PDGF-R and anti-C-Kit acitivity.

QUESTIONS

1. **Not an alkylating agent: [AI 07; AIIMS 07]**
   a. Cyclophosphamide
   b. 5FU
   c. Busulfan
   d. Melphalan

2. **High dose of methotrexate is used in the treatment of : [AI 07]**
   a. Rhabdomyosarcoma
   b. Osteosarcoma
   c. Multiple myeloma
   d. Ewing's sarcoma

3. **All of the following Anticancer agents cause bone marrow depression except :**
   a. Chlorambucil **[AI 05]**
   b. Daunorubicin
   c. Doxorubicin
   d. Flutamide

4. **Which of the following drugs is 'Topoisomerase 1 inhibitor' ? [AI 05]**
   a. Doxorubicin
   b. Irinotecan
   c. Etoposide
   d. Vincristine

5. **Which is the most active single chemotherapeutic agent in the treatment of Leiomyosarcoma ? [AI 05]**
   a. Adriamycin
   b. Doxorubicin
   c. Methotrexate
   d. Cisplatin

6. **Ifosfamide is an: [AI 09]**
   a. Alkylating Agent
   b. Antimetabolite
   c. Folate antagonist
   d. Plant Alkaloid

7. **Which of the following anticancer drugs is cell cycle phase specific [AI 09]**
   a. Ifosfamide
   b. Bleomycin
   c. Cisplatin
   d. Chlorambucil

8. **Bleomycin toxicity is characterized by Hyperplasia of [AI 09]**
   a. Endothelial cells
   b. Type I Pneumocytes
   c. Type II Pneumocytes
   d. Alveolar macrophages

9. **'Hand Foot' syndrome can be caused by?**
   a. Cisplatin **[AI 09]**
   b. Capecitabine
   c. Vincristine
   d. Azathioprine

10. **Which of the following antibiotics is an anti tumour peptide? [AI 08]**
    a. Bleomycin
    b. Doxorubcin
    c. Valinomycin
    d. L. Asparaginase

11. **Mechanism of action of paclitaxel is**
    a. Inhibits DNA synthesis **[AIIMS 08]**
    b. Topoisomerase II inhibitor
    c. Inhibition of tubulin
    d. Stabilisation of tubules

12. **Leucovorin is given with: [AI 08]**
    a. Methotrexate
    b. Cytosine arabinoside
    c. 6-MP
    d. Thio Tepa

13. **Sustained neutropenia is seen with:**
    a. Vinblastin **[AIIMS 08]**
    b. Cisplatin
    c. Carmustine
    d. Cyclophosphamide

14. SIADH is caused by all except: [AIIMS 08]
a. Vincristine
b. Vinblastine
c. Actinomycin D
d. Cyslophosphamide

15. Tyrosine kinase inhibitors are most commonly used in? [AI 10, AIIMS 08]
a. GIST
b. Receptor mediated neuroendocrine tumors
c. Breast cancer
d. RCC

16. Which of the following is HER2 and EGF receptor antagonist? [AI 10]
a. Geftinib
b. Imatinib
c. Erlotinib
d. Lepatinib

17. Alkylating agents are: [PGI 09]
a. Ifosfamide
b. Chlorabucil
c. Paclitaxel
d. Nitrosoureas
e. Cytarabine

18. All are anticancer antibiotics except
a. Tetracyline [AIIMS 06]
b. Adriamycin
c. Mitomycin C
d. Spiramycin

19. Most chemoresistant tumors is :
a. Synovial sarcoma [AIIMS 06]
b. Soft tissue Sarcoma
c. Osteosarcoma
d. Fibrous histiocytoma malignant

20. Which of the following is an aromatase inhibitior? [AIIMS 06]
a. Tamoxifen
b. Letrozole
c. Danazole
d. Taxane

21. Which of the following chemotherapeutic agents is associated with secondary leukemia ? [AIIMS 06]
a. Vinblastin
b. Etoposide
c. Cisplatin
d. Bleomycin

22. A 45 year old woman underwent a modified radical mastectomy 4 years ago. She was treated for multiple bone metastases with cyclophosphamide, doxorubicin, and fluorouracil for 6 months. She is complaining of exertion on exercise, swelling of the legs, and swelling around eyes in the morning. On examination, she has bilateral rales in the lungs, S1, S2 audible, S3, S4 gallop present. Her BP is 149/117 mmHg, PR is 80/min, and RR is 18/min. What is the most likely cause for her cardiac condition ?
a. Systolic dysfunction CHF [AIIMS 06]
b. Drug induced cardiac toxicity
c. Metastasis cardiac disease
d. Pneumonia

23. Adjuvant chemotherapy is provein in : [AIIMS 06]
a. Colon Ca
b. Oesophagus Ca
c. Pancreatic Ca
d. Gastric Ca

24. The chemotherapeutic drugs most commonly administrated by continous infusion is : [AIIMS 05]
a. AraC
b. 5-FU
c. Cisplatin
d. Etoposide

25. Which of the following chemotherapeutic drug has selective action on hypoxic tumor cells : [AIIMS 05]

a. Mitomycin C
b. Cisplatin
c. Doxorubicin
d. 5 Flurouracil

26. The new agent pemetrexed, useful in breast cancer, belongs to which category of drugs :

a. Antitumor antibiotic **[AIIMS 05]**
b. Alkylating agent
c. Hormonal agent
d. Animetabolite

27. Chemotherapeutic drug can cause :

a. Only necrosis **[AIIMS 05]**
b. Only apoptosis
c. Both necrosis and apoptosis
d. Anoikis

28. The most common side-effect of chemotherapy administration is :

a. Nausea **[AIIMS 05]**
b. Alopecia
c. Myelosuppression
d. Renal dysfunction

29. Tumors most amenable (cured with) to chemotherapy : [PGI 07]

a. Chorio Ca
b. Embryonal rhabdomyosarcoma
c. Hepatocellular Ca
d. Thyroid Ca

30. All of the following are anticancer antibiotics except : [PGI 07]

a. Vancomycin
b. Actinomycin D
c. Bleomycin
d. Mithramycin
e. Mitoxantrone

ANSWERS, REFERENCES, EXPLANATIONS WITH INFORMATIVE ILLUSTRATIONS

1. **Ans. is b i.e. 5FU** *Ref. Harrison 17/e, p 520*

5FU is an antimetabolite.

Alkylating agents :

- Electrophile molecules that reacts with electron rich atom to form covolent bond.
- It includes :

  - Nitrogen mustard - Cyclophosphamide, ifosphamide
  - Nitrosoureas - carmustine, Lomustine, streptozotocin
  - Platins -carloplatin, cisplatin, oxaliplatin
  - Mechloretamine
  - Chlorambulcil
  - Melphalan
  - Procarbazin; Dacarbazine
  - Busulphan
  - ThioTEPA
  - Temozolamide
  - Altretamin.

- They are phase non specific (i.e. active in all phase of cell cycle).
- **Common toxicities of alkylating agents are :** Myelosuppression mucositis, second neoplasm, alopecia, gonadal dysfunction, pulmonary fibrosis.

2. **Ans. is b i.e. Osteosarcoma** *Ref. Devita 8/e p 428*

"High dose methotrexate therapy is mainly used in the treatment of highgrade lymphomas, ostegenic sarcomas, and acute leukemia." ... Devita

High Dose Methotrexate (HDM)

– Infusion of methotrexate given over 6-42 hours in doses of 500 mg/m^2 with careful attention to IV hydration, urinary alkalinization and adequate (not excessive) administration of leucovorin.

– Drug level should be monitored every 24 hrs.

– HDM should not be used in patient with impaired renal function.

Other uses of methotrexate:

– Choriocarcinoma	– Ankylosing spondylytis
– Acute lukemia	– Asthma
– Giant cell arthritis	– Breast ca
– Multiple sclerosin	– IBD
– Rheumatoid arthritis	– Sarcoidosis
– SLE	– Wegner granulomatosis

3. Ans. is d i.e. Flutamide *Ref. KDT 6/e, p 828; Harrison 17/e, p 527*

"Flutamide is a non steroidal drug having specific antiandrogenic, but no other hormonal activity."

Action : Active metabolite is 2-hydroxyflutamide. It *competitively block androgen* action on accessory organ as well as pituitary. Increase LH secretion by blocking feed back inhibition.

Used :	• Palliative effect may occur in advanced Ca prostate. • In female hirustism it is given along with oral contraceptives. • Combined use of orchidectomy plus flutamide is called total androgen blockade.
Side effect :	• Gynaecomastia • Breast tenderness • Liver damage • Nausea and hot flushes.

4. Ans. is b i.e. Irinotecan *Ref. KDT 6/e, p 825; Harrison 17/e, p 525*

Irinotecan is a anticancer drug which acts by inhibiting topoisomerase 1, the enzyme responsible for cutting and resealing of DNA strand.

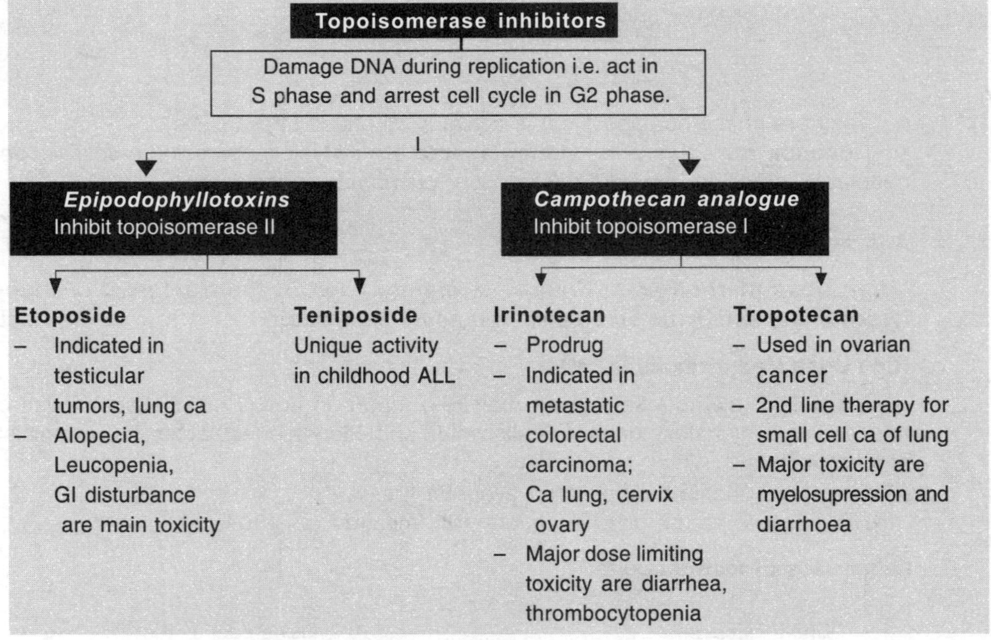

Remember : Topoisomerase is a enzyme that release or insert supercoil in DNA. ***On*** *binding with Topoisomerase inhibitors, Topoisomerase allow single strand break in DNA,* and not allow resealing after the strand has untwisted.

5. **Ans. is a and b i.e. Adriamycin; and Doxorubicin** *Ref. Devita 7/e, p 1630*

"Leiomyosarcoma is most responsive to doxorubicin, less sensitive to ifosfamide and is relatively unresponsive to cisplatin." ... Devita 7/e, p 1630

Now come to options : Adriamycin and doxorubicin are same drugs; adriamycin is infact a trade name of doxorubicin, *so it is not possible to choose one option.*

6. **Ans. is a i.e. Alkylating agent** *Ref. KDT 6/e 822; Harrison 17/e, p 421*

Already explained see answer no. 1

7. **Ans. is b i.e. Bleomycin** *Ref. Devita 8/e 491; KDT 6/e, p 830*

Bleomycin is an antineoplastic glycopeptide antibiotic isolated from fungus Streptomyces verticillus.

Cytotoxic effect results from formation of oxygen free radicals which then causes single and double stranded DNA breaks.

Effects are cell cycle specific with major effect in ***G2>M phase***

Drugs causing Cell cycle specific inhibition		
G1	:	Vinblastine, Vincristine.
S	:	Methotrexate, cytarabine, 6-Thioguanine, 6-Mercaptopurine, Hydroxyurea, mitomycin C, Doxorubicin, Daunorubicin.
G2	:	Daunorubicin, Bleomycin, Etoposide, Topotecan.
M	:	Vincristine, Vinblastune, Paclitaxel, Decetaxel

8. **Ans. is c i.e. Type II Pneumocytes**

Ref. Devita 8/e, p 2673; Fishmann; Pulmonary disease 4/e, p 1069

Hyperplasia/dysplasia of Type II pneumocytes is a characteristic feature of bleomycin toxicity

Bleomycin Induced Pulmonary Toxicity	
Probable Mechanism	**Histopathology**
• Direct toxicity through generation of active oxygen metabolities and activated neutrophils • Activation of alveolar macrophages Producing TNF α, TGF β and IL 1β • ↑ Collagen synthesis directly and via TGF β release	• Endothelial cell edema and blebing, • Necrosis of Type I Pneumocytes • Hyperplasis and Metaplasia of Type II Pneumocytes • Inflammatory infiltrate with PMN. • Proliferation of fibroblasts and fibrosis

Remember :
- Earliest sign of Bleomycin induced pulmonary damage is ↓ DLco.
- Diagnosed by bronchoalveolar lavage or lung biopsy.
- Oxygen therapy increase pulmonary toxicity of bleomycin.
- Bleomycin is not or rarely associated with myelosuppression.

Cancer drugs causing Pulmonary fibrosis / Infiltrate			
Antineoplastic drugs		**Other drugs**	
– Bleomycin	– Busulfan	– Acyclovir	– Azothioprine
– Cyclophosphamide	– Chlorambucil	– Sulfonamide	– Gold
– Melphalan	– Carmustine	– Amiadarone	– Methylsergide
– Vinca alkaloids	– Methotrexate (rarely)	– Nitrofurantoin	– Procarbazine
– Procarbazine (very rarely)			

9. **Ans. is a and b i.e. Cisplatin, Capecitabine** *Ref. Harrison 17/e, p 522-24*

Hand foot syndrome can be seen with both capecitabine and cisplatin. *However the incidence is much higher with capecitabine.*

So if same question is repeated go with capecitabine.

Antineoplastic agents associated with Hand Foot syndrome (in decreasing order)		
1. Capecitabine	2. Sorafenib	3. Doxorubicin
4. 5FU	5. Cytarabine	6. Cispatin

Other rare association

- Mitotane
- Cyclophosphamide
- Docetaxel
- Daunorubicin
- Etoposide
- Mercaptopurine
- Methotrexate
- Hydroxyurea
- Paclitaxel

10. **Ans. is a i.e. Bleomycin**

Ref. KDT 6/e, p 826; Harrison 17/e, p 525

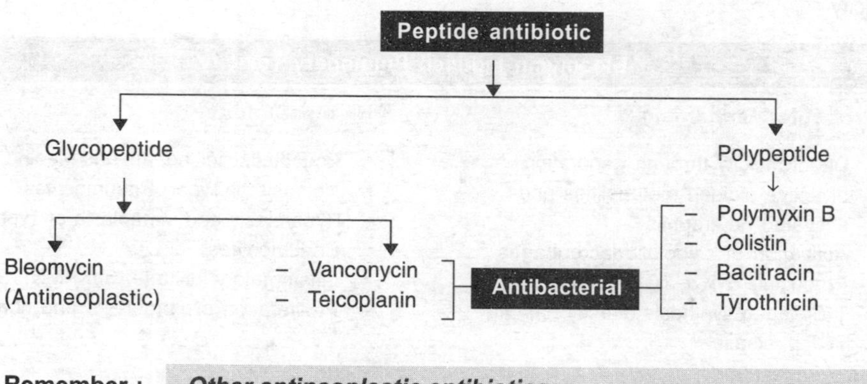

Remember : ***Other antineoplastic antibiotics***
- Actinomycin D
- Daunorubicin
- Mithramycin
- Doxorubin (Adriamycin)
- Mitomycin

11. Ans. is d i.e. Stabilization of tubules *Ref. KDT 6/e, p 825*

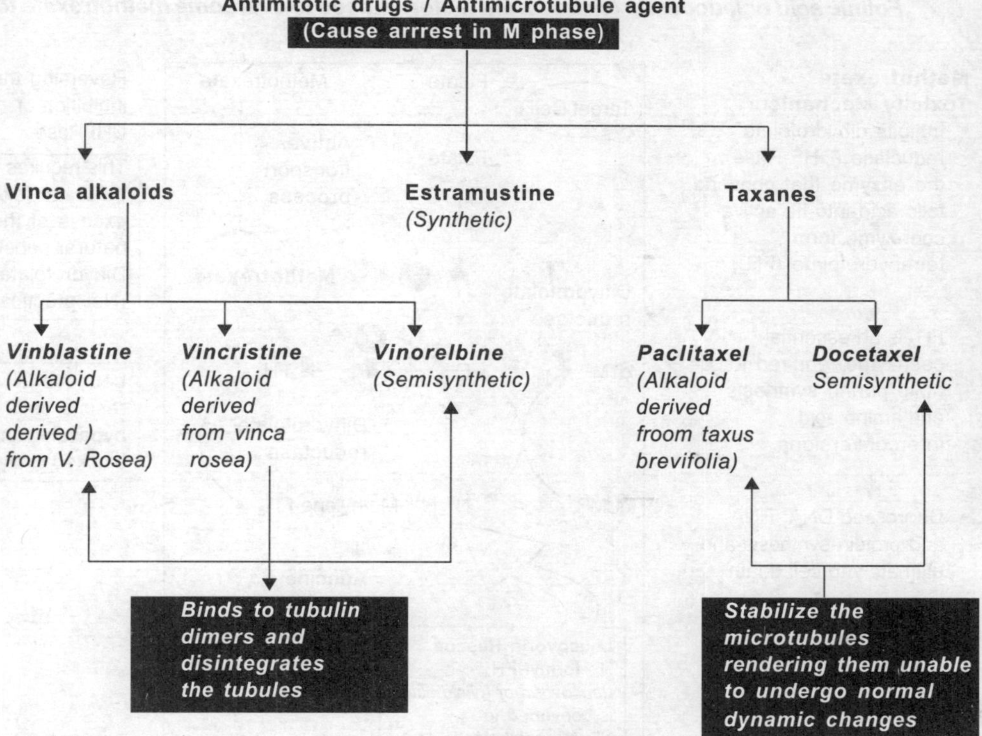

- All these drugs cause cell cycle arrest in ***metaphase.***
- *Isotretinoin is also derived from plant, but it is not antimitotic agent.*
- *Bleomycin is a antibiotic* derived from Streptomyces verticularis.

Remember : **Other anticancers derived from plants :**

– Podophyllotoxins	:	Etopside and teniopside
– Campothecans	:	Tropotecan and Irinotecan.

12. Ans. is a i.e. Methotrexate *Ref. KDT 6/e, p 592*

Folinic acid or leucoverin (cirtrovorum factor) is used to overcome methotrexate toxicity.

Methotrexate Toxicity Mechanism

- Inhibits dihydrofolate reductase (DHF Rase), the enzyme that converts folic acid into its active coenzyme form tetrahydrofolate (FH_4)

↓

FH_4 is an essential coenzyme required for de novo purine synthesis and amino acid interconversions

↓

- Depressed DNA, RNA and protein synthesis and ultimately to cell death

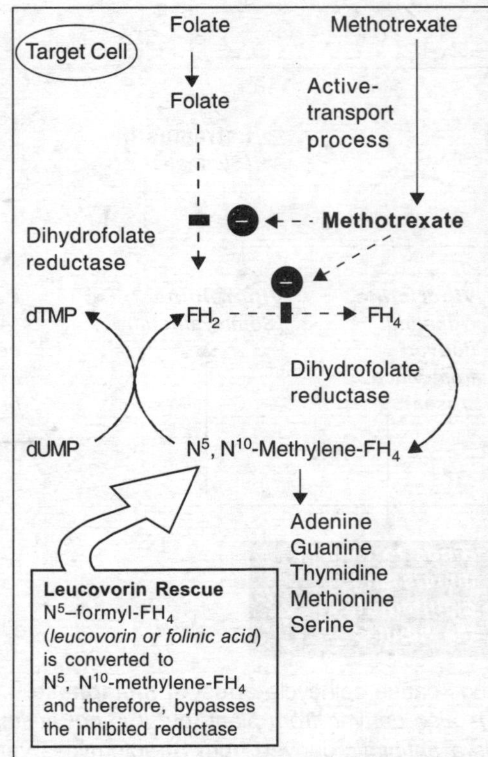

Reversing the inhibition of DHFRase

This requires a thousand fold excess of the natural substrate Dihydrofolate (FH2) (Not practical)

or

Leucoverin which rescue cells by bypassing the blocked Enzyme

Note: Leucoverin rescue both tumor and normal cells, so excess dose can result in loss of its antineoplastic effect and should be avoided

13. Ans. is c i.e. Carmustine *Ref. Goodman Gilman 11/e, p 1330*

Carmustine causes profound and delayed myelosuppression which takes 4-6 weeks to recover after a single dose. The myelosuppression leads to leukopenia and thrombocytopenia (may be prolonged)

Other toxicities of carmustine

- Leukemia
- Myocardial ischemia
- Delayed renal damage
- Reversible liver toxicity

Remember: Carmustine is a nitrosourea type alkylating agent. It is highly lipophilic and readily crosses blood brain barrier. Presently its main use is in brain tumor

14. Ans. is c i.e. Actinomycin D *Ref. Harrison 17/e, p 2222*

Drugs causing syndrome of inappropriate ADH secretion (SIADH)

- **D**esmopressin or Vasopressin
- **C**hlorpropamide
- **O**xytocin, high dose
- **V**incristine or vinblastine
- **C**arbamazepine
- **N**icotine
- **P**henothiazines
- **C**yclophosphamide
- **T**ricyclic antidepressants
- **M**onoamine oxidase inhibitors
- **S**erotonin reuptake inhibitors

Mnemonic: MOST Common drugs Can Produce Nausea, Vomiting

15. Ans. is a i.e. GIST *Ref. Devita 8/e, p 458*

FDA approved indications of Imatinib mesylate

1. First line treatment of ph^{+ve} (CML in blast crisis, **accelerated** phase, or chronic phase after failure of IFN α therapy)
2. First line treatment of kit (CD117) positive unresectable and/or metastatic malignant Gastrointestinal stromal tumor (GIST)
3. pH^{+ve} CML in chronic phase in pediatric patients after recurrence or resistant to IFN α therapy

Remember : Imatinib function in a selective manner by targeting PDGFR, c kit and Abl kinases

16. Ans. is d i.e. Lepatinib *Ref. Devita 8/e, p 458*

Tyrosine Kinase inhibitors

Drug	Target	Uses
Imatinib	Bcr-Abl ; PDGFR; C Kit	CML, GIST
Dasatinib	Bcr-Abl, Src family, C Kit EPHA$_2$; PDGFRβ	CML, pH+ve ALL
Nilotinib	Bcr-Abl, CKit, PDGFR	pH +ve CML
Gefitinib	EGFR	Non small cell lung Ca (NSCLC),
Erlotinib	EGFR	NSCLC Pancreatic Ca (in combination with gemcitabine)
Lepatinib	EGFR, HER-2	Breast Ca
Sunitinib	VEGFR-1,2,3, C Kit PDGFR, RET	GIST, advanced RCC
Sorafenib	VEGPR 2, 3, PDGFR, Raf, RET	Advanced RCC

GIST : Gastro Intestinal Stromal Tumor
RCC : Renal Cell Ca
NSCLC : Non small cell lung Ca

17. Ans. is a, b, d i.e. Ifosfamide, Chlorabucil, Nitrosoureas *Ref. Harrison 17/e, p 521*

Already explained see asnwer no.1

18. Ans. is a, d i.e. Tetracyline, Spiramycin *Ref. KDT 6/e, p 826*

Already explained see asnwer no.10

19. Ans. is a i.e. Synovial sarcoma *Ref. See below*

Role of Chemotherapy in Sarcoma

- Both postoperative (adjuvant) and preoperative chemotherapy (neoajuvant) have role in sarcoma.
- Chemotherapy is indicated in high grade soft tissue sarcoma of prediatric age group like *Rhabdomyosarcoma; Ewing's sarcoma; Malignant fibrous histocytoma.*
- In adult soft tissue sarcoma chemotherapy is disappointing. Slow growing cartilagenous sarcoma (chondro-sarcoma) are particularly resistant.
- For osteosarcoma chemotherapy has role in both adjuvant and neoadjuvant format.
- For synovial sarcoma chemotherapy has no role.

Treatment of synovial sarcoma is by Radical resection / Amputation.

20. Ans. is b i.e. Letrozole *Ref. Devita 7/e, p 462, 8/e, p 563, KDT 6/e 828*

Aromatase inhibitors

Inhibits aromatase, the enzyme responsible for final step of androgen to estrogen conversion

Aromatase inhibitors		
Non steroidal (reversible inhibition)		**Steroidal (irreversible)**
• Aminoglutethimide	(1st generation)	• Formestane (2nd generation)
• Rogletimide • Fadrazole	(2nd generation)	• Exmestane (3rd generation)
• Letrozole • Vorozole	(3rd generation)	• Anastrazole

Uses :

- Both letrozole and anastrozole are indicated as first line therapy for receptor positive metastatic breast Ca.
- Exmestane is used in the setting of tamoxifen refractory metastatic Ca.

Guys, I want to tell you one important thing at this point.

- Previously it was think that aromatase decrease estrogen level only in postmenopausal age group (due to non functional ovary). So, they are indicated only in post menopausal ca, but this is wrong.

- Most of the trials have suggested equal or only slightly lower efficacy of aromatase inhibitor in premenopausal age group. As a result some centers have began recommended them in both pre and post menopausal women.

21. Ans. is c i.e. Cisplatin *Ref. See Below*

"Cisplatin has been associated with the development of AML usually 4 or more years after treatment."

Cisplatin is a Platinum containing alkylating agent.

Toxicities of cisplatin are :

- Nausea and vomiting
- Nephrotoxicity manifest as decrease in GFR
- Neurotoxicity in the form of *stocking and glove* sensorimotor neuropathy
- Hearing loss
- Chronic vascular toxicity (Raynaud's syndrome, coronary artery disease)
- Myelosuppression is less when compared to other alkylating agent.

Amifostine provides protection against neurotoxicity and nephrotoxicity.

22. Ans. is b i.e. Drug induced cardiac toxicity

Ref. KDT 6/e, p 826; Harrison 17/e, p 525

The woman has suffered from delayed toxicity of doxorubicin, which manifest as CHF.

Cardiotoxicity of Doxorubicin (Adriamycin)	
Acute cardiotoxicity (Reversible)	**Delayed cardiotoxicity** (Irreversible)
• Arrythmias • Hypotension	• CHF secondary to cardiomyopathy • This is dose dependent and seen in about 10% of patient taking > 550mg/m^2

Cardiotoxic anticancer drugs	
Drug	**Toxicity**
Antracyclines (Doxorubicin and daunarubicin)	Reversible/acute cardiac toxicity in form of myocarditis with or with out pericarditis, delayed in the form of CHF
Mithoxantrone	Similar to anthracylines
Cyclophosphamide	Acute myopericarditis
Ifosfamide	Dose related CHF
Taxanes (paclitaxel and docetaxil)	Multiple cardiac effect including arrythmias
5 FU	Angina, ventricular arrhythmias, **MI**, cardiogenic shock.

23. Ans. is a i.e. Colon Ca *Ref. Harrison 17/e, p 518; Bailey & Love 24/e, p 225*

Adjuvant chemotherapy is indicated in	
• Breast carcinoma	• Colorectal carcinoma
• Osteogenic sarcoma	• Soft tissue sarcoma

Cancers in which drugs can be useful for treatment	
Acute leukemia in children	Ewing's sarcoma
Hodgkin's disease	Wilms' tumour
Histiocytic lymphoma	Burkitt's lymphoma
Skin cancer	Retinoblastoma
Testicular carcinoma	Choriocarcinoma
Embryonal rhabdomyosarcoma	

Cancers marginally responsive or unresponsive to chemotherapeutic agents	
Renal carcinoma	Pancreatic carcinoma
Bladder carcinoma	Hepatocellular carcinoma
Cancer of the oesophagus	Thyroid carcinoma
Squamous carcinoma of the lung	Malignant melanoma

24. Ans. is c i.e. Cisplatin *Ref. Devita 8/e, p 421*

Doses and Method of Cisplatin administration

Dose: Single IV of 50-75 mg/m^2 every 3 or 4 week.

Method: Drugs is given in 250 ml of normal saline as 1-4 hour infusion with 1 hour time frame being most common.

It is important to maintain patient hydration with atleast 2 lt of IV fluid to maintain good urine flow. Mannitol 125 mg may be mixed with drug to improve urine output. Furosamide and other renal tubule inhibitors should be avoided.

Cisplatin should not be mixed with any solution containing Mg^{2+}, Ca^{2+}, HCO^{3-} as they can inactivate the drug.

Remember: Cisplatin is also administered intraperitoneatly (IP). IP route is associated with increased efficiency in ovarian cancers.

25. Ans. is a i.e. Mitomycin *Ref. Katzung 8/e, p 939*

"Hypoxic tumor stem cells of solid tumors exist in an environment conductive to reductive reactions and are more sensitive to the cytotoxic action of mitomycin."

Mitomycin is best available drug for use an adjuvant to X-ray radiation to attack hypoxic tumour cells.

Remember :
- Mitomycin is a antibiotic acting as bioreductive alkylating agent that undergoes reduction in hypoxic environment to generate an alkylating agent that cross links DNA.
- Main toxicity is myelosuppression.

26. Ans. is d i.e. Antimetabolite *Ref. Harrison 17/e, p 526*

"Pemetrexed is a multitargeted antifolate analogue, that targets multiple enzyme involved in folate metabolism."

Pemetrexed : – **Cause cell cycle arrest at** *G_1 – S phase*
– **Active** *in breast ca, pancreatic ca, Mesothelioma, and many other solid tumors.*
– Main **toxicities** *include dose limiting myelosupression, mucositis and skin rash.*

Remember : *Newer antifolates :*		
	– Pemetrexed	– Raltitrexed
	– 5 FU	– Capecitabine

27. Ans. is c i.e. Both necrosis and apoptosis *Ref. Harrison 17/e, p 519*

"Cancer chemotherapeutic agents can cause both necrosis and apoptosis."
Anoikis refers to death of epithelial cells after removal from the normal milleu of substrate, particularly from cell to cell contact.

28. Ans. is a i.e. Nausea *Ref. Harrison 17/e, p 530*

"The most common side effect of chemotherapy administration is nausea, with or without vomiting."

On the basis of emetogenicity anticancers can be :

Highly emetogenic	Moderate emetogenic	Little or no emetogenic
– Mechlorethamine	– Doxorubicin	– Chlorambucil
– Nitrosoureas	– Dauno rubicin	– Melphalan
– Streptozocin	– Methotrexate	– Busulphan
– Cisplatin		
– Actinomycin		

Myelosuppression is 2nd most common side effect.

• In myelosuppression	:	Polymorphonuclear leukocytes most susceptible.
• Platelets	:	Moderately susceptible
• RBC	:	Least succeptible

29. Ans. is a and b i.e. Chorio Ca; and Embryonal rhabdomyosarcoma

Ref. Harrison 17/e, p 518

Already explained, see answer no. 23

30. Ans. is a i.e. Vancomycin *Ref. KDT 6/e, p 826*

Anticancer antibiotics

Drug	Source	Mechanism of Action
Anthracyclines *(Doxorubicin & Daunorubicin)*	Streptomyces peucetius var caesius	– Inhibitors of DNA and RNA synthesis. – Binding to membranes to alter ion transport – Free radical generation
Dactinomycin *(Actinomycin D)*	Streptomyces	– Binds DNA, inhibit DNA dependent RNA synthesis.
Plicamycin *(Mithramycin)*	Streptomyces Plicatus	– Decrease plasma calcium level
Mitomycin	Streptomyces caespitosus	– Generates alkyating agent in hypoxic medium that cross links DNA.
Bleomycin	Streptomyces verticuaris	– Binds to DNA, resulting in single and double strand and breaks inhibit DNA biosynthesis.

Vancomycin is not an anticancer drug.
Mithoxantrone is a synthetic antibiotic related to doxorubicin with lower cardiotoxicity.
..... *Harrison 16/e, p 476*

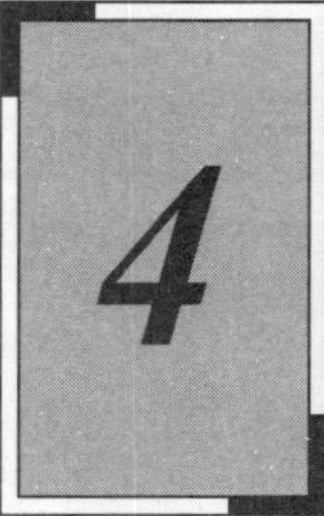

Multiple Tumour Syndrome

What's Important ?

- Components
- Type - I
- Type - II

MULTIPLE ENDOCRINE NEOPLASIA 1 = WERMER'S SYNDROME

- *Autosomal dominant*
- Peak incidence of symptoms is women with MEN-1 is during 3rd decade, while in man it is during 4th decade
- **Characterized** by neoplasia of parathyroid, pituitary, pancreatic islets and other neuroendocrine cell types (foregut carcinoid, pheochromocytoma, subcutaneous or visceral lipomas).
- **Hyperparathyroidism** is *MC* manifestation (cardinal sign of MEN 1 is parathyroidadenoma of multicentricity).
  - Diagnosed by elevated levels of serum calcium with normal or high PTH.
- **Pancreatic neoplasia** is 2nd *MC* manifestation.
  - Most commonly increase pancreatic hormone is *pancreatic polypeptides* > gastrin > insulin.
- In **pituitary, prolactinoma** is most common.
  - Diagnosed by increased prolactin (>200 mg/l) and MRI.
- **Defect :** In MEN 1, gene is located on chromosome 11q, 13 which encodes for ***tumour suppressor protein*** called *merin.*

MULTIPLE ENDOCRINE NEOPLASIA TYPE 2

	MEN 2A (Sipple syndrome)	**MEN 2B**
Components	• Medullary thyroid cancer (MTC) (*MC* component) • Hyperparathyroidism (hyperplasia or adenoma) • Pheochromocytoma (secrete Adr>NA) • **Subvariant are :** – Familial MTC – MEN 2A with hirschprung disease – MEN 2A with cutaneous lichen amyloidosis	• MTC (more aggressive than MEN 2A) • Pheochromocytoma • Mucosal neuromas • Intestinal anglioneuromatosis • Marfanoid features • Megacolon • Skeletal abnormalities
Defect	**RET oncogene** (cysteine codon)	**RET oncogene** (tyrosine kinase domain)
Transmission	Autosomal dominant	Autosomal dominant

NEUROFIBROMATOSIS

	Neurofibromatosis I	Neurofibromatosis II
Gene	*(Von Recklinghausen disease)* **NF-1** tumour suppressor gene on chromosome 17	*(Acoustic neurofibromatosis)* **NF-2** tumor suppressor gene on chromosome 22
Protein	Neurofibromin	Merlin or Schwanomin
Tumours	***CNS tumours*** a. Optic nerve gliomas (see in 15% of patient) b. Meningiomas c. Neurofibroma d. Astrocytomas e. Neurilemmomas f. Ependymomas ***Non CNS tumours*** a. Pheochromocytoma b. Rhabdomycosarcoma c. Leukemia (chronic myeloid leukemia) d. Wilm's tumour e. Juvenile Xanthogranuloma	a. B/L acoustic schwannomas (MC) b. Multiple meningiomas c. Gliomas typically ependymomas d. Schwannomas of cranial and spinal nerves

QUESTIONS

1. **Pancreatitis, pituitary tumor and pheochromocytoma may be associated with : [AI 05, 04, 00]**
   a. Medullary carcinoma of thyroid
   b. Papillary carcinoma
   c. Anaplastic carcinoma of thyroid
   d. Follicular carcinoma of thyroid
2. **36 year old female with symptoms of hyperparathyroidism, tumor in pancreas, adrenal cortical hyperplasia, pituitary adenomas, islet cell tumor with cutaneous angiofibromas. What is the diagnosis?**
   a. Men 1 **[AIIMS 07]**
   b. Men 2A
   c. Men 2B
   d. Men 2C
3. **All of the following may be associated with Von Hippel Lindua syndrome, except [AI 2009]**
   a. Retinal and cerebellar hemangioblastomas
   b. Gastric carcinoma
   c. Pheochromocytoma
   d. Renal cell carcinoma
4. **MEN I syndrome is most commonly associated with [AI 08]**
   a. Gastrinoma
   b. Insulinoma
   c. Glucucagonoma
   d. Somatistatinoma
5. **All of the following statements about Neurofibromatiosis are true, except [AI 09]**
   a. Autosomal Recessive Inheritance
   b. Cutaneous neurofibromas
   c. Cataract
   d. Scoliosis
6. **Lynch syndrome is associated with [AIIMS 09]**
   a. Breast Ca, Colon Ca, Ovary Ca
   b. Endometrial Ca, Colon Ca, Ovary Ca
   c. Breast Ca, Endometrial Ca, Ovarian Ca
   d. Breast Ca, Colon Ca, Endometrial Ca
7. **Multiple submucosal neuromas is most likely associated with : [AIIMS 05]**
   a. Medullary carcinoma of the thyroid
   b. Ovarian carcinoma
   c. Testicular teratoma
   d. Pancreatic beta cell carcinoma
8. **True about MEN IIb (Sipple syndrome) :**
   a. Pheochromocytoma **[PGI 06]**
   b. Hyperparathyroidism
   c. Mucocutaneous neuromas
   d. Medullary carcinoma

ANSWERS, REFERENCES, EXPLANATIONS WITH INFORMATIVE ILLUSTRATIONS

1. **Ans. is a i.e. Medullary carcinoma of thyroid**

Ref. Harrison 17/e, p 2361; Devita 8/e, p 1739

Combination of pancreatitis (due to hypercalcemia), pituitary tumour and pheochromocytoma suggest diagnosis of MEN-II A

- MEN-II is associated with medullary carcinoma of thyroid.

	MEN 2A (Sipple syndrome)	**MEN 2B**
Components	• Medullary thyroid cancer (MTC) (*MC* component) • Hyperparathyroidism (hyperplasia or adenoma) • Pheochromocytoma (secrete Adr>NA) • **Subvariant are :** – Familial MTC – MEN 2A with hirschprung disease – MEN 2A with cutaneous lichen amyloidosis	• MTC (more aggressive than MEN 2A) • Pheochromocytoma • Mucosal neuromas • Intestinal ganglioneuromatosis • Marfanoid features • Megacolon • Skeletal abnormalities
Defect	**RET oncogene** (cysteine codon)	**RET oncogene** (tyrosine kinase domain)
Transmission	Autosomal dominant	Autosomal dominant
Treatment	– Prophylactic thyroidectomy – Removal of 3 1/2 gland for parathyroid adenoma.	

Remember :
- MTC of MEN-2 is bilateral and multifocal.
- Mutation in RET of chromosome 10 is Germline ***missense*** mutation.
- For pheochromocytoma only the affected gland is removed or alternatively bilateral cortical sparing adrenalectomy can be performed.

2. **Ans. is a i.e. MEN-1** *Ref. Harrison 17/e, p 2360; Devita 8/e, p 1734*

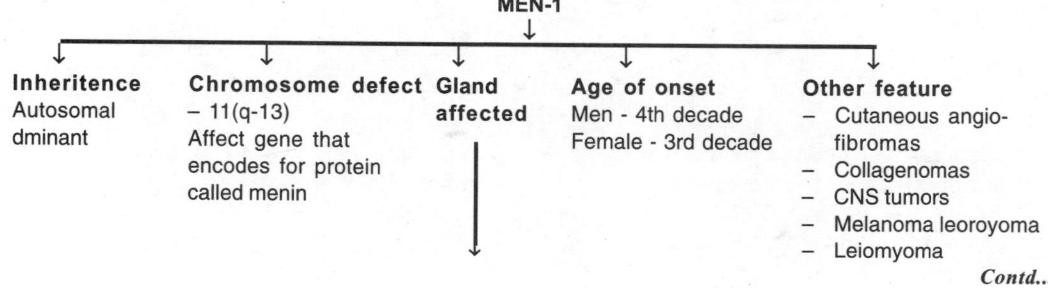

Contd...

Contd...

Parathyroid (MC) 90%	***Pancreatic endocrine tumor*** (80%)	***Pituitary tumor*** (60%)	***Adrenal*** (30%)	***Thyroid*** (20%)	***Carcinoid tumors*** (15%)
Multiple parathyroid adenomas resulting in primary parathyroidism – It is the MC and earliest detected abnormality in MEN-1	1. Pancreatic polypeptides producing tumor 2. Gastrinoma 3. Insulinoma 4. Glucagonoma 5. VIPoma	1. Prolactinoma 2. GH secreting tumor 3. Nonfunctional tumor	1. Benigm non-functional cortical adenoma 2. Cortical carcinoma	Thyroid adenoma	– Arise from gastric entero-chro-maffin like cells

3. **Ans. is b i.e. Gastric Carcinoma** *Ref. Harrison 17/e, p 2607*

Von Hippel lindau syndrome

- Autosomal dominant syndrome
- ***Components :***
  - Renal, hepatic, pancreatic and ependymal cyst
  - Pheochromocytoma
  - Hemangioblastomas of the retina, cerebellum, brain stem and spinal cord
  - Renal cell carcinoma (clear cell Ca)
  - Angiomatosis
  - Pancreatic endocrine tumour (non-functional)
  - Adenomas.
- **VHL gene** is tumour suppressor gene located on chromosome 3p 25 -26.
- Cerebellar capillary hemangioblastomas is the principal neurologic manifestation.
- 10% of hemangioblastoma are associated with polycythemia.
- *Feature differentiating VHL from MEN I or MEN 2 is hyperparathyroidism which rarely occurs in VHL.*

4. **Ans. a i.e. Gastrinoma** *Ref. Harrison 17/e p 2360; Devita 8/e, p 1734*

Already explained

5. **Ans. is a i.e. Autosomal recessive inheritance** *Ref. Nelson 18/e, p 2483; Robbin's 8/e, p 1342*

Neurofibromatosis is *neurocutaneous autosomal dominant disorder.*
It is of two types:

	NF1	NF-2
	(Von Recklinghausen disease)	*(Acoustic neurofibromatosis)*
Prevalance	More common	Less common
Gene	NF-1 tumour suppressor gene on chromosome ***17***	NF-2 tumor suppressor gene on chromosome **22**
Protein	***Neurofibromin***	***Merlin or Schwanomin***
Diagnostic criteria	Diagnosed when any two of the following are present : a. ***Six or more cafeau-lait macules*** b. Axilllary or inguinal freckling	Diagnosed when one of the following present : a. ***Bilateral eigth nerve masses*** consistent with acoustic neuroma b. A parent sibling or child with NF-2

Contd...

Contd...

	NF1	NF-2
Other abnormalities	c. Two or more iris ***lisch nodules*** d. Two or more neurofibromas or one plexiform neurofibroma e. Distinctive osseous lesion f. Optic gliomas g. A first degree relative with NF-1 **MC *associated abnormalities*** – Skeletal lesions in the form of erosive defects, – Scoliosis (MC orthopaedic abnormality) – Pseudoarthrosis of tibia etc.	c. Unilateral eight nerve mass or any two of the following: – Neurofibroma – Meningioma – Glioma – Schwannoma – Juvenile posterior subcapsular opacity *Bilateral acoustic neuromas are the most distinctive tumors in patients with NF-2.* **Tumours associated with NF-2** • Cafeau-laut spot and skin neurofibromas are less common than NF-1. ***Lisch nodules*** in iris are not found • Posterior subcapsular lens opacities seen in 50% of patients – B/L acoustic schwannomas (MC) – Multiple meningiomas – Gliomas typically ependymomas – Schwannomas of cranial and spinal nerves

Remember: Tumors associated with neurofibromatosis 1

CNS tumours	Non CNS tumours
a. Optic nerve gliomas (see in 15% of patient)	a. Pheochromocytoma
b. Meningiomas	b. Rhabdomyosarcoma
c. Neurofibroma	c. Leukemia (chronic myeloid leukemia)
d. Astrocytomas	d. Wilm's tumour
e. Neurilemmomas	e. Juvenile Xanthogranuloma
f. Ependymomas	

6. **Ans. b i.e. Endometrial Ca, Colon Ca, Ovary Ca** *Ref. Robbin's 8/e, p 821*

Lynch Syndrome (Hereditay nonpolyposis colorectal cancer)

- **A**utosomal dominant disorder due to defect in **D**NA **m**ismatch repair gene MSH-2, MIH-1
- As a consiquence of mismatch repair defciency, there is microstatelite instability.
- **Associated cancers:**
  - ***C**olorectum*
  - ***E**ndometrium*
  - ***G**astric Ca*
  - ***O**vary*
  - ***B**rain*
  - ***S**mall Bowel*
  - ***H**epatobiliary tract*
  - ***S**kin*

Mnemonic: A Dominant Man Subhash Chand BOSE Has Gastric Ca.

7. **Ans. is a i.e. Medullary carcinoma of the thyroid** *Ref. Harrison's 17/e, p 2361*

Both multiple submucosal neuromas and medullary carcinoma of thyroid are found in MEN 2A.

For more details, kindly see answer no. 1

8. **Ans. is a, c and d i.e. Pheochromocytoma; Mucocutaneous neuromas; and Medullary carcinoma** *Ref. Harrison's 17/e, p 2361*

	MEN-1	MEN-2A	MEN-2B
Pituitary	Adenomas		
Parathyroid	Hyperplasia +++	Hyperplasia+ Adenomas +	
Pancreatic islets	Hyperplasia ++ Adenomas ++ Carcinomas +++		
Adrenal	Cortical hyperplasia	Pheoch2romocytoma ++	Pheochromocytoma +++
Thyroid	None	C-cell hyperplasia +++ Medullary carcinoma +++	C-cell hypreplasia +++ Medullary carcinoma +++
Extraendocrine changes	None	None	Mucocutaneous ganglioneuromas Marfanoid habitus
Mutant gene locus	MEN-1	RET	RET

Thus, *MEN II-A = Sipple syndrome is associated with medullary carcinoma of thyroid,* (which does not produce hyperthyroidism, and ***patient*** are usually euthyroid).

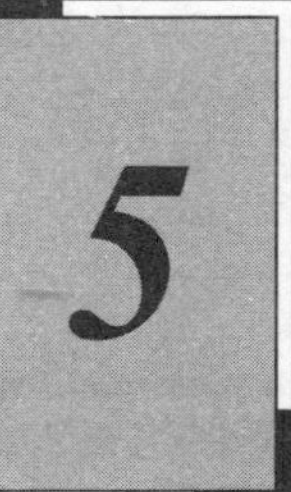

Paraneoplastic Syndromes

What's Important ?

- Hematological Syndrome
- Endocrinal Syndrome

Paraneoplastic syndromes are disorders ***caused by immune or other mechanism and are not due to direct effects of the tumour itself or metastases or opportunistic infections or complications of drug or radiation therapy.***

They are of following types :

1. ENDOCRINE SYNDROMES

Common Paraneoplastic Endocrine Syndromes		
Syndrome	**Mediators**	**Tumors Typically Associated with syndrome**
Hypercalcemia of malignancy	– Parathyroid hormone-related peptide (PTHrP) ***(MC)*** – Parathyroid hormone (PTH) (rare) – 125 dihydroxy vit. D – TGF a b; IL-I, IL-E, PG, TNF	Non-small cell lung cancer Breast cancer Renal cell carcinoma Head and neck cancer Myeloma, lymphoma leukemia
Syndrome of inappropriate antidiuretic hormone secretion	– Arginine vasopressin (AVP) – Atrial natriuretic peptide	Small cell lung cancer ***(MC)*** Head and neck cancer
Cushing's syndrome	– Adrenocorticotropic hormone – (ACTH) *ectopic* ***(MC)*** – Corticotropin-releasing hormone (CRH) - *ectopic*	Small cell lung cancer ***(MC)*** *Carcinoid syndrome* Thymic Ca pancreatic Ca. Pheochromocytoma
Acromegally	– Growth hormone-releasing hormone (GHRH) – Growth hormone (GH) *ectopic*	Carcinoid tumors Small cell lung cancer Pancreatic islet cell tumors
Gynecomastia	– Human chorionic gonadotropin (hCG) – Estrogen	Testicular cancer Lung cancer Carcinoid tumors of the lung and gastrointestinal tract
Non islet cell tumor hypoglycemia	– Insulin-like growth factor-2 (IGF-2)-*ectopic*	Sarcomas Mesothelioma; Hematoma

2. HEMATOLOGIC SYNDROMES

- Most common thrombotic conditions in cancer patient are ***deep venous thrombosis and pulmonary embolism.***
- Coexistence of peripheral migrating venous thrombosis with visceral carcinoma particularly pancreatic cancer is called ***Trousseau's syndrome.***

Paraneoplastic hematologic syndromes

Syndrome	Proteins	Cancers Associated
Erythrocytosis	Erythropoietin	Renal cancers, HCC Cerebellar hemangioblastomas
Granulocytosis	G-CSF GM-CSF IL-6	Lung cancer Gastrointestinal cancer Ovarian cancer, Hodgkin's disease Genitourinary cancer
Thrombocytosis	IL-6	Lung ca; GIT ca; Breast ca; Ovarian ca; Lymphoma
Eosinophilia	IL-5	Lymphoma; Leukemia; Lung ca
Thrombophlebitis	Unknown	Lung cancer ***(Non migratory)*** Pancreatic cancer; Gastrointestinal cancer; Breast cancer; Genitourinary cancer; Ovarian cancer; Prostate cancer; Lymphoma

3. PARANEOPLASTIC NEUROLOGIC SYNDROME

Paraneoplastic Syndrome of Brain and Spinal cord

Syndrome	Neoplasm
Limbic encephalitis	**(MC)** SCLC, testicular cancer, breast, colon, bladder, lymphoma
Brainstem encephalitis	SCLC
Cerebellar degeneration	SCLC, Ovary, uterus, Hodgkin's lymphoma
Opsoclonus/myoclonus (Dancing eye-dancing feet syndrome)	Neuroblastoma, lung, breast
Necrotizing myelopathy	SCLC, lymphoma

Paraneoplastic Syndrome of Peripheral nerve

Neuropathies	
Sensory neuronopathy	SCLC **(MC),** breast, ovary, prostate
Motor neuronopathy	Lymphoma
Axonal neuropathies	Lung, breast, stomach, lymphoma, leukemia, thymoma, multiple myeloma
Autonomic neuropathies	
Enteric neuropathy	Thymoma, SCLC
Demyelinating neuropathy	
Anti-MAG	MGUS, IgM M-protein in 85%
Multifocal motor neuropathy	
POEMS	MGUS, IgM M-protein in 20%
CIDP	Multiple myeloma
GB syndrome &	MGUS, IgM or IgG-protein in 15% lymphoma
branchia plexus	Lymphoma

Paraneoplastic Syndrome of Muscle :

Necrotizing myopathy	Adenocarcinoma and Non small cell cancer of lung, breast, alimentary tract
Dermatomyositis	Ovarian, nasopharyngeal ca Small cell carcinoma of lung

Others

Carcinoma associated retinopathy (CAR)	–	SCLC ***(MC)***, melanoma, gynaecologic malignancies.
Stiff person syndrome (SPS)	–	Breast cancer, SCLC
Guillain Barre syndrome	–	Hodgkin's disease

4. NEUROMUSCULAR SYNDROMES

Lambert Eaton Myasthenic Syndrome :

- Disorder of ***presynaptic component*** of neuromuscular transmission in which IgG *antibodies directed against P/Q voltage gated calcium channels (VGCC)* in motor nerve terminal.
- Most common with small cell lung carcinoma less often with lymphoproliferative disorder.
- **Weakness** is symmetric proximal and most prominent in lower limbs, diplopia, ptosis, may occur.
- **Tendon reflex** are either decreased or absent at rest but may increase after exercise.
- Most useful **diagnostic test** is repetitive nerve stimulation in *which compound muscle action potential amplitude increase by at least 100%* after rapid repititive nerve stimulation.

Myasthenia gravis :

- Seen with thymoma
- **Antibodies** are directed against acetyl choline receptor.

QUESTIONS

1. **Hypercalcemia associated with malignancy is most often mediated by :**
   a. Parathyroid hormone (PTH) **[AI 05]**
   b. Parathyroid hormone related protein (PTHrP)
   c. Interleukin-6(IL-6)
   d. Calcitonin
2. **Which of the following is not non-metastatic complication of malignances:**
   a. Cushings syndrome **[AIIMS 05]**
   b. Cerebral cortical degeneration
   c. Cerebellar degeneration
   d. Polymyositis
3. **Migratory thrombophlebitis seen in :**
   a. Pancreatic Ca **[PGI 06]**
   b. Bladder Ca
   c. Stomach Ca
   d. Breast Ca
   e. Liver Ca
4. **Which of the followng tumor secretes erythropoietin** **[PGI 10]**
   a. Pheochromocytoma
   b. Hepatoma
   c. Renal cell ca
   d. Adrenal adenoma
   e. Breast Ca

ANSWERS, REFERENCES, EXPLANATIONS WITH INFORMATIVE ILLUSTRATIONS

1. **Ans. is b i.e. Parathyroid hormone related protein (PTHrP)** *Ref. Harrison 17/e, p 619*

Hypercalcemia of malignancy is the most common paraneoplastic endocrine syndrome.
It is of 2 types :

Humoral hypercalcemia of malignancy (HHM) (MC)	Local ostelytic hypercalcemia (LOH)
Mediators :	***Mediators :***
• Parathyroid hormone related protein (PTHrP) (MC)	TGF a, β
• Parathyroid hormone (rare)	IL-I
• 1, 25 dihydroxyvitamin D (in lymphoma)	IL-6
• PTHrP binds to PTH receptors in bone and kidney	TNF
Tumors associated	**Tumors associated**
Non small cell lung cancer ***(MC),***	Breast, myeloma, lymphoma, leukemia
Breast; kidney ; head and neck; bladder	

Treatment of Hypercalcemia	
Mild to moderate	***Severe***
• Hydration • Diuretics + bisphosphonate pamidronate • In case of LH give glucocorticords	• As in mild to moderate hypercalemia + salmon calcifonin or if not effective add plicamycin and gallium nitrate

2. **Ans. is b i.e. Cerebral cortical degeneration** *Ref. Harrison 17/e, p 623*

Nonmetastatic complication means paraneoplastic syndromes.

Paraneoplastic syndromes of the Nervous system		
Focal encephalitis	***Syndromes of the spinal cord***	***Syndromes of dorsal root ganglia***
Cortical encephalitis	Subacute necrotizing myelopathy	Sensory neuronopathy
Limbic encephalitis	Motor neuron dysfunction	
Brainstem encephalitis	Myelitis	
Cerebellar dysfunction	Stiff-person syndrome	
Paraneoplastic cerebellar degeneration		
Opsoclonus-myoclonus		
Multiple levels of involvement	**Syndromes of the peripheral nerve**	**Syndromes of visual system**
Encephalomyelitis, sensorimotor neuropathy autonomic dysfunction	Chronic and subacute sensorimotor sensory neuronopathy, Vasculitis of nerve and muscle Peripheral nerve hyperexcitability Autonomic neuropathy	Cancer-associated retinopathy (CAR) Melanoma-associated retinopathy (MAR) Uveitis

Remember :
- Cushing syndrome is **most commonly caused by ectopic** ACTH production.
- **Most common** carcinoma causing Cushing syndrome is small cell lung carcinoma.

3. **Ans. is a, c, d, i.e. Pancreatic Ca; Stomach Ca; Breast Ca** *Ref. Devita 7/e, p 2195*

"The greatest risk of migratory thrombophlebitis is with pancreatic cancer; however it may be seen in variety of adenocarcinoma including breast, ovarian and prostate cancer." *..... Devita 7/e, 2195*

Migratory thrombophlebitis = (Trousseau's syndrome) also seen in gastrointestinal (stomach, colon) cancer. *..... Bailey & Love 25/e, p 1067*

Diagnosis :
- Impedance plethysmography or bilateral compression ultrasonography
- Elevation of D-dimer is less sensitive in cancer patients.

Treatment of paraneoplastic thrombophlebitis ..... *Harrison 17/e 622*
- IV low molecular weight heparin for 5 days and warfarin started with in 1-2 days. The goal is to keep INR around 2-3
- In patients where heparin is contraindicated IVC filter (Green-field filter) may be placed.

Remember : Thrombophlebitis (not migratory thrombophlebitis) is seen in :

Mnemonic = GLBL
- **G**enito urinary cancer
- **L**ung cancer
- **B**rain tumor
- **L**ymphoma

4. **Ans. is a, b, c, d, e i.e. Pheochromocytoma; Hepatoma; Renal cell Ca; Adrenal adenoma; and Fibromyoma of uterus.** *Ref. Harrison 16/e, p 569*

Tumor causing erythrocytosis :
- **M**eningioma
- **A**drenal adenoma
- **R**enal cell ca
- **C**erebellar hemangoblastoma
- **H**epatoma
- Uterine **F**ibromyoma
- **P**heochromocytoma.

Mnemonic – **MARCH F**or **P**olice

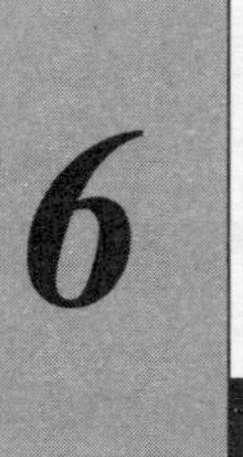

Oncologic Emergencies

What's Important ?

- Hypercalcemia
- Tumour Lysis Syndrome

Oncologic Emergencies		
Structural- obstructive oncologic emergencies by space occupying lesion	Metabolic or Hormonal emergencies = paraneoplastic syndromes	Treatment related emergencies

STRUCTURAL - OBSTRUCTIVE ONCOLOGIC EMERGENCIES BY SPACE OCCUPYING LESION

1. Superior vena-cava syndrome

- Caused by lung cancer (MC ***small cell and squamous cell type***), lymphoma and metastasis from testicular and breast carcinomas.
- ***Characteristic physical findings*** *are dilated neck veins, increased number of collateral veins covering the anterior chest wall, cyanosis, edema of fore arms and chest.*
- Most significant chest ***radiographic finding*** is *widening of superior mediastinum* (MC on right side).
- Most reliable ***diagnostic test*** is CT scan.
- Life threatening complication of superior mediastinal mass is tracheal obstruction.

SVC Syndrome

Underlying Cause	Treatment
Non small cell lung cancer and other metastatic tumours	Radiation therapy
Small cell carcinoma of lung or lymphoma	Chemotherapy
All other cases	Surgery

2. Pericardial - effusion / tamponade

- Caused by lung cancer *(MC)*, breast cancer, leukemia and lymphoma irradiation.
- Most frequent **physical findings :** *pleural effusion, sinus tachycardia, jugular venous distension, hepatomegaly, peripheral edema and cyanosis.*
- Most helpful **diagnostic test :** Echocardiography.

Treatment : *Pericardiocentesis with or without sclerosing agent.*

3. **Intestinal obstruction**
   - **Caused** by colorectal or ovarian carcinoma and metastasis from lung, breast, melanoma.
   - Most common **symptom** - pain (usually colicky).
4. **Urinary obstruction**
   - **Caused** by prostatic or gynecologic malignancies particularly cervical carcinoma or metastatic from other primary sites.
   - Most common symptom - *Flank pain*
5. **Malignant biliary obstruction**
   - **Caused** by primary carcinoma of pancreas, ampulla of vater, bile duct or by metastasis from gastric, colon, breast, lung cancer.
6. **Spinal cord compression**
   - Most common site ***thoracic spine.***
   - Caused by lung ca *(MC)* and metastasis from lung, breast prostate, multiple myeloma, lymphoma, melanoma, renal cell carcinoma and genitourinary cancers. Neuroblastoma, Ewing sarcoma and rhabdomyosarcoma are commonest cause in children.
   - Most common initial **symptom** - *localized back pain and tenderness.*
   - ***Earliest radiologic finding*** of vertebral tumour is *erosion of the pedicles* (the "winking owl" sign).
   - **Diagnosis** is made by *MRI scan with contrast.*
   - Initial **TOC** is radiation therapy plus glucocorticoids.
   - **Indication of surgery :**
     - Unknown etiology
     - Failure of radiation therapy
     - Radioresistant tumour (melanoma and renal cell cancer)
     - Pathologic fracture dislocation
     - Rapidly evolving neurologic symptoms.
7. **Increased intracranial pressure**
   - Most common cancers metastasize to brain are lung, breast cancer and melanoma.
   - Cancer having high incidence of **intracranial bleeding** are *melanoma, germ cell tumour and renal cell cancer.*
   - ***Best initial treatment*** for all symptomatic patients with brain metastases - Dexamethasone.
8. **Neoplastic meningitis**
   - Caused by *primary tumour of CNS* and *metastases* from melanoma, breast, lung cancer, lymphoma (including AIDS associated) and acute leukemia.
   - ***Elevated CSF protein*** level is nearly always present (except in HTLVI-associated adult T cell leukemia).

   Treatment : Intrathecal chemotherapy using methotrexate, cytarbine or thiotepa.
9. **Seizures :** Most common cause is ***metastatic disease*** to the CNS.
   Treatment : is ***diphenyl hydantoin*** ..... *Harrison 16/e, p 580*

Remember : Prophylactic anticonvulsant therapy is not recommended unless patient is at very high risk for late seizures as in melanoma primary hemorrhagic metastases, (treatment is radiosurgery).

10. **Intracerebral leukocytostasis (Ball's disease) : Caused** by acute leukemia particularly myelogenous leukemia (not caused by CLL, CML).
    Treatment : Whole blood irradiation.
11. **Hemoptysis : Caused** by lung cancer and metastases from carcinoid, breast, colon, kidney, melanoma.
12. **Airway Obstruction :** Most commonly caused by lung cancer followed by oesophgeal, thyroid and mediastinal malignancies.

METABOLIC / HORMONAL EMERGENCIES = PARANEOPLASTIC SYNDROME

1. **Hypercalcemia**
   - Main factor leading to hypercalcemia is either increased release of calcium from bone or an increased Ca^{2+} reabsorption from DCT.
   - Mostly **underlying cause** is secretion of PTHrP.

   Treatment : Hydration, Bisphosphonates (Zole dronic acid is DOC), Gallium nitrate, Calcitonin, Plicamycin (in refractory cases).
2. **SIADH** : Most common ***cause of hyponatremia in cancer patient.***
3. **Lactic acidosis** : Occur with leukemia, lymphoma or solid tumours causing altered liver functions.
4. **Hypoglycemia** : Most commonly caused by pancreatic islet cell tumors.
5. **Adrenal insufficiency** :
   - ***Caused by :***
     – Replacement of gland by metastases from lung, breast, colon, kidney cancer and lymphoma.
     – Removal of both glands hemorrhagic necrosis in association with sepsis or anticoagulation.
     – Impaired steroid synthesis by mitotane; Ketoconazole etc.

TREATMENT RELATED EMERGENCIES

1. **Tumour lysis syndrome**

   Associated with treatment of *Burkitt's lymphoma, ALL and other high grade lymphoma.*

   Characterized by :
   - *Hyperuricemia* – Due to destruction of malignant cells and rapid turnover of nucleic acid.
   - *Hyperkalemia* – Due to release of intracellular K^+ leading to arrythmia.
   - *Hyperphosphatemia and hypocalcemia* – Due to release of intracellular PO_4^{3-} which combine Ca^{2+} into bone, $CaPO_4$ gets deposited in renal tubules causing renal failure.
   - *Lactic acidosis* – Due to deranged oxidative metabolism.

   Treatment : Hydration, NaHCO3, Allopurinol, Rasburicase, recombinant urate oxidase Hemodialysis.
2. **Human antibody infusion reactions**
   - Occur after infusion of antibodies-such as rituximab.
   - **Characterized** by *fever, chills, nausea, headache.*

   Stop infusion and restart at half the initial infusion rate after the symptoms have abated.
3. **Hemolytic – Uremic syndrome :**
   - Most common agent causing this is ***Mitomycin.***
   - Most common cancer - gastric, calorectal and breast.
4. **Neutropenia and infection**
5. **Pulmonary infiltrate :**
   - Most common cause is as a consequence of treatment.
   - Also seen in case of *leukemia, lymphoma, breast* and other *solid cancers.*
6. **Typhilitis = Neutropenic enterocolitis**
   - ***Necrosis of caecum and adjacent colon*** occur during **treatment** of acute leukemia.
   - Surgical intervention should be considered if there is no improvement by 24h after start of antibiotic treatment.
7. **Hemorrhagic cystitis**
   - **Caused** by cyclophosphamide or ifosfamide due to ***metabolite acrolein.***
   - Best management is prevention (high urine flow + 2-mercaptoethane sulfonate i.e. mesna).

   Treatment :
   – High urine flow + irrigation of bladder with formalin; N. acetylcysteine.
   – Prostaglandins (Carboprost tromethamine); ligation of hypogastric arteries, urinary diversion or cystectomy done in extreme cases.

QUESTIONS

1. A patient with leukemia on chemotherapy develops acute lower abdominal pain associated with anaemia, thrombocytopenia and leucopenia. Which of the following is clinical diagnosis :
a. Appendicitis **[AI 06]**
b. Leukemic colitis
c. Perforation peritonitis
d. Neutropenic colitis

2. Which of the following are features of tumor lysis syndrome : [PGI 06]
a. Hyperuricemia
b. Hyperkalemia
c. Hyperphosphatemia
d. Hypercalcemia
e. Hypophosphatemia

ANSWERS, REFERENCES, EXPLANATIONS WITH INFORMATIVE ILLUSTRATIONS

1. **Ans. is d i.e. Neutropenic colit**is *Ref. Harrison 17/e, p 537*

Neutropenic Enterocolitis (Typhilitis)

- Neutropenic enterocolitis is an ***inflammation and necrosis of the caecum*** and surrounding tissue that may complicate treatment of acute leukemia.
- *Also seen in other forms of cancer treated* with taxanes.
- Patients develops ***right lower quadrant abdominal pain*** often with rebound tenderness and a tense distended abdomen *in a setting of fever and neutropenia.*
- Watery diarrhea and bacteremia are common and bleeding may occur.
- **CT scan** show *marked bowel wall thickness* particularly in caecum with bowel wall edema.

Treatment : – Includes rapid institution of **broad spectrum antibiotic and nasogastric suction.**
– *Surgical intervention* should be considered if their is ***no improvement by 24 hours.***

2. **Ans. is a, b, c i.e. Hyperuricemia; Hyperkalemia; Hyperphosphatemia**

Ref. Harrison 17/e, p 1736

Tumor lysis syndrome occur due to destruction of rapidly proliferating neoplastic cell.
It is characterized by :
- *Hyperuricemia* (due to turnover of nucleic acid)
- *Hyperkalemia* (as K^+ is main intracellular cation)
- *Hyperphosphatemia* with reciprocal depression in serum calcium *(hypocalcemia)*
- *Lactic acidosis.*

- Most common cause is ***treatment of Burkitt's lymphoma,*** ALL, high grade lymphomas, chronic leukemia (In CLL after treatment with fludarabine and cladribine) and rarely with solid tumors.

- *Factors correlate with risk of tumor lysis syndrome :*
  - Tumor burden
  - Renal function
  - Hyperuricemia
  - High serum level of LDH (> 1500 u/L).
- Standard preventive approach consist of allopurinol, urinary alkalinization by $NaHCO_3$, aggresive hydration.
- **Rasburicase** (recombinant urate oxidase) is given in *resistant cases,* it is contraindicated in G_6PD deficiency.
- If dialysis is required, hemodialysis is preferred mode.

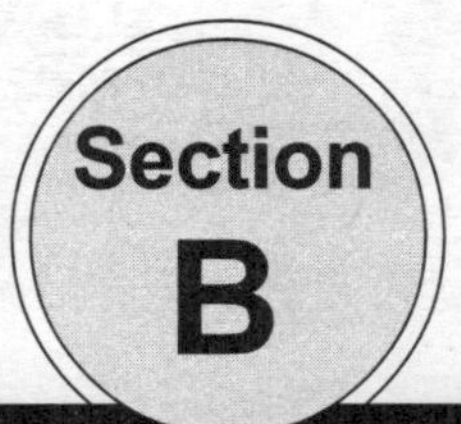

Skin, Bone and Soft Tissue Oncology

Skin Tumour

What's Important ?

- **Predisposing factors**
- **Treatment of melanoma**

MALIGNANT MELANOMA

- Malignant melanoma refers to malignant lesion **originating** in the melanoblast of skin at dermoepidermal junction but some lesions may be amelanotic.
- It is the MC cancer of **women** between **25 – 29 years.**

Origin	
In *pre-existing pigmented nevus* **(90%)** either in **junctional nevus** *(MC)*, compound nevus, Hutchinson's freckle, lentigo	Denovo in apparently normal skin (10%)

Risk factors	
– **Ultraviolet A and B** : *Most biologically relevant factor*	– Congenital nevi > 5% body surface area
– Previous melanoma	– Family history
– Dysplastic nevi syndrome	– 5 nevi > 5mm diameter / 50 nevi > 2mm diameter
– Sunburns during childhood and exposure to sunlight.	– Poor tanning ability
– White race	– Red hair / Blond hair
– Blue eyes	– Freckles
– Tanning salons	– Equatorial latitudes
– Psoralen sunscreen	– Xeroderma pigmentosa

Most common site for melanoma in **men** is on the **back and trunk** while in **women** ***MC*** site is *lower extremity.*

Clinicopathological classification

i. **Superficial spreading melanoma (SSM) :**
   - Most common type.
   - **Irregular border** is its characteristic.

- Some regress *spontaneously.*
- Most common **site** is *torso of men and lower leg, back of women.*

ii. **Lentigo Maligna Melanoma (LMM) / Hutchinson's melanotic freckle :**
- *Least common* and *least malignant* type.
- Occur nearly exclusively in older individuals (*6-8 th decade*) on chronically sun exposed, skin.
- Most common site is, *face.*
- Some may *regress spontaneously.*
- It is characterized by irregular margin.

iii. **Nodular Melanoma (NM) :**
- *Most malignant (worst prognosis)* type.
- Most common **site** is *head, neck and trunk.*
- Generally develop *de novo* not in pre-existing nevus.

iv. **Acral - lentiginous Melanoma (LM) :**
- Commonest type of lesion in coloured people. It is *not influenced by UV* radiation from sunlight.
- Most common site is sole (under great toe-nail), palm, subungual areas and mucocutaneous junctions.
- Hutchinson's sign is seen (pigmentation encroaching posterior nail fold).

v. **Amelanotic Melanoma : It is most virulent of all varieties of melanoma even more than nodular melanoma.**

Spread

- Most common route of metastasis is lymphatic (the **first site** of metastatic disease is to the *first regional lymph node* group).
- Most common site of **systemic** metastasis is *liver.*

Remember : In malignant melanoma of eye there is no lymphatic spread.

Staging :

1. **Clark's level of invasion :**

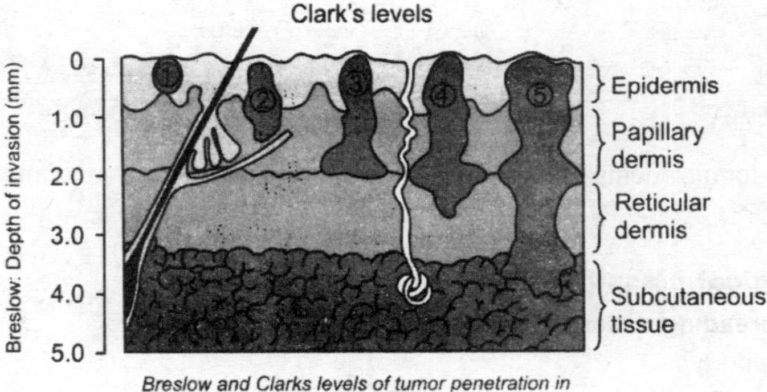

Breslow and Clarks levels of tumor penetration in relation to the normal layers of skin

Prognostic factors :

Prognostic factors in primary melanoma (stage I and II)

- **Breslow tumour thickness - most important**
- Tumour ulceration
- Clark's level of invasion
- Patient age- older patient have thicker tumours
- Patient Gender - better in female
- Growth pattern
- Desmoplastic neurotropic melanoma tumour type
- Tumour mitotic rate, microvessel density, vertical growth phase
- Anatomic location of primary tumour - prognosis of acral, trunk, head and neck is poor than melanoma of extremities (forearm and leg).

Prognostic factors in regionally metastatic melanoma (stage III)

- Number of metastatic nodes
- Nodal tumour burden
- Primary tumour ulceration
- Satellite nodules and in transit metastases.
  This question is of 1997 year when satellitosis comes under stage II but now satellitosis comes under stage III. So, we have mentioned two answer.

Prognostic factors in distant metastatic melanoma (Stage IV)

- Site of *Distant metastases*
- *Number of metastatic* sites
- Serum *Lactate Dehydrogenase* levels
- Performance status.
- *Patient factor for good prognosis* : Normal appetite; absence of nausea, vomiting or fever ; unimpaired performance status; female gender.
- Biochemical and serological markers : LDH, MIA (melanoma inhibitory activity), polypeptide S-100b.

Treatment

- It is radioresistant.
- *Surgery* is treatment of choice :
  - Any suspected melanoma should be removed by excisional biopsy and if biopsy specimen reveals melanoma, a formal excision with adequate margin is done.
  - Lesion < *1 mm* in depth excise with 1cm margins.
  - Lesion between *1mm and 4 mm* thickness should be excised with 2cm margins.
  - Lesion deeper > *4mm* should be excised with 2-3cm margin and may require resection of underlying fascia
  - Biopsy of sentinel lymph node is done.
  - Patients with clinically palpable lymph nodes or a positive sentinel lymph node biopsy should undergo formal lymph node dissection of entire drainage basin.
  - *Chemotherapy* : CVD (Cisplatin, Vinblastine, Dacarbazine), interperon alfa 2β, interleukin-2 this combination is called as biochemotherapy.

Remember : Local recurrence is defined as any melanoma that occurs within 5 cm of scar of previously excised lesion.

SQUAMOUS CELL CARCINOMA (SCC) / EPITHELIOMA / EPIDERMOID CARCINOMA

It is a carcinoma of the cells of epidermis that usually migrate outwards to the surface. It orginate from prickle cell layer. Usually present above 40 years.

- It is **second** MC skin cancer in **light skinned** racial group and MC skin cancer in **darkly pigmented** racial groups.
- Most common **causative factor** in white is *sunlight* (also for basal cell carcinoma).
- Most common **site** *ears, cheeks, lower lip and back of hands.*

Predisposing factors

- *Senile keratosis.*
- Chronic skin lesions eg lupus vulgaris, cutaneous TB, syphilis.
- Xeroderma pigmentosum.
- Exposure to sunlight or irradiation.
- Chronic irritation (leukoplakia; chronic ulcer called as Marjolin's ulcer following burn, venous ulcer, old scar).
- Viral infections HIV, HPV-16.
- Very rarely SCC arise from basal cell carcinoma known as *Baso-squamous carcinoma.*
- *Contact with tars and hydrocarbons.*
- *Erythroplasia of queyrat.*
- Actinic keratosis / solar keratotic intraepidermal SCC/SCC in situ.
- Fair complexion, poor tanning ability and sunburn.
- Immunosuppression after organ transplantation.
- Psoralens and ultraviolet A light *(PUVA) for psoriasis.*
- Patient exposed to arsenic particularly bowen's disease.

Most common **type** of SCC is ulcerative type.

Microscopically mass of keratin is surrounded by normal - looking squamous cells, presenting with the characteristic prickle cell' appearance which are arranged in concentric manner as seen in 'onion skin'. This whole appearance is called "cell nest or epithelial pearl".

Main presenting **symptom** of SCC is nodule or ulcer.

Edge of ulcer is raised and everted with indurated base (pathognomonic sign of epithelioma).

Treatment : ..... *Devita 7/e, p 1733*

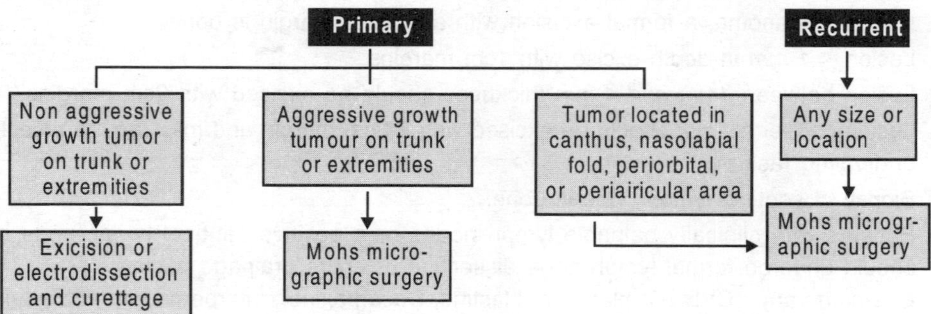

BASAL CELL CARCINOMA (BCC)/ RODENT ULCER

- It is the MC **skin cancer.**
- It is locally invasive carcinoma of **basal layer of epidermis** with no lymphatic spread and rare hematogenous spread.
- Tumour is *often multiple.*

Risk factors

i. Ultraviolet light particularly **UVB**
ii. Mutation in regulatory genes
iii. Exposure to ionizing radiation
iv. Immunosuppression (lymphoma, leukemia, transplantation, HIV)
v. Elder white male
vi. Prolonged administration of arsenic usually in form of liquor arsenicals.

- **Most common** histologic **subtype** of BCC is Nodular BCC.
- Lesion usually appear on face (around inner and outer canthus of eye).
- Typical lesion appear as small, translucent or shiny "pearly" elevated nodules with central umbilication and rolled pearly edges.
- Microscopically cells on periphery of is lands have ***'palisade'*** arrangement.
- Occasionally BCC arise from *basal cells of hair follicles and sweat glands.* Such tumours are mostly seen in the **scalp and adolescents** are usual victims. Such tumour is called *'turban tumor' or 'epithelioma adenoides cysticum.*
- ***Most invasive*** subtype is morpheaform (fibrosing) BCC.
- ***Least invasive*** subtype is superficial BCC.

Treatment :

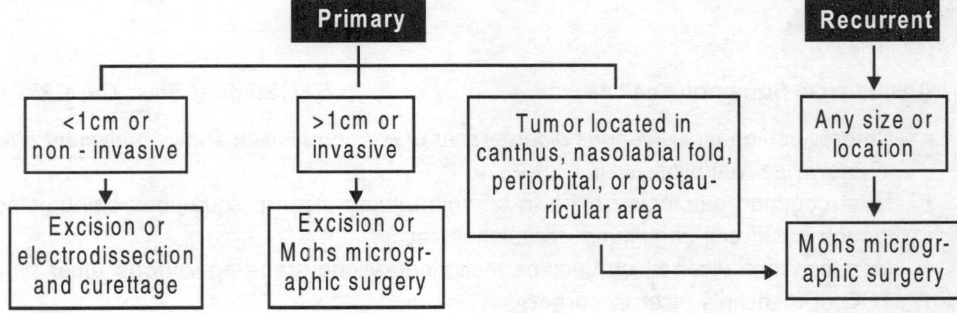

Remember:

- Mohs micrographic surgery is the treatment of choice for all recurrent and infiltrative BCC, particularly if tumour is located on the face.
- Radiotherapy is best suited for older patients particularly those with extensive lesions on the ear, lower limbs or eyelids. RT is not indicated for recurrent or morpheaform lesions.
- Excisional surgery, electrodissection curettage and cryosurgery are used to treat circumscribed, non-infiltrating BCC.

ANSWERS, REFERENCES, EXPLANATIONS WITH INFORMATIVE ILLUSTRATIONS

1. **The most common malignancy found in Marjolin's ulcer is : [AI 06]**
   a. Basal cell carcinoma
   b. Squamous cell carcinoma
   c. Malignant fibrous histiocytoma
   d. Neurotrophic malignant melanoma

2. **Biopsy from a mole on the foot shows cytologic atypia of melanocytes and diffuse epidermal infiltration by anaplastic cells, which are also present in the papillary and reticular dermis. The most likely diagnosis is : [AI 05]**
   a. Melanoma, Clark level IV
   b. Congenital melanocytic nevus
   c. Dysplastic nevus
   d. Melanoma, Clark level III

3. **Which of the following is true about melanoma? [PGI Dec 05]**
   a. Amelanotic melanoma is associated with worst prognosis
   b. Complete excisional biopsy is the treatment
   c. Thin lesion has good prognosis
   d. Back is most common site in female
   e. Junctional naevus is associated with maximum risk.

4. **All of the following statements about malignant melanoma are true except :**
   a. Lymphatic spread **[PGI June 08]**
   b. Lymph node biopsy is always done
   c. Biopsy to be done when sentinael lymph node is involved
   d. Microsatellitism may be present.

ANSWERS, REFERENCES, EXPLANATIONS WITH INFORMATIVE ILLUSTRATIONS

1. **Ans. is b i.e. Squamous cell ca** *Ref. Surgical Short Case 3/e, p 22*

- Chronic benign ulcer *(venous ulcer or scar of old burn)* which shows *malignant change* is known as Marjolins ulcer.
- Most common carcinoma arise in chronic benign ulcer is squamous cell carcinoma though basal cell carcinoma occasionally occur.
- Most common ulcer which become malignant is long **standing venous ulcer.**
- TOC of marjolin's ulcer is **surgery.**

Remember : *Marjolin's ulcer is radio resistant.*

2. **Ans. is a i.e. Melanoma, Clark level IV**

Ref. Surgical Short Case 3/e, p 26

It is typical histological appearance of malignant melanoma Clark level IV.

Staging of malignant melanoma

Clark's level of Invasion :

Level I (in situ)	–	All tumour cells are *above the basement membrane.*
Level II	–	tumour extends into *papillary but not the reticular dermis.*
Level III	–	tumour reach *interface* between papillary and reticular dermis.
Level IV	–	tumour cells *reach reticular dermis.*
Level V	–	tumour cells *invade the subcutaneous fat.*

Important points about melanoma

- **Most common** type of malignant melanorma – **Superficial spreading melanoma**
- **Least common** type of malignant melanoma **– Lentigo maligna melanoma**
- **Most malignant type** – Nodular type
- **Least malignant type** – Lentigo maligna melanoma
- **Most common** site of **Lentigo maligna** melanoma: *face*
- **Most common** site of malignant melanoma in **men** – back and trunk
- **Most common** site of malignant melanoma in **women** – Lower extremity
- **Most common** site of *superficial spreading* melanoma is torso of ***men and lower leg, back of women***
- **Most common** site of **nodular** melanoma is head neck and trunk
- **Most common** site of **Acral lentiginous** melanoma is under great toe nail (sole)
- **Most common** site of **desmoplastic** melanoma is head, neck and upper back
- Malignant melanoma shows **neurotropism** is **desmoplastic melanoma.**

3. **Ans. is (a, b, c and e), i.e. Amelanotic melanoma is associated with worst prognosis, Complete excisional biopsy is the treatment: Thin lesion has good prognosis; Junctional naevus is associated with maximum risk**

(Ref. Surgical short case 3/e, p 25-29, Devita 7/e, p 1759-1760, Sabiston 18/e 771)

Let us consider each option

Option a

Amelanotic Melanoma: It is most virulent of all varienties of melanoma even more than nodular melanoma. These melanoma does not produce melanin, so are difficult to recognize.

Option b

- Excisional biopsy is Treatment of choice for melanoma or suspicious lesion
- Lesion < 1 mm in depth   Excise with 1 cm margins.
- Lesion 1-4 mm in thickness   Excise with 2 cm margins.
- Lesion > 4 mm in thickness: Excise with 2 -3 cm margin with resection of underlying fascia.
- Biopsy of sentinel lymph node is done.
- Patient with clinically palpable lymph nodes or a positive sentinel lymph node biopsy should undergo lymph node dissection.
- Incisional biopsy in indicated for larger lesions or lesions located in close vicinity to important structures.

Option c

- Thickness of lesion is the most important prognostic factor in Stage I and Stage I and stage II. For stage III number of nodes become more important.

Option c

- Most common site of malignant melanoma in men: back and trunk
- Most common site of malignant melanoma in women: Lower extremity
- Most common site of desmoplastic (which shows neurotropism) melanoma is head and neck and upper back

Option e

- Junctional nerve has no malignant potential
- Following naevi increase the risk of malignancy:
  - Spliz naevus
  - Spindle cell naevus
  - Dysplastic naevus
  - Giant congenital pigmented naevus

4. Ans. is (a, b, c, d) i.e. All options are correct (*Ref. Bailey 25/e p 616*)

Let consider each option

Option 'a'

- Most common route of metastasis of melanoma is lymphatic
- Most common site of distant metastasis is liver

Option b and c

- Sentinel lymph node biopsy is on integral part of melanoma management and staging
- Sentinel lymph node is & identified by preoperative lymphomgiography and intraoperative lymph node sampling.
- If a lymph node in the vicinity of melanoma is enlarged biopsy of that node is also taken (so option c is also correct)

Option d

- Microsatellites are discrete tumour nests that are separated from main tumour mass by normal reticular dermal collagen or subcutaneous fat.
- Microsatellites are associated with increased frequency of regional lymph node metastasis

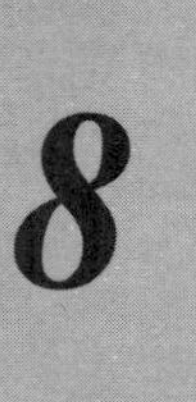

Bone Tumour

What's Important ?

- **Predisposing factors**
- **Treatment of melanoma**

CLASSIFICATION

A. Primary

Histologic type	*Benign*	*Malignant*
Hematopoietic (40%)	—	Myeloma ***(MC)***
	—	Reticulum cell sarcoma
Chondrogenic (25%)	Osteochondroma	Chondrosarcoma
	Chondroma	
	Chondroblastoma	
	Chondromyxoid fibroma	
Osteogenic (20%)	Osteoid osteoma	Osteosarcoma
	Benign osteoblastoma	Parosteal osteogenic sarcoma
Unknown origin (10%)	Giant cell tumor	Ewing's tumor
	—	Malignant giant cell tumor
	—	Adamantinoma
	(Fibrous) histiocytoma	(Fibrous) histiocytoma
Fibrogenic (5%)	Fibroma	Fibrosarcoma
	Desmoplastic fibroma	—
Notochordal (3.1%)	—	Chordoma
Vascular (1.6%)	Hemangioma	Hemangioendothelioma
	—	Hemangiopericytoma
Lipogenic (< 0.5%)	Lipoma	—
Neurogenic (< 0.5%)	Neurilemoma	—

B. Metastatic – More common

Remember :
- Most common **skeletal malignancy** is *metastatic bone tumours.*
- ***Most common*** **bone tumour in** pediatric **age group is *osteosarcoma.***
- ***Most common*** **bone tumour** <10 years **of age is *Ewing's sarcoma.***
- **Overall** *MC* **primary bone tumour is multiple myeloma.**
- ***Most common*** **bone tumour in** adults **is *Osteosarcoma.***
- ***Most common*** **tumour in** elders **is *Metastatic/Secondary bone tumour.***

- **Benign but occasionally aggressive bone tumours are :**
  - GCT
  - Chondroblastoma
  - Chondromyxoid fibroma
  - Osteoblastoma
  - Langerhan's Histiocytosis.

Etiology

Cause of most bone tumor is unknown.

- *Conditions predisposing for bone tumors are :*
  - Li-Fraumenni] ↑ risk of osteosarcoma
  - Retinoblastoma]
  - Paget's disease
  - Radiation
  - Bone infarct
  - Osteomyelitis

Spread

- Bone tumours, unlike carcinomas, disseminate almost exclusively through the blood.
- Most common site of hematogenous spread is lung followed by bone.
- Early lymphatic spread to regional nodes has only ***rarely*** been reported. Lymphatic involvement, is a poor prognostic sign.
- Skip metastases defined, as a tumor nodule that is located within the same bone as the main tumor but not in continuity with it.
  - Skip metastases are ***most often seen with high-grade sarcomas***. They develop by the embolization of tumor cells with in the marrow sinusoids.
  - These lesions are a *prognosticator of poor survival.*

Diagnostic evaluation

Imaging :

- ***X-ray:*** First investigation for any bone pathology.
  - Poorly delineated border or margin less border and periosteal reaction are indicative of malignancy.
- ***CT :*** for accurate determination of intra and extraosseus extension.
  - It accurately depicts the *transverse relationship* of a tumor.
  - CT should include entire bone and adjacent joint.
- ***MRI :*** MRI provides most accurate contrast discrimination of bone sarcomas. Single best study for determining intraosseus extension and is investigation of choice

  ... Devita 8/e p 1800
  - MRI is ideal for imaging the medullary marrow.
  - Especially helpful in detection of small bone lesion.
  - For evaluating conditions when radiography is negative and bone scan is positive.
  - Determining extent of infiltrative tumor and detecting skip metastases.
- ***Bone scans :*** Determine metastatic disease, intraosseous extension of tumor.
  - *Skip metastases* are not detected by bone scans.
- ***Angiography***
  - To determine vascularity of tumor.
  - Specially useful for tumors of proximal tibia, where vascular anomalies are common.

Isotope scanning :

- ***Thallium scans :*** Thallium 201 accumulates in musculoskeletal tumor.
- ***PET :*** under evaluation. Role is considered in metastatic disease.

Staging : AJCC & UICC (International Union Against Cancer) TNM Staging

Primary tumor (T)	
TX	Primary tumor cannot be assessed
T0	No evidence of primary tumor
T1	Tumor (maximum dimension) ≤ 8 cm at time of diagnosisc.
T2	Tumor (maximum dimension) > 8 cm at time of diagnosis
T3	Skip metastases – two discontinuous tumors in the same bone with no other distant metastases.
Regional lymph nodes (N)	
NX	Regional lymph nodes cannot be assessed
N0	No regional lymph node metastasis
N1	Regional lymph node metastasis to be considered equivalent to distant metastatic disease.
Distant metastasis (M)	
M X	Distant metastasis cannot be assessed
M X	No distant metastasis
M 1	Distant metastasis
M 1 a	Lung-only metastases
M 1 b	All other distant metastases including lymph nodes.

BENIGN TUMORS

A. **Bone forming benign tumors :** Neoplastic cell produce bone which is usually deposited as woven trabeculae (except osteoma) and is variably mineralized.

1. **Osteoid osteoma :**
   - *Definition :* Benign bone tumor which is less than 2cm in greatest dimension.
   - *Age :* 5 to 25 years
   - *Sex :* M > F
   - *Site :* any bone except skull; Cortex > Medulla.
     Diaphysis of long bones (tibia, femur). Tibia is most commonly involved.
   - Presented with nocturnal nagging pain, *relieved by salicylates.*
   - It is not premalignant.
     – *Diagnosis :* - Generally by X-ray : Radiolucent nidus (= actual tumor) surrounded by zone of sclerosis (reactive bone formation).
       - In rest 25% cases : CT diagnostic.
       - Double density sign on bone scan.
     – *Treatment* : Enbloc excision of nidus along with sclerotic bone; curettage or percutaneous CT guided ablation of nidus. Some lesion spontaneously resolve after skeletal maturity.

2. **Osteoblastoma :**
   – Histologically resemble osteoid osteoma.
   – Consist of vascular osteoid and new bone.

- Locally destructive, progressively growing lesion with predilection for vertebrae and flat bone (Jaw).
- Never involves epiphysis.
- Presents with dull, aching pain which not respond to salicylates.
- *X-ray* : radiolucent expansile bone lesion with minimal reactive new bone formation.
- *Treatment :* Curettage and bone grafting or block excision.

Remember : Malignant transformation is remote in both osteoid osteoma and osteoblastoma except, when treated with radiation which promotes this dreaded complication.

3. **Osteoma**
   - Bosselated, round to oval sessile tumor projected from subperiosteal or endosteal surface of cortex.
   - Composed of sclerotic well formed bone.
   - Most common **site** skull and facial bones.
   - *Usually solitary;* multiple osteomas seen in Gardner's syndrome.
   - *Age :* Middle aged
   - Generally slow growing and asymptomatic but can cause obstruction of sinus cavity, impinge on brain or eye.
   - Not premalignant and do not transform into osteosarcoma.
   - Generally no treatment given but excision may be done if cause cosmetic problems.

B. **Cartilage forming benign tumors :**

1. **Osteochondroma/exostosis**
   - *Definition* : Hyaline cartilage - capped mushroom shaped outgrowth which is attached to underlying skeleton by bony stalk.
   - Overall it is the MC benign bone tumor.
   - It is of two types :

Features	Solitary osteochondroma	Multiple osteochondroma
Pattern	Sporadic Occur due to aberrations at growth plate	Hereditary (autosomal dominant) Basic defects is in remodelling. Also called as multiple hereditary exostosis or diaphyseal aclasis
Age	Late adolescence and early adulthood	Childhood
Clinical features	Painless swelling around joint; complication is pain	Dwarfism, limb length inequality, deformities Pressure effects of exostosis
X-ray	Well defined bony growth made up of cortical bone and marrow (in continuity of bone) emerging from metaphysis. Cartilage cap not seen.	Trumpet shaped metaphysis & bony projection from it .
Treatment	Excision when cause symptoms or rapid growth occurs.	Excision of that exostosis which cause symptoms
Risk of malignant transformation	Less	More

- *Sex* : M > F
- *Gene* : Inactivation of EXT gene
  Molecular genetics suggest that it is a neoplasm. ..... *Robbin's 7/e, p 1296*

- *Site* : Develop only in bones of endochondral origin. Metaphysis near the growing and growth plate of long tubular bones especially around knee (distal femur).
- Growth usually stop at the time of growth plate closure or after maturity.
- Rarely (1%) of cases, convert into chondrosarcoma or other sarcoma.
- Cartilaginous cap thickness of more than 1cm should arouse suspicion of malignancy.

Treatment

Usually no treatment in required. Complete surgical excision is indicated in:

a. ***J**oint interference:* If tumor is large and obstructing the joint movements.
b. *Painful **b**urisitis:* Inflammation of bursa between the tumor and surrounding tissue.
c. **M**alignant cange (1-2%)
d. **P**ressure on neighbouring vessels and nerves
e. **F**racture of bony stask

Mnemonic : Priyanka Jain My Best Friend.

2. **Chondromas**
   - *Definition :* Tumor of hyaline cartilage encapsulated by fibrous tissue growth plate cartilage that subsequently proliferate and slowly enlarge.
   - It is of two types :

Enchondromas	Subperiosteal or Juxtacortical chondromas
Arise within medullary cavity	Arise from surface of bone

- **Enchondromas :**

  Most common *intraosseus cartilage tumours.*

  Most common tumor of hand bones.

  Age : 20-50 years

  Site : Usually solitary

  Metaphyseal region of short tubular bones of hands and feet.

  Association : A. **Ollier disease -**
  - Non hereditary, multiple enchondromas or enchondromatosis, seen in child hood. Chances of sarcomatous, transformation is more than solitary enchondromas.
  - Presents with bony deformity, short stature etc.

  B. **Maffucci syndrome :** Enchondromatoses with soft tissue ***hemangiomas.***
  - They are at risk of developing ovarian carcinoma and brain gliomas.
  - There is greater degree of cellularity and cytologic atypia in olliver and maffucci which mimics chondrosarcoma.

  Clinical features : *Mostly asymptomatic / swelling without much pain* occasionally painful and pathologic fracture.

  X-ray : Unmineralized nodules of cartilage producing expanding lytic lesion surrounded by rim of radiodense bone (O ring sign).

  Overlying cortices thinned out

  Matrix shows, punctate or stippled calcification, so flicks or wisp of calcification within lucent area is pathognomic.

  Treatment : Currettage with or without grafting (if cavity is big).

Remember : Enchondromas of long bones may change into chondrosarcoma more frequently than that of small bones. Appearance of pain is important sign of malignancy.

3. **Chondroblastoma :**
   - Chondroblastoma is a cartilagenous benign tumor characteristically containing multiple calcium deposits.
   - *Age* : Young adult, M < F
   - *Site* : Around epiphysis.
   - It also involve apophyses (epiphyseal equivalent i.e. iliac crest).
   - Bones around knee and humerus are most commonly affected.
   - Usually painful because of their location.
   - *Radiologically* : There is well defined geographic lytic lesion, surrounded by zone of sclerosis and mottled calcification may be seen.
   - *Microscopically :*
     - Characteristic "chicken wire pattern" of mineralization.
     - Large collection of chondroblasts surrounded by the immature fibrous tissue.
   - *Treatment :* Curretage and bone grafting.

4. **Chondromyxoid fibroma :**
   - *Age* : Adolescents and young adults
   - *Sex* : Male preponderance
   - *Site* : Long tubular bones of lower limb
   - *Location* : Metaphysis
   - *Clinical presentation* : **Mostly asymptomatic** and the lesion is usually discovered by accident or after a pathological fracture.

Radiological appearance : Rounded or ovoid radiolucent area placed eccentrically in the metaphysis that is delineated from the adjacent bone by a *rim of sclerosis.*

Histological appearance : Three types of tissue can usually be identified :

1. Patches of myxomatous tissue with *stellate cells.*
2. Islands of *hyaline cartilage.*
3. Areas of *fibrous tissue* with cells of varying degrees of maturity.

In contrast to other benign cartilage tumours, the neoplastic cells in chondromyxoid fibroma *show varying degrees of cytologic atypia.*

There may be small foci of calcification and scattered non neoplastic, osteoclast type giant cells.

Treatment :
- *Excision* **with autogenous bone grafting (TOC).**
- Curettage and bone grafting.

MALIGNANT TUMORS

1. **Osteosarcoma :**
   - Osteosarcoma is a high-grade, malignant spindle cell tumor that arises, with in a bone.
   - Its distinguishing characteristic is the production of 'tumor' osteoid or immature bone directly from a malignant spindle cell stroma.
   - Osteosarcoma typically occurs during childhood and adolescence with peak incidence between 10 and 19 years of age.
   - Osteosarcoma is the MC ***primary bone tumor in children and adolescence but in children younger than 10 years Ewing's sarcoma is*** most common.

Pathology : Classified into :

- Osteoblastic type
- Chondroblastic type
- Telangiectatic type
- Giant cell type
- Small cell type
- MC subtype is primary, solitary metaphysal, intramedullary and poorly differentiated gene mutation is of RB and p53 gene.

Predisposing factors

- The ***MC*** known ***risk factor*** is radiation exposure MC.
- Hereditary risk factors are hereditary retinoblastoma, Li-Fraumeni syndrome.
- When osteosarcoma occurs in patients older than 40 years, it is usually associated with a exostosis, or polyostotic fibrous dysplasia.
- In elderly Paget's disease, bone infarct and prior irradiation are known predisposing factors.

Clinical features

- Show bimodal age distribution : 75% occur in patients younger than 20; Smaller second peak occur in elders M > F.
- Pain is the MC ***complaint.***
- Lower end of femur ; upper end of tibia and the proximal humerus are the ***MC sites.***
- Night pain gradually develops and becomes a ***hallmark of skeletal involvement***.
- Physical examination demonstrates a firm, soft mass in the region of metaphysis which is fixed to the underlying bone with slight tenderness.
- No effusion is noted in the adjacent joint, and motion is normal.
- Incidence of pathologic fracture is less than 1%.
- Systemic symptoms are rare.

Investigations

Radiological features **:** Typically findings are :

- Increased intramedullary radiodensity (due to tumor bone or calcified cartilage).
- An area of radiolucency (due to nonossified tumor).
- A pattern of permeative destruction with poorly defined borders.
- Cortical destruction, periosteal elevation, and extraosseous extension with soft tissue ossification.
- **Codmann triangle :** A traingular area of ***sub periosteal new bone formation*** is seen at the tumor cortex junction.
- **Sun-ray appearance :** Due to growth of tumor in to the overlying soft tissue with subsequent ossification.

Serum Alkaline Phosphate (SAP)

- SAP level is an important biologic marker of tumor activity in patients with osteosarcoma.
- Levels elevated in 45% to 50% of patients.

Biopsy : An open biopsy is performed to confirm the diagnosis.

CT chest : To exclude lung metastasis.

Prognostic factors

- The *most significant pretreatment variable* is anatomic site. Patients with pelvic and axial lesions had a lower survival rate than those with tumors of the extremities.
- Tumor size, patient age, and degree of malignancy did not correlate with survival.

..... Devita 7/e, p 1660

- Presurgical SAP levels are useful prognostic markers, the higher the AFP serum levels, the greater the risk for relapse.
- *Most significant post treatment prognostic factor* is response to chemotherapy.

Variants of classic osteosarcoma

- Osteosarcoma arising in the ***jawbone,*** the most common variant, is characterized by well-differentiated cells with a low metastatic potential.
- Periosteal osteosarcoma are the most common variants of classic osteosarcoma arising in the ***extremities.***

a. Parosteal osteosarcoma :

- In contrast to classic osteosarcoma, which arises within a bone, parosteal osteosarcomas arise on the surface of the bone (juxtacortical).
- Generally occurs in older individuals.
- It has a better prognosis that classic osteosarcoma.
- ***Distal femur*** is MC site.
- ***Wide excision*** of the tumor is the treatment of choice.

b. Periosteal osteosarcoma :

- Periosteal osteosarcoma is a rare cortical variant of osteosarcoma that arises superficially on the cortex, (juxtacortical) most often on the tibia shaft.
- *Treatment* : En bloc resection should be performed when feasible, amputation is rarely indicated.

c. Paget's sarcoma :

- In approximately 1% of patients with Paget's disease, a primary bone sarcoma will develop.
- The average patient age is 64 years, and the MC site is the pelvis, femur, and humerus.
- Treatment is similar to that recommended for adolescent patients with osteosarcoma without metastatic disease.

Treatment

Surgery :

- Limb salvage TOC whenever possible and unless contraindication exist.
  - Reconstruction options include :
    - Arthrodesis
    - Osteoarticular allograft
    - Endoprosthetic reconstruction
    - Allograft-prosthesis reconstruction

***Chemotherapy* :** – It is given both before (neoadjuvant) and after (adjuvant) surgery.
– Effective drugs are Doxorubicin, cisplatin, methotrexate, ifosfamide.

***Radiotherapy* :** – Highly radioresistant, only indication is palliation of pain.

2. Chondrosarcomas :

- Chondrosarcomas are the second MC primary malignant spindle cell tumors of bone.
- Chondrosarcomas are the MC ***malignant tumors of the sternum scapula*** and hand bones. ..... *Campbell 10/e, p 833*
- Its basic neoplastic tissue is cartilage without evidence of direct osteoid formation.
- The classic chondrosarcomas are central (arising within a bone) or peripheral (arising from the surface of a bone) and can effect any site of bone.
- **76%** of primary chondrosarcomas arise centrally.
- Secondary chondrosarcomas most often arise from benign tumors (pain is most important symptom signifying malignancy).
- Metastasize hematogenously to lung and bones

Clinical characteristics

- One half of all chondrosarcomas occur in persons older than 40 years of age (**M**C malignant primary bone tumor in 40-60 yr. age group).
- The MC sites are the pelvis (**31%**), femur (**21%**) and shoulder girdle (**13%**).
- Peripheral chondrosarcomas may become large without causing pain, and local symptoms develop only because of mechanical irritation.
- Pelvic chondrosarcomas are often large and present with referred pain to the back of thigh, sciatica secondary to sacral plexus irritation, urinary symptoms from bladder neck involvement.
- An adult with a plain radiograph suggestive of a 'benign' cartilage tumor but associated with pain most likely has a chondrosarcoma.

Radiographic diagnosis

- This is the MC malignant bone tumor that may appear radiographically benign.
- Central chondrosarcomas have two distinct radiologic patterns. One is a small, well-defined lytic lesion with a narrow zone of transition and surrounding sclerosis with mottled calcification, and endosteal scalloping *second type;* has no sclerotic border and is difficult to localize.
- The ***key sign*** of malignancy is ***endosteal scalloping***.

Prognosis

- Histologic tumor grade is an ***important predictor*** of local recurrence and metastases.
- Peripheral chondrosarcoma have ***good prognosis*** than central lesions.

Treatment

- The treatment of chondrosarcoma is surgical removal.
- Resection guidelines for high-grade chondrosarcomas are similar to those for osteosarcoma.

3. Giant cell tumour / GCT

- GCT is locally aggressive, recurrent tumor with a low metastatic potential.
- It consists of spindle-shaped and ovoid cells uniformly interspersed with multinucleated giant cells.

Pathologic Characteristics

- Mononuclear cells are proliferating component of the tumour ***(not multinucleated giant cells).***
- Nucleus of both stromal cells and giant cells is identical.
- Necrosis, hemosiderin or hemorrhage is often noted. Neither of these have a relationship to malignant potential or local recurrence rate.
- *Malignancy*
  - Although GCTs are ***rarely malignant*** de novo they may undergo transformation and demonstrate malignant potential.
  - Between 8.6% to 22% of known GCT become malignant after local recurrence.
  - Each recurrence increases the risk of malignant transformation of typical GCT.

Clinical features :

Age : 20-40 years

Sex : F > M

Site : Usually solitary; 80% of GCTs in the long bones occur after skeletal maturity, and 75% of these develop around the knee joint.

- Pain, mass (may be pulsatile), local tenderness, and decreased motion in the adjacent joint are the MC clinical symptoms.

Radiographic evaluation :

- Tumor typically arise from epiphysis.
- GCTs are ***eccentric lytic*** lesions without matrix production with a characteristic Soap bubble appearance.
- No calcification.
- ***None or minimal sclerosis*** around tumor.
- Tumor usually does *not enter the adjacent joint.*

Treatment

Surgery *:* TOC

- Resection is curative in 90% of these tumors, whereas curettage, with or without bone grafts, has a recurrence rate of 40% to 75%.
- *Primarily resection* is recommended for GCT of the proximal radius and fibula, distal ulna, tubular bones of the hand and foot, coccyx, sacrum, and pelvic bones.
- *Amputation* is reserved sfor massive recurrence, malignant transformation or infection.

Radiation : Is reserved for specific lesions, usually lesions of the spine that cause bone destruction in a confined area and can lead to spinal cord compression and severe deformity.

Cryosurgery

- Cryosurgery has been used more successfully for GCT *than for any other type of bone tumor.*

- Cryosurgery is effective in eradicating the tumor while preserving joint motion and avoiding resection or amputation.
- The *major complications* of cryosurgery are necrosis of the adjacent bones, which are liable to develop a late pathologic fracture.

4. Chordoma

Chordoma is a locally malignant tumor arising from ***notochondral remnants*** in the midline of the neural axis and involving the adjacent bone.

Age : > 40 years

Site : The ends of the spine are the MC sites. The sacrococcus and the base of the skull (35%) near the sphenooccipital area are most commonly involved.

Histologically : The physaliferous cell is ***pathognomonic.***

This tumor is highly fatal because of the high rate of *local recurrence and local complications.*

Treatment :
- The ***first surgical procedure*** has the *best chance of cure.* Inadequate surgery results in local recurrence, with little chance of subsequent surgical removal.
- Because local recurrence is common with chordomas, radiation therapy is an intergral treatment modality, *particularly for tumors of the base of the skull and sphenooccipital region.*

5. Ewing sarcoma

- Ewing's sarcoma and primitive neuroectodermal tumor are closely related, malignancies, that may occur as osseous or soft tissue tumors.
- It is the most frequent chest wall tumor in children.
- It is the second most common (MC being osteosarcoma) primary bone tumor in pediatric patients, accounting for approximately 4% of pediatric malignancies.
- Femur is the ***most frequent primary site*** for Ewing's sarcoma followed by pelvis, tibia, fibula, or the bones of the feet.
- Cytogenetics : MC chromosomal abnormality is **t (11: 22)**

Pathology

- Arise from medullary cavity, and invades cortex and periosteum, producing soft tissue mass.
- Ewing's sarcoma and primary neuroectodermal tumors are counted among the small blue round cell tumors of childhood.
- Tumors of the Ewing's sarcoma family are characterized by the presence of highly cellular aggregates of tumor cells compartmentalized by widely separated strands of fibrous tissue.
- The *most frequent sites of metastases* are the lungs and other bones.
- These tumors typically demonstrate Homer-Wright pseudorosettes on light microscopy.

Clinical presentation

- Localized pain is typically the ***first symptom.***
- Pain progresses from intermittent to more constant, *often awakening the patient from sleep.*
- ***Fever*** is present in 28% of patients with Ewing's sarcoma at the time of diagnosis.
- Characteristically exhibits bone to bone metastases.

Radiographic evaluation

- Lesions that originate in the long bones characteristically involve the diaphysis, with extension towards the metaphyses.
- ***Lytic lesion without any new bone promotion.***
- Parallel, lamellated periosteal new bone formation (onion skin lesion) may be present.
- ***Radionuclide bone scans*** should be obtained, both to define more precisely the extent of disease at the primary site and determine whether bone metastases are present.

Treatment

- *Local control* must be achieved by either high-dose radiotherapy or resection.
- *Extremity lesions* amendable to limb-sparing resections are treated predominantly with resection after an initial 12 to 15 week phase of induction chemotherapy.
- *Central pelvic or spinal* lesions are frequently treated with radiation alone.

Prognostic Factors

- Radiographic and histologic response to initial chemotherapy are *strong predictors* of treatment outcome.

Commonest sites of important bone tumor

Tumour	*Site*
Osteosarcoma	Lower end of femur
Osteoclastoma	Lower end of femur
Chondrosarcoma	Pelvis
Secondary tumors	Lumbar vertebrae
Multiple Myeloma	Lumbar vertebrae
Ewing sarcoma	Femur
Osteoid osteoma	Tibia
Chondroma	Short tubular bones of hand
Chordoma	Sacrum and cervical spine
Osteoblastoma	Vertebrae
Osteoma	Skull and facial bones
Osteochondroma	Distal femur
Admantinoma	Mandible

Metastatic cancer to bone

- More common than primary bone malignancy
- Most likely site of primary in female is breast, while in males it is prostate. Bones involved in descending order: vertebrae > Proximal femur >pelvis> ribs > sternum > proximal humurus

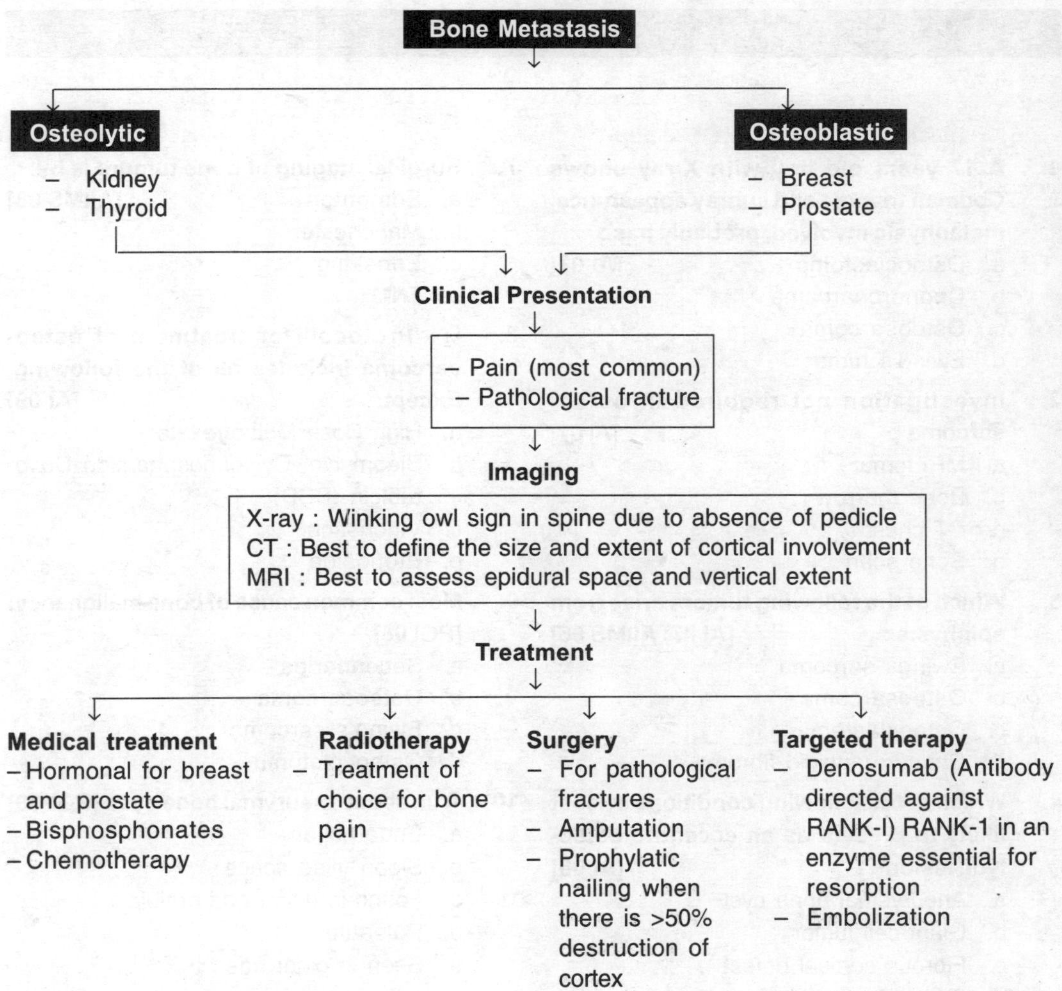
Bone Metastasis
Osteolytic
– Kidney
– Thyroid
Osteoblastic
– Breast
– Prostate
Clinical Presentation
– Pain (most common)
– Pathological fracture
Imaging
X-ray : Winking owl sign in spine due to absence of pedicle
CT : Best to define the size and extent of cortical involvement
MRI : Best to assess epidural space and vertical extent
Treatment
Medical treatment
– Hormonal for breast and prostate
– Bisphosphonates
– Chemotherapy
Radiotherapy
– Treatment of choice for bone pain
Surgery
– For pathological fractures
– Amputation
– Prophylatic nailing when there is >50% destruction of cortex
Targeted therapy
– Denosumab (Antibody directed against RANK-l) RANK-1 in an enzyme essential for resorption
– Embolization

QUESTIONS

1. **A 17 years old boy with X-ray shows Codman triangle and sunray appearance, metaphysic involved, probably has :**
   a. Osteoclastoma **[AI 07]**
   b. Chondrosarcoma
   c. Osteosarcoma
   d. Ewing's tumor

2. **Investigation not required in osteo-sarcoma :** [AI 07]
   a. MRI femur
   b. Bone marrow
   c. CT chest
   d. Bone scan

3. **Which of the following tumors arise from epiphysis : [AI 07; AIIMS 06]**
   a. Ewings sarcoma
   b. Osteosarcoma
   c. Osteoclastoma
   d. Chondro myxoid fibroma

4. **Which of the following conditions is least likely to present as an eccentric osteo-lytic lesions : [AI 06]**
   a. Aneurysmal bone cyst
   b. Giant cell tumor
   c. Fibrous cortical defect
   d. Simple bone cyst

5. **All the statement are true about exostosis except:**
   a. It occurs at growing end of bone
   b. Growth continues after skeletal maturity
   c. It is covered by cartilagenous cap
   d. Malignant transformation may occur

6. **Expansile lytic osseous metastases are characteristic of primary malignancy of :**
   a. Kidney **[AI 06]**
   b. Bronchus
   c. Breast
   d. Prostate

7. **Surgical staging of bone tumors is by:**
   a. Edmonton **[AIIMS 08]**
   b. Manchester
   c. Enneking
   d. TNM

8. **'T– Protocol' for treatment of osteo-carcoma includes all of the following, Except: [AI 09]**
   a. High Dose Methotrexate
   b. Bleomycin, Cyclophosphamide Doxo-rubicin (BCD)
   c. Vincristine
   d. Etoposide

9. **Most common cause of bone malignancy: [PGI 08]**
   a. Secondaries
   b. Osteosarcoma
   c. Ewing's sarcoma
   d. Osteoclastoma

10. **True about aneurymal bone cyst: [PGI 09]**
    a. Endothelial
    b. Blood filled space
    c. Found in upper end of tibia
    d. Pulsatile
    e. Seen in older age

11. **Bone metastasis seen in: [AI 01]**
    a. Skull
    b. Pelvis
    c. Vertebrae
    d. Small bones of hand
    e. Proximal part of long bones of upper limb.

12. **All of the following are the causes of sudden increase in pain in osteochondroma, except : [AIIMS 06]**
    a. Sarcomatous change
    b. Fracture
    c. Bursitis
    d. Degenerative change

13. A 15 year old boy is injred while playing cricket. X-rays of the leg rule out of a possible fracture. The radiologist reports the boy has an evidence of aggressive bone tumor with bone destruction and soft tissue mass. The bone biopsy reveals a bone cancer with neural differentiation. Which of the following is the most likely diagnosis ? [AIIMS 06]

a. Condrablastoma
b. Ewing's sarcoma
c. Neuroblastoma
d. Osteosarcoma

14. The differential diagnosis of lesion, histologically resembling giant cell tumor in the small bones of the hands or feet, includes all of the following except : [AIIMS 06]

a. Aneurysmal bone cyst
b. Fibrosarcoma
c. Osteosarcoma
d. Hyperparathyroidism

15. A 50 year old lady presented with a 3 month history of pain in the lowe third of the right thigh. There was no local swelling; tenderness was present on deep pressure. Plain X-rays showed an ill defined intra medullary lesion with blotchy calcification at the lower end of the right femoral diaphysis, possibly enchondroma or chondrosarcoma. Sections showed a cartilaginous tumor. Which of the following histological features [if seen] would be most helpful to differentiate the two tumours ? [AIIMS 06]

a. Focal necrosis and lobulation
b. Tumour permeation between bone trabeculae at periphery
c. Extensive myxoid change
d. High cellulararity

16. Which one of the following bone tumors typically affects the epiphysis of a long bone ? [AIIMS 05]

a. Osteosarcoma
b. Ewing's sarcoma
c. Chondroblastoma
d. Chondromyxoid fibroma

17. Which of the following is the most common cause of sclerotic skeletal metastasis in a female patient ?

a. Carcinoma breast [AIIMS 05]
b. Carcinoma ovary
c. Endometrial carcinoma
d. Melanoma
d. Synovial sarcoma

18. True about ameloblastoma : [PGI 06]

a. Cystic lesion
b. Rapidly growing
c. Malignant disease
d. MC site is tibia
e. Present in children

19. Radiological features of the osteosarcoma : [PGI 06]

a. New bone formation
b. Sun Ray appearance
c. Codman's triangle
d. Soap bubble appearance
e. Onion peel appearance

20. Metastatic tumor least common in :

a. Pelvis [PGI 08]
b. Ribs
c. Small bone of lower limb
d. Vertebra
e. Skull

21. Which of the following is a pulsatile tumor? [AIIMS May 10]

a. Osteosarcoma
b. Chondrosarcoma
c. Osteoclastoma
d. Ewing's sarcoma

ANSWERS, REFERENCES, EXPLANATIONS WITH INFORMATIVE ILLUSTRATIONS

1. **Ans. is c i.e. Osteosarcoma**

Ref. Maheshwary 3/e, p 218; Grainger Radiology 4/e, p 1882

Guy's I dont think that there is any confusion in this answer now just revise Osteosarcoma at glance.

Osteosarcoma

- 2nd Most common bone tumor, most common primary bone tumor in children.
- Most common predisposing factor is radiation exposure.
- Most common site (in order) lower end of femur; upper end of tibia; proximal humurus.
- Most common part of bone involved - metaphysis.
- **Treatment** : Limb salvage surgery when even possible is treatment of choice.

Radiological features of Osteosarcoma

- An area of irregular destruction in the metaphysis of long bone. The medullary changes are minimal initially although a non specific laminar periosteal reaction may be evident.
- As the tumor reaches the cortex, it transverses it and ultimately destroys it. The soft tissue mass enlarges and may show ill defined cloud like tumor bone within it.
- New bone formation.
- **Periosteal reaction :** As the tumor lifts the periosteum, it incites an intense irregular periosteal reaction (in osetomyelitis periosteal reaction is smooth).
- **Codman's trangle :** A triangular urea of subperiosteal new bone formation (seen in other conditions also)
- **Sunray appearance :** sunburst appearance – Due to growth of tumor cells in overlying soft tissue with subsiquent ossification.

Remember : MRI is best for staging and detection of tumor mass in soft tissue.

2. **Ans. is b i.e Bone marrow biopsy**

Ref. Devita 7/e, p 1638; Grainger Radiology 4/e, p 1884; Campbell 10/e, p 734 - 735

In osteosarcoma biopsy of mass (not marrow) is required.

Radiographic evaulation of Bone tumor

- ***Plane radiograph :*** First in investigation for any bone pathology. Should be done in two planes: Anteroposterior and lateral
- ***CT :***
  - For accurate determination of intra and extraosseus extension.
  - CT should include entire bone and adjacent joint.
- ***MRI :*** Single best study for bone sarcomas.
- ***Bone scan :*** Determine metastatic disease.
- ***Angiography :*** To determine vascularity of tumor.

In osteosarcoma it is essential to exclude the presence of lung metastases with CT for purpose of staging before initiating therapy.

3. **Ans. is c i.e. Osteoclastoma** *Ref. Apley 8/e, p 177; Campbell 10/e, p 802*

"Learn the commonest site of bone tumor by heart as they are regularly being asked."

Bone Tumor		
Epiphysis	*Metaphysis*	*Diaphysis*
– Chondroblastoma – Osteoclastoma – Clear cell chondro-sarcoma	– Osteosarcoma – Chondrosarcoma – Enchondroma – Simple bone cyst – Aneurysmal bone cyst – Brodies abscess (not a tumour) – Histiocytosis (ages 5 to 30)	– Ewings sarcoma (Ages 5 to 25) – Multiple myeloma – Osteoid osteoma – Lymphoma (Adult) – Admantioma – Fibrous dysplasia (ages 5 to 30) – Chondromyxoid fibroma

4. **Ans. is d i.e Simple bone cyst** *Ref. Chapman 3/e, p 24*

Eccentric Radiolucent Bone Lesion

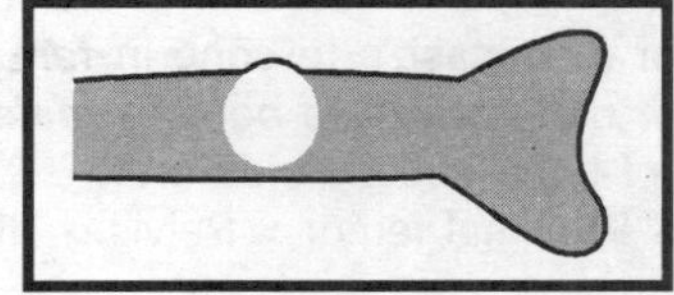

Causes of Eccentric Radiolucent Bone Lesion

Aneurysmal bone cyst : In the unfused metaphysis or metaphysis and epiphysis following fusion of the growth plate. Well-defined endosteal margin. ± thin internal strands of bone.

Giant cell tumor : Typically subarticular after epiphyseal fusion.

Enchondroma : Occur in the tubular bones of the hands and feet. Internal ground glass appearance ± calcification within it.

Non-ossifying fibroma (fibrous cortical defect) : Frequently in the distal tibia or femur and produces an eccentric expanded cortex.

Chondromyxoid fibroma : 75% in the lower limbs (50% in the proximal tibia).

5. **Ans. is b i.e. Growth continues after skeletal maturity**

Ref. Robbin's 7/e, p 1296; 8/e p 1227

In osteochondroma growth usually stop at the time of growth plate closure or after maturity.

Osteochondroma / Exostosis

- *Definition* : Hyaline cartilage-capped mushroom shaped outgrowth which is attached to underlying skeleton by bony stalk.
- Overall it is the MC benign bone tumor.
- *Sex* : M > F
- *Gene* : Inactivation of **EXT** gene
- *Site* : Develop only in bones of endochondral origin, Metaphysis near the growing and growth plate of long tubular bones especially about knee (distal femur).
- *Growth usually stop at the time of growth plate closure or after maturity.*
- Rarely (1%) of cases, convert into chondrosarcoma or other sarcoma.

6. Ans. is a i.e. Kidney

Ref. Devita 8/e, p 2510; Harrison 17/e, p 613; Maheshwari 3/e, p 224 - 225

- ***Osteolytic secondaries*** seen in primary malignancy of :
  - Kidney (Expansile secondaries)
  - Lung
  - Thyroid
- ***Osteoblastic secondaries*** clasically seen in prostate and breast carcinoma .

  ..... Campbell 10/e, p 848
- Most common cause of ***osteoblastic*** secondaries in *Males* : Prostate
- Most common cause of **osteoblastic** secondaries in *female* : Breast *(Breast also produces osteolytic secondaries).*
- ***Other tumour metastasize to bone produce mixed lytic and blastic lesion. They are:***
  - Seminoma
  - Neurogenic tumors
  - Carcinoid
  - Uterus, ovary
  - Gastointestinal Tract : Colon / stomach
  - Osteosarcoma, Ewing's sarcoma
- Most common tumor metastasize to bone in ***female*** is Ca breast
- Most common tumor metastasize to bone in ***male*** is Ca lung.
- Most common site of bone secondaries are :

  Lumbar vertebrae > Proximal femur > Pelvis > Rib > Sternum > Proximal humurus > Skull
- ***Least common*** bones involved are small bones of hand.
- Metastases to small bones of hand orignates in cancer of lungs, kidney or colon.

  ..... Robbin's 7/e p 1303
- Metastases from lung cancer have typical appearance *"Bite taken out of the cortex".*

7. Ans. is c i.e. Ennekin *Ref. Devita 8/e, p 1798; J Ebenezar 4/e, 617*

Enneking et.al. developed surgical staging system for musculaskeletal sarcoma in 1980, It is based on the GTM classification: Grade (G), Location (T), and metastasis including lymphnode involvement (M).

Enneking's Staging

Stage	Grade	M	Site
IA	Low (G1)	M_0	Intracompartmental (T1)
IB	Low (G1)	M_0	Extracompartmental (T2)
IIA	High (G2)	M_0	Intracompartmental (T1)
IIB	High (G2)	M_0	Extracompartmental (T2)
III	Any G	M_1	Any T

In 1983 AJCC recomended a different staging system for bone tumors, which after several changes (Latest one in 2002) is unversally followed.

A JCC staging is similar to Enneking's staging, however AJCC uses three grades (G1, G2, G3) and four stages.

8. Ans. is d i.e. Etoposide *Ref. Principles and practice of pediatric oncology*

Etoposide is not included in the 'T-10' protocol for osteosarcoma.

T-10' Protocol for Osteosarcoma		
HDMTX + VCR + DOX + BCD ± CDDP (Depending on Response)		
• HDMTX	:	High Dose Methotrexate
• VCR	:	Vincristine
• BCD	:	Bleomycin, Cylophosphamide,
	:	Dactinomycin (Actinomycin D)
• Dox	:	Doxorubicin
• CDDP	:	Cisplatin

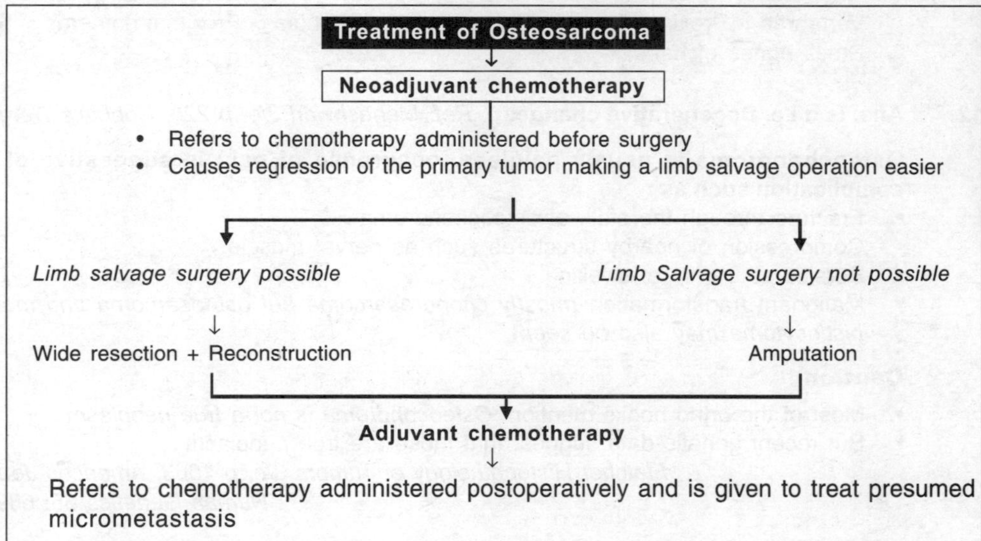

9. Ans. is a i.e. Secondaries *Ref. Robinson's 8/e, p 1235*

Metastatic tumors are the most common form of skeletal malignancy.

Remember :
- MC primary malignant tumor of bone : Osteosarcoma
- MC benign bone tumor: Osteochondroma

Commonest site of primary in metastatic bone tumor	
Adult	**Children**
– Prostate	– Neuroblastoma
– Breast	– Wilm's tumor
– Kidney	– Osteosarcoma

10. Ans. is b, c i.e. Blood filled space; Found in upper end of India *Ref. Ebnezar 4/e, p 629*

Aneurysmal bone cyst

- Benign lesion eccentrically situated in the metaphysal ends of long bones.
- It grows outward and is located subperiosteally.

- ***Age*** : 10-30 years, M>F
- ***Pathology*** : Multiloculated blood filled cyst spaces. Wall is formed by fibroblast, multinucleated osteoclast like giant cells and reactive woven bone.
- ***Clinical fatures*** : Pain and swelling after mild trauma. Joint movement may be decreased.
- ***Radiographs*** : Radiolucency in metaphysis which extended outwards eccentrically, ***with periosteal new bone formation.***
- ***Treatment*** : Surgery with curretage and bone grafting is treatment of choice.

11. Ans. is a, b, c, d, e i.e. All are correct *Ref. Harrison's 17/e, p 613*

Site of Metastatic bone Ca

Vertebrae > Proximal femur > Pelvis > ribs > Sternum > Proximal humerus > Skull > Small bones of hand.

12. Ans. is d i.e. Degenerative changes *Ref. Maheshwari 3/e, p 225; Robbin's 7/e, p 1296*

Osteochondroma is usualy painless, occurence of pain is suggestive of some complication such as :

- Fracture through the stalk of osteochondroma.
- Compression of nearby structures such as nerve, muscle.
- Bursitis as the tip of swelling.
- Malignant transformation *(mostly chondrosarcoma but osteosarcoma and malignant histiocytoma may also be seen).*

Caution !

- Most of the ortho books mention *'Osteocondroma is not a true neoplasm'.*
- But recent genetic data suggest that those are true neoplasm

..... Fletcher Histopathology of Tumors 3/e, p 1063; American Journal of Human Genetics 65; 689 - 698

13. Ans. is b i.e. Ewing sarcoma

Ref. Maheshwari 3/e, p 221; Robbin's Histopathology of Tumors 3/e, p 1600

"Ewing's sarcoma and other primitive neuro ectodermal tumors (PNET) shows neural differentiation."

Ewing's sarcoma

- 2nd most common primary bone tumor in pediatric patient.
- Majority of patients are seen in 2nd decade.
- Femur is the ***MC*** bone affected and diaphysis is the ***MC*** part.
- It may show multicentric origin.
- Clinically mimics osteomyelitis (pain, swelling, fever). Pathologic fracture may be present.
- Microscopically tumor shows homewright pseudo rossettes.

Other options :

Neuroblastoma : – May show neurological differentiation. Bone metastasis is also seen. But it is usually seen < 5 year of age and lesion are bilateral.

– Osteosarcoma and chondroblastoma do not show neurologic differentiation.

14. Ans. is b i.e. Fibrosarcoma *Ref. Fletcher 3/e, p 1625*

On histology osteoclastoma has to be differentiated from conditions which may have giant cells. They are:

- Aneurysmal bone cyst
- Non-ossifying fibroma
- Osteosarcoma with giant cells
- Brown tumor of hyperparathyroidism
- Osteosarcoma with giant cells
- Metastic bone tumors with giant cells

Note : **Fibrosarcoma is a fibroblastic collagen producing sarcoma of bone. Microscopically they are composed of malignant fibroblast arranged in** *"herring tone pattern".*

15. Ans. is b i.e. Tumour permeation between bone trabeculae at periphery
Ref. Fletcher 3/e, p 1605

Differentiation of chondroma from a well differentiated condrosarcoma is extremly difficult.
Following points are suggestive of chondrosarcoma :

Radiograph : Thinning of cortex in long bones. However in small bone this is not enough to make the diagnosis of chondrosarcoma. Extensive destruction of cortex is the only sure sign.
Gross examination : Myxoid quality or cystification of the matrix.
Microscopic : Permeation of surrounding structures is the best single criterion to differentiate chondrosarcoma from an enchondroma.

16. Ans. is c i.e. Chondroblastoma *Ref. Apley 8/e p 177; Campbell 10/e, p 734, 802*

Already explained

17. Ans. is a i.e. Carcinoma breast ***Ref. Harrison 16/e, p 561 - 562***

Already explained

18. Ans. is a i.e. cystic lesion *Ref. Robbin's 7/e, p 782; Compbell 19/e 840*

Ameloblastoma arise from odontogenic eipithelium. It is commonly cystic and has benign course.

Admantinoma (Ameoblastoma) = Eves disease

- Locally malignant epithelial tumor arising from mandible (in areas of molar and ramus) or diaphysis of tibia (i.e. Middle portion).
- Occurs between 10-35 years.
- Mostly cystic, slow growing and locally invasive with benign course in most case.
- Patients present with ***gradually enlarging swelling*** with only minimal pain.
- ***Radiological features :*** Multiple sharply demarcated lesion. The radiolucent lesions are seperated by areas of dense sclerotic bone giving the characterstic ***"HONEY COMB"*** appearance.
- ***Histology :*** Tumours reveals islands of epithelial cells present in fibrous stroma.
- ***Treatment :*** Local excision with substantial margin of bone .

Other option :

- ***Osteosarcoma :*** Tumor presents at upper end of tibia and is rapidly growing.

- ***Osteofibrous dysplasia*** **:** Also present with radiological features similar to admantinoma but usual age of presentation is 10-15 year.

19. Ans. is a, b and c i.e a. New bone formation; Sun Ray appearance; and Codman's triangle *Ref. Maheshwari 3/e, p 218*

• *Codman's Triangle*	– *Osteosarcoma*
• Onion peel appearance	– Ewings sarcoma
• Honey comb appearance	– Admantinoma
• Soop bubble appearance	– Osteo clastoma
• Mottled calcification	– Chondroblastoma

20. Ans. is c i.e. Small bones of lower limb

Ref. Harrison 17/e, p 613; Devita 7/e, p 2370

Most common bone involved in secondary bone tumour (decreasing order).

- **V**ertebrae (lumbar)
- **F**emur (proximal)
- **P**elvis
- **R**ibs
- **S**kull

Mnemonic **: V**ascular **F**actors **P**revent **R**upture of **S**arcoma

21. Ans. is c i.e. Osteoclastoma

See below

Pulsatile primary tumor of bone: Osteoclastoma
Pulsatile bone metastasis: Thyroid ca, renal cell ca
Pulsatile tumor of ear: Glomus tumor

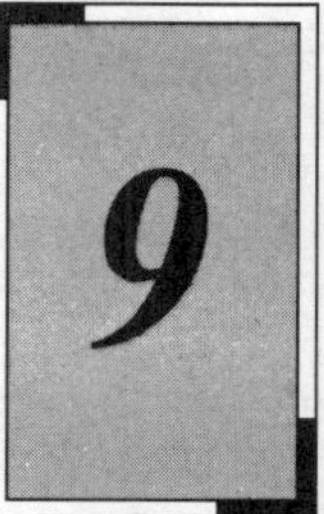

9 Soft Tissue Tumour

What's Important ?

- Spread
- Prognostic Factors

BENIGN SOFT TISSUE TUMOR

Lipoma :

Commonest and most benign of all tumor. Can occur any where so called as ***universal tumor or ubiquitous*** tumor.

Commonest site are subcutaneous tissue of :

i. The trunk
ii. The nape of neck
iii. The limbs

Varieties *: There are three types :*

1. *Encapsulated lipoma* - Commonest type
2. *Diffuse variety = Pseudolipoma* - Not a typical tumor but an over growth of fat in the region specially neck.
3. *Multiple lipomas = Lipomatosis*

Complications :

- Myxomatous degeneration
- Saponification
- Calcification
- Pain in neurolipoma
- Malignancy - Very rare.

Presentation : Painless soft swelling.

Examination :

- Edge of swelling are soft and compressible and often slips from finger called as *slip sign.*
- Transillumination test may be positive and this is the only non cystic condition in which transillumination test is positive.
- Lipoma is freely mobile over deeper structures.

Treatment :

– Lipoma should always be excised.
– Incision is made along the langer line.

SOFT TISSUE SARCOMA

- ***Malignant soft tissue*** tumor are called as soft tissue sarcoma.
- Soft tissue sarcoma affect all age group. 15% are found in children, 40% occur after age of 55.
- Sarcoma are 4th most common tumor of childhood.
- Most common ***site*** of soft tissue sarcoma is lower extremity.
- In ***trun***k ***MC*** site is retroperitoneum.
- Overall most common subtyope is malignant fibrous histiocytoma. ... *Schwartz 9/e, p 1284*

Etiology and Genetics

- ***Environmental factors :*** Sarcoma may arise in previous scar tissue due to prior operation, burn, fracture.
  - Chemical carcinogens in soft tissue sarcoma are polycyclic hydrocarbons, asbestos, and dioxin.
- ***Iatrogenic factor :*** Previous irradiation ↑ risk of soft tissue sarcoma.
- ***Immunologic factors :*** Congenital or acquired immunodeficiency, including therapeutic immunosuppression increase the risk.
- ***Genetic factor :*** Genetic diseases associated with soft tissue sarcoma are :

Hereditary Condition	Associated Sarcoma
• Neurofibromatosis type I (von Reckling hausen's disease)	• Malignant peripheral nerve sheath tumour
• Retinoblastoma	• Soft tissue, Osteogenic
• Li-Fraumeni syndrome	• Soft tissue, Osteogenic
• Gardner's syndrome	• Fibrosarcoma, desmoid tumor
• Werner's syndrome (adult *progeria*)	• Soft tissue
• Gorlin's syndrome (nevoid basal cell carcinoma syndrome)	• Fibrosarcoma, rhabdomyosarcoma
• Carney's triad	• Gastrointestinal stromal tumor
• Tuberous sclerosis (Bourneville disease)	• Rhabdomyoma, rhabdomyosarcoma

Remember : Malignant transformation of a benign soft tissue tumor is extremely rare with the exception of neurofibroma which predisposes for neurofibrosarcoma and malignant schwanoma.

Pathology : Classification

On the basis of tissue they recapitulate	
Tissue	**Soft tissue tumor**
Adipose tissue	Lipoma, Liposarcoma
Fibrous tissue	Nodular fascitis, fibromatoses, fibrosarcoma
Fibrohistiocytic tumor	– Fibrous histiocytoma, xanthoma, dermatofibrosarcoma protuberans
Skeletal muscle	– Rhabdomyoma, Rhabdomyosarcoma
Smooth muscle	– Leiomyoma, Leiomyosarcoma
Vascular tumor	– Hemangioma, Lymphangioma, Hemangio endothelioma, Angiosarcoma
Perivascular tumor	- Malignant glomus tumor - Malignant hemangiopericytoma
Miscellaneous	- Ewing sarcoma - Clear cell sarcoma

Histology : 3 cell types are recognised.

Cell type	Tumor type
• Spindle cell	Fibrous, fibrohistocytic, smooth muscle, schwann cell
• Small round cell	Rhabdomyosarcoma, Primitive neuroectodermal tumor
• Epitheloids	Smooth muscle, epitheloid sarcoma

Grading

- It is one of the ***most important prognostic factor.***
- Pathologic feature that determine grade are cellularity, degree of differentiation, pleomorphism, *necrosis* (reflects rate of growth) and number of mitosis.
- ***Mitotic activity and degree of necrosis*** is are *most important determinant of grading.*
- ***Miscellaneous tumor*** (Epitheloid sarcoma, ewings sarcoma) have no normal tissue counterpart So, they can not be graded.

Spread

- ***Mostly hematogenously*** to lung. In case of ***abdominal sarcoma*** liver is most common site.
- ***Lymphatic spread*** is seen in : *... Devita 8/e, p 1747*

  – Rhabdomyosarcoma
  – Clear cell sarcoma
  – Malignant fibrous histiocytoma
  – Epitheliod sarcoma
  – Angiosarcoma
  – Fibrosarcoma (Rare)
  – Synovial cell sarcoma

  Highest incidence of lymphatic metastasis is in embryonal rhabdomyosarcoma.

Clinical presentation

- Most common ***symptom*** is asymptomatic mass which is usually painless.

Diagnosis

Imaging study :

- MRI is best investigation for suspected sarcoma of ***extremities*** or head and neck. Best for detection of recurrence too.
- Spiral CT is best investigation for sarcoma of ***trunk.***
- PET – For detection of ***metastatic*** disease.
- For patient with high grade lesion or size > 5 cm CT chest, should also be advised.

... Schwartz 9/e, p 1285

Biopsy :

- ***Core needle biopsy or tru-cut biopsy*** for large palpable *superficial* tumor.
- For *large deep* tumor and those adjacent to vital structure incisional biopsy is diagnostic method of choice.
- For ***superficial small*** (<3cm) - Excisional biopsy should be performed.
- ***FNAC*** - Not a useful biopsy technique for initial diagnosis of sarcoma.

... CSDT 13/e, p 1223

Staging

Histologic grade (G)	Tumor size (T)	Node status (N0)	Metastases (M)
Well differentiated (GI) Moderately differentiated (G2) Poorly differentiated (G3)	≤ 5 cm (T1) ≥ 5 cm (T2) Superficial facial involvement (Tb)	Not involved (N0) Involved (N1)	Absent (M0) Present (M1)

Prognostic factors

- In *early stage* tumor grade is most significant; ***in advanced stage*** grade and size becomes equally significant. *... Devita 8/e, p 1781*
- ***Truncal*** location is associated with bad prognosis.
- ***Liposarcoma*** has better prognosis in comparison to other types.

Treatment :

a. ***Sarcoma of extremity :***

Stage I	Low grade tumors	Surgical resection
Stage II	≤ 5 cm high grade tumor	Surgical resection ± radiation
Stage III	> 5 cm, high grade or nodal disease	Surgical resection + radiation ± Chemotherapy
Stage IV	Distant metastatic disease	Chemotherapy ± surgical resection

High risk sarcoma (large size > 8cm, deep seated, High grade) are treated by combined chemoradiotherapy.

Most active chemotherapeutic agent are Doxorubicin and Ifosfamide.

b. ***Non extremity sarcoma :***

- Retroperitoneal sarcoma - Most common retroperitoneal sarcoma is ***liposarcoma.***
  - Primary ***surgical resection is best*** modality of treatment.
- Head and Neck sarcoma - Angiosarcoma is most common type.
  - Treated by ***surgical excision with adjuvant radiotherapy.***

QUESTIONS

1. **With regard to the malignant behavior of leio-moyosarcoma, the most important criterion is :**
   a. Blood vessel penetration by tumour cells **[AI 06]**
   b. Tumour cells is lymphatic channels
   c. Lymphocyte infiltration
   d. The number of mitoses per high power field
2. **Which one of the following soft tissue sarcomas frequently metastasizes to lymph nodes ? [AI 05]**
   a. Fibrosarcoma
   b. Osteosarcoma
   c. Embryonal rhabdomyosarcoma
   d. Alveolar soft part sarcoma
3. **The tissue of origin of kaposi sarcoma is: [AIIMS 05]**
   a. Lymphoid b. Neural
   c. Vascular d. Muscular
4. **All of the following soft tissue sarcoma have propensity for lymphatic spread except : [AIIMS 05]**
   a. Neurofibrosarcoma
   b. Synovial sarcoma
   c. Rhabdomyosarcoma
   d. Epitheliod sarcoma
5. **Synovial sarcoma all are true except:**
   a. Originates in synovium **[AI 10]**
   b. Seen in young age group
   c. Occurs at extra-articular sites more often
   d. Seen in sites such as knee and foot

ANSWERS, REFERENCES, EXPLANATIONS WITH INFORMATIVE ILLUSTRATIONS

1. **Ans. is d i.e. The number of mitoses per high power field**

Ref. Devita 7/e, p 1593, 8/e p 1752

"Grading of leiomyosarcoma can be quite difficult; mitotic activity appears to be the best indicator of malignancy along with tumour location and size."

Important points about Leiomyosarcoma

- Malignant tumour composed of cells showing distinct smooth muscle feature.
- Most common site of GI leomyosarcoma is rectum.
- Can arise in any location but more than half are located in retroperitoneal or intraabdominal sites.
- ***Lower extremity*** leimyosarcoma usually arise in the thigh.
- Leomyosarcoma may arise in large vessels, the most common arterial site is ***pulmonary artery.***
- Typical cells of leomyosarcoma is elongated.
- Localization of muscle antigens (Desmin and Actin) by means of immunohistochemistry is diagnostic method.
- Prognosis is poor.

Remember : ***Pathologic features that determine the grade of sarcoma are :***

– Cellularity	– Differentiation
– Pleomorphism	– Number of mitosis
– Histological type	– Necrosis

2. **Ans. is c i.e. Embryonal rhabdomyosarcoma**

Ref. Harrison 16/e, p 559; Devita 8/e, p 1747

"Lymphnode metastasis is rare except in synovial and epitheliod sarcoma, clear cell sarcoma, angiosarcoma and rhabdomyosarcoma." *... Harrison 16/e, p 559*

Spread of soft tissue sarcoma :

- *Mostly hematogenous* : MC site lung parenchyma
  Retroperitoneal sarcoma and GIST metastasize hematogenously most commonly to liver.
- **Lymphatic metastosis is seen in :**
  Rhabdomyosarcoma
  (maximum in embryonal rhabdomyosarcoma) *... Devita 7/e, p 1593*
  Angiosarcoma
  Clear cell sarcoma
  Epithelial sarcoma
  Fibrosarcoma (rarely)
  Malignant fibrous histiocytoma
  Synovial cell sarcoma
  Mnemonic = **RACE F**or **MS**

Remember :
- Soft tissue sarcoma tends to grow along plane (i.e. tissue plane) and compress the surrounding tissue to form pseudocapsule.
- ***Highest incidence of lymphatic*** metastasis is in embryonal rhabdomyosarcoma.
- Presence of nodal metastasis is designated as stage IV disease.

3. **Ans. is c i.e. Vascular** *Ref. Harrison 17/e, p 1186*

"Kaposi sarcoma is a multicentric neoplasm of vascular origin consisting of multiple vascular nodules appearing in skin, mucous membrane and viscera."

Features of Kaposi sarcoma

- Develop in patient with HIV infection and in organ transplant patient.
- Can develop at any stage of HIV infection, even in presence of normal CD-4 count.
- Occur due to excess proliferation of spindle cells that are believed to vascular origin. *... Harrison 16/e, p 1098*
- Human herpes virus -8 is supposed to be etiologic agent of Kaposi sarcoma.
- ***Clinically*** kaposi sarcoma often appear in sun exposed areas, particularly tip of nose. The initial lesion is a small raised reddish purple nodule on skin.
- ***LN*** involvement does not signify poor prognosis.

Diagnosis

- Diagnosis of KS is based upon biopsy of a suspicious lesion
- Histologically there is a proliferation of spindle cells and endothelial cells, extravasation of red cells, hemosiderin-laden macrophages.

Treatment

- Observation and optimization of retroviral therapy.
- **Single or limited number of lesion :**
  - Radiation
  - Intralesional vinblastine
  - Cryotherapy.
- **Extensive disease :**
  - ***Initial therapy :***
    - a. Interferon α (if CD4+ T cells > 150/µl)
    - b. Liposomal daunorubicin
  - ***Subsequent therapy :***
    - a. Liposomal doxorubicin
    - b. Paclitaxel
  - ***Radiation treatment***

4. **Ans. is a i.e. Neurofibrosarcoma** *Ref. Harrison 16/e, p 559*

Already explained

5. **Ans. is a i.e. Originates in synovium** *Ref. Devita 8/e, p 1754*

The term synovial sarcoma is a misnomer as the tumor does not originate from synovial tissue.

Synovial Sarcoma	
Age :	Young adults
Site :	Para-articular areas of tendon sheaths and joints. 50% are seen in lower limb (especially knee) remainder are seen in upper limb, head and neck, abdominal wall.
Pathology :	Tumor is composed of two types of cells: Epithelial cells with a surrounding spindle or fibrous components
Chromosomal abnormality:	They contain a characteristic translation t (X : 18). This translocation has become the gold standard for diagnosing synovial sarcoma
Clinical presentation:	As mass in affected area
Treatment:	Adequate excision and adjuant radiotherapy with or without adjuvant chemotherapy.

NOTES

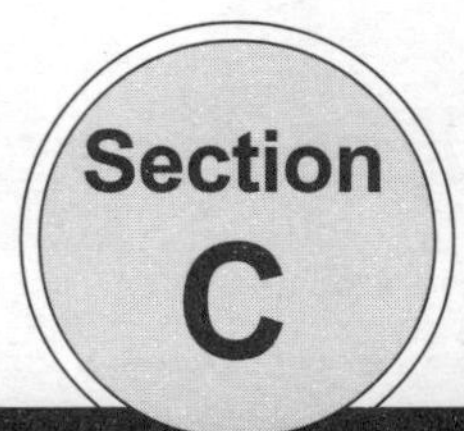

General Oncology

Unit IX	Brain Tumour
Unit X	Head and Neck Tumour
Unit XI	Lung and Pleural Tumour
Unit XII	Heart and Mediastinal Tumour
Unit XIII	GIT Tumour
Unit XIV	Hepatobiliary Tumour
Unit XV	Genitourinary Tumour
Unit XVI	Hematological Tumour
Unit XVII	Endocrinal Tumour

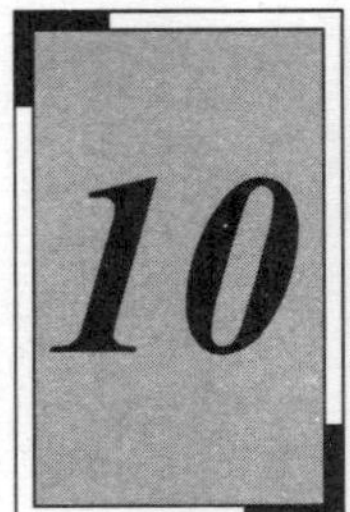

Brain Tumour

What's Important ?

- Spread
- Tumour showing calcification
- Medulloblastoma
- Craniopharyngioma

- Brain tumor can be primary or metastatic from systemic cancer. Metastatic tumor are far more common than primary CNS tumor.

WHO Classification of CNS tumor

1. **Neuroepithelial tumor:**
   - Astrocytoma
   - Oligodendroglioma
   - Ependymoma
   - Oligoastrocytoma
2. **Choroid plexus tumor**
3. **Neuronal tumor**
   - Ganglioglioma
   - Neurocytoma
4. **Pineal parenchymal tumor:**
   - Pineocytoma
   - Pineoblastoma
5. **Embryonal tumor:**
   - Medulloblastoma
   - Ependymoblastoma
6. **Tumor of cranial or spinal nerve:**
   - Schwannoma
   - Neurofibroma
7. **Tumor of Meninges:**
   - Meningioma
8. **Mesenchymal tumor:**
   - Hemangiopericytoma
   - Chondrosarcoma
   - Rhabdomyosarcoma
   - Malignant fibrous histiocytoma

9. **Uncertain histogenesis:**
   - Hemangioblastoma
10. **Hematopoietic neoplasm:**
    - Malignant lymphoma
    - Plasmacytoma
11. **Germ cell tumor:**
    - Seminoma
    - Yolk sac tumor
    - Choriocarcinoma
    - Teratoma
12. **Sellar tumors:**
    - Pituitary adenoma
    - Craniopharyngioma
13. **Cyst / Tumor like lesion:**
    - Rathke cleft cyst
    - Epidermoid cyst
    - Dermoid cyst

RADIOLOGICAL CLASSIFICATION (More important for diagnosis)

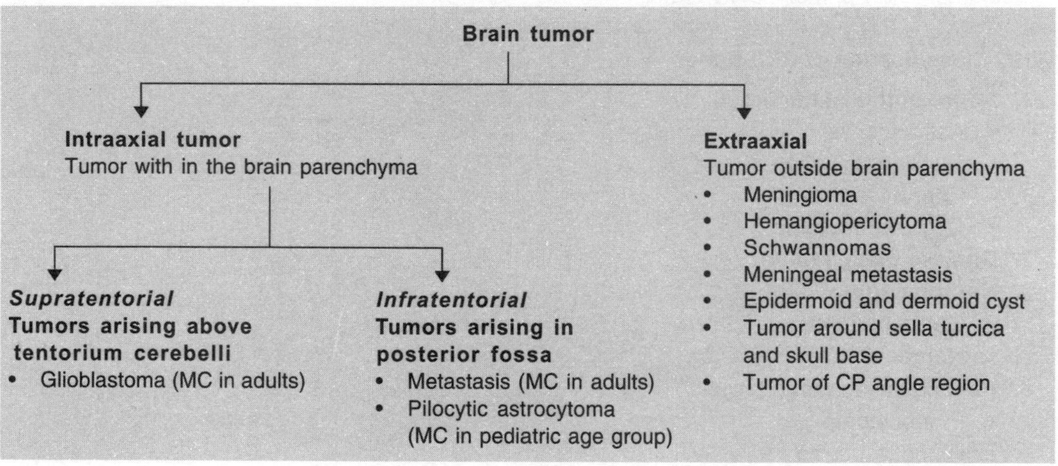

PEDIATRIC BRAIN TUMORS

Infratentroial tumor (MC) (posterior fossa)	Supratentorial tumors	Midline
– Medulloblastoma – Cerebellar astrocytoma – Brain stem glioma – Ependymoma	– Low grade astrocytoma – High grade astrocytoma	– Craniopharyngioma – Chiasmal glioma – Pineal region tumor

- Astrocytoma is most common brain tumor of childhood.

Before going to individual details let us consider clinical features and diagnosis of brain tumor in general.

Etiology

- Exposure to ionizing radiation increase risk of gliomas.
- Recently few studies have concluded that over use of cellular phones increase risk, but some studies found no correlation.
- Hereditary syndromes associated with brain tumors are :

  Mnemonic : **L**ala Lajpat **R**ai **N**ever **W**ants **T**o **G**o **T**amil**N**adu

Syndrome	Gene (Locus)	Nervous system neoplasm
Von Hippel-Lindau	VHL (3p)	Hemangioblastoma of retina, cerebellum and spinal cord; pheochromocytoma
Li-Fraumeni	p53(17p)	Malignant glioma
Retinoblastoma	RBI (13q)	Retinoblastoma, pineoblastoma, malignant glioma
Neurofibromatosis type 1(von Recklinghausen's disease)	NF1 (17q)	Neuroma, schwannoma, meningioma, optic glioma
Werner syndrome (Multiple endocrine neoplasia 1)	MEN1 (11q)	Pituitary adenoma, malignant schwannoma
Turcot syndrome	APC (5q)	Medulloblastoma, malignant glioma
Gorlin (basal cell nevus)	PTCH (9q)	Medulloblastoma
Tuberous sclerosis	TSC1 (9q) TSC2 (16p)	Astrocytoma
Neurofibromatosis type 2	NF2 (22q)	Schwannoma, glioma, ependymoma

Clinical presentation

Pediatric age :

- ***Child under 1 year***
  - Commonly have supratentorial tumor. *MC* are choroid plexus tumor and teratoma.
  - Present with vomiting, unsteadyness, lethargy and irritability.
    ... Nelson 17/e, p 1702
  - Signs include macrocephaly, ataxia, hyper-reflexia
  - Papilledema is usually absent as head of young child can expand.
- ***1–10 years***
  - Commonly have infratentorial tumor. MC being medulloblastoma.
  - Present with morning headache, visual symptoms, seizures and focal neurologic deficits.
  - Older children with infratemporal tumor present with symptoms and signs of hydrocephalus.
  - Morning vomiting may be the only symptom of posterior fossa ependymomas.
  - Children with brain stem tumor present with facial and extraocular muscle palsies.
- ***> 10 years***
  - Again commonly have supratentorial tumor with astrocytoma being most common.

Adult : • *Primary tumor present with one of the three syndrome in addition to location specific symptoms:*

1. *Subacute progression of focal neurologic deficit :* Results from compression of neuron or white matter. Sudden onset focal neurologic deficit may be the presenting feature due to hemorrhage.

Tumor frequently associated with hemorrhage are : High grade glioma, Metastatic melanoma and Choriocarcinoma.

2. *Seizures :* Tumor that invade or compress the cerebral cortex (eg. Meningioma).
3. *Non focal neurologic deficit :* Such as headache, dementia, personality change or gait disorder. Reflects increase ICT and diffuse tumor spread, e.g. Frontal lobe tumor present with dementia, personality change.

Remember :
- Presence of Malaise, weightloss and fever suggest metastatic tumor.
- Headache of brain tumor worsens with recumbency.
- Elevated ICP may cause papilledema although it is not present in infant or patient > 55 years.
- Karnofsky performance scale is usefull in assessing and following patient with brain tumor.

- **Location specific symptoms**

Frontal tumor	: Personality change, loss of initiative, abulia, contralateral weakness (posterior frontal tumor)
Temporal tumor	: Seizures, memory impairment, dysnomia, fluent (Wernicke) aphasia
Parietal tumor	: Sensory and perceptual function disturbances
Occipital tumor	: Contralateral homonymous hemianopsia or other complex visual disturbances B/L tumor can produce cortical blindness
Brain stem tumor	: Most common brain stem tumor is Pontine glioma which usually presents with cranial nerve VI and VII palsies ... *Devita 8/e, p 1979*
Tumors in medulla	: Defects in cranial nerves IX, X and XII, dysphagia and dysarthria

Diagnosis

Imaging

- MRI with contrast (gadolinium) is best, most sensitive and imaging modality of choice for both pediatric and adult brain tumor.
- MRI spine should also be done for tumor at high risk of spread through CSF. MRI spine has replaced myelography as imaging modality of choice for this purpose.
- ***CT :*** Is the imaging of choice when there is suspicion of acute hemorrhage in tumor or in patient where MRI is contraindicated.
- ***PET and SPECT :*** Useful to distinguish tumor recurrence from radiation necrosis.

Lumbar puncture

- Usually contraindicated in intracranial mass lesion due to increased ICP.
- Primary use is to exclude other diagnosis like infection
- *Malignant cells are not seen in CSF except in leptomeningeal metastases,* **primary CNS lymphoma, medulloblastoma, ependymomas** *as these tumour spread through CSF*
- Lumbar CSF is preferred over ventricular CSF for cytologic examination

... *CPDT 19/e, p 861*

Treatment

Surgery :

- Major objective is to resect and potentially *cure* the disease.
- When complete cure is not possible objective is *maximal bulk* reduction with minimal risk to patient.
- Patient with supratemporal tumor should always be given anticonvulsants before surgery. *Phenytoin, carbamazepine, valproic acid* equally effective.
- For all tumors except lymphoma, corticosteriod usually dexamethasone is given in postoperative period.

Radiation therapy :

- *Tolerance of brain* is a ***major limiting factor.***
- *Late radiation injury are the most serious complication* of therapeutic brain irradiation occur due to vascular endothelial injury or due to direct injury to oligodendrocytes.
- Corticosteroids improve or stabilize neurologic symptoms associated with effects of radiation.
- As definitive treatment for PNET and germ cell tumor.
- Postoperative radiation delay recurrence and prolong survival in gliomas.
- To halt tumor growth in schwannomas, meningiomas, pituitary tumor and craniopharyngiomas.
- As a palliative therapy in brain metastasis.

Chemotherapy :

- Role of chemotherapy in brain tumor is very limited except in primary CNS lymphoma for which chemotherapy is preferred treatment.
- Reason for this limited use is the fact that most cytotoxic drugs are not able to cross blood brain barrier.
- New techniques to deliver chemotherapy directly in the tumor are:
  1. ***BCNU*** **:** After surgical resection a implantable polyme Glidel water (which contain carmustine) is implanted in the surgical cavity, from there drug diffuses to surrounding brain.
  2. ***CED (Convection enhanced delivery)*** : Catheter is implanted directly to brain through which drugs is delivered.
  3. *Intravascular mannitol* : Result in cerebral endothelial shrinkage and disruption of blood brain barrier. Most widely used method ...*Devita 8/e p 1987*

Symptomatic treatment :

- *Glucocorticoids* : Decrease volume of edema
- *Anticonvulsant* : For cortical tumors
- *Prophylactic low dose heparin* : For gliomas and primary CNS lymphoma as they are associated with deep vein thrombosis.

IMPORTANT INDIVIDUAL TUMORS

Astrocytoma

- Most common primary brain tumor of both child and adult.
- On the basis of histological variation and severity they are divided into :

Grade I	Juvenile pliocytic astrocytoma, subependymal Giant cell astrocytoma, pleomorphic xanthoastrocytoma
Grade II	Diffuse astrocytoma = Fibrillary astrocytoma
Grade III	Anaplastic astrocytoma
Grade IV	Glioblastoma

- ***Pliocytic astrocytoma*** is MC childhood brain tumor.
- Pliocytic astrocytoma is usually located at ***cerebellum.***
- ***Glioblastoma = Glioblastoma multiforme*** show characteristic feature of necrosis *(leading to pseudopallisading)* and vascular or endothelial cell proliferation giving rise to glomeruloid body.
- ***Gliomatous cereberi*** is a condition in which multiple regions of brain are infiltrated by neoplastic astrocytes.
- ***Low grade astroctoma*** are best managed by surgery.
- Majority of adult are of astrocytoma of high grade.
- High grade astrocytoma specially those located in posterior fossa can ***metastasize along CSF pathway to spine.***
- As astrocytoma infiltrate adjacent normal brain, total surgical excision is not possible and treatment includes glucocorticoid, surgery followed by radiation therapy or chemotherapy (lamustine, carmustine are most effective chemotherapeutic agents).

... Harrison 17/e, p 2604

- Gliomatous cereberi is treated with whole brain radiation therapy or temozolamide.
- Over all prognosis is very poor in adult age group.

Oligodendroglioma

- Comprise ***15%*** of gliomas of adult and are MC in 4th and 5th decades (supratentorial).
- Found mostly in ***cerebral hemisphere*** with predilection for *white matter.*
- Characteristic feature is presence of ***anastomosing capillaries*** and calcification.
- Surgery in the form of stereotaxic biopsy is necessary to establish diagnosis.
- These tumor are less infiltrative than astrocytoma, permitting more complete surgical excision.
- These tumors have ***better prognosis*** than astrocytoma.
- Treatment is ***surgical resection*** where ever possible.
- They respond to ***systemic chemotherapy*** of PCV (procabazine, lomustine, vincristine).

Ependymoma

- In *adult* they are ***mostly located in spinal canal*** specially in lumbosacral region.
- In *pediatric age* group they are typically occur near the 4th ventricle.
- Ependymoma are particularly frequent in setting of neurofibromatosis type -2.
- Due to relationship of ependymoma to ventricular system, ***CSF dissemination*** is particularly prominent.
- Clinically pediatric ependymoma present with ***hydrocephalus.***
- *Prognosis of pediatric ependymoma is poor* as surgical resection is not possible.
- Clinical outcome of spinal ependymoma is better as surgical resection is usually possible.
- In adults the most frequent histological type myopapillary ependymoma.

Remember : Brain tumor metastases that spread to spinal cord by way of CSF is called drop metastases.

... Harrison 16/e, p 244

Gangliocytoma and Ganglioglioma

- These tumor contain mature appearing ganglion cells either entirely (gangliocytoma) or mixed with glial neoplasm (gangiogliomas).
- Most of these tumor are ***slow growing.***
- Gangliocytoma are well circumscribed mass with focal area of calcification usually found in floor of 3rd ventricle, hypothalamus or the temporal lobe.
- Ganglioglioma is mostly found in ***temporal lobe*** and often have a cystic component.
- Both of these mostly present with ***seizure*** disorder.
- ***Surgical resection*** is treatment of choice.

Medulloblastoma

- ***Highly malignant*** tumor found exclusively in ***cerebellum (in midline posterior and posterior vermis)***
- Occur predominantly in children and are ***most frequent malignant brain tumor of children***
- Peak incidence ***3 and 4 years*** of age. For adult peak age is between 20–35 years of age.

... Harrison 16/e, p 2455

- *PNET (primitive neuroectodermal tumors)* is a term applied for medulloblastoma like tumor but occuring either in adult or supratentorially in children. All of these are composed of small round blue cells.
- *Dissemination through CSF* is common leading to drop metastases.
- *Metastases* outside CNS affect bone, lymphnode, liver.
- Child usually present with features of increase ICP.
- *Adult with PNET* present with ataxia and unilateral dysmetria as lateral origin is more common.
- CT shows a well circumscribed mass that may be calcified. MRI reveals T1 dark lesion that may or may not enhance.
- ***Tumor dissemination is most important prognostic factor.***
- ***Surgery*** is treatment of choice if possible
- *Medulloblastoma is most radiosensitive brain tumor.* *... Devita 7/e, p 1867*
- ***Radiotherapy*** is given postoperatively and for tumors in which surgical resection is not possible.

Meningioma

- Predominantly benign tumors of adult derived from ***epitheloid cells*** on outer surface of arachanoid villi also known as arachnoid cap cells.
- Mostly occur ***along the sagittal sinus,*** over the cerebral convexities, in the cerebellar pontine angle and along the dorsum of spinal cord.
- Round encapsulated mass showing characteristic ***enplaque pattern of growth.***

... Robbin's 8/e, p 1338

- Tumor range from firm to fibrous to finely gritty and may show extreme ***calcification and psammoma bodies.***
- Xanthomatous degeneration, metaplasia (often osseous) and moderate nuclear polymorphism are common but have no prognostic significance.

- They may be found incidentally on CT or MRI scan or present with a focal seizure or symptom of raised ICP. On radiography meningioma show a typical radiographic tail.

Treatment :
- *Small asymptomatic* meningioma incidentally discovered in older patient can safely be followed radiographically.
- Large tumor can be resected
- If resection is not possible local external beam ***radiotherapy*** is appropriate.

Craniopharyngioma

- Arise from remnant of ***Rathke's pouch***. Arise near the pituitary stalk and commonly extend to the suprasellar cistern.
- Tumor is large cystic and ***locally invasive*** with characteristic appearance on skull X-ray and CT due to partial calcification.
- Most patient present ***before age of 20*** with signs of raised ICP, visual field abnormality; personality changes and cognitive deterioration.
- Treatment involves transcranial or transphenoidal ***surgical resection*** followed by post operative radiation of residual tumor.

Primary CNS lymphoma

- Accounts for 2% of extranodal lymphoma (***MC site of extranodal lymphoma is stomach***) and 1% of intracranial tumor.
- Most common CNS neoplasm in immunocompromised including those with ***AIDS.***
- Mostly associated with ***EBV*** infection.
- Majority of primary CNS lymphoma are B-cell origin ***most commonly large B-cell lymphoma type.***
- Spread to CSF is common.
- On imaging it appears as multicentric mass with ring enhancement in immunocompromised patient. In immunocompetent neuroimaging reveals uniformly enhancing mass lesion.
- Diagnosed by stereotaxic needle ***biopsy.***
- Prognosis is poor.

Treatment :
- Most Responding tumor to steroid however disease relapse as soon as steroid are stopped, so steroid use is *not permitted.*
- ***Definitive therapy :*** Chemotherapy incorporating high dose methotrexate followed by whole body irradiation.

TUMOR METASTATIC TO BRAIN

Site of primary	Brain metastases	Leptomeningeal metastases
Lung	40%	2%
Breast (specially ductal)	19%	41%
Melanoma	10%	12%
GIT	7%	13%
Genitourinary	7%	—

- Mechanism of Brain Metastases : ***Mostly hematogenous***

- Evaluation : On *MRI scan* brain metastases typically appear as *well demarcated spherical lesion* that are hypointense or isointense relative to brain on T1 image and bright on T2 image.

Treatment :
- Most Responding tumor to steroid however disease relapse as soon as steroid are stopped, so steroid use is *not permitted.*
- ***Definitive therapy :*** Chemotherapy incorporating high dose methotrexate followed by whole body irradiation.

NEUROCUTANEOUS SYNDROMES = PHAKOMATOSIS

These are syndromes which produces a developmental abnormalities of skin along with ↑risk of nervous system tumor. ***These includes :***

- Neurofibromatosis (described in multiple tumor syndrome)
- VHL syndrome (described in multiple tumor syndrome)
- Sturge Weber syndrome
- Tuberous sclerosis (Bourneville disease)
- Ataxia telangiectasia.

	Tubrous sclerosis (Encephalotrigeminal angiomatosis)	Sturge Weber Syndrome (ataxic dyskinetic syndrome)	Ataxia telangectasia
Components	• Adenoma sebacium (facial angiofibroma) • Ash leaf shaped macules • Shagreen patches • Depigmented nevis • Subependymal nodule • Subependymal giant cell • Ependymoma • Epilepsy • Mental retardation glaucoma	• Venous angiomatous masses in the lepto-meninges over the cortex • Ipsilateral cavernous heman-gioma, port-wine stain in the distribution of trigeminal nerve • Mental retardation, • Seizures • Hemiplegia • Radioopacities in skull • Pheochromocytoma • Secondary open angle due to ocular vascular malformation • Neurologic malignancy in minority of patient	• Gradual loss of purkinje cells in the cerebellum • Cerebellar ataxia • Defective lymphocyte maturation & proliferation • Lymphoma leukemia, Gliomas, carcinomas • IgA ± IgE deficiency • Sinopulmonary infection • Telangiectasias in skin & conjunctiva
Transmission Defect	• Autosomal dominant • Mutation of 9q and 16p • Defective tuberins protein	• Autosomal dominant	• Autosomal recessive • Mutated ATM gene (defect in DNA repair) on 11q 22-23

LEPTOMENINGEAL METASTASIS = CARCINOMATOUS MENINGITIS

- Seen in about 8% of patient with metastatic solid tumor
- Adenocarcinoma of breast, lung, GIT and melanoma are most common cause
- Metastasis to meninges is usually hematogenous
- **Clinical features:** Encephalopathy, cranial neuropathy, radiculopathy hydrocephalous

- **Diagnosis**
  - MRI is the imaging modality of choice which shows nodular tumor deposits or diffuse enhancement in meninges
  - Malignant cells in CSP is confirmatory
- **Treatment**
  - *Intrathecal chemotherapy. Effective agents include methotrexate, cytarabine thiotepa*
  - External beam radiotherapy in cases with large tumor deposit blocking CSF flow

Note: Glioblastoma multiforme has highest propensity to show extracranial metastasis and is the most common brain tumour which show extracranial metastasis in adults. In children, it is medulloblastoma

QUESTIONS

1. **A patient prevented with weakness in lower limb, bladder and bowel involvement. On MRI intradural middorsal enhancing lesion was found, likely diagnosis : [AI 07]**
   a. Meningioma
   b. Intradural lipoma
   c. Dermoid
   d. Neuroepithelioma

2. **Which of the following is the most common type of glial tumors : [AI 06]**
   a. Astrocytomas
   b. Medulloblastomas
   c. Neurofibromas
   d. Ependymomas

3. **Which of the following tumor is not known to increase in pregnancy : [AI 06]**
   a. Glioma
   b. Pituitary adenoma
   c. Meningioma
   d. Neurofibroma

4. **Which one of the following tumors shows calcification on CT scan : [AI 05]**
   a. Ependymoma
   b. Medulloblastoma
   c. Meningioma
   d. CNS lymphoma

5. **Which of the following brain tumors does not spread via CSF : [AI 04]**
   a. Germ cell tumors
   b. Medulloblastoma
   c. CNS lymphoma
   d. Craniopharyngioma

6. **Imaging modality of choice for detecting radiation induced cerebral necrosis: [AIIMS Nov 09]**
   a. PET scan b. Biopsy
   c. MRI d. CT

7. **All are true regarding pilocytic astrocytoma, except : [AIIMS May 09]**
   a. Seen in elderly above 80 years
   b. Seen in posterior fossa
   c. Good prognosis
   d. Most common primary brain tumor in children.

8. **Most common site of subependymal astrocytoma (giant cell) : [AIIMS Nov 07]**
   a. Trigon of lateral ventricle
   b. Foramen of Monro
   c. Temporal horn of lateral ventricle
   d. 4th ventricle

9. **Neurofibromatosis 1 is most commonly associated with : [AIIMS Nov 07]**
   a. Brain stem gliomas
   b. Optic pathway glioma
   c. Sub-ependymal pilocytic astrocytoma
   d. Glioblastoma multiforme

10. **Which of the following statements about cerebellar astrocytomas in paediatric age group is False : [AI 08]**
    a. These are usually Low grade tumors
    b. These tumors have a good prognosis
    c. These are more commonly seen in the 1st and 2nd decades
    d. These tumours are more common in females

11. **A 40-years old female patient presented with recurrent headaches. MRI showd an extra-axial, dural based and enhancing lesion. The most likely diagnosis is : [AIIMS 06]**
    a. Meningioma
    b. Glioma
    c. Schwannoma
    d. Pituitary adenoma

12. Which of the following brain tumours is highly vascular in nature ? [AIIMS 06]
a. Glioblastoma
b. Meningiomas
c. CP angle epidermoid
d. Pituitory adenomas

13. Which of the following techniques is the best for differentiating recurrence of brain tumor form radiation therapy induced necrosis : [AIIMS 05]
a. MRI
b. Contrast enhanced MRI
c. PET scan
d. CT scan

14. All of the following hereditary conditions predispose to CNS tumors, except : [AIIMS 05]
a. Neurofibromatosis 1 and 2
b. Tuberous sclerosis
c. Von-Hippel-Lindau syndrome
d. Xeroderma pigmentosum

15. Which of the following is the most common cause of a mixed cystic and solid suprasellar mass seen on cranial MR scan of a 10 years old child :
a. Pituitary adenoma **[AIIMS 05]**
b. Craniopharyngioma
c. Optic chiasmal glioma
d. Germinoma

16. A metastatic carcinoma in the brain of an adult, most often comes from primary in the : [AIIMS 05]
a. Stomach
b. Ovary
c. Oral cavity
d. Lung

17. Adenoma sebacium is a feature of :
a. Neurofibromatosis **[AIIMS 05]**
b. Tuberous sclerosis
c. Xanthomatosis
d. Incontinentia pigmenti

18. Which of the following carcinoma most frequently metastasizes to brain :
a. Small cell carcinoma lung **[AIIMS 05]**
b. Prostate cancer
c. Rectal carcinoma
d. Endomerial cancer

19. A 6 year old boy has been complaining of headache, ignoring to see the objects on the sides for four months. On examination, he is not mentally retarded, his grades at a school are good, and visual acuity is diminished in both the eyes. Visual charting showed significant field defect. CT scan of the head showed suprasellar mass with calcification. Which of the following is the most probable diagnosis : [AIIMS 05]
a. Astrocytoma
b. Craniopharyngioma
c. Pituitary adenoma
d. Meningioma

20. Most common location of spinal tumor:
a. Intramedullary **[AIIMS Nov 07]**
b. Intradural extramedullary
c. Extradural
d. Equally distributed

21. Prophylactic craniospinal irradiation is recommended in : [PGI 07]
a. Gemistocytic astrocytoma
b. Posterior fossa ependymoma
c. Meningioma
d. Medulloblastoma

22. True about primary CNS lymphoma:
a. Reticulin staining done **[PGI 09]**
b. Essentially B-cell type
c. a/w EBV
d. Indolent disease with good prognosis
e. Chemotherapy highly effective

23. Radiological features of Meningioma: [PGI 09]
a. Calcification
b. Erosion
c. Sutural diastasis
d. Osteosclerosis
e. Vascular erosion

24. A 48 yr old woman comes with bilateral progressive weakness of both lower limbs, spasticity and mild impairment of respiratory movements. MRI shows an intradural mid-dorsal midline enhancing lesion. What is the diagnosis? [AIIMS May 10]
a. Intradural lipoma
b. Meningioma
c. Neuroenteric cyst
d. Dermoid cyst

25. Chang staging is used for: [AIIMS May 10]
a. Retinoblastoma
b. Medulloblastoma
c. Ewing's sarcoma
d. Rhabdomyosarcoma

ANSWERS, REFERENCES, EXPLANATIONS WITH INFORMATIVE ILLUSTRATIONS

1. **Ans. is a i.e. Meningioma**
Ref. Sutton 7/e, p 1634, 1638, 1640; Grainger 5/e, p 1385

Intradural enhancing lesion in middorsal region is clearly suggestive of spinal cord meningioma.

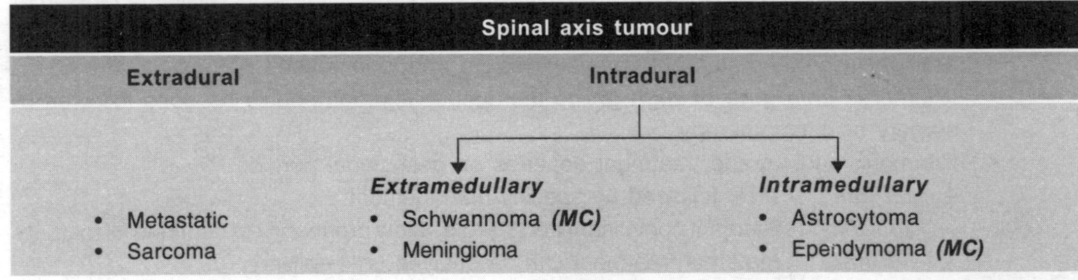

- Most of the spinal axis tumor are extradural metastatic lesions.
- Most of primary spinal axis tumour are intradural among which schwannomas and meningiomas are most common.
- Most primary spinal axis tumors produce symptoms and signs as a result of spinal cord and nerve root compression.
- Most primary spinal cord tumours involve the thoracic spinal canal followed by lumbosacral area.

Features	Meningioma	Schwannoma/Neurinoma
• Level	Thoracic	Any level
• Age	Middle age	Any age
• Sex	F > M	M = F
• Expansion of spinal cord or intervertebral foramen	Rare	Common
• MRI	Hyperintense on T_2 W	Isointense to spinal cord on T_1 and T_2 W

2. Ans. is a i.e. Astrocytomas *Ref. Harrison 17/e, p 2603*

- Astrocytoma (type of glial tumor) is ***MC*** brain tumor in both childs and adults.
- Majority of astrocytomas are of ***low grade in child hood and high grade in adult hood.***

Remember : ***Glioma :*** Tumors derived from glial cells, include :
- **Astrocytoma** (*MC*)
- **Oligodendroglioma**
- **Ependymomas (least common)**

In adults, diffuse astrocytoma is most common.

In children, pliocytic astrocytoma is most common.

3. Ans. is a. i.e. Glioma *Ref. CGDT 9/e, p 429*

"Although brain tumors are not specifically related to gestation; meningiomas, angiomas and neurofibromas are thought to grow more rapidly with pregnancy."

... CGDT 9/e, p 429

Pituitary adenoma may increase during pregnancy and become symptomatic

... Williams Obstetrics

Management of brain tumor during pregnancy
- Anticonvulsant and steroid to prevent seizure and to increased ICP.
- If tumor is ***enlarging or high grade*** therapeutic abortion should be done followed by surgery or chemotherapy.
- If tumour is low grade treatment depends on gestational period.
  - *1st trim* : MTP followed by specific management.
  - *2nd trim* : Start anticonvulsant and steroid, allow pregnancy to continue till maturity.
  - *3rd trim* : Maternal treatment can be delayed until delivery.

Remember : As in normal adult MC brain tumor in pregnancy is glioma.

4. Ans. is c i.e. Meningioma *Ref. Robbin's 7/e, p 1409; Sutton Radiology 8/e, p 1338*

"Meningioma range from firm and fibrous to finely gritty or they may be extremely calcified with psammoma bodies."

... Robbin's 8/e, p 1338

Although calcification is also seen in some cases of ependymomas but is more common in meningioma, hence answer.

Brain tumors showing calcification are :

- ***Gliomas :***
  - Astrocytoma (pliocytic astrocytoma, subependymal giant cell astrocytoma, pleomorphic xanthoastrocytoma).
  - Oligodendroglioma : Calcification seen 50% cases (serpiginous calcification).
- *Ependymoma* : Unusual.
- *Choroid plexus tumor (punctate calcification)* : Papilloma of choroid plexus.
- *Neuronal and mixed neuronal* - ***Glial tumors :***
  - *Gangliomas*
  - L'hermitte-Duclos disease
  - Dysembryoplastic Neuroepithelial Tumor
  - Central neurocytoma.
- *Pineal parenchymal tumors.*
- Tumor with neuroblastic/glioblastic elements or embryonal tumor or Primitive neuroectodermal tumor/PNET *Clump like calcification* (uncommon in medullo-blastoma).
- Tumor of sellar region (craniopharyngioma, calcification seen in over 75% cases).
- Germ cell tumor (Teratoma).
- Meningioma (*Homogeneous ball like calcification*/less regular or dense calcification) in 10-20% cases.
- Malignant mesenchymal – Hemangiopericytoma (*not frequently* shows calcification).
- Tumor of cranial and spinal nerves – Schwannoma.
- Metastatic tumors (very rare except from bone tumor, colonic carcinoma, after radiation treatment).
- Lipoma (bracket calcification), Hamartoma, pituitary adenoma.
- Dermoids (Arc-like).

5. **Ans. is d i.e. Craniopharyngioma** *Ref. Harrison 17/e, p 2602; Devita 8/e, p 1982*

Tumor showing CSF dissemination are :

Mnemonic : **G**wallior **Ca** **MELA**

- **G**erm cell tumors *... Robbin's 7/e, p 1409*
- **C**horoid plexus tumor
- **M**edulloblastoma
- **E**pendymoma *... Harrison 17/e, p 2605*
- Primary CNS **L**ymphoma
- High grade **A**strocytoma

Remember :
- Germinoma is MC ***germ cell tumor*** of brain.
- *Drop metastases* : Brain tumor metastases that spread to spinal cord by way of CSF is called *drop metastases.*

6. **Ans. is a i.e PET scan** *Ref. Harrison 17/e, p 2602*

"Positron emission tomography (PET) and single photon emission tomography (SPECT) have ancillary role in the imaging of brain tumor, primarily in distinguishing tumor recurrence from tissue necrosis."

In PET a positron labelled form of biologically relevant molecule is injected in the body and used to trace the biochemical behavior of that molecule through ***non invasive*** imaging. Tumor tissue shows increase glucose metabolism, which is decreased in necrotic tissue.

Though biopsy is the most specific investigation, it is not imaging modality so answer is PET scan.

Radiation toxicity in Brain

- Nervous system is vulnerable to injury by therapeutic radiation. Histologically there is demyelination, degeneration of small arterioles and eventually brain infarction and necrosis.

Radiation injury can be:

1. ***Acute radiation injury:*** This occur during or immediately after therapy with current protocols. It is rarely seen after eaternal beam radiation and most cases occur after stereotactic radiosurgery.

   Manifestations include headache, sleepiness and worsening of preexisting neurologic deficit.

2. **Early delayed radiation injury:**
   - Occurs with in 4 months of therapy
   - In children present with somnolence and ataxia
   - Lhermitte's phenomenon (an electricity like sensation evoked by neck flexion) can be the manifestation after cervical spine irradiation. MRI shows increased white matter T_2 signal
   - Symptoms often respond to glucocorticoids and usually resolve without residual deficit
   - These injuries do not increase the risk of late radiation injury

3. **Late delayed radiation injury:**
   - Seen after 4 months (generally 8-24 months) and produces permanent damage
   - Results in radiation necrosis, which if untreated may act as an expanding mass lesion.
   - It is very difficult to distinguish radiation necrosis from tumor recurrence. PET or SPECT scan are imaging modality of choice, but confirmation often require bioipsy
   - Clinically present with progressive dementia, often accompanied by gait apraxia, and urinary incontinence
   - There is accelerated atherosclerosis too
   - Progressive radiation necrosis is best treated by surgical resection, if the patient has life expectancy of atleast 6 months. In other cases glucocorticoids are the only treatment
   - Hypopituitarism frequently follows exposure of hypothalamus or pituitary to therapeutic radiation. Growth hormone is most sensitive while TSH is least sensitive to radiation therapy
   - Development of second neoplasm is another risk

7. **Ans. is a i.e. seen in elderly above 80 years** *Ref. Harrison 17/e p 2603*

Juvenile pilocytic astrocytoma is seen in children and young adults.

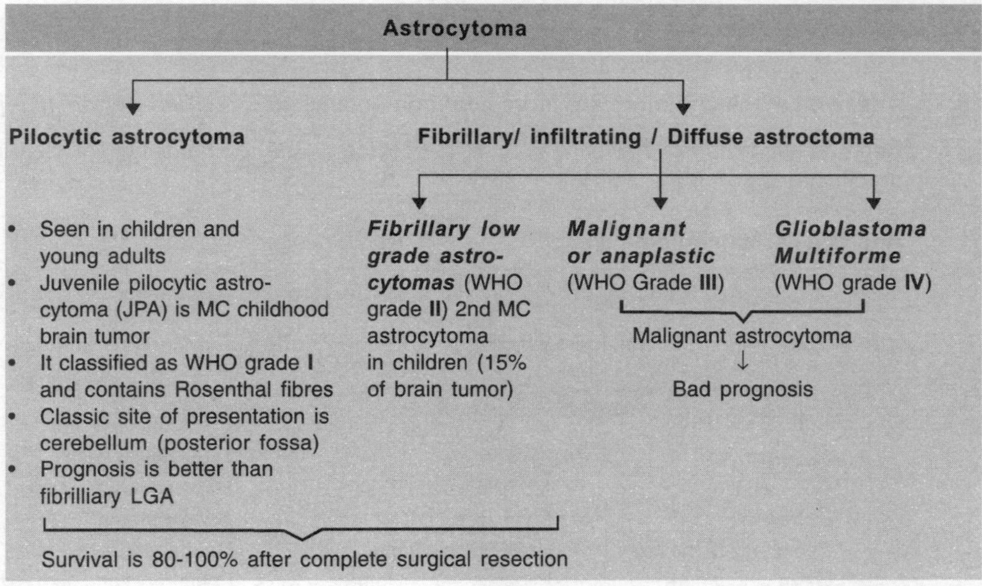

8. **Ans. is b i.e. Foramen of Monro**

See below

Glial tumor	Most common site
Juvenile pilocytic astrocytoma	Cerebellum
Subependymal giant cell astrocytoma	Foramen of monr
Oligodenroglioma	Cerebral hemisphere
Ependymoma	Filum terminate of spinal cord

Subependymal giant cell astrocytoma

- **Subependymal giant cell astrocytomas (SGCAs)** are a group of benign (WHO grade I[4]) astrocytomas and are seen with increased incidence in tuberous sclerosis (TS).
- They principally affect patients under 20, but are occasionally fouond in older people.
- The foramen of Monroe is the classic location
- Symptoms are usually a result of obstructive hydrocephalus because of mass effect around the ventricular system.

Imaging

CT: Calcification is common and haemorrhage is possible. Often shows marked contrast enhancement (differentiating feature from sub ependymal nodule)

MRI: Hypo to isointense on T1, hyperintense on T2

Treatment

The main treatment is surgical removal and is usually curative. Oral rapamycin (sirolimus) has also been trialled.

9. Ans. is b i.e. Optic pathway glioma *Ref. Devita 8/e p 1977*

Syndrome	CNS tumor
Neurofibromatosis Type 1	Schwannoma, optic glioma, astrocytoma and meningioma
Neurofibromatosis Type 2	Bilateral vestibular schwannomma, meningioma

10. Ans is d i.e. these tumors are more common in females *Ref. Nelson 18/e p 2130*

Cerebral astrocytoma or juvenile pilocytic astrocytoma (JPA) do not show any clear gender predilection.

11. Ans. is a i.e. Meningioma *Ref. Grainger Radiology 4/e, p 2328 - 2329*

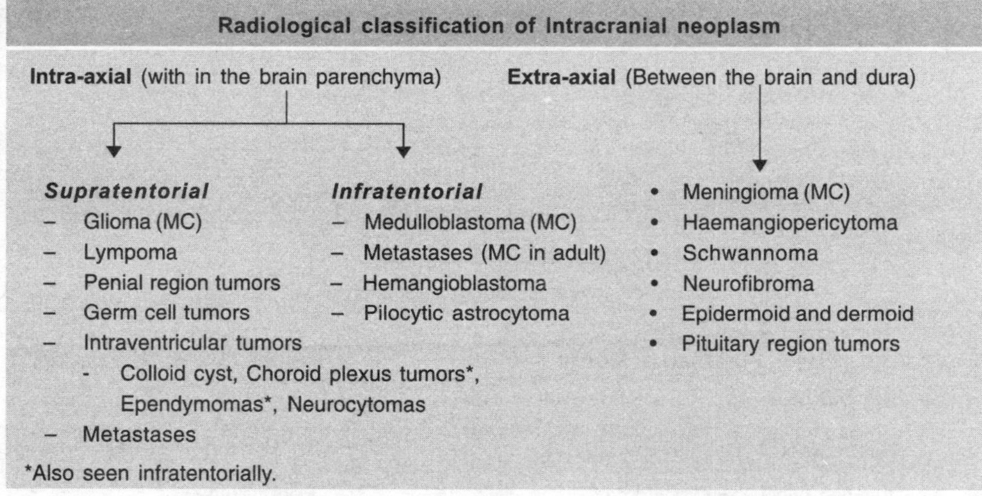

12. Ans. is a i.e. Glioblastoma *Ref. Grainger Radiology 4/e, p 2327*

Glioblastoma is WHO Grade IV tumor which characteristically shows necrolic and hemorrhagic foci. Vasogenic edema and contrast enhancement are shared features with anaplastic astrocytoma.

13. Ans. is c i.e PET scan *Ref. Harrison 17/e, p 2603*

Already explained

14. Ans. is d i.e. Xeroderma pigmentosum *Ref. Harrison 17/e, p 2603*

Hereditary syndromes associated with Brain tumors are :

Mnemonic : **L**ala **L**ajpat **R**ai **N**ever **W**ants **T**o **G**o **T**amil**N**adu

Von HIppel-**L**indau

Li-Fraumeni

Retinoblastoma

Neurofibromatosis type 1

Werner syndrome (Multiple endocrine neoplasia 1)

Turcot syndrome

Gorlin (basal cell nevus)

Tuberous sclerosis

Neurofibromatosis type 2

Remember : **Xeroderma pigmentosum :**
- **Inherited disorder with defective DNA repair genes.**
- Patient are at increased risk for developing skin cancer.

15. Ans. is b i.e. Craniopharyngioma *Ref. Harrison 17/e, p 2607; Sutton 7/e, p 1752*

Craniopharyngioma

- Craniopharyngioma is MC suprasellar tumor in children.
- Tumor is usually cystic with areas of ***calcification.***
- Mostly occur ***before age of 20.***
- Tumor is ***locally invasive.***
- Present with headache, vomiting, visual field abnormality, personality change and cognitive disorder.

Pituitary adenoma : is ***rare*** in childhood.

Optic chiasmal glioma and Germinoma : Occurring in childhood but cystic change is very rare.

16. Ans. is d i.e. Lung *Ref. Harrison 17/e, p 2608; Devita 7/e, p 2324*

"Lung is the MC origin of brain metastases both primary lung cancer (adenocarcinoma and small cell) ca and cancer metastatic to lung can metastasize to brain."

... Harrison 17/e, p 2608

Site of primary tumor	Brain Metastases	Tumor	Incidence
		Incidence of Brain metastases	
Lung	40%	Lung cancer	16%
Breast	19%	Renal cell cancer	10%
Melanoma	10%	Melanoma	7%
Gastrointestinal tract	7%	Breast cancer	5%
Genitourinary tract	7%	Colorectal carcinoma	1%
Other	17%		

Guys *! both incidence and site of primary are different thing,* incidence of brain metastasis in lung cancer is 16% that is 16% of patients will have brain metastases at time of diagnosis. *Site of primary indicates if metastatic brain tumor is found in 100 patients, 40 patients (40%) will have primary in lung.*

In this question there is no matter as it is the lung cancer which is most common in both the conditions.

17. Ans. is b i.e. Tuberous sclerosis *Ref. Harrison 17/e, p 2607*

Adenoma sebacium = *Facial angiofibroma are found in tuberous sclerosis*

Tuberous sclerosis (Bourneville disease)

- Characterized by cutaneous lesions, mental retardation and seizures.

- ***Cutaneous lesion include :***
  - **A**denoma sebacium
  - **S**hagreen patches (yellowish thickening of the skin over lumbosacral region of back)
  - **A**sh leaf hypopigmented macules
  - Depigmented **N**evi-.

***Mnemonic : Adenoma* Sebacium *And* Nevi.**

- Neural lesion include : Subependymal nodules that may be calcified
- *It ↑ risk of developing :*
  - Ependymomas
  - Rhabdomyoma of myocardium
  - Angiomyoma of Kidney, liver, adrenal and pancreas.
- Defect on both ***9q and 16q*** are associated with tuberous sclerosis, resulting in defective tuberin proteins.

Other options :

- ***Xanthomatosis :*** Widespread xanthomas specially on the elbow and knee that some times affect mucous membrane and are associated with metabolic disturbances. Also called xanthoma multiplex.

... Stedmann Dictonarry 27/e, p 1993

- ***Incontinentia pigmenti :*** Rare genodermatosis characterized by hyperpigmented lesions in linear, Zebra strippe and Bizarre configuration, following lines of blaschko. Occasionally accompany other developmental anomalies of eyes, teeth, nails and heart.

18. Ans. is a i.e. Small cell ca lung *Ref. Devita 17/e, p 2608*

Guys ! see one thing, these two questions (15 and 17) are not same, as in this question it is incidence which has been asked.

19. Ans. is b i.e. Craniopharygioma *Ref. Harrison 16/e, p 2607*

Remember :
- In child most common suprasellar mass - Craniopharyngioma.
- In adults most common suprasellar mass - Pituitary adenoma.

20. Ans. is c i.e. Extradural *Ref. Sutton 7/e, p 1634, 1638, 1640*

Already explained

21. Ans. is d i.e. Medulloblastoma

Ref. Devita 7/e, p 1844; Text book of radiation oncology Lebiel Phillips 2/e, p 489

"Prophylactic craniospinal irradiation is recommended in primary tumor showing high propensity to metastasize to CSF and Metastatic tumors of brain."

Prophylactic craniospinal irradiation	
Primary brain tumor	*Tumor with high risk of brain metastases*
• Medulloblastoma • Germ cell tumors such as Germinoma • Glioblastoma • Anaplastic ependymomas.	• Non hodgkin lymphoma • ALL • Small cell Ca of lung

... Devita 7/e, p 1861

Remember :
- Dose is 30 Gy given in 10 daily fraction of 3 Gy each over 2 weeks.
- Hodgkin lymphoma has no propensity to cause CSF metastases.

22. **Ans. is a, b and c i.e. Reticulin staining done, Essentially B-cell type, a/w EBV**

Ref. Robbins 8/e, p 1337

Primary CNS lymphoma

- Most common CNS neoplasm in immunocompromised individuals
- ***Morphology:*** Often multifocal, nodal, marrow or extracranial spread is rare and delayed complication
- Mostly B-cell origin and nearly all tumors are latently infected by EBV. ***Diffuse large cell B-cell lymphoma*** is the most common histologic type
- Overall primary lymphomas of the CNS are ***aggressive with*** relatively poor response to chemotherapy
- Reticulin stains demonstrate that the infiltrating cells are separated from one another by silver staining material. This pattern referred to as "***hooping***" is characteristic of primary brain lymphoma

23. **Ans. is a, d and e i.e. Calcification, Osteosclerosis, Vascular erosion**

Ref. Sutton 7/e, p 1634, 1638, 1640; Grainger 4/e, p 2328

Radiological findings of Meningioma

- ***Abnormal vascular markings:*** Meningioma is most common cause of pathological vascular markings in the skull vault
- ***Enlarged foramen spinosum*** on the side of lesion
- ***Invasion of bone*** cause localized bony hyperostosis / mixed osteoblastic and osteolytic less commonly. It may show sunray spicules and local bone expansion with pneumatization so called blistering
- ***Calcification*** in the tumor
- Signs of ***increased intracranial*** tension
- Enlarged meningeal grooves

24. **Ans. is a i.e. Meningioma** *Ref. Sutton 7/e, p 1634, 1638*

Already explained see answer no. 1

25. **Ans is b i.e. meduloblastoma** *Ref. Devita 8/e, 2008-2009*

A modified version of Chang staging is currently used for meduloblastoma.

- In this modified version T stage has made less relevant than the extent of residual disease.

- M stage remains a crucial staging component. It includes
  - M_0: No tumor dissemination
  - M_1 : Presence of tumor cells in the CSF
  - M_2 : Presence of gross tumor nodules in the intracranial, subarachnoid, or ventricular space.
  - M_3 : Gross tumor nodules in the spinal subarachnoid spaces
  - M_4 : Systemic metastasis
- Chang staging therefore requires the assessment of these potential sites and include CSF examination, MRI spine. Bone scan, chest-x-ray and bilateral bone marrow biopsies in patients with M_2 and M_3 disease.

Remember:

Duke's staging	Colorectal Ca
Gleason's taging	Prostatic Ca

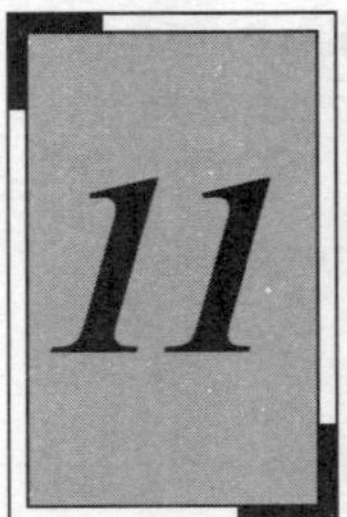

11 Tumour of Ear

What's Important ?

- Clinical Features
- Diagnosis

GLOMUS TUMOUR

- Non chromaffin producing paragangliomas.
- Most common *benign neoplasm of middle ear*
- Most common site in middle ear : ***hypotympanum***
- It consist of paraganglionic cells derived from ***neural crest.***
- It is *non encapsulated, extremely vascular* and ***locally invasive*** tumour; commonly affect ***middle aged females.***
- It usually ***arise*** from dome of jugular bulb as glomus jugulare or from promontory along the course of tympanic branch of IX cranial nerve *(Jacobson's nerve)* as glomus tympanicum.

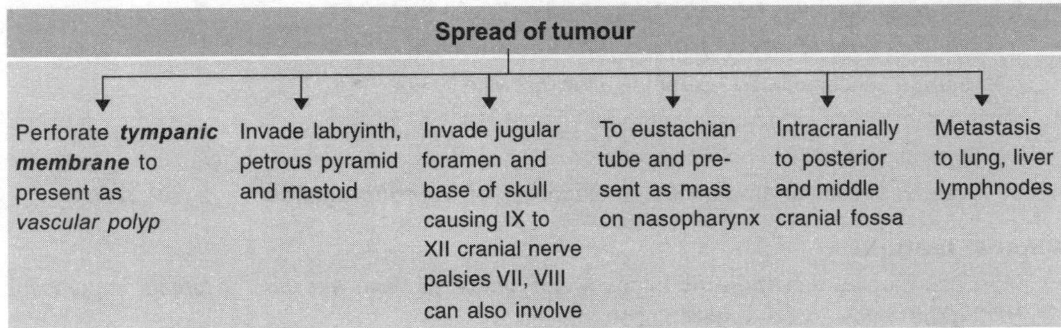

Clinical features

- **When tumour is intratympanic :**
  1. Earliest symptoms are **deafness** (conductive*) and* **tinnitus** *(*pulsatile and of swishing character, synchronous with pulse and can be temporarily stopped by carotid pressure*).*
  2. *Otoscopy shows* **red reflex; rising sun appearance**, tympanic membrane *appears* **bluish and bulging.**
  3. **Brown's sign** *may present (*pulsation of tympanic membrane *that is inhibited by positive pressure applied to the tympanic membrane by pneumatic otoscope).*

4. **Pulsation sign** *is positive (when ear canal pressure is raised with seigle's speculum, tumour pulsates vigorously and then blanches, reverse happens with release of pressure).*

- **When tumour present as polyp :**
  1. History of profuse bleeding from the ear either spontaneously or on attempts to clear it.
  2. Dizziness, vertigo, facial paralysis, earache, otorrhea.
- **Audible bruit :** Heard by stethoscope over mastoid at all stages.
- Some glomus tumour secrete catecholamines and produce headache, sweating etc.

Diagnosis

- **CT scan head :** To distinguish glomus jugulare from glomus tympanicum by identification of corticojugular spine, which is eroded in glomus jugulare ***(PHELP SIGN).***
- ***Gadolinium enhanced MRI*** is used to delineate the extent of tumour.
- ***Four vessel angiography :*** For pre-operative assesment of tumours requiring therapeutic embolization as glomus tumor can have tremendous blood supply via ascending pharyngeal artery

Treatment

- ***Surgery*** : TOC is *Lateral cranial base surgical removal* with preoperative embolization, if the lesion doesn't involve carotid siphon and has not spread by distant metastasis.
- ***Radiation*** : Used for inoperable, residual tumours, recurrences after surgery or for older individual where extensive skull base surgery is not indicated.
- ***Embolisation*** : Is the sole treatment in inoperable patients who have received radiation.
- ***Radiosurgery*** : For tumor <3 cm *... Devita 8/e p 2020*

ACOUSTIC NEUROMA / VESTIBULAR SCHWANNOMA / NEURILEMMOMA OR EIGHTH NERVE TUMOUR

- It is the most common ***intracranial schwannoma.***
- It constitutes ***80% of all cerebellopontine angle*** tumour.
- It is ***benign***, encapsulated, extremely slow growing tumour.
- Most common site of acoustic neuroma :
  - *Superior vestibular nuclei > inferior vestibular nuclei > Cochlear nuclei.*
  - Bilateral vestibular shwannoma is diagnostic of ***Neurofibromatosis – 2 (NF 2).***

Clinical features

- Most schwnomas are ***sporadic*** tumours and almost all have *mutation of tumour suppressor* **NF 2 gene** *which encodes* **merlin protein.**
- **Age :** 40-60 years.
- **Earliest symptom** : cochleovestibular symptoms (deafness, tinnitus).
- Most common symptom : ***Progressive unilateral sensorineural (retrocochlear) hearing loss*** often accompanied by tinnitus.
- There is **marked difficulty in understanding speech out of proportion to the puretone** hearing loss. *This is characteristic of acoustic neuroma.*
- May also present with sudden hearing loss.
- True vertigo is seldom seen.

- Earliest cranial Nerve to be involved **V nerve.**
- Sensory fibres of VII N. are affected ***early*** than motor fibres. *There is hypoaesthesia of posterior meatal wall, called as* **Hitselberger's sign.**
- IV, VI, IX, X XI, XII cranial nerve can also be involved.
- Features of brainstem, cerebellar involvement and raised intracranial tension also present.

Diagnosis

- ***Audiological test :*** Show features of retrocochlear hearing loss.
- ***Acoustic reflex :*** Shows stapedial reflex decay.
- ***Vestibular test :*** Caloric test usually show diminished or absent response but may be normal if tumour is very small.
- Complete neurological examination including *fundoscopy.*
- ***Radiological test :***
  - Plain X-ray.
  - MRI with gadolinium contrast - *gold standard – Best investigation.*
  - CT scan - Shows erosion and widening of internal auditory meatus.
  - Vertebral angiography has been replaced by MRI
- Evoked response Audiometry (BERA)
- Electric response audiometry delay of > 0.2msec in wave V between two ears is significant.
- Pure tone and speech audiometry

Treatment

- ***Surgery :*** Treatment of choice :
  - *Middle cranial fossa approach* - If tumour is *small with hearing* present
  - *Suboccipital approach* - Large tumour with some hearing
  - *Translabyrinthine approach* - Large tumour with no hearing
- ***Radiosurgery :*** < 2.5 cm
- ***Gamma knife surgery (form of stereotactic radiosurgery).*** Used in patients who refuse surgery or *have contraindications to surgery* or *those* with *residual tumour.*

QUESTIONS

1. **Acoustic neur1oma arises from :**
   a. Superior vestibular part of VIII CN
   b. Inferior vestibular part of VIII CN
   c. VII CN **[AI 10, AIIMS Nov 09]**
   d. Cochlear part of VIII CN

2. **A 70 year old male presents with loss of sensation in external auditory meatus (Histelberg's sign positive). The likely diagnosis is : [AI 08]**
   a. Vestibular schwannoma
   b. Mastoiditis
   c. Bells palsy
   d. Middle ear cholesteatoma

3. **Investigation of choice of acoustic neuroma:**
   a. CT without contrast **[AIIMS May 08]**
   b. CT with contrast
   c. MR without contrast
   d. MR with contrast

4. **True about acoustic neuroma : [PGI 08]**
   a. Malignant tumour
   b. Arises form vestibular nerve
   c. Involves cochlear nerve also
   d. Upper pole displaces IX, X, XI nerves
   e. Lower pole displaces trigeminal cranial nerve

ANSWERS, REFERENCES, EXPLANATIONS WITH INFORMATIVE ILLUSTRATIONS

1. **Ans. is a i.e. Superior vestibular nuclei** *Ref. Dhingra 4/e, p 111; Devita 8/e, p 2017*

Schwannoma can be arise from any cranial nerve but most common ***nerve involved is superior vestibular division of VIII nerve*** (rarely from the cochlear division) > V, VII nerve.

- Most common ***site*** of vestibular schwannoma is superior vestibular division and rarely from the cochlear division.
- Acoustic neuroma is ***benign***, encapsulated, extremely slow growing tumor occuring in 40 - 60 years.
- Acoustic neuroma is most common ***cerebellopontine angle tumour.***
- IOC is *contrast enhanced* (using gadolinium DTPA) MRI.
- Treatment of choice is surgery.

Mnemonic : ANS (Acoustic Neuroma - Superior division)

Remember :
- Schwannoma also affect other cranial nerves V > VII > IX, X, XI.
- Acoustic neuroma occur in late childhood/adults and may be bilateral when associated with familial neurofibromatosis.
- First and second cranial nerve lack schwann cell sheath, therefore they are not potential sites of schwannoma.

2. **Ans. is a i.e. Vestibular Schwannoma** *Ref. Dhingra 4/e, p 111*

Hitzelberg sign is typical of vestibular Schwannoma

Presentation of Acoustic Neuroma		
Cochleovestibular symptoms	***Cranial nerve involvement***	***Brainstem involvement***
(Earliest symptoms) ***Cochlear*** • Progressive U/L sensorineural (retrocochlear) hearing loss *(MC symptom)* • Tinnitus • Difficulty in understanding speech ***Vestibular*** • Imbalance • Unsteadiness • Vertigo	• **V** *(earliest nerve to be involved)*. Reduced corneal sensitivity & numbness of face • **VII** hypoesthesia of posterior meatal wall, loss of taste sensation, reduced lacrimation • **IX** and **X** - dysphagia, hoarseness • XI, XII, III, IV and VI can also affected	• Ataxia • Cerebellar involvement (past pointing, intention tremor, Dysdiadokinesia spontaneous nystagmus, ipsilateral ataxia) • Increased ICT (Headache nausea, vomiting) • Diplopia due to VI nerve and papilloedema with blurred vision • Hydrocephalus

3. **Ans. is d i.e. MR with contrast** *Ref. Devita 8/e, p 217*

Already explained

4. **Ans. is b and c i.e. Arises form vestibular nerve; and Involves cochlear nerve also**
Ref. Dhingra 4/e, p 110 -145 fig. 19.1; Devita 8/e, p 2017

- **Most common site of vestibular Schwanoma :** *Vestibular division of VIII nerve at the transition point between central* and peripheral myelin located near the medial end of internal auditory canal (IAC).
- First it fills IAC and then expand in to posterior fossa.
- Its upper pole compress V nerve while lower pole compress IX, X, XI nerves. If it grows more it compress brain stem and cerebellum.

12 Nasopharyngeal Tumour

What's Important ?

- Clinical Features
- Treatment

NASOPHARYNGEAL FIBROMA/JUVENILE NASOPHARYNGEAL ANGIOFIBROMA

- Most common ***benign tumour*** of nasopharynx.
- Most common **site** is *posterior part of nasal cavity* close to the margin of sphenopalatine foramen.
- Seen almost exclusively in males of ***10-20 years*** (*testosterone dependent*).
- ***Locally invasive*** tumour consist *of endothelium lined vessels with no muscle coat.*
- The major blood supply is from **internal maxillary artery.**

Clinical features

- Depend on spread of tumour to nasal cavity, paranasal sinuses, pterygomaxillary fossa, infratemporal fossa, cheek, orbits (through inferior orbital fissure), cranial cavity (*MC* site is ***middle cranial fossa***).
- Most common symptom - *Profuse and recurrent epistaxis.*
- **Other features :**
  - Progressive nasal obstruction, denasal speech.
  - Conductive hearing loss and serous otitis media.
  - *Pink or purplish mass* obstructing one or both chonae in nasopharynx.
  - Broadening of nasal bridge; proptosis; ***frog-face deformity;*** swelling of cheek; ***involvement of II, III, IV, VI cranial nerve.***

Diagnosis

- Soft tissue lateral film of nasopharynx and X-ray of paranasal sinuses, base of skull.
- **CT scan of head** *with contrast enhancement* is now the IOC. It shows extent, bony destruction or displacements and anterior bowing of the posterior wall of maxillary sinus (called as *antral sign) which is pathognomic of angiofibroma.*
- MRI especially for soft tissue extension.
- Carotid angiography
- Biopsy is ***contraindicated.***

Treatment

- ***Surgical excision is*** treatment of choice.
- *Preooperatively embolization* and *estrogen therapy or cryotherapy or radiotherapy reduce blood loss in surgery.*
- ***Approach :*** - Transpalatal approach done for ***tumour confined to nasopharynx.***
  - Lateral rhinotomy done for larger tumours involving nasal cavity, paranasal sinuses.
  - ***Other approach :*** - Transpalatine + Sublabial (Sardana' approach)
    - Extended Denker's approach.
- Recurrence is not uncommon after surgery.

NASOPHARYNGEAL CARCINOMA

Uncommon in India except in North - East region where people are predominantly of mongoloid origin.

- It is MC tumour of head and neck which give rise to secondaries with occult primary.
- Most common ***site*** is *fossa of rosenmuller* in the lateral wall of nasopharynx.
- Most common ***type*** of nasopharyngeal carcinoma - ***Squamous cell carcinoma***

Etiology

- **Genetic :** Mostly seen in Chinese
- **Viral :** Epstein Barr virus has identified in tumour epithelial cells (not lymphocytes) of most undifferentiated and Nonkeratinizing squamous cell carcinoma.
- **Environmental :** Burning of incense or wood (polycyclic hydrocarbon); smoking of tobacco and opium; air pollution; nitrosamines from dry salted fish along with vitamin C deficient diet.

Clinical features

- Most common ***manifestation*** *is cervical lymphadenopathy since nasopharynx is richly supplied by Lymphatics.*
- Most common ***cranial nerve palsy*** in nasopharyngeal carcinoma is **VI cranial nerve.**

Spread of Tumour	Findings
• Cervical nodes	– Upper and mid jugular; posterior triangle nodes enlargement
• Eustachian tube	– Serous / suppurative otitis media; tinnitus; dizziness
• Nose and orbit (even involve CN II at apex)	– Nasal obstruction and discharge; epistaxis; proptosis; blindness
• Foramen lacerum and ovale	– Ophthalmic symptoms and facial pain *(CN III, IV, V, VI)*
• Parapharyngeal space	– *Cranial nerve palsies IX, X, XI, XII;* ***Horner's syndrome;*** trismus
• Retropharyngeal nodes	– Neck pain and stiffness
• Distant metastases	– Secondaries in lung, liver, bone

Remember :

- Presence of ***unilateral serous otitis media*** in an adult should raise suspicion of nasopharyngeal growth.
- **Trotter's triad :** Seen in Nasopharyngeal cancer. Includes *conductive deafness; ipsilateral tempoparietal neuralgia due to CN V; palatal paralysis due to CN X.*
- Unlike other squamous cell carcinoma, it can metastasize to posterior triangle (level V) in the absence of jugular lymph node involvement.
- Site of clinically occult primary cancer : tonsillar fossa, tongue base, pyriform sinus, nasopharynx.

Diagnosis

- Most important is examination of postnasal space by nasopharyngeal mirror or nasopharyngoscope.

Treatment

- ***Irradiation is*** treatment of choice.
- Radical neck dissection is required for persistent nodes when primary has been controlled.
- Systemic chemotherapy is used as palliation for distant metastases or radiation failure.

QUESTIONS

1. A 70 year old male presents with hearing loss and tinnitus. On examination he was observed to have a conductive type of deafness and a dull tympanic membrane on the right side. Lymph nodal enlargement of 3 × 3 cm was noted in the posterior triangle of neck. Tympanogram revealed a type B wave. The most likely diagnosis is : [AI 08]

a. Middle ear tumor
b. Nasopharyngeal malignancy
c. Acoustic neuroma
d. TB of middle ear

2. Radiotherapy is the primary treatment for: [AIIMS 09]

a. Supraglottic C_a T_3 N_0
b. Subglottic C_a T_3 N_0
c. Glottis C_a T_3 N_1
d. Nasopharyngeal C_a T_3 N_1

3. Wood workers and associated sinus Ca:

a. Adeno Ca **[PGI 06]**
b. Sq. Cell Ca
c. Anaplastic Ca
d. Melanoma

4. Common about tumors of PNS and Nasal Ca : [PGI 06]

a. Sq cell Ca is the MC type
b. Adeno Ca is the MC type
c. Melanoma
d. Lymphoma

5. Nasopharyngeal carcinoma true are all except: [AI 10]

a. Bimodal age distribution
b. EBV
c. Nasopharyngectomy treatment of choice
d. Can present with ophthalmoplegia

ANSWERS, REFERENCES, EXPLANATIONS WITH INFORMATIVE ILLUSTRATIONS

1. **Ans. is b i.e. Nasopharyngeal malignancy** *Ref. Dhingra 4/e, p 232, 26*

This is a case of otitis media (conductive deafness with type B wave on tympanogram secondary to nasopharyngeal Ca (nodal enlargement in posterior triangle).

Presence of unilateral serous otitis media in an adult always raise the suspicion of nasopharyngeal growth, as nasopharyngeal Ca is the most common tumor of head and neck which give rise to secondaries without any oblivious primary growth.

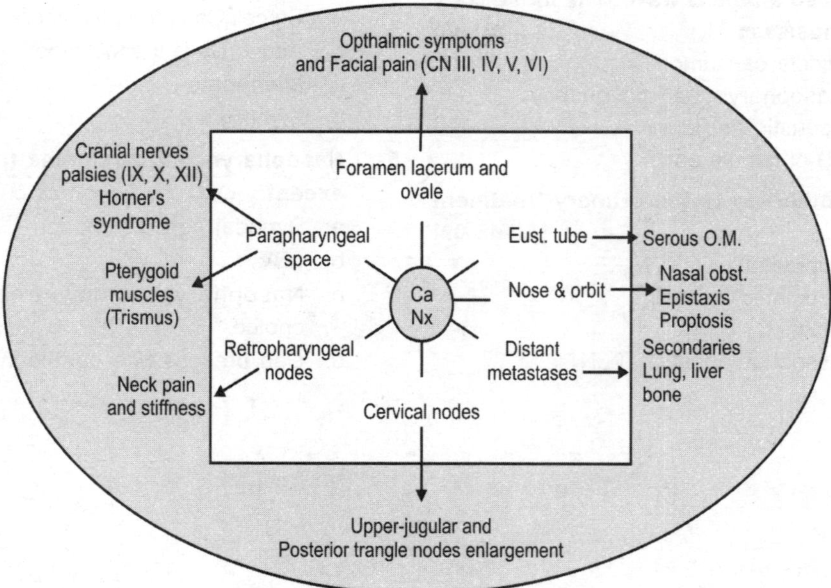

Routes of spread and clinical features of nasopharyngeal cancer

2. **Ans. is d i.e. Nasopharyngeal Ca T_3 N_1** *Ref. Devita 8/e p 856*

The treatment of almost all malignancies of the nasopharynx is by radiation therapy since complete surgical resection is usually not feasable.

Irradiation technique: Following areas are included in radiotherapy for tumor limited to nasopharynx or have minimal soft tissue extension.

- Nasopharynx proper
- Posterior ethmoid sinus
- Cavernous sinus
- Pterygold fossa
- Oropharyngeal wall upto the level of mid tonsillar fossa
- Retropharyngeal nodes
- Posterior 2 cm of nasal cavity
- Entire sphenoid sinus and basooccipital bone
- Base of skull

- Posterior 1/3rd of maxillary sinus
- Neck nodes on both side

With IMRT (intensity modulated radiotherapy), dose delivered to parotid and temporal lobe can be reduced.

Sequelae of Radiotherapy

Acute:
- Sore throat, begins at the end of 2nd week of therapy and persist for 2-3 months
- Loss of taste and papetite
- Obstruction to eustachian tube and otitis media

Long term: Xerostomia

3. **Ans. is a i.e. Adenocarcinoma** *Ref. Dhingra 4/e, p 195 - 197*

Etiology of Malignant neoplasm of Paranasal sinuses.

- **Hardwood furniture industry :** It causes adenocarcinoma of ethmoid and upper nasal cavity.

  Mnemonic : **NEHA**
- **Nickel refinery :** Cause Squamous cell and Anaplastic carcinoma.

  Mnemonic : **ANS**
- *Leather work*
- *Exposure to mustard gas*
- *Snuff rich in nickel and chromiun.*

Carcinoma of ethmoid sinus

- Primary malignancy is not common.
- Early features include nasal obstruction, blood stained nasal discharge and retroorbital pain.
- **Treatment :**
  - In early cases, preoperative radiation followed by lateral rhinotomy and total ethmoidectomy.
  - If cribriform plate is involved, craniofacial resection is done.

Remember :
- Most common ***site*** *of malignant neoplasm is maxillary antrum.*
- Most common ***variety of sinus malignancy is squamous cell variety.***
- Melanoma.

4. **Ans. is a i.e. Sq. Cell Ca is MC Type**

Already explained

5. **Ans. is c i.e. Nasopharyngectomy treatment of choice** *Ref. Dhingra 4/e, p 232 - 235*

Treatment of choice for nasopharyngeal Ca is radiotherapy. Another confusing option is option 'a'

Nasopharyngeal Ca is usually seen in 6th or 7th decade but may be seen in younger age group. So, there is bimodart distribution.

13 Laryngeal Tumour

What's Important ?

- Predisposing Factors
- Spread
- Treatment

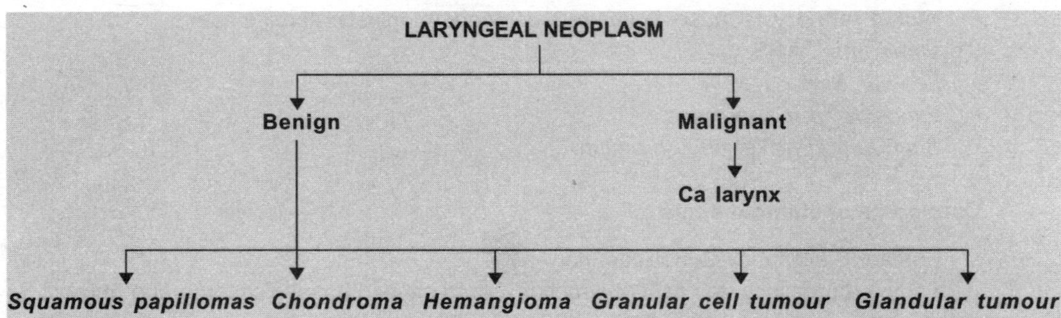

SQUAMOUS PAPILLOMAS

Most common ***benign tumour.***

Two types :

a. **Juvenile papillomas = Recurrent respiratory papillomatosis**
   - Viral in origin, caused by ***HPV types 6 and 11.***
   - *Multiple lesions* involving infant and young children, *presenting with hoarseness and stridor.*
   - Most common site – vocal fold is first and predominant site. ... *CSDT 12/e, p 971*
   - ***Treatment :***
     - Recurrence after removal is common.
     - *Micro endoscopic CO_2 laser excision of papillomas at fixed interval (2, 4 and 6 month) according to individual need* ***is*** *treatment of choice.*
     - **Interferon alfacon :** *1 adjuvant therapy in patient with severe disease.*
     - *Other adjuvant are* ***podophyllin*** *(most effective), Vit A derivative, Hematoporphyrin derivative.*

b. **Adult onset papilloma**
   - Single, smaller in size and less aggressive and ***does'nt recur*** after surgery.

- Age : 30 - 50; M > F.
- Arise from ***anterior half of vocal cord or*** anterior commisure.
- Treatment is same.

HEMANGIOMA

Infantile hemangioma involves the ***subglottic area*** and presents with stridor in first 6 months of life.

- Tends to ***involute spontaneously*** but a tracheostomy may be needed to relieve respiratory obstruction.
- **Treated** by CO_2 laser.

Adult hemangioma involves ***vocal cord*** or supraglottic larynx.

- *Most are* ***cavernous type*** and can't be treated with laser.
- *No treatment for asymptomatic, larger ones are treated by steroids or radiation therapy.*

CANCER LARYNX

- More prevalent in India.
- **Age** : 40 - 70; M > F

Etiology

- *Tobacco smoking and alcohol are most important.* Combination of alcohol and smoking ↑ the risk ***15 fold.***
- Previous neck irradiation.
- *Occupational exposure* to ***asbestos, mustard gas*** and petroleum products.

Histopathology

- 90 - 95% of CA larynx are ***squamous cell ca.***
- *Cordal lesions* are ***well differentiated*** while supraglottic ones are anaplastic.

Classification

According to site Ca larynx is divided into :

a. **Supraglottic cancer** (Include epiglottis, false cord, ventricles, aryepiglottic fold, arytenoids)
   - Less common
   - *Majority of lesion is on epiglottis, false cords or ventricular bands followed by aryepiglottic folds (laryngeal aspect only); arytenoids.*
   - **Spread :**
     - Locally to invade vallecula, base of tongue and pyriform fossa.
     - *Lymphatic* **:** Nodal metastases occurs early; upper and ***middle jugular nodes*** are often involved.
     - *Extralaryngeal spread increase risk of nodal metastases.*
   - **Symptoms :**
     - ***Pain on swallowing is the*** most frequent ***initial symptom.*** *... Devita 7/e, p 698*
     - *Mass in neck* may be the ***first sign.***
     - ***Hoaresness*** *is a late symptom.*

- *Pain may referred to ear* by way of ***vagus nerve*** and ***auricular nerve of arnold.***
- Late symptom include foul breath, dysphagia and aspiration.

b. Glottic cancer (include true vocal cord and anterior commisure)

- It is the MC ***site of Ca larynx.***
- Mostly originates on *free edge and upper surface of anterior 1/3 of true vocal cord* followed by middle 1/3rd.
- **Spread :**
  - *Locally* to anterior commissure than to opposite cord (conus ***elasticus initially acts as barrier for subglottic spread).***
  - ***Fixation*** of vocal cord indicates spread of disease to thyroarytenoid muscle and is bad prognostic sign.
  - ***Lymphatic*** : As vocal cord is free of lymphatics, nodal metastasis is never seen in cordal cancer, unless the disease spread beyond membranous cord.
- **Symptom :**
  - ***Hoarseness*** is MC and earliest symptom and because of this glottic cancer is ***detected early.***
  - Pain and sore throat is a symptom of advanced lesion.

c. Subglottic cancer

- *Least common site.*
- Subglottic region extends from glottic area to lower border of cricoid cartilage.
- **Spread :**
  - Locally around anterior wall to opposite side or down wards to trachea. Upward spread to vocal cord is late and *hoarseness in not an early symptom.*
  - **Lymphatic metastases :** To prelaryngeal, pretracheal (Delphian node) and lower jugular nodes.
- **Symptoms :**
  - *Earliest and most prominent symptom* is ***stridor,*** *but it appears only in advanced stage.*
  - Hoarseness is late feature.

Diagnosis

- ***Indirect laryngoscopy :***
  - Lesions of *suprahyoid epiglottis* are usually exophytic while that of infrahyoid epiglottis are ulcerative.
  - Lesion of *vocal cord* appear as ***raised nodule.***
  - Lesion on anterior commissure appear as ***granulation tissue.***
  - Lesion of subglottic region appears as raised ***sub mucosal nodule.***
- ***Examination of neck :***
  - To check extra laryngeal spread.
  - To detect Nodal metastasis.
- ***Radiography :***
  - X-ray soft tissue lateral view neck.

- X-ray chest for co existent lung disease.
- Contrast laryngograms have been replaced by CT.
- **CT-** *Very useful investigation* to find extent of tumor, invasion of preepiglottic or paraepiglottic space.
- **MRI :** It is less suitable for Ca larynx than CT due to motion artifacts associated with longer scanning times.

- ***Direct laryngoscopy*** : To see hidden areas of larynx which include :
  a. Infrahyoid epiglottis
  b. *Anterior commisure*
  c. *Subglottis*
  d. *Ventricles*
- **Supravital staining and biopsy :** ***Toulidine*** blue is applied to laryngeal lesion and then washed with saline. Carcinoma in situ and superficial carcinoma *take dye while leukoplakia does not.*

Staging ... *Devita 8/e, p 847*

The AJCC staging system for primary tumors of the larynx is as follows :

Primary Tumor (T)	
TX	Primary tumor cannot be assessed
T0	No evidence of primary tumor
Tis	Carcinoma in situ
Supraglottis	
T1	Tumor limited to one subsite of supraglottis with normal vocal cord mobility
T2	Tumor invades mucosa of more than one adjacent sub-site of supraglottis or region outside the supraglottis, without fixation of larynx.
T3	Tumor limited to larynx with vocal cord fixation and or invades any of the following : postcoricoid area preepiglottic tissues, paraglottic space, and/or minor thyroid cartilage erosion (e.g., inner cortex).
T4a	Tumor invades through the thyroid cartilage and/or invades tissues beyond the larynx.
T4b	Tumor invades prevertebral space, encases carotid artery or invades mediastinal structures
Glottis	
T1	Tumor limited to one (T1a) or both (T1b) vocal cord(s) (may involve anterior or posterior commisure) with normal mobility
T2	Tumor extends to supraglottis and/or subglottis, or with imaired vocal cord mobility
T3	Tumor limited to the larynx with vocal cord fixation, and/or invades paraglottic space, and/or minor thyroid cartilage erosion (e.g., inner cortex)
T4	Same as supraglottis
Subglottis	
T1	Tumour limited to subglottis
T2	Tumor extends to vocal cords with normal or impaired mobility
T3	Tumor limited to larynx with vocal cord fixation
T4	Same as supraglottis

Treatment

A. Glottic = Vocal cord carcinoma

Ca in situ : Endoscopic removal by ***CO2 laser*** is *treatment of choice*. If recurrences are present radiotherapy is given.

Small T_1 : CO_2 Laser ... *Devita 7/e, p 699*

T_1 and T_2 : *Radiotherapy* is treatment of choice for T_1 and small T_2. Partial laryngectomy in case of radiation failure and large tumour

T_3, T_4 : ***For large volume disease.*** *Total laryngectomy with radical neck dissection* for clinically positive nodes, with post operative radiation.

In low volume disease radiation therapy with chemotherapy is given.

> **Remember :** Most frequent sites of local reccurence are around tracheal stoma in the base of tongue, and in the neck nodes.

B. Supraglottic cancer

T_1 – Radiotherapy

T_2 – Supraglottic laryngectomy with or without neck dissection

T_3 and T_4 – Total laryngectomy with neck dissection and postoperative radiotherapy.

C. Subglottic cancer

T_1 and T_2 – Radiotherapy

T_3 and T_4 – Total laryngectomy and postoperative radiotherapy.

Complication of treatment

- **Surgery** : Speech loss after laryngectomy.
- **Radiation** : Laryngeal edema is MC complication after radiation for glottic or supraglottic lesion.

Vocal rehabilitation after laryngectomy

- Oesophageal speech : – Rough and loud voice but understandable
- Artificial larynx : – Electrolarynx
  – Trans oral pneumatic device.
- Tracheo oesophageal speech.

QUESTIONS

1. **The most common and earliest manifestation of carcinoma of the glottis is :**
   a. Hoarseness **[AI 05; AIIMS 04]**
   b. Hemoptysis
   c. Cervical lymph nodes
   d. Stridor

2. **A patient presents with carcinoma of the larynx involving the left false cords, left arytenoid and the left aryepiglottic folds with bilateral mobile true cords. Treatment of choice is: [AIIMS 07]**
   a. Vertical hemilalryngectomy
   b. Horizontal partial hemilaryngectomy
   c. Total laryngectomy
   d. Radiotherapy followed by chemotherapy

3. **A middle aged male comes to the outer patient department (OPD) with the only complaint of hoarseness of voice for the past 2 years. He had been a chronic smoker for 30 years. On examination, a reddish area of mucosal irregularity overlying a portion of both cords was seen. Management would include all except : [AIIMS 05]**
   a. Cessation of smoking
   b. Bilateral cordectomy
   c. Microlaryngeal surgery for biopsy
   d. Regular follow-up

4. **A case of carcinoma larynx with the involvement of anterior commissure and right vocal cord, developed perichondritis of thyroid cartilage. Which of the following statements is true for the managements of this case ? [AIIMS 06]**
   a. He should be given radical radiotherapy as this can cure early tumours
   b. He should be treated with combination of chemotherapy and radiotherapy
   c. He should first receive radiotherapy and if residual tumour is present then should under go laryngectomy
   d. He should first undergo laryngectomy and then post -operative radiotherapy

5. **True about laryngeal ca is/are: [PGI 05]**
   a. Glottis is the MC site
   b. Commonly metastasize to cervical lymphnode
   c. Lesions seen at the edge of vocal cord
   d. Laryngeal compartment acts as barrier

6. **Select correct statements about Ca larynx : [PGI 02]**
   a. Glottic Ca is the most common
   b. Supraglottic is least common
   c. Lymphatic spread is most common in subglottic Ca
   d. T1 tumour is best treated by radiotherapy
   e. Smoking predisposes

ANSWERS, REFERENCES, EXPLANATIONS WITH INFORMATIVE ILLUSTRATIONS

1. **Ans. is a i.e. Hoarseness** *Ref. Dhingra 4/e, p 285; Devita 8/e, p 846*

"Hoarseness of voice is an early sign because lesion of cord affects its vibratory capacity." *... Dhingra*

Cancer site	Symptom
Supraglottic	Pain on swallowing (earliest), mass in neck, hoarseness is delayed
Glottis	Hoarseness (earliest), pain, dysphagia, airway obstruction suggest advance cancer
Subglottis	Stridor or airway obstruction Hoarseness is late feature

Remember : Most common site of Ca larynx is free edge or upper margin of anterior 2/3 of vocal cord.

2. **Ans. is b i.e. Horizontal partial laryngectomy**

This is a case of T_2 supraglottic carcinoma

Treatment of Supraglottic cancer

T_1 lesions—respond well to radiation. They can also be excised with CO_2 laser

T_2 lesions—voice conserving supraglottic partial hemilaryngectomy with or without neck dissection if lung function is good, otherwise radiotherapy can be given to the primary cancer and the nodes

T_3 and T_4 lesions—often require total laryngectomy with neck dissection and post op radiotherapy

3. **Ans. is b i.e. Bilateral cordectomy** *Ref. Dhingra 3/e, p 367; Devita 7/e, p 699*

In a smoker, hoarseness of voice with reddish area overlying both cord suggest leukoplakia or keratosis or early carcinoma.
Bilateral cordectomy is not recommended in leukoplakia.

Leukoplakia or keratosis

- Mostly involves *upper surface of one or both cords.*
- Appear *as white to reddish warty growth* over cord.
- Mostly present with ***hoarseness.***
- As lesion is precancerous ***treatment is stripping of the vocal cord*** or endoscopic removal by CO_2 laser and subjecting tissue for histology.
- Regular observation and follow up is necessary.
- *Smoking* and other *laryngeal irritant should be eliminated.*

4. **Ans. is d i.e. He should first undergo laryngectomy and then post-operative radiotherapy.** *Ref. Dhingra 4/e, p 284 - 285; 3/e, p 372*

Perichondritis suggest invasion of thyroid cartilage or T_4 lesion for which treatment is total laryngectomy with post operative radiotherapy.

Treatment of Ca larynx		
Stage	***Site***	***Treatment***
T_1	All site	External beam radio therapy
T_2	Glottic and subglottic lesion	Radiotherapy
	Supraglottic lesion	Supraglottic laryngectomy
T_3 and T_4	All sites	Total laryngectomy with neck dissection for clinically positive nodes with post operative radiotherapy

Indication of Total laryngectomy in Ca larynx *... Dhingra 4/e, p 286*

- T3 lesions (i.e. with *cord fixed*)
- All *T4* lesions
- *Invasion* of thyroid or cricoid cartilage
- Bilateral *arytenoid* cartilage involvement
- Lesions of *posterior commissure*
- *Failure* after radiotherapy or conservation surgery
- *Transglottic cancers* i.e. tumors involving supraglottis and glottis across the ventricle, causing fixation of the vocal cord.

Remember : Total laryngectomy is contraindicated in patients with distant metastasis.

For staging, kindly see theory portion.

5. **Ans. is a, b, c and d i.e. Glottis is the most common site; Commonly metastasize to cervical lymphnode; Lesions seen at the edge of vocal cord; and Laryngeal compartment acts as barrier** *Ref. Dhingra 4/e, p 285*

Laryngeal carcinoma			
	Supraglottis	***Glottis***	***Subglottis***
Site	• Epiglottis (Both supra and infrahyoid) • Aryepiglottic folds (laryngeal aspect only) • ***Ventricular bands*** (or false cord) • Ventricles	• True cords (anterior commisure, posterior commisure)	• Subglottis up to lower border of cricoid cartilage
Frequency	25-30%	• 70% (MC)	• 1-2 %

Contd...

Contd...

	Supraglottis	*Glottis*	*Subglottis*
Nodal metastasis	• Occurs early to upper and deep cervical nodes	Very rare	• Occur to pre-tracheal, pre-laryngeal nodes
Differentiation	• Poor	• Well	• Moderate
Most common symptom	• Pain on swallowing or	• Hoarseness	• Stridor neck mass
Prognosis	• Poor	• Best	• Good

Remember : Most common site of Ca larynx is free edge or upper margin of anterior 2/3 of vocal cord.

6. **Ans. is a, d and e i.e. Glottic ca is the most common; T1 tumour is best treated by radiotherapy; and Smoking predisposes** *Ref. Dhingra 4/e, p 283*

Predisposing factor far Ca larynx :

- **C**hronic Laryngitis
- **A**lcohol
- **L**eukoplakia
- **A**sbestosis
- **R**adiation
- Mustard **G**as
- **E**xposure to petroleum products
- **S**moking

***Mnemonic* : CA LARGES**

Tumour of Salivary Gland

What's Important ?

- Types
- General Features

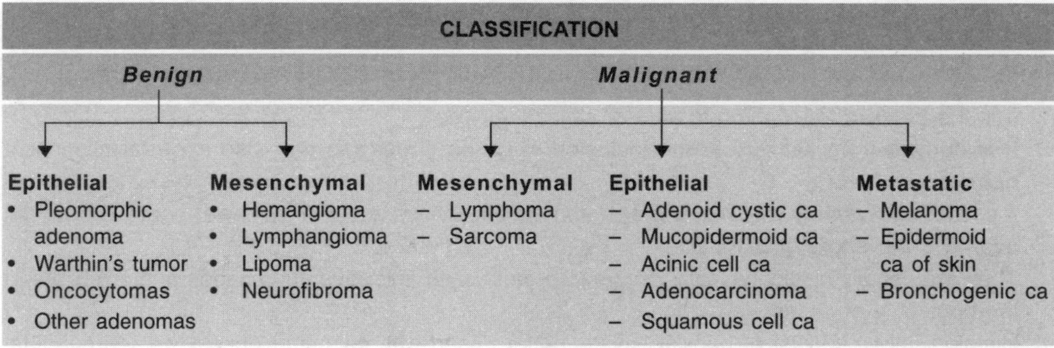

General features

- ***Most*** salivary gland tumor are benign, pleomorphic adenoma being most common.
- CT and MRI scanning (more sensitive) are the ***most helpful*** imaging techniques.
- ***Open surgical biopsy is contraindicated*** as this may seed the tumor to surrounding tissue.
- FNAC is a safe alternative to open biopsy and is the ***investigation of choice*** for salivary gland swelling.
- Treatment is excision not enucleation as tumor has microscopic extension outside capsule.
- Major salivary gland involved more commonly than minor salivary glands.
- Most common *Benign tumour of parotid in children* is ***hemangioma.***
- *Malignancy varies inversely* with the ***size of gland*** (90% of minor salivary gland tumours are malignant).
- Most common ***site of minor salivary gland tumor*** *is oral cavity principally on hard palate.*
- Majority of salivary gland tumours are radioresistant.
- Parotid gland accounts for 80% of all neoplasm, 15% arise from submandibular, and 5% arise from sublingual and minor salivary gland.

PLEOMORPHIC ADENOMA (MIXED TUMOUR)

- It is the MC benign salivary gland tumour. It is the MC tumour of major salivary gland.
- Most common site is ***parotid gland*** and it is the MC tumour of parotid gland.
- Most common site in parotid gland is ***tail (superficial lobe).***
- It is slow growing lobular tumour affecting women around 40 years.
- It consist of epithelial and mesenchymal (myoepithelial) cells.
- It is encapsulated but it sends pseudopods into surrounding glands. So *enucleation is not done* as a treatment.
- Present as painless swelling with typical site at below the lobule of ear.
- Usually not involve the facial nerve and infiltration of nerve is a sure indication of caracinomatous change.
- Malignant transformation occur in approximate 3 - 5% of cases which is apprehended by rapid growth, pain, stony hard tumour, fixed to masseter deeply or to skin superficially, enlarged cervical nodes, restriction of jaw movement.
- **Treatment of parotid tumour :** Superficial parotidectomy (***Patey's operation***).
- **Treatment of submandibular gland tumour :** *Excision of whole gland with particular care to preserve lingual and hypoglossal nerves.*
- **Treatment of palatal growth :** Incision is made over tumor and excision is done.

PAPILLARY CYSTADENOMA LYMPHOMATOSUM (WARTHIN'S TUMOR/ ADENOLYMPHOMA)

- It is the ***second*** MC *benign tumour of salivary glands.*
- It is derived from salivary tissue inclusion in lymph nodes (so can also arise from cervical nodes).
- It occurs ***exclusively in parotid gland*** and almost always occur in the lower portion of parotid overlying the *angle of mandible.*
- They are usually cystic, typically occurs in ***men*** in sixth and seventh decades and are bilateral in about 10% of cases.
- Histologically it consist of papillary-cystic pattern lined with columnar oncocytes and cuboidal cells with marked lymphoid component.
- ***Smoking*** ↑ its risk.
- *It never involves facial nerve.*
- It shows **hot spot *in 99Tc^{M} scan*** which ***is diagnostic.***
- *Treatment of choice* is ***superficial parotidectomy.***

Remember : – *It is the only salivary gland tumour which is more often seen in* ***men.***
– *Beside Warthins other tumours of parotid shows cold spot in 99Tc^{M} scan.*

MALIGNANT TUMOURS

Adenoid cystic carcinoma (Cylindroma)

- It is the MC ***cancer of minor salivary gland***
- It is poorly encapsulated infiltrating tumour arise from the ducts so also arise from accessory salivary glands *(called as* cylindroma*)* and trachea, bronchi, paranasal sinuses pharynx, lacrimal glands.
- It is as common in submandibular as in parotid gland.

- It has tendency to ***invade perineural space and lymphatics*** which causes pain (may be prominent and early symptom) and VII nerve paralysis.
- TOC is ***radical parotidectomy*** with largest cuff of grossly normal tissue around the boundaries of tumour. Postoperative radiation is given if margins of resected specimen are not free of tumour.

Remember : Unlike other salivary gland tumors it is ***more radiosensitive.***

Mucoepidermoid carcinoma

- It is MC *malignant salivary gland tumour in both adults and children* ... *CSDT 13/e p 258*
- MC site is parotid and it is the MC malignant tumour of parotid.
- It is MC ***radiation induced*** neoplasm of salivary gland.
- It consist of mixture of squamous cells, mucous - secreting cells, intermediate cells and clear or hydropic cells.
- ***It is divided into :***

Low grade type	High grade type
• Well circumscribed mass having cystic mucinous material • ***Mucin*** producing cells predominate • More common (usually in children) • ***TOC*** superficial or total parotidectomy	• Grossly infiltrative and has less tendency to cyst formation (hard tumour) • ***Squamous*** cells predominate • Less common • Total parotidectomy ± radical neck dissection

- Greater the epidermoid element more malignant is the behaviour of tumour.
- It usually not cause facial paralysis.

Acinic cell adenocarcinoma

- Rare tumor with low grade malignancy affecting women mostly.
- Tumor occurs ***almost exclusively in the parotid gland.***
- Present as round or ovoid solitary encapsulated tumor.
- Histologically tumor is characterized by highly cellular structure with relative absence of stroma.
- Tumor tends to involve the regional lymph nodes.
- Treatment is ***radical excision.***

Papillary adenocarcinoma

- Extremely rare tumor which can grow large.
- Histologically characterized by hemorrhage and necrosis.

Squamous cell carcinoma

- Seen mostly in ***submandibular gland.***
- Tumor arises from squamous ***metaplasia*** of the lining epithelium of the ducts.
- This is ***only tumor*** which ***responds*** to *radiotherapy* so, irradiation therapy is usefull.

Metastatic carcinoma

- Tumor that most commonly metastasize to the parotid gland are ***epidermoid carcinoma of skin*** and malignant melanoma.

Carcinoma ex-pleomorphic adenoma

- Carcinoma arising from pleomorphic adenoma
- **Sudden rapid growth** in previously stable parotid mass is commonest presentation
- Histologically malignant cell can take the form of any epithelial malignancy except acinic cell
- This carcinoma has predilection for **nodal involvement**
- Treatment include radical surgical resection with postoperative radiotherapy

QUESTIONS

1. **Acinic cell carcinomas of the salivary gland arise most often in the : [AI 06]**
   a. Parotid salivary gland
   b. Minor salivary glands
   c. Submandibular salivary glands
   d. Sublingual salivary glands
2. **Mixed tumors of the salivary glands are : [AI 06]**
   a. Most common in submandibular gland
   b. Usually malignant
   c. Most common in parotid gland
   d. Associated with calculi
3. **In which one of the following head and neck cancer perineural invasion is most commonly seen : [AI 05]**
   a. Adenocarcinoma
   b. Adenoid cystic carcinoma
   c. Basal cell carcinoma
   d. Squamous cell carcinoma
4. **Warthin's tumour is : [AIIMS 05, 03]**
   a. An adenolymphoma of parotid gland
   b. A pleomorphic adenoma of the parotid
   c. A carcinoma of the parotid
   d. A carcinoma of submandibular salivary gland
5. **True statement[s] about salivary gland tumours: [PGI 07]**
   a. Pleomorphic adenoma can arise in submandibular gland
   b. Warthin's tumour arises from submandibular gland
   c. Pleomorphic adenoma is most common tumour of submandibular gland
   d. Acinic cell ca is most malignant
   e. Frey's syndrome can occur after parotid surgery
6. **Following are the indications for radiotherapy in salivary gland tumor [PGI 09]**
   a. Facial nerve involvement
   b. High grade
   c. Perineural invasion
   d. Recurrency

ANSWERS, REFERENCES, EXPLANATIONS WITH INFORMATIVE ILLUSTRATIONS

1. **Ans. is a i.e. Parotid salivary gland**

Ref. Short case by S. Das 3/e, p 79; Schwartz 8/e, p 539

Acinic cell carcinoma is a low grade malignant tumor occur almost exclusively in parotid gland.

Remember : All salivary gland tumor are most common in parotid gland *except adenoid cystic carcinoma* (most common in minor salivary gland) and ***squamous cell carcinoma*** (most common is submandibular gland).

Important points about Acinic cell carcinoma :

- Affect exclusively *parotid gland*
- *Low grade* malignancy
- *Hypercellular* tumor with ***relative absence of stroma***
- Treatment is ***radical excision.***

2. **Ans. is c i.e. Most common in parotid gland** *Ref. Bailey & Love 25/e, p 761*

In total 80-90% of tumors of parotid gland are benign the most common tumor being pleomorphic adenoma = Mixed tumor.

Remember : ***The old Mnemonic***
- **80% of salivary gland tumor occur in parotid.**
- **80% of parotid gland tumor are pleomorphic adenoma.**

Other options :
- Only 7% of pleomorphic adenoma occur in submandibular salivary gland.
- Malignant change is seen in only 3-5% of cases, chance is more for old tumor

3. **Ans. is b i.e. Adenoid cystic carcinoma**

Ref. Short Case by S Das 3/e p 79; Schwartz 9/e, p 506

Perineural invasion is the most constant microscopic finding in adenoid cystic carcinoma.

Adenoid cystic carcinoma (Cylindroma)
- Most common minor salivary gland tumor.
- ***Characterized*** by its tendency to invade perineural space and lymphatics and thus causes ***pain*** (which may be prominent and early symptom) and ***VII nerve paralysis.***
- ***Skip lesions*** along nerves are common and local extension beyond gross tumor leading to late recurrence.
- It is ***treacherous tumor*** as it appears benign even when it is malignant.
- Treatment of choice is ***radical parotidectomy*** *irrespective of its benign appearance under the microscopy.*
- Distant metastases to lung, brain and bone.

4. **Ans. is a i.e. An adenolymphoma of parotid gland** *Ref. CSDT 13/e, p 257*

- Warthin's tumour or papillary cystadenoma lymphomatosum is 2nd MC benign tumour account for 10% of parotid tumours.
- It arise **exclusively** from parotid gland.
- It almost always occur in ***older males.***
- Most common ***site is tail of parotid.***
- It is *bilateral* in ***10%*** cases.
- It consist of papillary cystic pattern lined with cuboidal and columnar cells with core of lymphoid tissue.
- Treatment of choice is superficial parotidectomy but because of its benign nature and since it can be easily diagnosed cytologically, *surgical removal is not always necessary especially in older or unhealthy person.*

5. **Ans. is a and e i.e. Pleomorphic adenoma can arise in subhmandibular gland; and Frey's syndrome can occur after parotid surgery**

Ref. Surgical Short Case 3/e, p 82; Bailey & Love 25/e, p 762

Frey's syndrome (gustatory sweating) **is an universal sequelae following parotid surgery.**

Complications of parotid gland surgery include :

- Haematoma formation
- Infection
- Transection of the facial nerve and permanent facial weakness; sialocele
- Facial numbness
- Frey syndrome
- Numbness of ear lobe due to greater auricular nerve transection
- Sialocele

6. **Ans. is a, b, c, d i.e. All options are correct** *Ref. Devita 8/e, p 868*

Radiotherapy is indicated for malignant recurrence not for benign recurrence.

Indication of radiotherapy in salivary gland tumours

- Low grade neoplasm with close or positive margin
- Facial nerve involvement
- Multiple regional node metastasis
- High grade histology
- Deep lobe involvement
- Perineural invasion
- Recurrence malignant tumors.

Remember :
- Treatment of choice for pleomorphic adenoma is superficial parotidectomy (patey's operation).
- FNAC is investigation of choice for any salivary gland swelling.
- As such pleomorphic adenoma is radioresistant.

Tumour of Oral Cavity and Oropharynx

What's Important ?
- Commonest Site
- Premalignant Lesion
- Treatment

- Most common cancer of oral cavity in World : ***Ca tongue***
- Most common cancer of oral cavity in India : ***Buccal mucosa > Anterior tongue***
- Most common type of oral cancer is squamous cell carcinoma.

Etiology and Risk factors

- Smoking of tobacco
- Spiritis (alcohol)
- Sepsis
- Sharp jagged tooth and ill fitting dentures
- Syndrome of plummer vinsion (iron deficiency anemia)
- Syphillic glossitis
- Sideropenic dysphagia
- **Premalignant conditions :**
  - Leucoplakia
  - Erythroplakia
  - Chronic hyperplastic candidiasis
- **Risk is doubtful :**
  - Oral lichen planus
  - Discoid lupus erythematosus
  - Dyskeratosis congenita.

Investigation

- Incisional biopsy is recommended in all cases.
- FNAC done for lump in neck especially suspicious lymph nodes.
- MRI when available is IOC.

Staging

Irrespective of site same staging is recommended for all oral cavity tumours.

T stage :	
T1	Tumor 2cm or less in greatest dimension
T2	Tumor more than 2cm but not more than 4cm in greatest dimension
T3	Tumor more than 4cm in greatest dimension
T4 *Lip*	Tumor invades adjacent structures (eg, through cortical bone, tongue, skin)
T4 *Oral cavity*	Tumor invades adjacent structures (eg, through cortical bone, into deep [extrinsic] muscle of tongue, maxillary sinus, skin
N stage	
NX	Regional lymph nodes cannot be assessed
N0	No regional lymph node metastasis
N1	Metastasis in a single ipsilateral clinically positive node, 3cm or less in greatest dimension
N2	***Metastasis in :***
	N2a Single ipsilateral lymph node more than 3cm but not more than 6cm in greatest dimension
	N2b Multiple ipsilateral lymph nodes, none more than 6cm in greatest dimension
	N2c Bilateral or contralateral lymph nodes, none more than 6cm in greatest dimension
N3	Metastasis in a lymph node more than 6cm in greatest dimension
M Stage	
MX	Presence of distant metastasis cannot be assessed
M0	No distant metastasis
M1	Distant metastasis

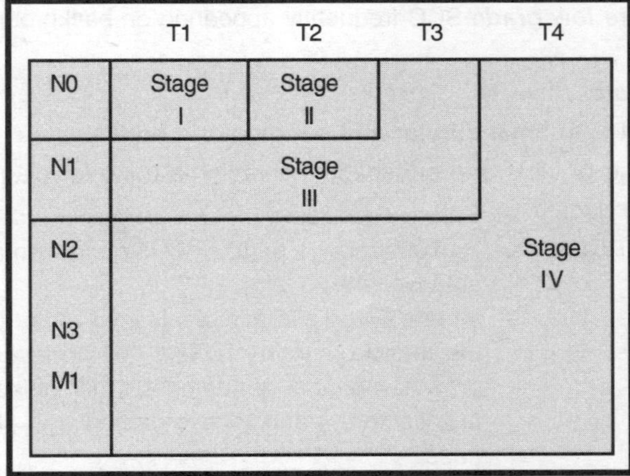

CLASSIFICATION

- According to site oral cavity carcinoma is divided into :

Carcinoma Lip

- Most common site is vermilion of lower lip and MC type is squamous cell Ca.
- Typically seen in **males** of 40 - 70 year (MF = 15 : 1).
- There is definite correlation between lip cancer and exposure to ***sunlight.***

- Non healing ulcer or growth is a common presentation.
- It is locally malignant, Lymph node metastases develop late.
- **Treatment**
  - Surgery is preferred for lower lip lesion upto 2 cm in diameter that do not involve the commissure ... *Devita 8/e p 830*
  - Radiation is preferred for lesion involving the commissure, for lesion over 2 cm in length, and for upper lip carcinoma ... *Devita 8/e p 830*
  - Advanced lesion with bone, nerve or node involvement frequently requires a combined approach.
  - Surgical treatment involve V or W shaped excision with lateral tumor free margin of 5 mm.

Reconstruction of Lip

- Necessory when more than 1/3rd of lip is excised
- **Commonly used flaps are:**
  - Abbe-Estander Flap (= Sair advancement technique)
  - Karapandzic flap
  - Webster or Benard flap (For very large defect)

Carcinoma cheek

- Most common site is the ***angle of mouth*** or the line of occlusion of upper and lower teeth. It may be ***multicentric.***
- Most malignant tumor are ***low grade*** SCC frequently appearing on background of leukoplakia or lichen planus.
- Typically occur in ***old male.***
- Lymphatic spread is first to **submandibular and subdigastric nodes.**
- Wedge biopsy from edge of ulcer and orthopentomography is done for diagnosis.
- **Treatment :**

Stage I *(T1N0)* :	– Surgical exicision
Stage II *(T2N0)* :	– Radiotherapy to primary lesion and also nodes if bone is not involved. – If bone (Maxilla /mandible) is involved or growth infiltrates the muscle, surgery is TOC, which involves excision of growth, marginal or segmental mandiblectomy (or partial maxillectomy) and reconstruction with skin or mucosal, flaps.
Stage III and IV :	– Radical surgery followed by postoperative RT with reconstruction

Reconstruction : For cheek reconstruction mucosal flaps are used :

Mucosal flaps		
In males - Forehead Flap based on *anterior branch of superficial temporal artery* can be used	***In females*** - Deltopectoral flap based on perforating branch of *internal mammary artery* is used	***PMMC flap*** (pectorais major myocutaneous flap) It is *most widely used flap* for head and neck reconstruction

Carcinoma Tongue

- Most common site of carcinoma tongue is ***middle of lateral border*** or ventral aspect of tongue.
- Most common variety is ***ulcerative***. It is divided into two types :

1. ***Carcinoma oral tongue (subsite of oral cavity)***
   - Commonly seen in men in age of ***50-70 years.***
   - Most common complaint is ***mild irritation*** of tongue. *... Devita 8/e p 834*
   - Most carcinoma occur on middle and posterior thirds of oral tongue.
   - The first nodes involved are subdigastric and submandibular nodes.
   - For diagnosis Wedge biopsy taken from edge of ulcer of tongue but in *proliferative growth, punch biopsy is taken.*
   - **Treatment :**

Tx	– *Excisional biopsy* or local resection. CO_2 laser can also be used for small T1 also
T1 and small T2	– *Partial glossectomy* with primary closure.
T2 and T3	– *Partial glossectomy* followed by postoperative radiotherapy
T4	– Combined surgery (total glossectomy, mandibulectomy, neck node dissection one or both side, laryngectomy) and post operative radiation.

Remember : – Preoperative radiation is given only if nodes are fixed.
– **Most common** and serious toxicity of oral radiotherapy is xerostomia.

- **Management of recurrence :**
  - Recurrence mostly develops ***within 2 years.***
  - It is differentiated from radiaton induced necrosis by the absence of necrosis.
  - Radiation failure is managed by glossectomy.
  - Surgery failure is managed by radiation usually but if recurrence is limited to mucosa it is managed by surgery and if recurrence is in the soft tissue of neck no treatment is successful and palliation is indicated.

Remember : Commondo's operation is indicated when carcinoma is fixed to mandible with infiltration of floor of mouth. It consist of Hemimandibulectomy and removal of floor of mouth and radical neck dissection.

2. ***Carcinoma of posterior one third or base of tongue (subsite in oropharynx)***
   - It remains asymptomatic for long time and patient present with metastases in cervicalnodes.
   - ***Earlier symptoms :*** Sore throat, feeling of lump in throat and slight discomfort on swallowing.
   - The first nodes involved are subdiagastic (level II), spread is then along the Jugular chain to the midjugular level III and lower jugular (level IV nodes).
   - **Treatment :**
     - ***T1 and T2 with N0 or N1 :*** Surgical excision with block dissection is preferred and if neck dissection specimen reveals a stage more than N1, postoperative radiation is added.

- ***T3 and T4 lesion :*** Surgical excision with mandibular resection, neck dissection and postoperative radiation.
- ***T4 lesion which also extend into Anterior 2/3 of tongue or valleculae :*** Total glossectomy and laryngectomy in addition to block dissection with or without chemotherapy.
- ***For advanced cancers, or in patient with poor health :*** only palliation with radio or chemotherapy.

Remember :
- Posterior 1/3 tongue has very less cornification but has abundant lymphatics so it cause massive lymphadenopathy.
- Blind spot in oral cavity : (i.e. Where carcinomatous lesion is not visible)
  - *Posterior 1/3 of tongue*
  - *Retromolar trigone*
  - *Gingolabial sulcus.*

Alveolus / gingiva and hard palate

- Alveolar mucosa overlies the bone of the mandible and maxilla. Retromolar trigone lies behind the third molar
- Carcinoma in these location is characterized by early involvement of bone
- **Clinical Features:**
  - Patient usually present to dentist with ill fitting dentures, pain, loose teeth or a sore that will not heal. Retromolar trigone lesion can cause referred pain to external auditary canal and preauricular area. Invasion to pterygoid muscle produce trismus
- **Treatment:**

  T1 and T2 – Surgery, radiation for superficial lesion involving large area

  T3 and T4 – Surgery with postoperative radiation

Note:

Type of presentation of oral cavity tumor	Treatment
• Mucosal lesios with mandibular approximation, ***freely mobile***	– Wide local excision with removal of adjacent periosteum
• Mucosal lesions with isolated adherence to the mandible ***lingual*** aspect	– Lingual sagittal marginal mandibulectomy
• Mucosal lesion with isolated adherence to mandible ***gingival*** aspects	– 'Rim' - coronal marginal mandibulectomy
• Gross cortical invasion involving alveolar ***margin, inferior alveolar nerve*** involvement	– Segmental mandibulectomy

QUESTIONS

1. **The commonest site of oral cancer among Indian population is : [AIIMS 05]**
   a. Tongue
   b. Floor of mouth
   c. Alveobuccal complex
   d. Lip
2. **Carcinoma tongue most frequently develops from: [PGI 08]**
   a. Tip
   b. Lateral margin
   c. Dorsal portion
   d. All portions equally
3. **The most common pre-malignant condition of oral carcinoma is : [PGI 07]**
   a. Leukoplakia
   b. Erythroplakia
   c. Lichen planus
   d. Submucosal fibrosis
4. **A patient present with carcinoma of right lateral border of tongue with level III lymph nodes on left side of a size of 4 cm. Staging is : [AIIMS 07, 06]**
   a. No
   b. N_1
   c. N_2
   d. N_3
5. **In which of the following head and neck cancer lymph node metastasis is least common: [AIIMS 08]**
   a. Tongue
   b. Buccal mucosa
   c. Hard palate
   d. Lower alveolus

ANSWERS, REFERENCES, EXPLANATIONS WITH INFORMATIVE ILLUSTRATIONS

1. **Ans. is c i.e. Alveobuccal complex** *Ref. ASI 1/e, p 348*

Frequency of various cancer of oral cavity in India are :

- ***Buccal mucosa 38%***
- Anterior tongue 16%
- Lower alveolus 15%.

So, Most common site of oral cancer among Indian population is buccal mucosa or in this question Alveobuccal complex, can be taken as correct option.

Remember : Most common site of oral cancer in world : Tongue

Most common malignant tumor of adult *males in India* – ***Oral cancer***
Most common malignant tumor of *female in India* – ***Carcinoma cervix***
Most common malignant tumor of *female in World* – ***Carcinoma breast***
Most common malignant tumor of adult *males in World* – ***Lung carcinoma.***

2. Ans. is b i.e. Lateral margin *Ref. Dhingra 4/e, p 211*

"Most common site of carcinoma tongue is middle of lateral border or the ventral aspect of the tongue. followed by tip and dorsum."

Cancer	Most common site
Lip	Vermillion of lower lip
Tongue	Lateral border
Cheek	Angle of mouth
Nasopharyngeal carcinoma	Fossa of rosenmuller
Larynx	Glottis

3. Ans. is a i.e. Leukoplakia *Ref. Bailey & Love 25/e, p 735*

Lesions and conditions of the oral mucosa associated with an incresed risk of malignancy.

Premalignant conditions	Conditions increasing risk	Risk is doubtful
– Leukoplakia *(MC)*	– Oral submucosal fibrosis	– Oral lichen planus
– Erythroplakia	– Syphilitic glossitis	– Discoid lupus erythematosus
– Chronic hyperplastic candidiasis	– Sideropenic dysphagia	– Dyskeratosis congenita

Important points of leukoplakia

- Defined as ***clinical white patch*** that can't be characterized clinically or pathologically as any other disease.
- Features suggestive ***malignant change*** in leukoplakia are induration, speckled or nodular appearance.
- Chances of malignant changes in leukoplakia increases with *increases in age of lesion and age of patient.*
- Most common ***site*** is buccal mucosa and oral commisures.
- Tobacco smoking and chewing are main etiological factor.
- If patient stops smoking for 1 year, it will disappear in 60% of cases.
- ***All lesion*** must be biopsied and send for histology.
- **Treatment :**

Degree of dysplasia	Treatment
– Mild to moderate epithelial dysplasia	Follow up at 4 month interval
– Severe dysplasia or carcinoma in situ	Surgical excision or CO_2 laser exicison

Remember : Incidence of malignant change in erythroplakia is 17 fold higher than leukoplakia.

4. **Ans. is c i.e. N_2** *Ref. Dhingra 4/e p 213*

Guy's don't get confuse by level of nodes, as N stage in TNM staging of oral cavity ca depends only on size of nodes not level.

N stage		
NX	Regional lymph nodes cannot be assessed	
N0	No regional lymph node metastasis	
N1	Metastasis in a single ipsilateral clinically positive node, 3cm or less in greatest dimension	
N2	***Metastasis in :***	
	N2a	Single ipsilateral lymph node more than 3cm but not more than 6cm in greatest dimension
	N2b	Multiple ipsilateral lymph nodes, none more than 6cm in greatest dimension
	N2c	Bilateral or contralateral lymph nodes, none more than 6cm in greatest dimension
N3	Metastasis in a lymph node more than 6cm in greatest dimension	

5. **Ans. is c i.e. Hard palate** *Ref. Internet*

Incidence of lymph node metastasis in head and neck cancer *(In decreasing order)*

- Tongue
- Floor of mouth
- Lower alveolus
- Buccal mucosa
- Upper alveolus
- Hard palate
- Lip

Lymph nodes site	Lymph node level	Primary cancer site
Submental group	Level I	Cental part of lower lip, tip of tongue and central part of floor of mouth
Submandibular gland	Level I	Inner angle of eye, side of nose, ***cheek,*** angle of mouth, whole of upper lip, outer part of lower lip, gums, sides of anterior 2/3 of tongue.
Upper jugular nodes	Level II	Oral cavity, oropharynx, hypopharynx, larynx, salivary gland
Mid jugular	Level III	Oral cavity, oropharynx, hypopharynx, larynx, thryoid
Lower jugular nodes	Level IV	Oropharynx, hypopharynx, larynx, cervical esophagus, thyroid
Accessory nerve nodes	Level V	Nasopharynx, scalp
Supraclavicular nodes	Level V	Breast, lung, gastrointestinal tract
Anterior compartment group	Level VI	

16 Lung and Pleural Tumour

What's Important ?

- Paraneoplastic Syndromes
- Histologic Types

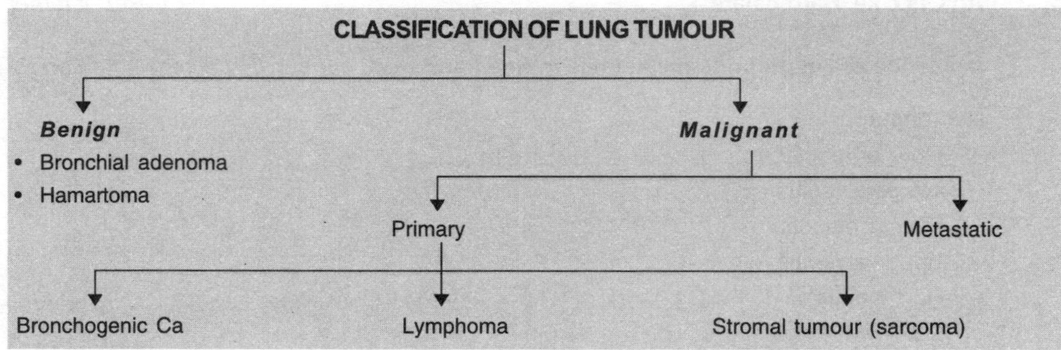

BRONCHOGENIC CARCINOMA

- Tumours arising from respiratory epithelium of bronchi, bronchioles and alveoli.
- *Most common* of all lung neoplasm.
- Lung cancer is the most common ***malignancy*** of humans and also most *leading cancer causing death.* Incidence of lung cancer is increasing.

Etiology and risk factors

Smoking – Risk increase *both* in active (13 times) and passive (1.5 times) smoking. Main carcinogen are nitrosamines, polycyclic aromatic hydrocarbons such as benzopyerene. 87% of lung Ca are associated with smoking.

Women have higher susceptibility to carcinogenic effect of smoking.

Industrial hazards – Important elements associated with lung cancer are *Uranium; Nickel; Asbestos; Cobalt; Cadmium.*

Air Pollution – *Radon* in air ↑ risk of lung carcinoma.

Scars in lung – Scars in lung mostly old infarct may progress to lung ca *mostly Adenocarcinoma.*
Diet: Vitamin A deficiency increase risk while carrots and tomatoes appear to have protective effect.

Radiation: Thoracic radiation increase the risk.

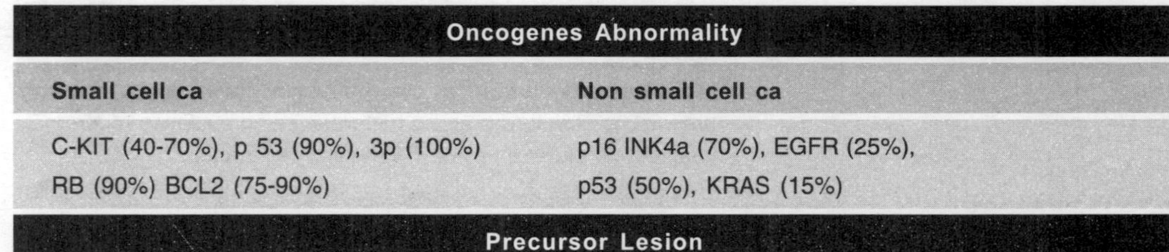

Oncogenes Abnormality	
Small cell ca	**Non small cell ca**
C-KIT (40-70%), p 53 (90%), 3p (100%) RB (90%) BCL2 (75-90%)	p16 INK4a (70%), EGFR (25%), p53 (50%), KRAS (15%)

Precursor Lesion

1. Squamous dysplasia and ca in situ
2. Atypical adenomatus hyperplasia
3. Diffuse idiopathic pulmonary neuroendocrine cell hyperplasia

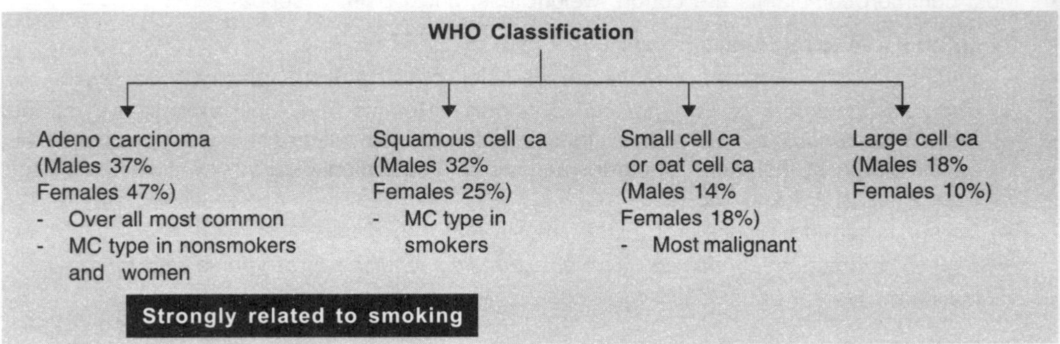

Remember : ***Bronchoalveolar*** is a special *subtype of adenocarcinoma* arising from peripheral airways.

Morphology and Pathology

Bronchogenic ca arise mostly in and about ***hilus of lung except*** bronchoalveolar ca and some adenocarcinoma.

- **Adenocarcinoma :**
  - Located somewhat *peripherally* arise from smaller airways.
  - *Grows slowly* than other types. Precursor lesion is atypical adenomatous hyperplasia.
  - Less frequently associated with history of smoking.
  - Most cells contain *mucin* and majority are positive for thyroid transcription factor 1 (TTF 1)
- **Squamous cell carcinoma :**
  - Arise from larger *central bronchi.* However incidence of peripheral SCC is increasing.
  - Histologically characterized by presence of keratinization
  - Metastasize late but *locally aggressive.*
  - *Strongly* related to smoking.
  - Focal areas of necroses and hemorrhage in bulk tumour .
- **Small cell ca :**
  - Highly malignant, Cells are small with little cytoplasm called ***"oat cell".***
  - *Strongly* related to smoking.
  - Basophillic staining of vascular wall (***Azzopardi effect***) is seen frequently.

- **Bronchoalveolar carcinoma:**
  - Occurs in terminal bronchoalveolar regions as solitary or multiple nodules
  - Histologically tumour is characterized its by growth along preexisting structure (Lepidic pattern) with no evidence of stromal, vascular or plural invasion or alveolar destruction
  - Ultrastructurally they contain mucin secreting bronchiolar cells, clara cells, or rarely type II pneumocytes
- **Large call ca :** – Probably represent *highly undifferentiated* squamous cell or adenocarcinoma.

Clinical features

- Most common complaints are cough, weight loss, chest pain, dyspnea
- **Symptoms due to regional spread :**
  - Tracheal obstruction; oesophagial compression causing dysphagia; RLN paralysis.
  - *Pancoast syndrome (= Superior sulcus tumor)* - Results from local extension of tumour (*usually squamous cell Ca*) growing in apex of lung with involvement of C8-T2 spinal nerves causing pain in ipsilateral shoulder and ulnar distribution of arm often with radiologic destruction of 1st and 2nd rib.
  - *Horner syndrome :* Ipsilateral miosis, ptosis and anhydrosis.
  - *SVC syndrome, Precordial and cardiac extension resulting in arrythmia and tamponade.*
  - Malignant pleural effusion.

Metastasis

Adrenal is *most common* site of metastasis > liver > brain. *... Robbins 8/e, p 723*

Remember : *Bronchoalveolar* ca may spread *transbronchially* by aerosolisation.

Paraneoplastic syndromes

Cardiovascular	**Gastrointestinal**	**Hematological**
Thrombophlebitis Non bacterial thrombotic endocarditis	Carcinoid syndrome (carcinoid and small cell)	Leukoerythroblastosis Anemia Thrombocytosis/penia Leukoerythroblastosis
Neuromuscular	**Metabolic**	**Dermatologic**
Dementia (adenocarcinoma) Optic neuritis, retinopathy Limbic encephalitis Autonomic neuropathy (small cell) Myasthenic (Eaton-Lambert syndrome *(small cell)* Polymyositis	Inappropriate **ACTH** *(small cell)* Inappropriate **ADH** (small cell) **Hypercalcemia** (squamous cell carcinoma) (d/t ectopic PTH) Inappropriate gonadotropins Hypoglycemia *Cushing syndrome*	Acanthosis nigricans Dermatomyositis Ichthyosis Hypertrichosis Hyperkeratosis

Other :

- Hypertrophic pulmonary osteoarthropathy (squamous cell, large cell, and adenocarcinoma).
- Nephrotic syndrome, fever.

Diagnosis and Staging

- **Tissue diagnosis :** Tumour tissue can be obtained by *bronchial* or *transbronchial* biopsy through fiberoptic bronchoscopy; by percutaneous biopsy of enlarged node.
- Integrated PET-CT scan is the best imaging modality for diagnosis and staging.

... Devita 8/e, p 909

- **Staging :** Lung cancer staging consist of :
  - *Anatomic Staging :* Which decides *resectability* (whether the tumour can be removed completely by standard surgical procedure or not) It depends on *location* and *size* of tumor.
  - *Physiologic Staging :* Which decides *operability* (whether the patient can tolerate surgical procedure or not) Depends on *cardiopulmonary function* of patient.
  - *Staging of non small cell carcinoma :* TNM Staging should be used.

Stage	TNM Descriptors
IA	T1 N0 M0
IB	T2 N0 M0
IIA	T1 N1 M0
IIB	T2 N1 M0
IIIA	T3 N1 M0
	T1 – 2 - 3 N2 M0
IIIB	T4 N0 – 1 - 2 M0
	T1– 2 - 3 N3 M0
IV	Any T any N M1

Tumor (T) Status descriptor	
T0	No evidence of a primary tumor
Tx	Primary tumor cannot be assessed, or tumor proven by the presence of malgnant cells in sputum or bronchial washing but not visualized by imaging or bronchoscopy
TIS	Carcinoma in situ
T1	Tumour <3 cm in greatest dimension, surrounded by lung or visceral pleura, without bronchoscopic evidence of invasion more proximal than lobar bronchus (i.e. not in main bronchus)
T2	Tumor with any of following : > 3cm in greatest dimension ; involves main bronchus, ≥ 2cm distal to the carina; invades visceral pleura; associated with atelectasis or obstructive pneumonitis extending to hilum but does not involve entire lung.
T3	Tumor of any size that directly invades any of the following : chest wall (including superior sulcus tumors), diaphragm, mediastinal pleura, parietal pericaddium; or tumor in main bronchus < 2 cm distal to carina but without involvement of carina; or associated atelectasis or obstructive pneumonitis of entire lung.
T4	Tumor of any size that invades any of the following : mediastinum, heart, great vessels, trachea, oesophagus, vertebral body, carina; or tumor with a malignant pleural or pericardial effusion, or with a malignant pleural or pericardial effusion, or *with satellite tumor nodule within the ipslilateral primary-tumor lobe of the lung.*

Lymph node (N) involvement descriptor	
NX	Regional lymph nodes cannot be assesed
N0	No regional lymph node metastasis
N1	Metastasis to ipsilateral peribronchial and / or ipsilateral hilar lymph nodes, and intrapulmonary nodes involved by direct extentsion of the primary tumor.
N2	Metastasis to ipsilateral mediastinal and / or subcranial lymph nodes
N3	Metastasis to contralateral mediastinal, contralateral hilar, ipsilateral or contralateral mediastinal, scalene, or supraclavicular lymph
Distant metastasis Descriptor	
MX	Presence of distant metastasis cannot be assessed
M0	No distant metastasis
M1	Distant metastasis present

*Tumour nodule in ipsilateral non primary tumor lobe of lung is classified as M1

– *Staging of small cell lung carcinoma :* A simple two system is used :

a. *Limited -stage disease :* Seen in **30%** of patient. Defined as disease confined to *one hemi thorax and regional lymph nodes* including mediastinal, contralateral hilar and ipsilateral supraclavicular.

b. *Extensive disease :* Seen in **70%** of patient. Defined as disease exceeding the boundaries of limited disease Contralateral supraclavicular node; RLN involvement; SVC obstruction can be part of limited disease while cardiac tamponade, malignant pleural effusion and B/L pulmonary parenchyma involvement comes under extensive disease.

Resectability and Operability

In Patients with non small cell Ca contraindications to resection are :

ABSOLUTE	RELATIVE
Distant metastasis *(except solitary brain or adrenal metastasis)*	Metastasis higher than midtracheal lymph nodes
Malignant pleural effusion; Cardiac tamponade	Pericardial involvement
Bilateral endobronchial tumor (curable by radiotherapy)	Recurrent laryngeal nerve paralysis; Horner syndrome
Contralateral lymph node metastasis (curable by radio therapy)	Main pulmonary artery involvement
SVC syndrome *(due to metastatic tumor)* MI with in *3 months;* Uncontrolled major arrhythmias	SVC syndrome *(due to primary tumor)* MI with in *6 months*
Significant pulmonary hypertension	FEV_1 < 50% and insufficient pulmonary reserve for resection
Tumor *within 2 cm of carina* (curable by radiotherapy)	

In patient with resectable tumor but with borderline lung function exercise test is performed to estimate max O_2 consumption (V max O_2). V max $O_2 \geq 15$ ml/kg predicts high risk of post operative complication.

Treatment

Non-small cell ca

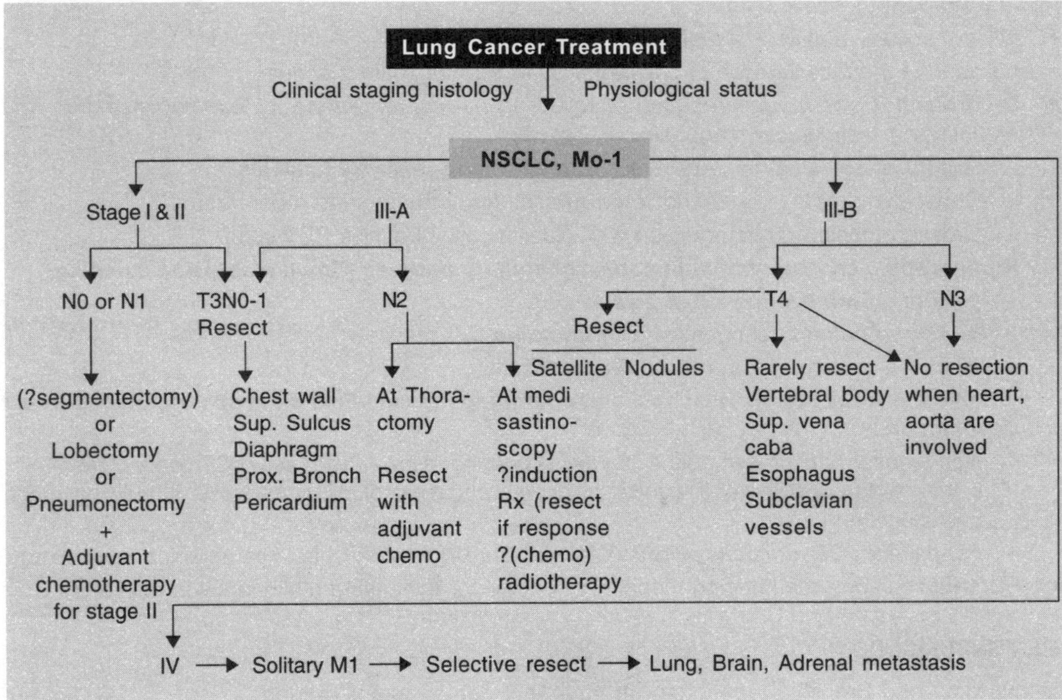

Selected special cases of stage IIIA :

- *Tumor with chest wall invasion (T-3)* - En bloc resection of tumor with chest wall and postoperative RT.
- *Pancoast tumor (T-3)* - Preoperative RT followed by En bloc resection of lung and chest wall with consideration of postoperative RT or intraoperative brachytherapy.
- *Involvement of proximal airways (Tumor with in 2 cm of carina)* - Pneumonectomy or sleeve resection with preserving distal airways.

Chemotherapeutic agents effective in NSCLC are:

- Carboplatin or cisplatin
- Paclitaxel or docetaxel
- Gemcitabine
- Bevacizumab (anybody against VEGF)
- Eritonib (inhibitor of EGPR kinase)

Small cell ca

- *Limited stage disease :* Combination CT + Chest RT; Consider resection of peripheral tumor.
- *Extensive stage :*
  - Combination CT; RT for palliation.
  - Most widely used chemotherapy combination is etopaside + cisplatin or carboplatin

Occult and stage 0 carcinoma

Situation when malignant cells are identified on sputum but chest radiography appears normal. Treatment is *removal of tumor* and conservation of lung parenchyma.

SOLITARY PULMONARY NODULE (COIN LESION)

- Defined as X-Ray density surrounded by normal aerated lung with circumscribed margin of any shape with *size < 6 cm.*
- **10%** of solitary nodule are *malignant.*
- **CT** scan *is the investigation of choice for evaluation of solitary nodule.*
- *If no diagnosis is made presence of following risk factor will be in favor of resection and establishing histological diagnosis :*
  - History of smoking – Age ≥ 35 years growth of relatively large lesion.
  - Chest symptoms – Associated atelectasis, pneumonitis, adenopathy.
  - Growth of lesion on comparison with older X ray – Positive PET scan.
- ***Radiographic criteria of benign nature of solitary nodule : (Small stable and calcified)***
  - *Lack of growth* over period of *2 year.*
  - *'Bulls eye pattern'* (suggestive of ***granuloma***).
  - *"Popcorn pattern"* (***hamartoma***) of calcification.
- ***When older X ray are not available and characteristic calcification is absent, management depends on :***
  - *Non smoker patient with age ≤ 35 year should be followed* with serial CT every 3 month for a year than once yearly if significant growth occur histological diagnosis should be made by resection.
  - *For patient ≥ 35 years and all with history of smoking* nodule should be *resected* for histology.
- **FDG PET** scan is the imaging modality of choice for evaluating malignancy in coin lesions

BENIGN TUMOURS

Hamartoma and Bronchial adenoma are important benign tumor of lung.

a. **Bronchial Adenoma :**

- ***Slow growing*** endobronchial tumor, mostly *central.*
- Represent **50%** of all benign tumor.
- Most of bronchial adenoma are *carcinoids.* *... Harrison 17/e p 562*
- Usually present as *recurrent haemoptysis* as they are hyper vascular, they can also bleed during biopsy.
- Bronchial adenoma must be *dealt as potentially malignant.*
- ***Surgical excision*** is the primary treatment of all bronchial adenoma.

b. **Hamartoma :**

- They represent normal pulmonary tissue components in disorganized fashion.
- *Popcorn calcification* is pathognomic for hamartoma.
- If popcorn calcification is not found lesion should be resected.

METASTATIC PULMONARY TUMORS

- Usually present as ***solitary*** pulmonary shadow. Tumors most prone to metastasis to lung include colon Ca, RCC, Breast Ca.
- Even in patient known to have extrathoracic neoplasm a *solitary nodule should be approached as lung cancer.*

- CT is the most effective method for imaging lung metastasis.
- Important tumors whose pulmonary metastasis can be resected are :
  - Colon
  - Rectum
  - Uterine
  - Cervix
  - Breast
  - Kidney
  - Bladder tumor.

LUNG CANCER SCREENING

- Historically X-ray chest and sputum cytology were used to screen lung cancer in high risk patients. But there was no benefit and these had been withdrawn.
- Recently low dose CT (LDCT) has become available as screen mode and once again prompting interest for screening of lung cancer.

QUESTIONS

1. **In a 56 year old chronic smoker there was a mass in bronchus which is successfully resected. This mass is most likely to be positive for: [AIIMS 2009]**
   a. Cytokeratin
   b. Vimentin
   c. Epithelial membrane cadherin
   d. Leukocyte
2. **Which of the following has no infectious etiology: [AIIMS 2009]**
   a. Nasopharyngeal ca
   b. Hepatocellular ca
   c. Non small cell lung ca
   d. Gastric ca
3. **Which of the following statements about small cell carcinoma is true? [AI 2009]**
   a. Bone metastasis is uncommon
   b. Peripheral in location
   c. Chemosensitive tumor
   d. Paraneoplastic syndrome with ↑PTH is common
4. **Most common site of metastasis in lung Ca: [AIIMS May 07]**
   a. Liver b. Adrenal
   c. Bone d. Brain
5. **A 65 year old miner has lost 7 kgs weight within two months, has presented with cough, and blood streaked sputum. He was treated for pulmonary tuberculosis 10 years ago. He also has drooping of his left eyelid for one month. On physical examination, there is ptosis of the left eye and papillary miosis. Chest X-ray revealed round opacification in the left upper apical lobe. What is the most probable diagnosis : [AIIMS 06]**
   a. Secondary tuberculosis
   b. Adenocarcinoma
   c. Squamous cells carcinoma
   d. Asbestosis
6. **Lung to lung metastasis is seen in :**
   a. Adenocarcinoma of lung **[AIIMS 05]**
   b. Squamous cell carcinoma of lung
   c. Small cell carcinoma
   d. Neuroendocrine tumor of lung
7. **True about carcinoma bronchus is :**
   a. 75% are SCC **[AI 2010]**
   b. Cavitation is most common in oat cell type
   c. Perihilar lymphadenapathy is most common in oat cell type
   d. Peripheral nodule is more commonly seen in squamous cell ca.
8. **Ture about Lung Carcinoma : [PGI 09]**
   a. Adenocarcinoma most common
   b. Squamous cell Ca most common
   c. Originates from type-II pneumocytes
   d. Oat Cell (Neuroendocrine cells)
   e. Sq. cell carcinoma peripherally located.

ANSWERS, REFERENCES, EXPLANATIONS WITH INFORMATIVE ILLUSTRATIONS

1. **Ans. is a i.e. Cytokeratin.**

Ref. Tumor Diagnosis by Awatif, 2/e, p 630-640, Fishman 4/e 848

Cytokeratin positivity is seen in almost all non small cell ca due to their epithelial origin

..... *Fishman Pulmonary disease, 4/e, 1848*

Immunophenotype of various bronchogenic carcinoma

Adenocarcinoma : 80% express TTF-1, and CK7, 60% express CEA and over 90% express Ber Ep4.

Bronchoalveolar carcinoma : Mucinous type is TTF-1 negative, exhibit linear staining for laminin and type IV collagen

Non-mucinous type is TTF-1 positive while laminin and type IV collagen staining is absent.

Small cell ca : Tumor express one or more epithelial cell markers (cytokeratin, epithelial membrane antigen, CET)

CD-56 and TTF-1 are often positive, and the lesion may also stain for one or more neuroendocrine marker (neuron specific enolase, chromogranin, leu-7, VIP)

Squamous cell ca : The cells show diffuse staining with cytokeratins and they show no staining with CD-56 or neuroendocrine markers.

Clear cell variant shows intracytoplasmic glycogen (PAS-diastase) and are positive for ck-14.

Note: Leukocyte common antigen (LCA), CD30 and other B, T cell marker are the immunohistochemical stains most frequently used to exclude lymphoma

..... *Fishmann*

2. **Ans. is c i.e. Non small cell lung ca** *Ref. Harrison 17/e, p 552*

Lung ca is not associated with any infectious agent

Other choice

Nasopharyngeal ca	:	Ebstein barr virus
Hepatocellular ca	:	Hepatitis B virus
Gastric ca	:	Helicobacter pyori

3. **Ans is c i.e. Chemosensitive tumor** *Ref. Harrison 17/e p 561*

Small cell lung ca is chemosensitive disease

Feature	Small cell carcinoma	Non small cell carcinoma
Location	• ***Central***	Peripheral
Metastasis	• ***Highly metastatic lesion*** with widespread metastasis at time of diagnosis	Less metastatic than small cell carcinomas

Contd...

Contd...

	• Common site of metastasis include brain, bone (Osteolytic) liver and adrenals • Osteolytic	
Paraneoplastic syndrome	• *ACTH* • *AVP (Vasopressin)* • *Calcitonin* • *Neurologic*	• PTH
Response to chemotherapy	*Superior Response* *Overall regression rate is 60-80%* Rate of complete regression 30%	*Inferior Response* *Shrinkage in 30-50%* Complete response is very rare

4. **Ans. is b i.e. Adrenal** *Ref. Robbin's 8/e, p 723*

Most common site of metastasis from Ca lung are adrenal > livers brain.

Spread of Lung carcinoma

Direct : To invade contiguous structures such as mediastinum, pleura, great vessels, heart, esophagus, diaphragm, metastasis within lung occur as a result of aerosolization, embolization.

Lymphatic : Usually precedes systemic dissemination.
Most lymphatic drainages of lung ultimately reach *right superior mediastinum and right supraclavicular nodes,* so they are prone to involve.

Hematogenous : Most common **site** of distant metastases is adrenal followed by liver, brain and bone. In bone osteolytic secondaries are more common.

5. **Ans. is c i.e Squamous cell carcinoma** *Ref. Robbin's 8/e, p 725; Harrison 17/e, p 553*

Guy's this is case of Horner's syndrome secondary to superior sulcus squamous Cell ca.

Features	Adenocarcinoma	SCC
Cell of origin	Mucous glands	• Bronchial epithelium
Incidence	Most common lung ca in females	• More common in males
Smoking	Less frequent association	• Almost 100% association
Pathology		
Morphology	Located peripherally	• Tends to grow in central bronchi
Histology	Characterised by presence of keratinization and / or intracellular bridge	• Shows formation of gland or secretion of inulin

Contd...

Contd...

Clinical features		
Cough	+++	++
Hemoptysis	+/–	+
Bronchial obstruction	Less common	Common
Horner syndrome (due to compression of cervical chain by apical lobe tumor	Less common	Common
Pancoast syndrome (due to compression of C_8, T_1, T_2)	Less common	Common

Pancoast's Syndrome (= Superior sulcus syndrome)

- It resultls from local extension of tumor (usually squamous cell ca) growing in apex of lung with involvement of C8-T2 leading to shoulder pain that characteristically radiates to ulnar distribution of arm often with radiologic destruction of 1st and 2nd rib.
- Often Pancost syndrome and Horner syndrome (Ptosis, miosis, anhydrosis, enopthalmos) co-exist.
- Results from SCC of the extreme apex either in left or right lung in the superior sulcus (a shallow furrow on the surface of lung).

Treatment

- Preoperative RT and cisplatin and Etoposide followed by En bloc resection of lung and chest wall with consideration of postoperative RT or intraoperative brachytherapy.

Remember:
- Horner syndrome and SVC syndrome are also caused by local extension of tumor.
- Pancost tumor is associated with favourable prognosis.

6. **Ans. is a i.e. Adenocarcinoma** *Ref. Schwartz 8/e, p 560; Robbin's 8/e, p 725*

Lung to lung metastasis is seen in bronchoalveolar carcinoma which is an atypical subtype of adenocarcinoma.

Bronchoalvelaor carcinoma spread aerogenously to forming ***satellite tumours*** in lung and may spread ***transbronchially to contralateral lung.***

Bronchoalveolar carcinoma

- Carcinoma arising from terminal airways (terminal bronchioles or alveoli).
- It is thought to arise from surfactant producing clara cells or from type II pneumocytes.
- The key histologic feature is their growth along the pre-existing structures without distruction of alveolar architecture (lepidic growth pattern).

7. Ans. is c i.e Perihilar Lymphadenopathy *Ref. Grainger 4/e, p 468*

Feature	Type of bronchogenic Ca associated
Massive hilar or mediastinal lymphadenopathy	Small Cell Ca
Mediastinal invasion	Small Cell Ca
Perihilar mass	Small Cell Ca
Peripheral nodule	Adenocarinoma (72%) > large cell tumor (63%)
Cavitation	Squamous cell ca
Collapse/Consolidation	Squamous cell ca

Remember: – *Collapse, Consolidation, Presence of hilar enlargement are the cardinal signs of central tumor.*

Features suggestive of pneumonia secondary to obstructing neoplasm:
- Presence of pneumonia in a patient in the cancer age group, confined to one lobe, that remain unchanged for more than 3 weeks.
- Alteration in shape of collapsed, consolidated lobe, in case of lobar collapse fissure may show a bulge (**Golden S sign**) as a result of underlying mass
- Presence of visible mass or irregular stenosis
- Presence of enlarged hilar nodes
- Presence of mucous filled dilated bronchi

8. Ans. is a and d i.e. Adenocarcinoma most common, Oat Cell (Neuroendocrine cells)
Ref. Robbins 8/e p 727

Presence of neuroendocrine markers such as chromogranin, synaptophysin, and CD-57 suggest derivation of oat cell tumor from neuroendocrine progenitor cells of lining bronchial epithelium. *... Robbins*

Types of Bronchogenic Ca (in decreasing order)

Males	Females
– Adenocarcinoma (37)	– Adenocarcinoma (47%)
– SCC	– SCC
– Large cell ca	– Small cell ca
– Small cell ca (14%)	– Large cell ca (10%)

Heart and Mediastinal Tumour

What's Important ?

- **Paraneoplastic Syndromes**
- **Classification of Mediastinal Masses**
- **Thymoma**

Primary tumors of heart are rare. 75% of primary heart tumor are benign with myxoma being most common.

MYXOMA

- Most common ***primary*** cardiac tumour.
- Age : **30 - 60;** F > M
- Sporadic or familial or part of syndrome that includes **NAME** syndrome (pigmented **n**evi, **a**trial myxoma, **m**yxoid neurofibroma, **e**phelides; **LAMB** syndrome (**l**entigenes, **a**trial **m**yxoma and **b**lue nevi).

Pathology :

- Consist of ***myxoma cells*** embedded in a stroma rich in glycosaminoglycans.
- Most common **site :** – Left atria (for sporadic)
  – Ventricle for (familial and syndromic)
- Most commonly orginates from ***inter arterial septum*** in vicinity of fossa ovalis.

Clinical feature :

- Mostly *mimics that of* ***mitral valve disease*** (either obstruction or regurgitation).
- Ventricular myxoma present as subaortic or subpulmonic stenosis.
- Symptoms are of ***sudden onset*** or ***positional*** in nature.
- On auscultation "Tumor plop" a low pitch sound audible during ***early*** or ***middiastole.***
- ***Constitutional signs includes :*** Fever, weight loss, cachexia, malaise, athralgia, rash, clubbing, raynauds phenomenon, anemia, polycythemia, hypergammaglobulinemia, leucocytosis, increase ESR, thrombocytopenia, thrombocytosis.

Diagnosis : Trans thoracic and transesophageal echocardiography (IOC).

Treatment :– *Excision*
– Chance of recurrence is more in familial cases.

SARCOMA

- Most common ***primary malignant*** tumor of heart.
- Mostly involve ***right side*** of heart.
- *Prognosis* is very poor.

SECONDARY TUMOR (More common)

- More common than primary tumors of heart.
- Most common site - Pericardium
- Most common site of primary : *Male* - Ca lung
  - Ca breast.
- Tumor with *highest risk of cardiac metastases* - Malignant melanoma.
- Pericardium is most likely to be induced.

Treatment :

- As most patient has widespread disease, treatment is mainly symptomatic.
- *Malignant pericardial effusion* - treated by pericardiocentesis with instillation of sclerosing agent (e.g., Tetracycline).

MEDIASTINAL TUMOURS

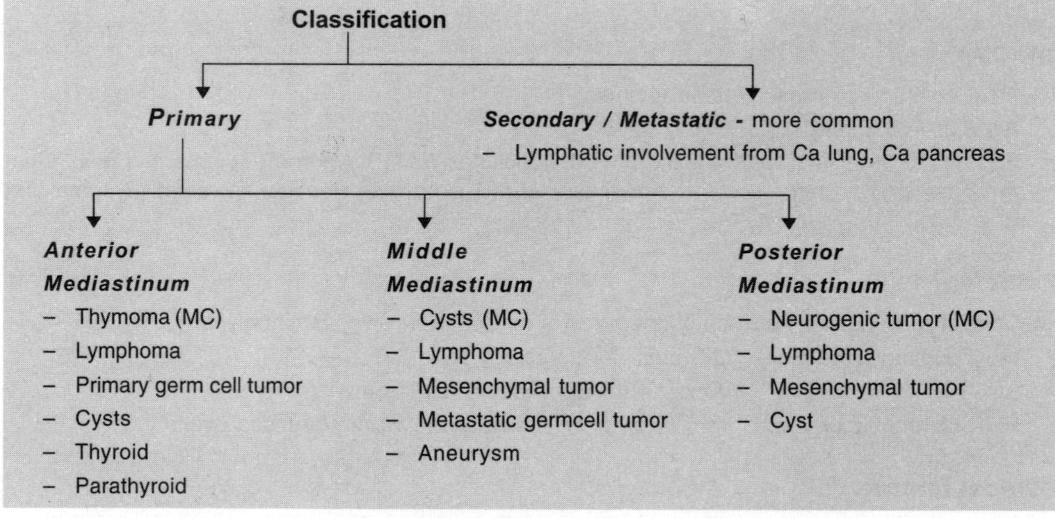

- Most common tumor of mediastinum ***in adult*** : Metastatic
- Most common *primary* tumor of mediastinum ***in adult*** : Thymoma
- Most common tumor of mediastinum in ***pediatric age group*** : Neurogenic
- ***CT scan*** is most useful technique in evaluating mediastinal masses.

THYMOMA

- Most common neoplasm of thymus.
- Most common **site** is *anterior mediastinum.*
- They can be non invasive (with intact capsule) or invasive which penetrate through the capsule into surrounding structure

Clinical feature :

- ***Mostly asymptomatic*** (found during chest X-ray), but may cause dysphagia, dyspnoea, SVC syndrome and variety of paraneoplastic.
- **Paraneoplastic syndromes :**

Autoimmune	Hematological	Neuromuscular disorder
– SLE – Rheumatoid arthritis – Polymyositis – Sarcoidosis	– Cytopenias – Red cell aplasia – Hypogammaglobulinemia – Erythrocytosis	– *Myasthenia gravis* (**MC** paraneoplastic syndrome) – Neuromuscular disorder – Myotonic dystrophy. – Myositis

Diagnosis :

- **CT :** Investigation of choice (IOC).
- **Definitive diagnosis** only on histological study of tissues.

Staging :

- ***Masoaka staging*** system is used.

Treatment :

"Treatment of choice is total thymectomy which is performed through median sternotomy."

- *Posterior lateral thoracotomy or clamshell (bilateral anterior thoracotomy) or trapdoor incision* are used for resection of *advance stage thymoma.*
- *Larger thymoma (> 5 - 6 cm) with evidence of invasion,* are being treated with combined agent induction chemotherapy.
- *Myasthenia gravis* is treated with thymectomy and anti-cholinesterase drugs.

NEUROGENIC TUMORS

- Most common mediastinal mass in both adults and children ... *CSDT 13/e p 332*
- In young children (< 4 years) they are invariably malignant
- Most common *site* : ***posterior mediastinum.***
- Mostly arise from ***nerve sheath*** (schwannoma and neurofibroma) and are mostly *benign.*
- ***MRI*** is necessary to *determine their extension to spinal canal.*
- ***Treatment :***
  - ***Complete resection*** is *treatment of choice.*
  - Approach is through ***posterolateral*** thoracotomy.
  - For < 6 cm lesion ***thoracoscopic*** approach can be sufficient.

CYSTIC LESION

- Arise from ***pericardium*** (Most common), bronchi, oesophagus or thymus.
- Pericardial cyst are also called ***spring water*** or mesothelial cyst.
- Mostly *located* near ***cardiophrenic angle on right side.***

GERM CELL TUMOR

- Mostly metastatic.
- Most common type ***seminoma.***

- **Treatment :** *Combination chemotherapy* and *multimodality therapy* (surgery and radiation therapy).

Approach for Exposure of mediastinum	
– Median sternotomy	- Anterior mediastinum
– Posterolaleral thoracotomy	- Posterior and middle mediastinal mosses
– VATS	- All mediastinal compartment (small masses)
– Bilateral anterior thoracotomy	- All mediastinal compartments.

QUESTIONS

1. **Thymoma is associated with: [AI 2008]**
   a. Myasthenia gravis
   b. Hypergammaglobulinemia
   c. SLE
   d. Multiple sclerosis
2. **Most common tumor in the posterior mediastinum is : [AI 2008, PGI 09]**
   a. Neurofibroma
   b. Teratoma
   c. Lymphoma
   d. Bronchogenic cyst
3. **A patient presents with mediastinal mass with sheets of epithelial cells giving arborizing pattern of reactivity alongwith interspersed lymphoid cells. The probable diagnosis would be :**
   a. Thymoma **[AIIMS May 08]**
   b. Thymic carcinoid
   c. Primary mediastinal lymphoma
   d. Non-Hodgkin lymphoma
4. **Myxoma is most likely to occur in :**
   a. Left atria **[PGI June 08]**
   b. Right atria
   c. Left ventricle
   d. Right ventricle
5. **True statement is /are: [PGI-09]**
   a. Thymoma is the most common mediastinal tumor
   b. Lymphoma is the most common anterior mediastinal tumor
   c. Thymoma is associated with polycythemia
   d. Germ cell tumor responds best to chemotheropy

ANSWERS, REFERENCES, EXPLANATIONS WITH INFORMATIVE ILLUSTRATIONS

1. **Ans. is a i.e. Myasthenia Gravis** *Ref. Devita 8/e, p 977*

Paraneoplastic syndromes of Thymoma	
• ***Autoimmune disorders***	• ***Endocrine disorder***
– SLE – Polmyositis – Rheumatoid arthritis – Ulcerative colitis – Hashimoto's thyroiditis – Myocarditis	– Hyperthyroidism – Hyperparathyroidism – Addison's disease – Panhypopitutarism
• ***Hematological***	• ***Neuromuscular***
– Red cell aplasia – Hypogammaglobulinemia – T-Cell deficiency – Pancytopenia – Megakaryocytopenia – Erythrocytosis	– Myasthenia gravis ***(MC)*** – Myotonic dystrophy – Polymyositis – Lambert eaton syndrome

Contd...

Contd...

- ***Miscellaneous***
  - Hypertrophic osteoarthropathy
  - Minimal change nephropathy
  - Pemphigus

Remember :
- Myasthenia gravis is most common paraneoplastic syndrome of thymoma seen in 30-50% of patient.
- *Thymoma is most common disorder associated with myasthenia.*
- Thymoma compress superior mediastinum which manifest as **SVC syndrome.**

2. Ans. is a i.e. Neurofibroma *Ref. CSDT 13/e, p 332; Devita 8/e, p 974*

Mediastinal Masses

- **Neurogenic** (MC *posterior mediastinal mass*) : – Neurofibroma
  - Schwanoma
- **Thymic** (Anterior mediastinal mass) : – Thymoma (MC *anterior mediastinal mass*)
  - Thymic carcinoma
- **Cysts** (All three compartments) : – Pericardial (MC *middle mediastinal mass*)
  - Bronchogenic
  - Enteric
- **Lymphoma** (Anterior, middle and rarely posterior) : – Hodgkin's disease
  - Histocytic lymphoma
- **Germ cell tumor** (*primary* in *anterior mediastinum* and *metastatic* in *middle and posterior*) : – Seminoma
  - Non seminoma
- **Mesenchymal tumors** (all three compartments)
- **Aneurysms** (Middle and posterior).

3. Answer is a i.e. Thymoma *Ref. Devita 8/e p 976*

Presence of epithelial cells along with *lymphoid cells is suggestive of type B thymoma.*

World Health Organization Classification System for Thymic Epithelial Tumors

Tumor Type	Cells	Clinicopathologic Classification	Histologic Terminology
A	Spindle or oval	Benign thymoma	Medullary
B	Epithelioid or dendritic	Malignant thymoma (Category I)	Cortical, organoid
–B1			Lymphocyte-rich; predominately cortical
–B2			Cortical
–B3			Well-differentiated thymic carcinoma

Contd...

Contd...

AB	Benign thymoma	Mixed
C	Malignant (Category II) thymoma	Nonorganotypic; thymic carcinoma, epidermoid keratinizing and nonkeratinizing carcinoma, sarcomatoid carcinoma, clear cell carcinoma, basaloid carcinoma, mucoepi-dermoid carcinoma, undifferentiated carcinoma.

4. **Ans. is a i.e. Left atria** *Ref. Harrison 17/e, p 1494*

Important points about Myxoma

- Age 30-60, F > M
- Sporadic (MC); familial; syndromic (associated with LAMB syndrome, NAME syndrome)
- Most common site ***left atria*** (for sporadic)
- Most common site ***ventricle*** (for familial and syndromic)
- Most common site of *origin* - ***Inter atrial septum***
- Most common symptom - ***Mimics mitral stenosis***
- Investigation of choice - Transophageal ***echo***
- **Treatment** - Excision

Remember : Most common tumor of heart is not myxoma rather it is secondary metastases from lung (in males) and breast (in females).

5. **Ans. is a Thymoma is the most common mediastinal tumor** *Ref. Devita 8/e p 975*

Thymoma is the MC mediastinal mass in adults
Neurogenic tumor are MC mediastinal mass in pediatric age group

Option D

Treatment of Mediastinal Germ Cell Tumor

Tumor	Treatment
Teratoma (MC germ cell tumor in mediastinum)	Surgery
Seminoma	
– Small	Radiotherapy
– Bulky or advanced	Chemotherapy followed by radiotherapy
Nonseminomatous germ cell tumor	Chemotherapy

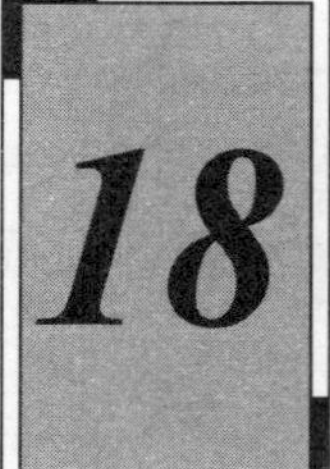

18 Oesophageal Tumour

What's Important ?

- Risk Factors
- Types
- Site

Classification	
Benign	*Malignant (more common)*
– Leiomyoma ***(MC)***	– Adenocarcinoma ***(MC)***
– Granular cell tumor	– Squamous cell Ca
	– Malignant melanoma
	– Sarcoma
	– Carcinoids
	– Secondary tumor

LEIOMYOMA

- Most common ***benign tumor*** of Oesophagus.
- Most common **site** *lower 1/3rd.*
- Mostly asymptomatic.
- *Barium swallow* is IOC.
- *Biopsy* is ***contraindicated*** as there is risk of hemorrhage and adhesion develop between tumor and mucosa, which makes removal of tumor difficult.
- ***Thoracoscopic or laparoscopic enucleation*** is treatment of choice. *... CSDT 13/e, p 442*

CARCINOMA OF OESOPHAGUS

- Age : > 50 years; Sex - M > F

Etiology and risk factors

Squamous cell ca	Adeno ca	
– Smoking	– Barret's esophagus	*Premalignant*
– Nitrites	– Chronic GERD	
– Ingestion of lye / corrosives	– Smoking	
– Chronic Achalasia		
– Alcohol		
– Extreme hot tea		
– Dietary deficiency of Mo, Vit A, Zn		
– Caustic ingestion		
– Radiation induced strictures		
– Congenital hyperkeratosis (Tylosis palmaris)	*Premalignant condition*	
– Radiation induced stricture		
– Plummer vinson syndrome		
– HIV infection		

Pathology

- **Type** – Squamous Cell Ca ***(MC)*** and Adeno Ca.
- **Site** – *Squamous Cell Ca* is the predominant type in upper and middle third of oesophagus. *... Devita 8/e, p 999*
  - *Adeno Ca* mostly arise in distal 1/3rd.
  - **Overall *MC* site of Ca oesophagus :** Lower/distal 1/3rd
    Middle 1/3rd of osophages is commonest site of SCC

Spread

- **Direct extension** – Intramurally with in oesophagus.
  – Extramurally to near by structures.
- **Lymphatic** – ***Upper*** 1/3rd metastasize to cervical LN.
  – ***Middle*** 1/3rd metastasize to mediastinal, paratracheal and tracheo bronchial nodes.
  – ***Lower*** 1/3rd metastasize to gastric and celiac group of nodes.
- **Hematogenous** – Lung, bone, liver and adrenal gland.

Clinical presentation

- ***Dysphagia:*** Most common symptom and suggest advance Ca. Initially dysphagia is for solids then for liquids, and in the end patient is even unable to swallow their saliva.
- Weight loss, weakness, anemia.
- Constant pain indicates extramural invasion.
- ***Coughing on swallowing*** indicates cancerous tracheoesophageal fistula.
- **Hoarseness :** Due to RLN palsy is a sign of advanced and incurable disease.

Diagnosis

- **Endoscopy :**
  a. *Esophagoscopy* is the diagnostic method of choice to determine whether mass is present and biopsy to establish tissue diagnosis
  Targeted biopsy can be enhanced by the use of chemoendoscopy techniques which uses dyes such as indigo carmine, Lugol's solution, methylene blue, and toulidine blue
  b. *In Lesion of upper 2/3rd bronchoscopy* is also indicated as the lesion may have invaded tracheobronchial tree.

- **Imaging study :**
  a. *Ba swallow :* – Narrowing of lumen with proximal dilation and shouldering (= Rat tail appear)
  – Upper border of tumor is horizontal and resemble shelf.
  b. *Chest X-ray:* A column of air in esophagus (due to tracheoesophagial fistula) with pneumonitis or pleural effusion is seen.
  c. *Endoscopic ultrasound :* Best method for ***preoperative staging*** of primary lesion and locoregional lymphnodes.
  d. *Abdominal ultrasound :* For liver metastasis.
  e. All patient should undergo CT abdomen, chest and pelvis, so as to evaluate the extent of disease

Treatment : **Curable :**

A. Surgery :

- *Surgical resection* is **treatment of choice.**
- *Contraindication for resection are :*
  – Tumor > 10cm
  – Horner syndrome
  – Direct spread to tracheobronchial tree or aorta
  – Paralysis of diaphragm
  – Vocal cord paralysis
  – Malignant pleural effusion
  – Tracheo esophageal fistula.
- *Resection involves : Subtotal esophagectomy, stomach proximal to left gastric vessel, spleen in cases of adenocarcinoma.*
- *Approaches for resection :*
  – Transhiatal which includes laparotomy and cervical approach.
  – **Transthoracic :**
    - Ivor lewis approach = Right thoracoabdominal approach
    - Left thoracoabdominal approach
    - Three incisional en bloc oesophagestomy = Mc KEOWN approach
- *Restoration of continuity* is achieved by transposition of stomach and oesophago gastric anastomosis.

For T_1 disease and high grade dysplasia endoscopic mucosal resection can be employed as treatment.

B. ***Chemotherapy :*** Chemotherapy never cures the disease but can shrink the tumor. Squamous cell ca are more sensitive than adenocarcinoma.

Palliative therapy :

- *Goal* of palliation is *relief of dysphagia.*
- *Gastrostomy* should *never be carried* out as the palliation.

... Bailey & Love 24/e, p 1012

- Surgical resection with external beam radiotherapy may be used.
- *Intubation* of oesophagus with celestin tube, Akinson tube.

Malignant tracheosophageal fistula :

Best treatment is expandable metal stent.

Prognosis

Five year survival rate is : – 9% for patient with squamous cell carcinoma.
– 20% for patient with adeno carcinoma.

QUESTIONS

1. **Predisposing factors for esophageal cancer are all except: [AIIMS Nov 2009]**
   a. Mediastinal fibrosis
   b. Diverticula
   c. Caustic alkali burn
   d. HPV

2. **Transhiatal esophagectomy was planned for adenocarcinoma of lower end of esophagus. The approach would be in the following order: [AIIMS Nov 2007]**
   a. Abdomen-Neck
   b. Abdomen-Thorax-Neck
   c. Neck-Thorax-Abdomen
   d. Abdomen-Thorax

3. **Stain used to find carcinoma while doing endoscopy:: [AIIMS May 2009]**
   a. Toluidine blue
   b. Gentian violet
   c. Hematoxylin and eosin
   d. Methyl red

4. **Barrets oesophagus is commonly associated with one of the following :**
   a. Adenocarcinoma **[AIIMS 06; PGI 97]**
   b. Squamous cell carcinoma
   c. Sarcoma
   d. Gastrointestinal stromal tumour

5. **Most common site for squamous cell ca esophagus is : [PGI 08]**
   a. Upper third
   b. Middle third
   c. Lower third
   d. Gastro-esophageal junction

6. **In Barret's oesophagus - true is : [PGI 06]**
   a. Metaplasia
   b. Peptic stricture
   c. Paraoesophageal hernia
   d. Squamous carcinoma

7. **Predisposing factor for oesophageal Ca:**
   a. Tylosis **[PGI 05]**
   b. Achalasia
   c. Barrets esophagus
   d. Hiatus hernia
   e. Corrosive ingestion

8. **Malignant tracheosophageal fistula is best treated by : [PGI 05]**
   a. Radiotherapy
   b. Chemotherapy
   c. Stenting
   d. Tube
   e. Surgical correction

9. **Barrett's esophagus shows: [AIIMS May 10]**
   a. Intestinal dysplasia
   b. Intestinal metaplasia
   c. Squamous cell metaplasia
   d. Columnar cell metaplasia

ANSWERS, REFERENCES, EXPLANATIONS WITH INFORMATIVE ILLUSTRATIONS

1. **Ans. is a i.e. Mediastinal fibrosis** *Ref. Harrison 17/e, p 570*

Etiologic factors for Esophageal cancer

- Excess *alcohol* consumption
- Cigarette *smoking*
- Other ingested carcinogens :
  - Nitrates (Converted to nitrites)
  - Smoked opiates
  - Fungal toxins in pickled vegetables.
- Mucosal damage from physical agents :
  - Hot tea
  - Lye ingestion / corrosives
  - Radiation-induced strictures
  - Chronic achalasia.
  - Caustic injury esophageal diverticula
  - Esophageal deverticula
- Host susceptibility
  - Esophageal web with glossitis and iron deficiency (i.e., Plummer-Vinson or paterson-Kelly syndrome).
  - Congenital hyperkeratosis and pitting of the palms and soles (i.e., tylosis palmaris et.plantaris).
- Dietary deficiency of molybdenum, zinc, vitamin A
- Celiac sprue
- Chronic gastric reflux *(i.e., Barrett's esophagus)* ***for adenocarcinoma.***
- Prior aerodigestive malignancy
- ***HPV Infection:*** HPV infection contributes in the pathogenesis of oesophagial squamous carcinoma in high incidence areas of Asia and Africa.

2. **Ans. is a i.e. Abdomen Neck** *Ref. Devita 8/e, p 1006; Maingoti's 11/e p 381-320*

Types of Oesophagectomy

Feature	*Transhiatal Oesophagectomy (THE) (safest)*	*Transthoracic Oesophagectomy (TTE) (Ivor-Lewis approach) (most common)*	*Triincisional En Bloc Oesophagectomy (EBE) (Mc KEOWN technique)*
Incisions	Upper midline abdomen Left neck	Upper midline abdomen Right posterolateral thoracotomy	Right thoracotomy Midline laparotomy Left neck
Anastomosis	Cervical oesophago-gastric	Intrathoracic oesopha-gogastric at or above the level of azygous vein	Cervical oesophogo-gastric
Lymphadenectomy	Neck, lower chest and abdomen	Thoracic, abdominal	Radical thorax, abdominal
Advantages	Less anastomotic leak rate (3%)	Lowest anstomotic leak rate	Allows loca! excision of enveloping tumour

Contd...

Contd...

Feature	*Transhiatal Oesophagectomy (THE) (safest)*	*Transthoracic Oesophagectomy (TTE) (Ivor-Lewis approach) (most common)*	*Triincisional En Bloc Oesophagectomy (EBE) (Mc KEOWN technique)*
	Less morbid cervical leak Less operative time	Complete staging possible	Improves survival if patient has ≤ 6 lymph nodes
Disadvantages	High rate of post-operative strictures, injury to great vessels and nearby structure Incomplete lymph node dissection, so staging can't done Not done if tumor invades pericardium, aorta or tracheo-bronchial tree	Thoracic leak can lead to intrathoracic infection, sepsis and death Pneumonia, effusion, respiratory failure, atrial fibrillation, MI, GERD causing Barretts oesophagus leading to recurrent and metachronous cancers	Anastomotic leak rate is high EBE> THE> TTE MC postoperative complications are pulmonary Morbidity and mortality is high EBE> TTE> THE

Remember: Vagal sparing Oesophagectomy/VSE: Same as THE but without vagotomy so pyloroplasty is not needed. In all other oesophagectomy vagotomy is done so pyloroplasty is indicated.

- **Advantage is better gastric function**

Minimal Invasive Oesophagectomy/MIE: Same as THE but done with thoracoscope-laparoscope technique

- **Advantage is less pain and short hospital stay**

3. **Ans is a i.e. Toulidine Blue** *Ref. Devia 8/e p 1001*

Diagnostic accuracy of endoscopic biopsy technique can be enhanced by use of chemoendoscopic techniques, which uses dyes such as indigo carmine, Lugol's solution, methylene blue and toulidine blue to highlight topographic features and epithelial changes.

Other techniques to enhance diagnostic capability of endoscopy
- Narrow band imaging: Both diagnostic and therapeutic
- Autofluorescence Imaging

4. **Ans is a i.e. Adenocarcinoma** *Ref. Harrison 17/e, p 1852; Bailey and Love 25/e p 1022*

Barret's Oesophagus
- ***Metaplasia of lower oesophageal squamous epithelium*** to intestinal like columnar epithelium in response to chronic GERD
- More common in men
- Normally the oesophagus is lined by squamous epithelium, in Barrets oesophagus the junction of squamous oesophageal mucosa and columnar gastric mucosa *moves proximally*
- When intestinal metaplasia occurs there is an increased risk of adenocarcinoma (25 times) *Ref... Bailey 25/e p 1022*
- **Classification:**
  A. Clinical
  - Classical long segment Barret's (3 cm or more columnar epithelium)

- Short segment Barret's (Less than 3 cm of columnar epithelium)
- Cardia metaplasia (*Intestinal metaplasia at the oesophagogastric junction without any macroscopic change at endoscopy)*

B. Pathological
- Gastric type
- Intestinal type - Most common
- Junctional type - Resemble gastric cardia

- **Investigation** Endoscopic biopsy is diagnostic (intestinal metaplasia with goblet cells in any length of oesophages is diagnostic)
- **Treatment**
  - Treat underlying GERD
  - Chemoprevention by proton pump blockers
  - Ablation by laser, photodynamic therapy
  - Argon-beam plasma coagulation

5. **Ans. is b i.e. Middle third** *Ref. Robbin's 7/e, p 807; Devita 8/e, p 1000*

Location of squamous cell ca :
- Upper 1/3 rd – 20%
- Middle 1/3rd – 50%
- Lower 1/3rd – 30% *... Devita 7/e, p 866*

Other important point about Oesophageal ca
- Most common ***site of Adeno ca*** : Lower 1/3rd
- Most common ***site of squamous cell ca*** : Middle 1/3
- Most important **risk factor for squamous** cell ca : Smoking
- Most important ***risk factor for adenocarcinoma*** : Barret esophagus and GERD.
- Most common ***type*** : Squamous cell ca > Adenocarcinoma
- Most common ***type in India*** : Squamous cell ca > Adenocarcinoma
- Most common ***site in world*** : Lower 1/3rd; while MC ***site in India*** : Middle 1/3 rd

6. **Ans. is a i.e. Metaplasia** *Ref. Bailey and Love 25/e p 1022*

Already explained, kindly see answer no. 4

7. **Ans. is a, b, c and e i.e. Tylosis; Achalasia; Barrets esophagus; and Corrosive ingestion**

Already explained, see answer no. 1 *Ref. Harrison 17/e p 570*

8. **Ans is c i.e. Metal stenting** *Ref. Bailey, 25/e, p 1035*

- Malignant trachea-oesophageal fistula is sign of incurable disease
- Some have advocated surgical bypass and oesophageal excision but this is a major procedure. An expandable metal stent is probably the best treatment
- Stent is placed through endoscope under fluoroscopic guidance

9. **Ans. is b i.e. Intestinal metaplasia** *Ref. Robbins 8/e p 770*

Barret's oesophagus is a complication of chronic GERD that is characterized by intestinal metaplasia within the esophageal squamous mucosa.

Diagnosis of Barrett esophagus requires both endoscopic evidence of abnormal mucosa above the gastroesophageal junction and histologically documented intestinal metaplasia. Intestinal metaplasia which is defined by the presence of Globlet cells is necessary for the diagnosis of Barret's oesophagus.

Note: There is confusion in ***option 'd'*** (columnar metaplasia). Guy's in Barret's esophagus there is metaplasia to intestinal type columnar cells.

So, intestinal type could be the better choice, hence answer.

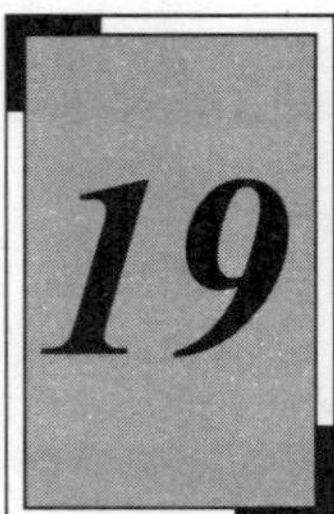

19 Gastric Tumour

What's Important ?

- Spread
- Early gastric carcinoma

GASTRIC ADENOCARCINOMA

- Most common tumor of stomach.
- Age - older age group (mean age 63); M > F.
- Gastric carcinoma is second most common (after lung ca) cause of cancer deaths.

Etiology and Risk factors

Acquired factors	Genetic factors	Precursor lesion
• *Nutritional* – High salt consumption – High nitrate consumption – Low dietary vitamin A and C – Poor food preparation (smoked, salt cured) – Poor drinking water (well water) • *Occupational* : – Rubber workers – Coal workers • *Cigarette smoking* • *Helicobacter pylori infection* • *Epstein-Barr virus* • *Radiation exposure* • *Prior gastric surgery for benign gastric ulcer disease.*	• *Type A blood group* • *Pernicious anemia* • *Family history* • *Hereditary nonpolyposis colon cancer* • *LI-Fraumeni syndrome*	• *Adenomatous gastric polyps* • *Chronic atrophic gastritis* • *Dysplasia* • *Intestinal metaplasia* • *Menetrier's disease* • Stomach remnant

Remember : Incidence of gastric adenocarcinoma is *decreasing* while carcinoma of gastric cardia is increasing now a days

Pathology

- **Site :** Most common site (in ↓ order) :
  - Proximal third (oesophagiogastric junction and cardia)

  - Pylorus and antrum (30%)
  - Fundus and body (20%). *... Harrison 17/e, p 572*

- ***Lesser curvature*** is more commonly involved then greater curvature.
- Pathological feature that has *greatest impact on survival* is depth of invasion.
- **Macroscopically** gastric cancer is divided in to 5 types :
  1. *Ulcerating carcinoma (25%) :*
     - Tumor extends through all layers of stomach. Resemble peptic ulcer but the edges are shallow in contrast to overhanging edges of benign ulcer.
  2. *Polypoid carcinoma (25%) :*
     - Large bulky intraluminal growth that tends to metastasize late.
  3. *Superficial spreading carcinoma (early gastric ca) (15%) :*
     - Carcinoma confined to mucosa and submucosa with or without lymphatic involvement.
     - This type has best prognosis.
  4. *Linitis plastica = Leather bottle stomach (10%)*
     - Tumour involved all the layer of stomach with marked desmoplastic reactions.
  5. *Advanced Ca (55%) :* Big tumor that is found partly with in and partly out side stomach.
- **Microscopy** : Lauren classification divides gastric carcinoma into :
  1. *Intestinal type :* (53%)
     - Resemble colonic carcinoma. Cells are differentiated and show expanding growth pattern.
     - Prognosis relatively good.
  2. *Diffuse type : (33%)*
     - Gastric type mucosa cells which do not form glands and show infiltrative growth, prognosis poor.
     - *Associated with loss of E-codherin* *... Robbins 8/e p 785*

Spread

- ***Local extension*** to near structures either directly (to duodenum) or by way of submucosal lymphatics (to oesophagus)
- ***Lymphatic :***
  - Tumors located at gastroesophageal junction have maximum chance of nodal metastases.
  - Most common node involved is *left gastric artery node.*
  - Spread along the intrathoracic lymphatic channel leads to metastases in *left supraclavicular node* (virchow node) *i.e. Troiser sign, left axillary nodes* (Irish node).
- ***Transperitoneal spread :*** Spread along the lymphatics of falciform ligament transperitoneally results in periumblical tumor deposits called as "sister marry Joseph nodes".
- ***Hematogenous :*** Most common site are liver > lung > bone.

Clinical features

- *Earliest symptoms* is **vague post prandial heavyness** which is usually neglected by patient.
- *Weight loss* is the most common symptom and represent advanced disease.
- Other symptoms are : Early satiety, hematemesis.

- *Ascites, jaundice or palpable mass* indicates ***incurable disease***.
- *Transverse colon* is ***most frequent site*** of malignant fistulization and obstruction from gastric primary tumor.
- A large krukenburg tumor or a large peritoneal implant in the pelvis (blumer's shelf) can cause ***rectal obstruction***.
- Enlarge virchow node or Sister Marry Joseph nodule may be the first sign.
- *Migratory thrombophlebitis* (Trouseau's sign) and deep vein thrombosis are paraneoplastic effects.

Investigations

- ***Tumor markers :*** CEA level correlates well with *tumor size and aggressiveness.*
- ***Endoscopy :*** – Best method (IOC) to diagnose gastric cancer.
  – Biopsy (*minimum 6* biopsy can be taken simultaneously).
- ***CT scan :*** CT of abdomen and pelvis is important part of staging.
- ***Laparoscopy :*** *Indicated in patients who have localized gastric ca after initial CT scan.* Purpose is to check any CT occult small volume metastases which is sign of inoperability.

Staging

- Two staging systems ***(AJCC and Japanese staging)*** are used :
- *American Joint Committee on Cancer Staging of Gastric Cancer, 2002*

Definition of TNM

Primary tumor (T)	
Tx	Primary tumor cannot be assessed
To	No evidence of primary tumor
Tis	Carcinoma in situ; intraepithelial tumor without invasion of the lamina propria
T1	Tumor invades lamina propria or submucosa
T2	Tumor invades muscularis propria or subserosa
T2a	Tumor invades muscularis propria
T2b	Tumor invades subserosa
T3	Tumor penetrates serosa (Visceral peritoneum) without invasion of adjacent structures
T4	Tumor invades adjacent structures
Regional lymph nodes (N)	
Nx	Regional lymph nodes cannot be assesed
No	No regional lymph node metastasis
N1	Metastasis in 1-6 regional lymph nodes
N2	Metastasis in 7-15 regional lymph nodes
N3	Metastases in more than 15 regional lymph nodes
Distant metastasis (M)	
Mx	Presence of distant metastasis cannot be assessed
Mo	No distant metastasis
M1	Distant metastasis

AJCC staging correctly tells about prognosis while Japanese staging correctly tells about exact extent of disease. *... Devita 8/e, p 1050*

Treatment

A. **Surgery :** Surgical resection is the *only curative* treatment. Goal of surgical resection is resection of whole tumor (Ro resection).

- ***Signs of inoperability are :***
  - Growth fixed to pancreas
  - Rectovesical deposit
  - Transperitoneal extension (Sister Marry Joseph nodes or krukenburg tumor)
  - Secondaries in liver
  - Enlarged fixed celiac mass
  - Enlarged supraclavicular nodes
  - Malignant ascites.
  - The standard operation for gastric ca is radical subtotal gastrectomy

... Schwartz 9/e p 933

- ***Stage I = Early gastric cancer***
  - *Endoscopic Mucosal resection (EMR)* : For well differentiated *superficial lesion smaller than 3 cm* in diameter, which are located in an easily accessible area.
  - *Limited surgical resection (LSR)* : For patient with < 3cm ulcerated intramucosal tumor and those with non ulcerated intramucosal tumor of any size. Procedure involves full thickness mural excision without nodal dissection.
  - *Gastrectomy with nodal dissection* : For patient with early gastric ca who can not be treated with EMR or LSR. Procedure involves removal of stomach along with removal of level 1 nodes, entire greater omentum and lesser omentum.

- ***Stage II and Stage III disease***
  - *For mid and distal half tumors:* Resection involves total or distal gastrectomy with enblock removal of omentum, a 3 - 4 cm cuff of duodenum, subpyloric lymphnodes and in some cases excision of left gastric artery and near by nodes.

    ... CSDT 13/e p 503
  - *For tumor of proximal half and for extensive tumors (linitis plastica)* : Total gastrectomy and splenectomy is required.
  - *For tumors of cardia* : Esophagogastrectomy plus splenectomy.

- ***Advanced disease :*** Palliative resection is indicated only when stomach is still moving and life expectancy is greater than 1 - 2 month.

B. **Chemotherapy** *:* Indicated *only in advanced disease*

Agent used are :
- 5FU (MC used)
- Cisplatin
- Mitomycin C and doxorubicin.

C. **Radiotherapy :** No role in either local or advanced gastric carcinoma. *Use is limited to palliation of symptoms such as bleeding or controlling pain* secondary to local tumor infiltration. However, *intraoperative radiotherapy* using ***electron beams*** can be used.

Prognosis

- 5 year survival rates is only 12%. However, for early gastric Ca 5 yar survival rate is 90%.
- Most important prognostic indicators are lymphnode involvement and depth of tumor invasion.

GASTRIC STROMAL TUMOR

- Previously called leiomyoma or leiomyosarcoma
- ***Stomach*** is MC site of *GI leiomyoma or leiomyosarcoma.*
- These are submucosal growth that are usually asymptomatic but may cause intestinal bleeding.
- Originates from ***interstitial cell of cajal.***
- Mostly *arise* from ***proximal stomach.***
- Spread is mostly hematogenous to liver, lung and bone.
- *Surgery* is the only **treatment** and tumor is *resistant to radio therapy.*

GASTRIC LYMPHOMA

- *Stomach* is MC *site* of ***extranodal lymphoma.***
- 2nd MC primary malignancy of stomach. In stomach most common site of lymphoma is antrum.
- Almost *all are non-hodgkins lymphomas* and are generally classified as ***B-cell mucosa associated lymphoid tissue*** arising from mucosa or superficial submucosa.
- Risk increased after H.Pylori infection.
- Mostly present in 6th decade with epigastric pain, weight loss and bleeding.
- **Diagnosis** is made by *endoscopic biopsy.*
- Preoperative staging should include a CT scan and bone marrow biopsy.
- ***Endoscopic ultrasound*** is most sensitive technique for perigastric lymphatic involvement.

Treatment

– *For low grade lymphoma* :
  - H. pylori *antibiotics* should be given for those who are H.pylori positive.
  - For H. pylori negative patient and antibiotics resistant tumour radiotherapy is treatment of choice.

– *High grade lymphoma* – Should be treated with CHOP therapy.

– *Large size (stage III and Stage IV)* : Combination chemotherapy is treatment of choice.

Remember : Surgery is indicated only for emergency situation such as bleeding, perforation.

QUESTIONS

1. The most common cause of gastric outlet obstruction in india is : [AI 06]
a. Tuberculosis
b. Cancer of stomach
c. Duodenal lymphoma
d. Peptic ulcer disase

2. When carcinoma of stomach develops secondarily to pernicious anemia, it is usually situated in the : [AI 06]
a. Pre-pyloric region
b. Pylorus
c. Body
d. Fundus

3. Which one of the following is the most significant risk factor for development of gastric carcinoma : [AI 06]
a. Paneth cell metaplasia
b. Pyloric cell metaplasia
c. Intestinal cell metaplasia
d. Ciliated metaplasia

4. False about Gastric lymphoma is: [AIIMS May 08]
a. Stomach is the most common site
b. Associate with H. pylori infection
c. Total gastrectomy with adjuvant chemotherapy is the treatment of choice
d. 5 yr survival rate after treatment is 60%

5. Sister Mary Joseph nodules are found in: [AIIMS May 09, 10]
a. Gastric Ca
b. Pancreatic Ca
c. Lung Ca
d. Ovary Ca

6. True about gastric Ca includes all of the following except: [PGI June 09]
a. H. pylori associataion is present
b. D2 gastrectomy include total gastrectomy
c. Surgical non curative lesion should not be resected
d. Pt under total gastrectomy shouold be given Vit. B12
e. Haematemesis present in majority of Pt

7. True about Gastric Ca includes all except:
a. Lesser curvature is more commonly invovled **[AIIMS 07]**
b. Intestinal type is more common
c. Most patient present with advanced ca
d. Fundus is the most common site

8. All of the following are indications for surgery in gastric lymphomas except :
a. Bleeding **[AIIMS 05, 02]**
b. Perforation
c. Residual disease following chemotherapy
d. Intractable pain

9. True about gastric cancer are all except:
a. Incidence increasing worldwide
b. Incidence of proximal gastric cancer is increasing **[PGI 05]**
c. Surgically curable
d. Most patient present with curable disease
e. Depth of lesion is more important prognostically than size

10. True about gastric lymphoma: [PGI-09]
a. Non Hodgkins lymphoma commonest variety
b. Diagnosis made by biopsy
c. Chemoresistant
d. Essentially B-cell type
e. H. pylori have direct relation

ANSWERS, REFERENCES, EXPLANATIONS WITH INFORMATIVE ILLUSTRATIONS

1. **Ans. is b i.e. Cancer of Stomach** *Ref. Endoscopy 1998 Jun; 30(5); 484-486*

Malignancy is the most common cause of gastric outlet obstruction even in developing countries.

Study was conducted in Department of Gastroenterology M.L.N. Medical college Allahabad.

Causes of gastric outlet obstruction

- Gastric cancer ***(MC)***
- Secondary to peptic ulcer
- Adult pyloric stenosis : Treated by pyloroplasty
- Pyloric mucosal diaphragm : Treated by simple exicision

2. **Ans. is d i.e. Fundus**

Ref. Sleisenger & Fordtrans text book of Gastrointestinal disease 7/e, p 813

"Diffuse corporal Atrophic gastritis (DCAG) is an autoimmune destruction of fundic glands. It is the pathologic process in patients with pernicious anemia. It is exhibits achlorhydria. or hydrochlorhydria, hypergastrenemia, antral G cell hyperplasia, circulating parietal cell and intrinsic factor antibodies."

The incomplete (colonic) type of intestinal metaplasia also occur in DCAG. Atrophic glands with extensive intestinal metaplasia are confined to fundus and are risk factor for gastric carcinoma.

Remember : H. pylori injection is associated with adenocarcinoma of body.

3. **Ans. is c i.e. Intestinal metaplasia** *Ref. Schwartz 9/e, p 930*

Premalignant conditions for gastric carcinoma

- Intestinal metaplasia
- Adenoma
- Atrophic gastritis
- Aberrant pancreas.
- Hyperplastic polyp (Mentrier's disease)
- Chronic ulcer
- Stomach remnant

Intestinal Metaplasia :
- Gastric carcinoma often occurs in an area of intestinal metaplasia.
- Risk of gastric carcinoma is directly proportional to intestinal metaplasia.
- Most cases are associated with **H. pylori infection.**
- It is a ***reversible condition*** and mostly regresses after H.pylori treatment.

4. **Ans. is c i.e. Total gastrectomy**

Ref. Sabiston 18/e, p 1271; Ann Surg 2004 July; 240(1): 28-37

Gastric Lymphoma
- Stomach is MC site of extranodal and GI lymphoma
- Common in 6th decade, M : F = 2 : 1

- MC symptom is epigastric pain and loss of appetite
- Risk increased after H. pylori chronic gastritis and HIV infection
- Diagnosed by endoscopic biopsy

Treatment of Primary Gastric Lymphoma

- They are NHL that originate in stomach and are divided into:

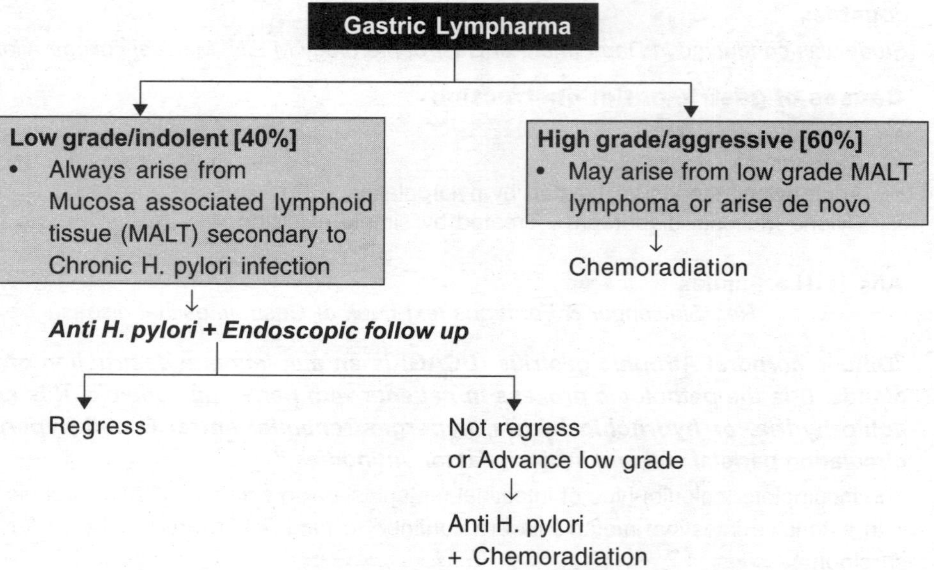

- Though surgery can result in excellent 5 year survival (even over 90%), it is associated with many complications
- Surgery is reserved for localized, residual disease after non surgical therapy or for rare patient with complication
- Chemotherapy for low grade is COP and CHOP regine is used high grade

5. **Ans. is a i.e. Gastric** *Ref. Bailey 25/e, p 1070*

Sister Joseph's nodule represent gastric Ca that has been metastasized to umbilicus via abdominal cavity.

Clinical presentation of gastric Ca

- ***Earliest symptom:*** Vague postprandial abdominal heavyness
- ***MC symptom:*** Weight loss which represent advanced disease
- Ascites, jaundice, palpable mass represent incurable disease
- Enlarged Virchow node ***(Troisier's sign)*** or *Sister Marry Joseph nodule* may be the first sign
- A large ***Krukenberg's tumor*** (secondary ovarian tumor) or a large peritoneal implant in pelvis ***(Blumer's shelf)*** can cause rectal obstruction
- Thrombophlebitis (***Trousseau's sign)*** and deep vein thrombosis are paraneoplastic effects

6. **Ans. is e i.e. Hematemesis is present in most cases**

Ref. Sabiston 18/e 1266, Bailey 25/e 1074, 1071, 1067

Let us consider each option

Option 'a' ... *Harrison 17/e p 572*

H. pylori infection increase risk of Gastric cancer by causing chronic gastritis, loss of gastric acidity and bacterial growth in stomach

Option 'b' ... *Sabiston 18/e p 1266*

D-2 gastrectomy means gastrectomy (whether subtotal radical or total) along with removal of N2 nodes or group II nodes. In gastric cancer lymphadenectomy depends upon the level on nodes involved

- Level I (Group 1) N1 or D1: Nodes within 3 cm of tumour
- Level II (Group 2) N2 or D2: Nodes along hepatic or splenic artery
- Level III (Group 3) N3 or D3: Most distant
  - *D1 resection refers to removal of Group 1 lymph nodes*
  - D2 resection includes removal of Group 1 and 2 nodes. Standard D2 gastrectomy also removes the peritoneal layer over pancreas and anterior mesocolon together with the nodes along the hepatic and splenic arteries and the crural nodes
  - D3 resection refers to D2 resection + removal of paraaortic lymph nodes

Option 'c'

Patient with incurable disease are not subjected to radical surgery

- ***Signs of inoperability are:***
  - Growth fixed to pancreas
  - Rectovesical deposit
  - Enlarged supraclavicular nodes
  - Transperitoneal extension (Sister Marry Joseph nodes or Krukenberg's tumor)
  - Secondaries in liver
  - Enlarged fixed celiac mass
  - Malignant ascites

Option 'd'

After gastrectomy there is loss of parietal cell mass which leads to vitamin B12 deficiency, so replacement should be given routinely

Option 'e'

- Hematemesis is very rare in gastric cancer
- Earliest symptom is postparandial heaviness
- Most common symptom is weight loss

7. **Ans. is d i.e. Fundus is the common site** *Ref. Harrison 17/e, p 572*

- **Most common site of gastric Ca (in ↓ order) :**
  - Proximal third (Oesophagiogastric junction and cardia)
  - Pylorus and antrum (30%)
  - Fundus and body (20%).

- Lesser curvature is more commonly involved than greater curvature.
- Microscopically intestinal type (53%) is more common than diffuse type (33%).

8. Ans. is d i.e. Intractable pain

Ref. Sliesenger & Fortdrans Gastrointestinal & Liver disese 7/e, Vol. I, p 846

Treatment of gastric lymphoma

- ***Ist line (for all stage) :*** *Radiotherapy + chemotherapy.*
- ***Surgery*** is *reserved* only for *urgent cases* (bleeding, perforation) in which gastrectomy is done, followed by chemotherapy.
- Surgical resection is also carried out for patients who respond to chemotherapy but have residual disease. ... *Blackwell Clinical Surgery 2/e, p 322*

Important point about gastric lymphoma

– Stomach is MC site of extranodal and GI lymphoma.
– Most common gastric lymphoma is ***MALToma.***
– H.pylori infection ↑ risk of gastric lymphoma.
– Treatment of choice is *combined radio* and *chemotherapy.*

9. Ans. is a and d i.e. Incidence increasing worldwide; and Most patient with curable disease *Ref. Devita 8/e, p 1048; Robbin's 8/e, p 785*

Let us consider *every option.*

Option 'a'	:	In many parts of world incidence of gastric ca is gradually decreasing because of change in diet, food, and other environmental factors. So, *option 'a'* is wrong. *... Robbins 8/e, p 785*
Option 'b'	:	One of the most striking epidemiological observation has been the increasing incidence of adenocarcinoma involving proximal stomach and distal esophagus. *... Robbins 8/e, p 785* This is probably due to increase GERD and obesity
Options 'c'	:	The only proven, potentially curable treatment for gastric cancer is surgical resection of all gross and microscopic disease.
Option 'd'	:	Less than 50% patients presents with curable disese. Weight loss is the *MC* symptom which represent advanced disease. *... Devita 8/e, p 1048* So, *option 'd'* is wrong.
Option 'e'	:	The morphological feature that has greatest impact on clinical outcome are depth of invasion and extent of nodal and distant metastasis. *... Robbin's 8/e, p 786*

Prognostic factors of Gastric Ca :

- ***Most important depth of invasion***
- ***Site*** (distal tumor has better prognosis than proximal).
- ***Histology*** (intestinal type has better than diffuse type).
- ***Morphology*** (superficial spreading type has better than ulcerative type).
- ***Nodal status*** (more the number of nodes grave is the prognosis).

10. Ans. is a, b, d, e, i.e. Non Hodgkins lymphoma commonest variety, Diagnosis made by biopsy, Essentially B-cell type, H. pylori have direct relation

Ref. Harrison 17/e, 573, Sabiston 18/e p 1271

- ***"Microscopically vast majority of gastric lymphoid tumors are non Hodgkin's lymphoma of B-cell origin"*** ... Harrison.

Refer Ans. 4 for details.

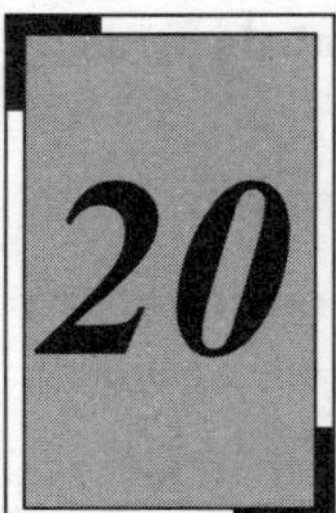

Tumour of Exocrine Pancreas

What's Important ?

- Diagnosis
- Clinical Features

CLASSIFICATION

Benign	*Malignant*
– Cyst adenomas	– Ductal adenocarcinoma = Pancreatic carcinoma (TIC)
– Intraductal papillary mucinous neoplasm	– Cystoadenocarcinoma
	– Acinar cell carcinoma

PANCREATIC CANCER

- Cancer with ***highest mortality*** rate (5 years. survival rate < 5%).
- **Age :** 60 – 65; Male > Female.
- *Cigarette smoking* is the ***most consistent*** risk factor.

... Devita 8/e, p 1087

Others risk factors include:

- Diabetes mellitus
- Chronic cirrhosis
- Pancreatitis
- High fat cholesterol diet
- Prior cholecystectomy
- Obesity
- Occupational (workers of nickel, polycylic aromatic hydrocarbons, silica dusts, organochlorine insecticides industries)

- ***K-ras*** is *most frequently* altered oncogene.
- ***p-16*** *i*s *most frequently* inactivated tumor suppressor gene followed by p 53; SMAD-4.

Pathology

Site :	Most common site is ***head*** (60%) followed by body (15%) and tail (5%). In 20% neoplasm diffusely involve whole gland.
Morphology :	– Hard stellate, grey white, poorly defined mass. – Characteristic feature is its *high invasiveness* and an intense *non-neoplastic host reaction composed of fibroblast, lymphocytes and extracellular matrix* called *desmoplastic reaction.* – *Carcinoma of head of pancreas* obstruct the distal CBD which leads to ***jaundice,*** *Ca of body and tail* do not compress CBD.
Microscopically :	– Tumor composed of moderately to poorly differentiated cells having an aggressive and deeply infiltrative growth pattern.
Spread :	Local – To near by structures. Distant – To lungs and bones.

Clinical features

Frequent	Infrequent
– Abdominal pain *(MC symptom)* – Weight loss – Jaundice *(MC physical sign)* – Migratory thrombophlebitis *(Trousseau sign)* – GI hemorrhage	– Glucose intolerance – Palpable gall bladder – Acute pancreatitis

Remember : 85% of cases are seen at a late incurable stage.

Diagnosis

Tumor marker – CEA and CA - 19 - 9 (More useful) are ***most consistently*** used tumor marker.

Imaging
- *Barium meal* - In ca head of pancreas there is ***widening of C-loop*** of duodenum called *pad sign.*
- *Endoscopic ultrasonography* – Imaging ***modality of choice*** for diagnosis.
- *Multidetector CT with dual phase imaging* - ***Modality of choice*** for staging of pancreatic carcinoma. ... *Devita 8/e, p 1094*

Treatment

A. Curative Surgery :

Complete surgical resection is *only curable treatment* but ***curative operations are possible (only in 10-15% of cases).***

- *Pancreaticoduodenectomy (whipples operation) or distal pancreatectomy* (preferred surgery for small lesion because of (preservation of exocrine pancreas and avoidance of brittle diabetes). Whipples operation includes removal of head of pancreas, duedenum, first 15 cm of the jejunum, common bile duct, gall bladder along with partial gastrectomy. Pancreatic and bilary anastomosis are placed 45 to 60 cm proximal to gastrojejunostomy.

B. Palliative:

Palliation in pancreatic Ca revolves around management of three clinical problems:

1. Pain: Main stay is oral narcotics, celiac plexus block can provide prolong pain relief.
2. Jaundice: Bile duct stent, choledochojejunostomy
3. Duodenal obstruction: Gastrojejunostomy

Chemotherapy: It is disappointing. *Gemcitabine is most effective drug.*

... Harrison 17/e, p 588

Immunotherapy: Antigen based and whole tumor cell vaccines are being under trial.

Prognosis : Median survival for unresectable tumor is 6 months.

PERIAMPULLARY CARCINOMA

Periampullary carcinoma refers to carcinoma arising from ampulla of vater, duodenal mucosa or the lower end of the common bile duct.

- ***Clinically*** present as obstructive jaundice.
- On Ba ***meal*** show inverted '3' sign.
- **Treatment :**
  1. – *Radical pancreaticoduodenectomy* (whipple's operation) when growth is mobile with no metastases and if general condition of patient is good.
     – In this operation growth along the 'c' loop of duodenum upto DJ flexure, removal of head of pancreas and partial gastrectomy followed by :
       - pancreaticojejunal anastomosis
       - gastrojejujnostomy
       - choledochojejunostomy
  2. *Cholecystojejunostomy* + *Entero enterostomy* - as palliative surgery; if growth is fixed.

QUESTIONS

1. **Radiological features of pancreatic carcinoma includes: [PGI 08]**
   a. Widened duodenal loop
   b. Elongation of oesophagus
   c. Dilation of CBD
   d. Dilation of pancreatic duct
   e. Fixation of gastric wall

2. **Which of the following statements about Pancreatic Carcinoma is not true: [AI 09]**
   a. Mutation in P53 gene is associated in 75% of cases
   b. Hereditary pancreatitis significantly increases the risk
   c. Median survival in locally advanced (Stage III) disease is 3-6 months
   d. Five year survival after curative pancreaticoduodenectomy is 15-20%

ANSWERS, REFERENCES, EXPLANATIONS WITH INFORMATIVE ILLUSTRATIONS

1. **Ans. is a, b, c, d, e i.e. All options are correct** *Ref. Sutton 7/e, p 788, 792 - 793*

Imaging in case of carcinoma pancreas

1. **Barium studies**
   a. *Oesophagus :* Elongation and straightening, usually by tumor of tail of pancreas.
   b. *Stomach :* Superior and anterior displacement with *widened retrogastric space*; *splaying, irregularity and ulceration* predominantly in the posterior wall resulting in ***fixation of gastric wall as well as abnormal peristalsis***.
   c. *Duodenum (Hypotonic duodenography) :* Widened 'c' duodenal loop *(also in acute pancreatitis not in chronic pancreatitis)* with mucosal irregularity; spiculation; nodularity; double contour of medial border of loop (also seen in chronic pancreatitis) and Frostberg's reversed 3 sign (also in acute pancreatitis).
2. **Percutaneous transhepatic cholangiogram :** Shows characteristic 'gloved finger' obstruction of intrapancreatic common bile duct.
3. **CT :** With contrast enhancement is the most effective technique for diagnosis and staging.
   Characteristic finding is obstruction with uniform dilatation of distal pancreatic duct in the absence of duct calculi and atrophy of distal gland : Also demonstrate vascular encasement or occlusion.
4. **MRI :** Main role is to distinguish tumor (less enhanced with gadolinium) from inflammatory masses associated with chronic pancreatitis and to determine local extent.
5. **USG :** To determine level of obstruction of bile duct and masses in pancreatic head. *'Ultrasound courvoisier sign that is distended gall bladder containing partial'* layering sludge.

Double duct sign (pathognomonic): Dilatation of common bile duct and main pancreatic head. Tumor is hypoechoic with irregular well defined margin.

6. **ERCP :** *Commonest finding* is complete block of pancreatic duct often accompanied by complete block of common bile duct. Also seen in chronic pancreatitis but side branches are dilated and beaded in chronic pancreatitis, while normal in carcinoma. Necrotic cavities containing contrast give 'scrambled egg appearance'.

2. **Ans. is c i.e. Median survival in locally advanced (Stage III) disease is 3-6 months**

Ref. Sabiston 18/e p 1616; Devita 8/e 1088-1089

Let's consider each option

Option 'a'

Genes involved in pancreatic Ca		
Gene	**Nature**	**Association**
K-ras	Oncogene	95%
P16	Tumor suppressor gene	90%
P53	Tumor suppressor gene	75%
DPC4	Tumor suppressor gene	55%

Option 'b'

Genetic syndromes associated with familial pancreatic Ca

- Hereditary pancreatitis
- HNPCC syndrome
- Peutz-Jeghers syndrome
- Atoxia telangiectasia

In hereditary pancreatitis there is mutation is PRSS1 (cationic trypsinogen) gene. Patient develop severe pancreatitis at a young age. (< 20 years) and have a 50-fold excess risk of developing pancreatic Ca.

Option 'c'

Median survival of patient with stage III tumor ranges from 8-12 months, where as that for patient with stage IV tumor is only 3-6 months ... *Sabiston*

Option 'd'

Outcome after curative surgery (pancreaticoduodenectomy)

- 5 year survival rate is 10-15% (15-25% in some centres)
- Most of these patients succumbs in next 5 year. So, 10 year survival rate is negligible.
- Over all 5 year survival rate in pancreatic Ca is below 5%

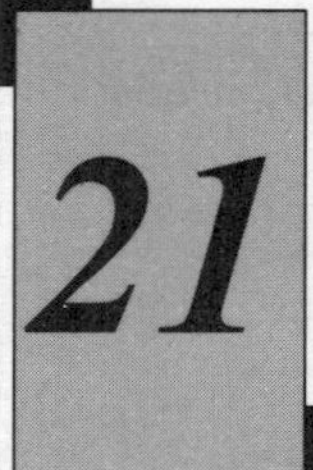

21 Tumour of Small Intestine, Appendix and Peritoneum

What's Important ?

- Types
- Pseudomyxoma Peritonei

- ***Rare,*** accounts for 3 - 6% of all GIT tumors.
- ***Benign tumor*** are more common.

Less incidence of cancer of small intestine in comparision of large intestine is due to following reasons:

- *Content of small intestine have faster transit time, so provide less time for exposure to carcinogens.*
- *pH is neutral to alkaline.*
- *Small bowel contain fewer stem cells, which are target of carcinogens.*
- *Presence of high lymphoid tissue which provides immunoprotection.*

CLASSIFICATION

Benign (more common)	***Malignant***
– Adenoma ***(MC)***	– Adenocarcinoma ***(MC)***
– Lipoma	– Carcinoid
– Angioma	– Lymphoma
– Hamartoma	– Sarcoma

MALIGNANT TUMOURS

- Most common is ***adenocarcinoma.***
- *Age :* 40 - 70 years.

Pathology

- **Site :** – *Adenocarcinoma : Duodenum* (MC) > Jejunum > ileum.
  – Lymphoma : *Ileocecum*; MC type is diffuse large B cell.

... Devita 7/e, p 1045

- **Morphology :** Tumor grows in napkin ring pattern or as polypoid exophytic masses.
- **Spread :** At the time of diagnosis most tumors have penetrated the bowel wall, invaded the mesentery and spread to regional nodes.

Clinical features

- *Most frequent symptom* is *vague abdominal pain, nausea* and *vomiting.*
- Half of patient present as an acute event mostly obstruction or perforation.
- Carcinoid and sarcoma are associated with acute GI hemmorhage.
- *Lymphoma are associated with higher rate of perforation.*
- Duodenal adenocarcinoma leads to early jaundice.

Diagnosis

- *Barium contrast study* ***(Small bowel enteroclysis study)*** *: Initial investigation of choice* for any patient complaining vague abdominal pain and weight loss.
- ***Findings of Barium follow through are :***
  - *Adenocarcinoma :* Annular lesion affecting very short segment of bowel.
  - *Lymphoma :* Non-obstructing narrowing of lumen. In contrast to adenocarcinoma, it is located distally.
  - *Sarcoma / GIST :* Present as punched out or filling defect (submucosal growth pattern) or *dumbbell type growth pattern.*
- *CT Scan :* More sensitive than Ba contrast study, staging can also be done.
- *Endoscopic visualization and Biopsy :* Most specific diagnostic technique.

Prognostic factors

Bad prognostic factors are :
- Positive surgical margins
- Extramural venous spread
- Presence of lymphnode metastasis
- Poor tumor differentiation.

Treatment

Site	Surgery
Duodenum	Pancreaticoduodenectomy (best) or pancreatic sparing duodenal resection.
Remaining SI	Complete surgical resection with negative margins.

Adjuvant chemotherapy increase survival. **5 FU** is most effective chemotherapeutic agent.

BENIGN TUMOR

Adenoma
- Mostly occur in region of ***ampulla of vater.***
- Patients with *familial adenomatous polyposis* are prone to develop adenoma.
- Usually present in 30-60 years old patient with occult blood loss, obstruction or intususception.
- It is a ***premalignant lesion.***
- Treatment is ***resection.***

NEOPLASM OF APPENDIX

- ***Benign*** : Adenoma; neuroma; lipoma; GIST
- ***Malignant*** : Carcinoid; adenocarcinoma

Carcinoid Tumor

- Most common malignant tumor of appendix.

Remember:
- *Most common* site of carcinoid tumor in GIT is ileum.
- Most appendicular carcinoid are benign.

Adenocarcinoma
- Very rare
- Spread rapidly to regional lymphnodes or implant on ovaries or peritoneal surface
- Mostly present as acute appendicitis or appendicular perforation
- Treatment is right hemicolectomy.

NEOPLASM OF PERITONEUM

Carcinoma Peritonei

- Common terminal event in many cases of *cancer of stomach, colon, ovary and may be seen in carcinoma breast, bronchus.*
- *Both parietal* and *visceral peritoneum* is *studded* with secondary growth and peritoneal cavity becomes filled with malignant cell containing ascitic fluid.
- ***Main form of peritoneal metastases are :***
  - Discrete nodules - Most common variety
  - Plaques - Varying in size and colour
  - Diffuse adhesion - Giving rise to frozen pelvis.

Treatment

Systemic chemotherapy or Intraperitoneal chemotherapy with cisplatin, Mitomycin or methotrexate after drainage of ascites.

Pseudomyxoma peritonei

- ***Locally malignant*** condition mostly after primary appendicular tumor with secondary ovarian implant. ... *Bailey & Love 24/e, p 1146*
- Peritoneal cavity is filled with large quantity of yellow jelly.
- Condition is ***painless*** and *shifting dullness or fluid thrills can not be elicited.*
- ***Diagnosis*** is suggested by US or CT and confirmed by operation.

Treatment :
- Removal of jelly with appendicectomy and oophorectomy with adjuvant intraperitoneal chemotherapy.
- Intracavitary radiotherapy for residual disease.

Mesothelioma

- Highly malignant tumor associated with ***asbestos*** exposure.
- Mostly occur in *pelvic peritoneum.*
- Tumor is ***radioresistant*** and treatment is multiagent chemotherapy.
- Prognosis is poor.

QUESTIONS

1. **GIST tumor marker is:** **[AIIMS 09]**
   a. CD 117
   b. CD 34
   c. CD 30
   d. CD 10
2. **Which of the following markers is specific for gastrointestinal stromal tumors:** **[AI-2010]**
   a. CD 117
   b. CD 34
   c. CD 23
   d. S 100
3. **Commonest site from where pseudomyxoma peritonei arise:** **[PGI June 06]**
   a. Ovary
   b. Appendix
   c. Pancreas
   d. Stomach
   e. Colon
4. **Primary small intestinal lymphoma is mostly :** **[PGI 07]**
   a. Hodgkin lymphoma
   b. Diffuse large B-cell lymphoma
   c. Burkitt lymphoma
   d. MALToma
5. **Causes of pseudomyxoma peritonei includes:** **[PGI 08]**
   a. Mucocele of appendix
   b. Mucinous cyst of ovary
   c. Ovarian dermoid
   d. Adenocarcinoma of colon
   e. Ovarian Ca

ANSWERS, REFERENCES, EXPLANATIONS WITH INFORMATIVE ILLUSTRATIONS

1. **Ans. is a i.e. CD 117** *Ref. Robbins 8/e p 790; Devita 8/e, p 1200*

Gastrointestinal stromal tumor

- Distinct group of GI tumors originating from interstitial cells of cajol
- CD 117 (Kit)+ mesenchymal tumors. Most of these tumors were misdiagnosed as leomyoma and leomyosarcoma
- GIST are most common mesenchymal tumors arising from the small intestine.
- All GIST have mutation in the ckit or PDGFRA tyrosins kinase.
- Usually seen in elder age group (sixth decade)
- In small intestine most common site is jejunum > ileum > duodenum
- Tumor are usually intraluminal or intramural (as opposed to small intestine)
- Most GIST have spindle cell histology
- Size and mitotic count are most important factor determining malignant potential

Diagnosis

- Most useful diagnostic ***marker is CKIT (CD 117)*** which is detectable in 95% of GIST
- ***Other markers are :***
  - CD 34 : 70% cases
  - Smooth muscle actin : 5%

Treatment

- Complete surgical excision is treatment of choice

Remember : Most common site of GIST is stomach ... *Robbins 8/e p 789*

True leomyoma and leomyosarcoma are very rare in GIT with the exception of oesophages

2. **Ans. is a i.e. CD 117** *Ref. Robbins 8/e p 790*

Already explained

3. **Ans. is b i.e. Appendix** *Ref. Bailey & Love 25/e, p 1003*

Pseudomyxoma peritonei

- Peritoneal cavity is filled with a yellow jelly.
- Associated with both mucinous and cystic tumors of *appendix and ovary.*
- Most cases arise from a primary appendicular tumor having secondary implant over ovary.
- ***Locally malignant*** condition and does not give raise to extraperitoneal metastases.
- Diagnosis is suggested by US and CT but *confirmed by Laparotomy.*
- Treatment is removal of jelly with appendicectomy with B/l oopherectomy (in females) with adjuvant intraperitoneal chemotherapy. Intracavitary radiotherapy is given for residual disease.

4. **Ans. is b i.e. Diffuse large B cell lymphoma** *Ref. Devita 8/e, p 1198*

Lymphoma arising in small intestine are :

- Diffuse large B-cell lymphoma – 55%
- MALT lymphoma – 20%
- Peripheral T-cell lymphoma – 15%
- Burkitt's lymphoma – 5%

Criteria for primary GI lymphoma is :

- Absence of palpable lymphadenopathy.
- Normal peripheral blood smear and bone marrow biopsy.
- Absence of mediastinal lymphadenopathy on chest X-ray.
- Disease grossly confined to small bowel with regional lymphadenopathy only.
- Absence of hepatic or splenic tumor involvement except via direct extension of primary tumor.

5. **Ans. is a, b Mucocele of appendix, Mucinous cyst of ovary** *Ref. Baily 25/e p 1005*

Causes of Pseudomyxoma Peritonei

- Mucocele of appendix
- Mucinous cystadenocarcinoma of appendix
- Ovarion cystadenoma
- Mucinous ovarian tumor.

22 Colorectal Tumour

What's Important ?

- Polyps
- Predisposing Factors
- Carcinogenesis

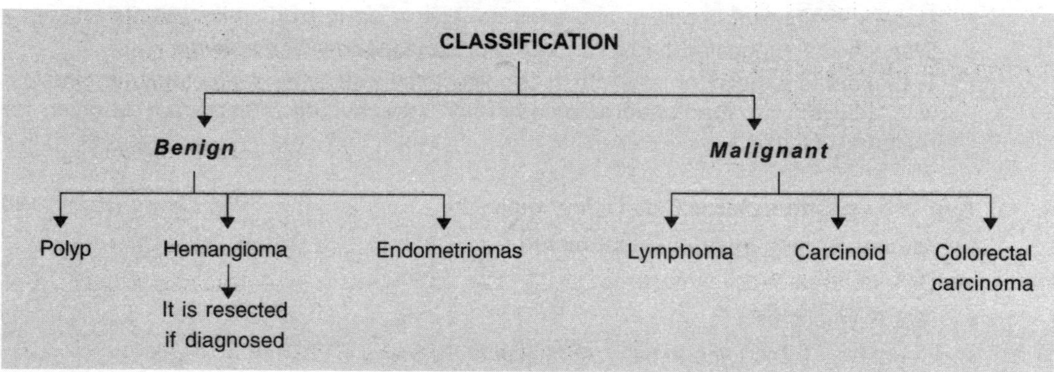

POLYP OF LARGE INTESTINE

Class	Variety
• *Metaplastic*	Hyperplastic polyp ***(MC)***
• *Inflammatory*	Inflammatory (pseudopolyp), benign lymphoid polyp
• *Hamartomas*	Juvenile polyp, peutz jeghers polyp
• *Neoplastic*	Adenoma (adenomatous polyp), adenocarcinoma, carcinoid ***(MC in rectum)***
• *Miscellaneous*	Lipoma, leiomyoma

- Polyps can be seen anywhere in GIT but are most common in colon.
- Approximately 50% of polyps occur in sigmoid colon or rectum.
- ***Inflammatory polyp*** seen in *inflammatory bowel disease and tuberous sclerosis.*
- Most polyps are asymptomatic and *MC complaint* is *intermittent bleeding.*
- Prolapse polyp is usually juvenile type polyp.
- ***Colonoscopy*** is *most reliable* way to diagnose colonic polyp.

- On ***barium enema,*** polyp appears as rounded filling defect with smooth, sharply defined margin.

Hyperplastic polyp

- Most common epithelial polyp of large intestine.
- ***No malignant potential*** but if harbour epithelial cell dysplasia (adenoma), or size >2 cm patient is at risk for carcinoma. *Ref. ... Schwartz 9/e p 1043*
- Most often found in left colon.
- Usually discovered incidentally in 6th and 7th decades.

Juvenile polyp (Cherry tumour)

- Most common site is rectum.
- Incidence is highest between 3 and 5 years. Bleeding is the commonest symptom.
- If occur in ***adults,*** it is known as *retention polyps.*
- It shows autoamputation.
- ***No malignant potential*** but juvenile polyposis syndrome (50-100 juvenile polyps) carry risk of carcinoma.
- It is associated with malrotation or Meckel's diverticulum.
- ***Colonoscopy*** is both diagnostic and therapeutic.

Peutz jeghers polyps

- Most common site is small bowel > colon.
- ***No malignant potential but*** patient with peutz Jeghers syndrome have an increased risk of carcinomas of pancreas, breast, lung, ovary, uterus, stomach, duodenum, and small intestine.

Adenomatous polyp / adenomas

- Most common type of adenomas is ***tubular.***
- It is a *premalignant* lesion.
- Most common site of ***tubular*** adenoma is ***colon*** while MC site of ***villous*** adenoma is ***rectum*** and rectosigmoid colon.
- ***Most worrisome adenoma*** is **s**essile, **v**illous adenoma greater than 4 cm and if sex is male.
- ***Villous*** adenoma are much more frequently symptomatic and cause overt rectal bleeding, mucoid secretion rich in protein and potassium causing hypoproteinemia and hypokalemia.
- Adenomas > 5mm in diameter are usually treated by polypectomy.

Lymphoma

- Most common non-carcinomatous malignant tumor of large bowel.
- Non-Hodgkin's B-cell lymphoma and kaposi sarcoma are two AIDS related cancers that affect the colon and rectum.

COLORECTAL CARCINOMA

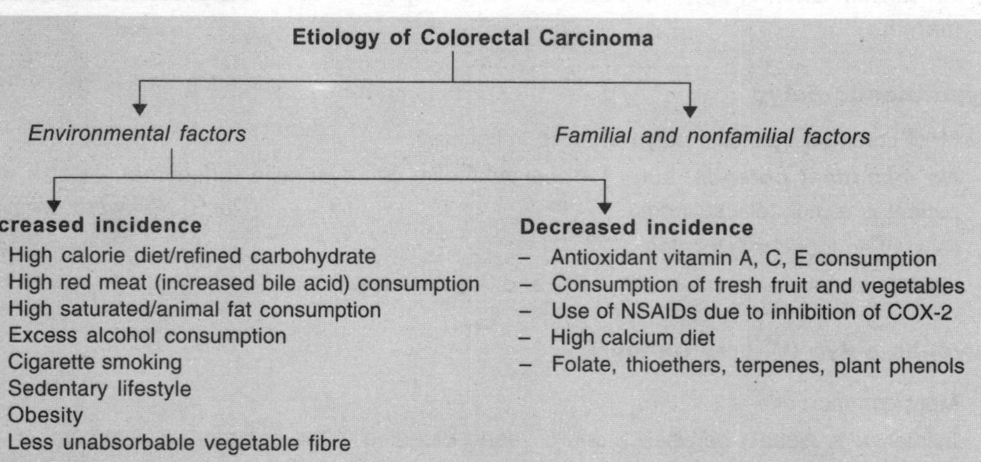

Familial factors of Colorectal cancer

Syndrome	*Altered gene*	*Components*
1. Familial adenomatous polyposis (FAP)	APC on 5q 2l	
• *Classic FAP* (Min. number of polyp = 100)		Frequency of progression to colon carcinoma is *100%*. Typically 500-2500 colonic' adenoma (usually tubular type). Can have polyp in stomach and small intestine also.
• *Attenuated FAP* (average of 30 polyp)		Most of polyp located in proximal colon
• *Gardner syndrome*		Classic FAP with multiple *osteomas* of mandible skull, long bones; *epidermal cyst; fibromatosis;* Abnormalities of dentition; higher frequency of duodenal, thyroid cancer; desmoid tumor; sebaceous cyst.
• *Turcot's syndrome* (Polyps are few & larger than classic FAP)		Adenomatous colonic polyposis; CNS tumor *(medulloblastoma* if APC gene mutated or *Glioblastoma* if MMR gene mutated).
2. Hereditary non polyposis colorectal cancer (HNPCC) syndrome or lynch syndrome	Defect in mis-match DNA repair gene (MMR)	Increased risk of colorectal cancer (usually not associated with pre-existing adenomas or have few adenomas) and endometrial, small intestine, renal, vesical, ovarian, hepatobiliary cancer.
3. Syndromes with Hamartomatous polyps SMAD 4/DPC-4 BMPRIA		
• *Juvenile polyposis syndrome*	SMAD 4/DPC-4 BMPRIA (polygenic)	Colonic polyp, gastric or small bowel polyp around lip, in buccal mucosa, periorbital; polyp
• *Peutz-Jeghers syndrome*	STKII (LKB1)	Git polyp; freckles i.e. *pigmentation* on hands, of sinus, bronchial, bladder; sex cord, lung, pancreatic tumor; increased risk of intussuscep-tion.
• Cowden syndrome	PTEN of chromo-some 10	Hamartomas of GIT, mucocutaneous region; intestinal polyp; facial trichilemeomas; acral keratoses; oral papillomas; thyroid and breast cancers
• Cronkhite-Canda syndrome	Non hereditary	GIT polyposis; ectodermal abnormalities (nail atrophy, skin pigmentation, alopecia)

Remember : Familial syndromes are usually autosomal dominant.

Non familial causes :

– Personal history of adenomatous polyp or colorectal cancer
– Inflammatory bowel disease [ulcerative colitis - 10%],
[crohn's colitis - rare]
– Radiation colitis
– Ureterosigmoidostomy
– Acromegaly
– Cronkhite - Canada syndrome.

Pathology

- Most common site of colorectal carcinoma is ***rectum.*** *... Bailey 25/e p 1179*
- Most common site of colon carcinoma is ***sigmoid colon.***
- Most common type of colorectal carcinoma is ***adenocarcinoma.***
- Most tumors are ***single*** and occur sporadically.
- Right sided colon carcinoma tend to have greater microsatellite instability.
- Carcinoma of colon particularly the right colon is more common in women and carcinoma of rectum is more common in men.
- **Microscopically :**
  – Colonic carcinoma present in four types :
    - 1 annular type
    - 2 tubular type
    - 3 ulcer type
    - 4 cauliflower
  – *Least malignant* is ***type - 4.***
  – Rectal carcinoma usually present as an ulcer.
  – Some colorectal carcinoma shows endocrine differentiation, signet ring appearance and squamous cell differentiation (usually in left colon).
  – Most common histological variety of rectal carcinoma is moderately differentiated.
  – ***Mucin*** production worsens the prognosis since mucin aids tumor extension.
- **Macroscopically**
  – Right sided tumor is large sized *polypoid* tumor and of left sided colon is annular encircling tumor producing *napkin - ring* constriction with heaped up, beaded, firm margin and ulcerated mid region.
  – Most colonic tumor have characteristic firm, hard consistency due to strong desmoplastic stromal response.

Clinical features

Right colon	Left colon	Rectum
• Unexplained weakness or *anemia* • *Occult blood* in faces • Persistent right abdominal discomfort mostly postprandial • Palpable abdominal *mass* • Obstruction is uncommon	• Since feces is semisolid here tumour occlude the lumen causing altered bowel habits • Hematochezia or *gross blood* in stool or bleeding per rectum • *Obstructive* symptoms • *Pain, tenesmus and bladder symptom in sigmoid* colon	• *Bleeding (earliest and MC s symptom)* • Sense of incomplete defecation, tenesmus and spurious diarrhoea with bloody slime • *Altered bowel habits* with early morning bloody diarrhoea tumour • Pain - late symptoms • Weight loss (hepatic metastases occur) • Intrarectal palpable tumour

Spread

- Most common form of tumor spread is *regional lymph node* metastases.
- In carcinoma rectum, lymphatic spread follows the blood supply of rectum when tumor lies in field of middle rectal vessels between 4cm and 8cm from the anus but most lymphatic spread occur in *upward direction* through superior rectal vessels to the para-aortic nodes of Gerota.
- *Transperitoneal metastasis* cause palpable deposit in pelvic cul-de-sac called as *BLUMER'S SHELF* (hard shelf).
- In carcinoma rectum local spread occur circumferentially (common in left colon also) rather than longitudinally.
- *Hematogenous* spread occur in liver, lung, ovary.

Diagnosis

1. *Carcinoma embryonic antigen (CEA) :* Glycoprotein found in cell membrane of many tissues including colo-rectal cancer. CEA is also detected in serum, urine and feces. It is not specific for colorectal cancer but is helpful in detecting metastases, recurrence after curative surgical resection.
2. *Barium enema :* It is most important radiographic means of diagnosing colon cancer. Cancer of left colon appears as "Apple core configuration" while of right colon shows constriction or intraluminal mass.

   It is the investigation of choice in patients in whom predominant change in bowel habit is the presenting symptom.
3. *Colonoscopy (Diagnostic) :* It picks not only primary carcinoma but also detect synchronous polyp or multiple carcinoma. Done in patients whose main symptom is bleeding, known polyps, doubtful barium enema.
4. *Digital rectal examination, prostosigmoidoscopy and biopsy.*
5. *Chest X-ray* should be done routinely.
6. *CT/MRI* (better) in detecting extramural extension in rectal cancer. Not done in colon cancer.
7. All patients with proven rectal cancer should have imaging of liver and chest preferably by CT; local pelvic imaging by endoluminal USG, CT or MRI.

Staging

Previously ***Duke's, Astler coller*** staging is done but now TNM staging is internationally accepted.

Staging of Colorectal cancer

Joint Committee Classification	*TNM*			*Dukes class*
Stage 0				
Carcinoma in Situ	Tis	N0	M0	
Stage I				
a. Tumour invades *submucosa*	T1	N0	M0	Dukes A
b. Tumour invades *muscularis propria*	T2	N0	M0	Dukes B1
Stage II				
a. Tumour invades into *subserosa* or into nonperitonealized pericolic or perirectal tissues	T3	N0	M0	Dukes B1orB2
b. Tumour perforates the visceral peritoneum or directly invades other organs or strucutres	T4	N0	M0	Dukes B2
Stage III				
Any degree of *bowel wall perforation with lymph node* metastasis				
a. One to three pericolic or perirectal lymph nodes involved	T1/T2	N1	M0	Dukes C1
b. One to three pericolic or perirectal lymph nodes involved	T3/T4	N1	M0	Dukes C2
c. 4 or more pericolic or perirectal lymph nodes involved	AnyT	N2	M0	
Stage IV				
Presence of distant metastasis	Any T	Any N	M_1	Dukes D

- *Overall the most important prognostic* indicator of colorectal carcinoma is the ***extent of tumor*** at the time of diagnosis the so called **stage.** *... Devika 8/e, p 1241*
- The *single most important prognostic* factor is ***number of positive nodes.*** *... Devita 7/e, p 1069*

Treatment

1. **Colonic carcinoma**

   Preoperative preparation : Full mechanical bowel preparation by dietary restriction to fluids for 48 hrs. before surgery; sodium picosulphate for purging; rectal washout / prograde lavage via nasogastric tube using water or balanced electrolyte solution; stoma site is decided; antiemboli stockings are fitted; prophylactic subcutaneous heparin and intravenous prophylactic antibiotics given at start of surgery.

   Operation : Wide surgical resection of tumor and its regional lymphatic drainage (e.g. right hemicolectomy in carcinoma caecum) followed by end to end anastomosis.

   Inoperable growth :
   - In upper part of left colon – Transverse colostomy is performed.
   - In pelvis colon – Left iliac fossa colostomy performed.
   - In ascending colon – Bypass using an ileocolonic anastomosis is best procedure.

Hepatic metastasis (1 to 3) in number :

- It is not a contraindication for resection of tumor.
- After recovery from colonic resection, hepatic resection is done (resection can *also done in lung metastasis*).
- In case of irresectable symptomatic hepatic metastasis (jaundice, ascites, hepatomgegally), local ablative treatment done (cryosurgery, radio-frequency or microwave coagulation, embolization, hepatic intra-arterial chemotherapy).

Adjuvant therapy for colon Ca :

Stage I	As surgery is sufficient no adjuvant is required.
Stage II	(Node negative disease) Adjuvant chemotherapy is recommended only in cases with advanced local Stage II disease (perforation, T4)
Stage III	(node positive disease) : Post operative adjuvant chemotherapy significantly prolong the survival. Regimen used are 5FU + Leucovorin, FOL-fox (oxaliplatin, fluorouracil, leucovorin).
Stage IV	Chemotherapy in the form of FOL-Fox is recommended.

Remember : For patients with ulcerative colitis or familial polyposis syndrome, who either have evidence of invasive carcinoma or are at significant risk for development of invasive carcinoma, total abdominal colectomy is the treatment

2. **Rectal carcinoma :** ***Surgery is TOC***

a. ***Resection of bowel :***

Low anterior (sphincter saving) resection	Combined abdominoperineal resection
For tumor of ***upper 2/3*** of rectum (more commonly done) Resection of tumor with at least 2 cm margin of normal bowel below lower edge of tumor with total mesorectal excision followed by stapled colo-rectal anastomosis.	For extensive tumor of ***lower third*** of rectum. Distal sigmoid, rectosigmoid, rectum and anus are removed followed by permanent end-sigmoid colostomy. It is *not performed in case of peritoneal seeding or fixation to bony pelvis.*

These surgery can also done by laparoscopy.

b. ***Local excision :*** done in small well differentiated mobile polypoid tumor which are often Duke's A (T_1) tumor.

c. ***Palliative procedures :*** Rectal excision is the best means of palliation and should be considered even in presence of liver metastasis

Local procedures	*Palliative colostomy*	*Hartman's procedure*
Palliation done by fulguration (electrocoagulation) or laser photo coagulation, in patient who are unfit for radical surgery	Done in gross infection of neoplasm or for obstructing rectal cancer that can't be resected (Diverting colostomy)	Done in old, feeble, poor risk unstable patient with obstruction or sepsis. Bowel with tumor is removed through abdomen with permanent colostomy but without excision of distal rectum which is sutured closed.

d. ***Radiotherapy :*** Used alone or in combination of surgery for small rectal cancers, reduce size of bulky fixed tumor, prevent recurrence and also used in treatment of recurrence.

e. ***Adjuvant chemotherapy*** (5 flurouracil and folinic acid) : Improve survival in node positive cases (stage III) and also stage II.

f. ***In extensive tumor / direct spread to contagious organs :*** Remove affected organ or pelvic exenteration (Brunschwig's operation in which removal of all pelvic organs with internal iliac and obturator lymph nodes) is done.

g. ***Liver resection*** in cases with hepatic metastases is done after resection of primary tumor.

QUESTIONS

1. **All of the following genes may be involved in development of carcinoma of colon except: [AI 09, AIIMS May 10]**
   a. APL
   b. Beta-catenin
   c. K-ras
   d. Mismatch repair gene
2. **Most important prognostic factor for colorectal carcinoma is: [AI 09]**
   a. Site of lesion
   b. Stage of lesion
   c. Age of patient
   d. Lymphnode status
3. **Treatment of Carcinoma left colon with acute obstruction: [PGI June 08]**
   a. Hartman's procedure
   b. Left colectomy with anastomosis
   c. Proximal colostomy anal anastomosis
   d. Extended right colectomy with ilieoanal anastomosis
   e. Primary anastomosis should never be attempted
4. **Which of the following is protective against carcinoma colon? [AI-09]**
   a. High fiber diet
   b. High fat
   c. High selenium diet
   d. Low protein diet
5. **Carcinoma of right colon can present as: [PGI Dec 06]**
   a. Anemia
   b. Mass in right iliac fossa
   c. Bleeding PR
   d. Alternate constipation and diarrhea
   e. Presents with obstruction
6. **Which of the following colonic polyps are not premalignant : [AI 07, 06; PGI 08; AIIMS 09]**
   a. Juvenile polyps
   b. Hamartomatous polyps associated with Peutz Jegher syndrome
   c. Villous adenoma
   d. Tubular adenoma
7. **Gardner's syndrome is a rare hereditary disorder involving the colon. It is characterized by :**
   a. Poplyposis colon, cancer thyroid, skin tumuors
   b. Poplyposis in jejunum, pituitary adenoma and skin tumours **[AI 05]**
   c. Polyposis colon, osteomas, epidermal inclusion cysts and fibrous tumours in the skin
   d. Polyposis of gastrointestinal tract, cholangio-carcinoma and skin tumour
8. **Which one the following conditions commonly predisposes to colonic carcinoma ? [AI 05]**
   a. Ulcerative colitis
   b. Crohn's disease
   c. Diverticular disease
   d. Ischemic colitis
9. **Peutz Jegher syndrome is characterized by mutation of: [PGI Dec 09]**
   a. Chromosome 18
   b. Chromosome 23
   c. Chromosome 19
   d. Chromosome 20
   e. It is an acquired disease
10. **Screening test which you would like to offer to a family with history of familial polyposis after genetic counselling ? [AIIMS 06]**
   a. Colonoscopy
   b. Sigmoidscopy
   c. Screening for APC gene
   d. CPC gene analysis

11. Which of the following is the investigation of choice for assessment of depth of penetration and perirectal nodes in rectal cancer :

a. Trans rectal ultrasound **[AIIMS 05]**
b. CT Scan pelvis
c. MRI Scan
d. Double contrast Barium enema

12. Pre-malignant conditions for colorectal Ca is / are:

a. Ulcerative colitis **[PGI 06]**
b. Amoebic colitis
c. Familial poliposis coli
d. Juvenile poliposis
e. Peutz-Jeghers syndrome

13. In case of elective surgery of Ca sigmoid colon, which of the following should be done : [PGI 05]

a. Mechanical bowel wash
b. Broad spectrum antibiotic given 48 hours before operation
c. Broad spectrum antibiotic at the time of operation
d. Gastric lavage E. LV Heparin

14. Regarding Ca colon true is / are : [PGI 07, 06]

a. Sigmoid colon involvement leads to obstruction
b. Right sided involvement causes bleeding PR commonly
c. FAP deforming predisposes
d. Liver metastasis is present in 1/3rd of cases
e. Bladder symptoms are common in ca sigmoid colon

15. Which of the following is true about colorectal carcinoma? [PGI 05, 06]

a. Right sided colon carcinoma is more common in women
b. Most common site of colon carcinoma is sigmoid colon
c. Right sided colon carcinoma presents as chronic anaemia
d. Not resectable in case of metastasis
e. Right sided Colon Ca has better prognosis than left sided carcinoma

16. True about rectal Ca: [PGI 05]

a. MC type is adenocarcinoma
b. Surgery is the treatment of choice
c. Surgical treatment indicated in spite of hepatic metastasis
d. APR done in lesions of upper zone

17. True about dietary factors in colorectal carcinoma: [PGI 06]

a. Low fiber diet
b. High fiber diet and high fat intake
c. Low fiber, high fat intake
d. Smoked fish
e. High fiber diet

18. True about Peutz Jegher's [PGI 09]

a. Polyps seen in other places such as nasopharynx, bladder
b. Polyps have no malignant potential as they are hamartomas in other sites
c. Polypectomy on colonoscopy is Rx of choice
d. Mucosal involvement present

19. Polyp not associated with risk of malignancy: [AIIMS May 10]

a. Juvenile polyp
b. FAP
c. Peutz Jeghers syndrome
d. Juvenile polyposis syndrome

20. Peutz Jeghers polyps present mostly in: [AIIMS May 10]

a. Rectum
b. Colon
c. Esophagus
d. Jejunum

21. Which of the following is not true about FAP? [AIIMS May 10]

a. AR inheritance
b. Screeing done by sigmoidoscopy
c. Polyps develop in late childhood
d. Epidermal cysts and osteomas may occur

ANSWERS, REFERENCES, EXPLANATIONS WITH INFORMATIVE ILLUSTRATIONS

1. **Ans. is b i.e. beta cetenin** *Ref. Devita 8/e p 1220, Robbins 8/e p 823*

Guy's to be frank all the given genes might be involved in colorectal Ca, but prevelance of β catenin involvement is very low (2%), hence can be considered as answer.

Pathogenesis of colo-rectal carcinoma

Normal epithelium	**APC / β catenin pathway**	***Microsatellite instability pathway***
↕		
Mucosa at risk (hyperproliferative epithelium, dysplastic foci)	Loss or mutation of APC gene ↓ β catenin accumulates which binds T cell factor or lymphoid enhancer factor ↓	• Lesion in DNA mismatch repair gene (MMR) • Most common is in MSH 2 and MLH 1 gene ↓ Mutation in genes regulating growth and apoptosis (TGF β, BAX, BRAF, TCF-4) ↓
↕		
Adenoma	Activation of Cmyc & cyclin D1 ↓ K ras mutation (Most frequently activated oncogene in colorectal Ca) ↓	Carcinoma
↕		
Carcinoma	Loss of SMADs, P53 ↓ Telomerase activation	Remember : Hereditary non-polyposis colorectal cancer, Turcot's syndrome (1/3rd cases) and Muir - Torre syndrome have defect in MMR gene

Remember: APC protein normally binds and promotes degradation of b catenin (a component of WNET signaling pathway) with loss of APC protein (seen in 80% sporadic colorectal Ca) there is accumulation of b catenin.
In mismatch repair pathway KRAS and p53 are not typically mutated, rather there is combination of microsatellite instability, BRAF mutation and methylation of MLH-L

Oncogenes and Tumor suppressor genes in colorectal Ca

Oncogenes	**Frequency**
K-ras	40%
N-ras	< 5%
PIK-3C	14-35%
β catenin	2-5%
neu	<5%
C-myc	<5%
Myb	<5%
Tumor suppressor genes	
p53	>60%
APC	>70%
SMAD-4	60%
SMAD-2	60%
Mismatch repair gene defect	**15%**

2. **Ans. is b i.e. Stage of lesion** *Ref. Devita 8/e p 1239; Robbins 8/e p 825*

Although many factors have been identified that have an impact on recurrence and survival, none exceeds stage in terms of prognostic significance *... Devita*

Involvement of regional lymphnode is the single most important factor

Prognosis Factors in Patients with Colorectal Cancer:

Factors	Effect of prognosis
Pathologic	
• *Surgical pathologic stage*	
- Depth of bowel wall invasion	Increased penetration diminishes prognosis
- Number of regional nodes involved	1-4 nodes is better than >4 nodes
• *Tumor morphology histology*	
- Degree of differentiation	Well-differentiated is better than poorly differentiated
- Mucinous (colloid) or signet ring cell histology	Diminishes prognosis
Scirrhous histology	
• Lymphovascular invason	Bad prognosis
• Perineural invasion	Bad prognosis
• Local inflammation and immunologic reaction	Good prognosis
• Tumor morphology	Better for Polypoid/exophytic than ulcerating/infiltrating
• Tumor DNA content	Increased DNA content (aneuploidy) bad prognosis
• Tumor size	No effect in most studies
Genetic	
• Loss of heterozygosity at chromosome 18q (DCC, DPC4)	Bad prognosis
• Loss of heterozygosity at chromosome {17q (p53)}	Bad prognosis
• Loss of heterozygosity at chromosome 8p	Bad prognosis
• Increased labeling index for p21WAF/CIPl protein	Good prognosis
• Microsatellite instability	Good prognosis
• Mutation in BAX gene	Bad prognosis
Clinical	
• Diagnosis in asymptomatic patients	Possibly improved prognosis
• Rectal bleeding as a presenting symptom	Improved prognosis
• Bowel obstruction	Diminishes prognosis
• Bowel perforation	Diminishes prognosis
• Tumor location	Better for left colon than for right colon tumors
• Younger age (<30)	Diminished prognosis
• Preoperative CEA	Diminished prognosis with a high CEA level
• Distant metastases	Markedly diminished prognosis

3. Ans. is (a, b and c) i.e. Hartman's procedure, left colectomy with anastomosis, proximal colostomy anal anastomosis *Ref. Maingot 11/e 649; Bailey 25/e p 1183*

Colon cancer with bowel obstruction

- Causes colicky abdominal pain, abdominal distension, vomiting, constipation and occasionally paradoxical diarrhea.
- X-ray or CT characteristically demonstrate features of large or small bowel obstruction depending on the level of obstruction and competency of ileocaecal valve
- Chances of caecal perforation is high if caecal diameter is ≥ 12 cm
- Every patient should undergo *rigid proctoscopy* followed by water soluble contrast enema to rule out Ogilvie's syndrome and to visualize colon up to the site of obstruction (not beyond the stenosis as hyperosmolar nature of contrast can increase intraluminal volume and trigger perforation)
- If level of obstruction in colon is proximal enough then resection with primary enterocolonic anastomosis is done (e.g. right hemicolectomy, extended right hemicolectomy or subtotal colectomy)
- If tumor is located on left side, than strategies are:

a. Subtotal colectomy
b. On table lavage with segmental colon resection, intraoperative colonoscopy and primary anastomosis
c. ***Three stage operation***
   1. Defunctioning loop colostomy (temporary transient colostomy)
   2. Resection and anastomosis
   3. Closure of defunctioning stoma
d. Two stage (e.g. Hartmann) procedure:
   - Consist of rectosigmoid resection with creation of terminal colostomy and blind rectal lstump in the first stage followed by colostomy take down and reanastomosis in a second operation
e. Recently, colonoscopic insertion of a self expanding metal stent has also emerged as treatment in emergency situation

4. Ans. is a high fiber diet

Ref. Devita 8/e, p 1234

Environmental factors for colorectal Ca

Increased incidence	*Decreased incidence*
– High calorie diet/refined carbohydrate	– Antioxidant vitamin A, C, E consumption
– High red meat (increased bile acid) consumption	– Consumption of fresh fruit and vegetables
– *High saturated*/animal fat consumption	– Use of *NSAIDs* due to inhibition of COX-2
– Excess alcohol consumption	– High calcium diet
– Cigarette smoking	– Folate, thioethers, terpenes, plant phenols
– Sedentary lifestyle	
– Obesity	
– *Less unabsorbable vegetable fibre*	

Remember :

- Coffee or tea consumption has no effect on incidence of colorectal carcinoma.
- *Fat :* ↑ synthesis of bile acids → carcinogen form by action of gut flora on bile acid → carcinogen cause abnormal colonic epithelial proliferation.
- *High fiber diet :* Dilute fecal carcinogen, decrease colon transit time and generate favorable luminal environment.

5. **Ans. is a and b i.e. Anemia; Mass in right iliac fossa** *Ref. Bailey 25/e, p 1181*

Clinical features of ascending colon and caecal carcinoma

- Anaemia (MC)
- Malena (Not fresh bleeding)
- Mars in right iliac fossa
- Ca caecum may present with intersusception

Note: Iron deficiency anemia in an older man or postmenopausal women is usually caused by GI carcinoma until proven otherwise.

6. **Ans. is a i.e. Juvenile polyps** *Ref. Robbin's 8/e, p 817-820*

Polyp is defined as tumours mass that protrudes into the lumen of gut. It is of two types:

Non-neoplastic / Benign polyp	*Neoplastic polyp*
Do not have malignant potential. Includes hyperplastic *(MC),* Hamartomatous (juvenile and peutz jegher polyp), Inflammatory (Pseudopolyp of inflammatory bowel disease) and lymphoid polyp But syndrome associated with Hamartomatous polyp (juvenile polyposis, peutz Jeghers, Cowden, cronkhite canada, Bannayan Ruvalcaba-Riley) have increased risk for colorectal cancer (which arise from concomitant adenomatous lesion not from hamartomatous polyps)	These are *precancerous.* Includes adenomatous polyp or adenoma seen in familial adenomatous polyposis syndrome (classic FAP, attenuated FAP, Gardner and Turcot syndrome); Hereditary non polyposes colorectal cancer i.e. Lynch I, II; Muir - Torre syndrome

- Most common site of polyp is ***sigmoid colon or rectum.***
- Most common symptom of polyp is ***intermittent bleeding.***
- Hyperplastic polyp usually occur in 5-6 decade but *Juvenile polyp is most commonly occur in 3-5* years and adenoma occur in 40 - 60 years.
- Most common type of adenomatous polyp is tubular adenoma.
- Maximum malignant risk is seen in adenoma which is :
  - Sessile
  - Villous type
  - Severe dysplastic
  - Size greater than 4 cm.

7. **Ans. is c i.e. Polyposis colon, osteomas, epidermal inclusion cysts and fibrous tumours in the skin** *Ref. Robbin's 8/e, p 821*

Components of Gardner syndrome

- Intestinal polyps
- Epidermoid cyst
- Thyroid tumor
- Osteomas of long bones, mandible and skull
- Dermoid tumor
- Dental abnormalities (unerupted or supernumery teeth

Remember : Similar to FAP most common site of polyp is colon.

8. **Ans. is a i.e. Ulcerative colitis** *Ref. Harrison 17/e, p 574*

Non familial causes of Colorectal carcinoma

- Personal history of adenomatous polyp or colorectal cancer.
- Inflammatory bowel disease [Ulcerative colitis - 10%]
  [Crohn's colitis - rare]
- Radiation colitis
- Ureterosigmoidostomy
- Acromegaly
- Cronkhite - Canada syndrome
- Streptococcal bovis bacteremia
- Schistosomal colitis
- Associated with barret's oesophagus; breast cancer; gallstones (usually for right colon); human papillomavirus 16, 18.

Remember :
- Tumor associated with ulcerative colitis has aggressive course.
- In ulcerative colites carcinoma develops from dysplastic site, not from pseudopolyp

9. **Ans. is c i.e. Chromosome 19** *Ref. Robbin's 8/e, p 817, Devita 8/e p 1236*

Peutz Jegher syndrome

- Autosomal dominant
- **Characterized by :**
  - Multiple *hamartomatous* polyp scattered through out GIT (MC in small bowel > colon > stomach), along with sinus, bronchial and bladder polyps.
  - Melanotic mucosal and cutaneous *pigmentation* around lip mucosa, face, genitalia, palmar surface of hand.
- Patient are at risk of *intusussception* which is most common cause of death in these patient. Polyps may cause bleeding also
- The polyps of this syndrome *do not have malignant potential but* patients have increased risk of developing carcinoma of colon pancreas, breast, lung, ovary and uterus.
- Defect is in STK 11 gene located on chromosome 19.
- ***Management:***
  - If surgery is required for complication an attempt should be made to remove as many polyp as possible with the aid of intraoperative endoscopy and polypectomy. Any polyp> 1.5 cm should always be removed.
  - For other cases, colonic survey by colonoscopy every 2 year. Screening for malignancies of breast, cervix, ovary.

10. **Ans. is b i.e. Sigmoidoscopy** *Ref. Harrison 17/e, p 576*

- The off springs of patients with polyposis coli, (*who often are prepubertal when the diagnosis is made in the parent)*, have a 50% risk for the development of this premalignant disorder and should be carefully screened by *annual flexible sigmoidoscopy until age 35.*
- **Proctosigmoidoscopy is a sufficient screening procedure,** because polyps tend to be evenly distributed from ceacum to anus, making more invasive and expensive techniques such as colonscopy or barum enema unnecessary.

- An alternative method for identifying carriers is testing DNA from peripheral blood mononuclear cells for the presence of mutated APC gene. The detection of such a germline mutation can lead to a definitive diagnosis before the development of polyps.

11. **Ans. is c i.e. MRI Scan** *Ref. Devita 8/e, p 1287*

Investigations for Rectal carcinoma

For diagnosis
- Best diagnosed by *sigmoidoscopy* (rigid not flexible) and Biopsy of tumour.
- Barium enema.

For staging
- ***TRUS - (Trans Rectal Ultrasonography)***
  - The depth of tumour invasion can be accurately determined by TRUS.
  - But it cannot detect cancer metastasis in lymphnode (though it can detect enlarged lymph node, but it cannot predict if cancer infiltration is present or not).
- ***CT***
  - Helpful for evalulation of cancer extension.
  - But again, CT also cannot tell clearly about lymph node invasion by cancer cell.
- ***MRI***
  - It has become the most useful investigation tool for rectal carcinoma.
  - It can very predict the invasion of tumour in Rectal wall as well as lymph node invasion with high accuracy.

12. **Ans. is a, c and e i.e. Ulcerative colitis; Familial poliposis coli; and Peutz-Jeghers.**

Familial polyposis Coli/Familial adenomatous polyposis

Ref. Harrison 17/e p 574, Maingot 11/e p 632

- It is ***autosomal dominant*** neoplastic disorder of intestine caused by mutation of adenomatous polyposes coli (APC) gene on chromosome 5q21.
- It exhibits adenomatous polyp of large bowel (usually) but also of stomach, periampullary area and small intestine.
- Males and females are ***equally*** affected.
- Frequency of progression of FAP to colon adenocarcinoma is 100% if prophylactic colectomy is not done.
- Adenomatous polyp start to develop in the late teens and early twenties and turns in to cancer by age 40-45.
- Nearly all FAP patients develop duodenal adenomas, and these patients are at risk for periampullary adenocarcinoma too.
- After colectomy carcinoma of antrum and duodenum is the main cause of cancer related deaths.
- ***Greater than 100*** colonic adenomas are diagnostic.
- Once the diagnosis is made, complete proctocolectomy with ileoanal anastomosis (more commonly done) or colectomy with ileorectal anastomoses (superior bowel function but 10% risk of rectal cancer) is done usually before 20 years age.

Remember : If diagnosis is made during adolescence operation deferred usually to age of 17 or 18 years.

13. **Ans. is (a and c), i.e. Mechanical bowel wash; broad spectrum antibiotic at the time of operation** *Ref. Bailey and Love 25/e, p 1181; Maingot 11/e, p 644*

Preoperative preparation in colorectal cancer:

- Full mechanical bowel preparation by dietary restriction to fluids (nil per orally) for 48 hours before surgery. Generally products based on either polyethylene glycol or sodium phosphate (contraindicaated in renal failure) are given
- Elder patient are prone to dehydration, so IV fluids are also given
- Sodium picosulphate for purging
- Rectal washout / prograde lavage via nasogastric tube using water or balanced electrolyte solution
- Stoma site is decided
- Antiemboli stockings are fitted
- Prophylactic subcutaneous heparin at least 2 hr before surgery and continued postop until patient obtain full ambulation
- Intravenous or oral or both prophylactic antibiotics given at start of surgery / 1-2 hr before incision and continued upto 36 hours
- Urinary cataheter / sents (if patient has history of colorectal or pelvi dissection)
- Nasogastric tube when patient present with obstruction / emergency operation
- Pain management by placing epidural analgesia
- Transfusion (minimum of 2 units blood should be arranged)

14. **Ans. is a, c and e i.e. Sigmoid colon involvement leads to obstruction; FAP deforming predisposes; and Bladder symptoms are common in ca sigmoid colon**

Ref. Bailey 25/e, p 1180 - 1181

Site of Colorectal Ca	Symptom
Caecum and ascending colon (Rt colon)	• Anemia • Mass in rt. iliac fossa/mimicking appendicitis • Intermittent obstruction due to intussuception
Transverse colon	• Anemia • Lassitude • May be mistaken as gastric Ca
Descending colon (Lt. colon)	• Pain • Palpable lump • Alteration of bowel habit • Distension
Sigmoid	• Pain • Tenesmus • Bladder symptoms
Rectum	• Bleeding PR • Sense of incomplete defecation • Altered bowel habbits

Note: 20% of patient have metastasis at the time of diagnosis.

15. Ans. is a, b, c, i.e. Right sided colon carcinoma is more ...; Most common site of colon carcinoma is sigmoid colon; Right sided colon carcinoma presents as ...; is ...

Ref. CSDT 13/e, p 659

"Resection of isolated (1 to 3) liver or lung metastases may result long-term (over 5 years) survival in 30-55% cases".

So, liver metastasis is not a contraindication for surgery in colorectal carcinoma.

Remember:

- Most common site of colorectal carcinoma is rectum
- Most common site of colon carcinoma is sigmoid colon
- Most common type of colorectal carcinoma is adenocarcinoma
- Cancer of rectum and sigmoid have poor prognosis in comparison to proximal right sided lesion due to their more infiltrative nature at the time of diagnosis. Overall righ sided colon Ca carries worse prognosis in comparison to left sided ... *Devita 1245,* Robbins 7/e p 866
- Carcinoma of colon particularly right colon is more common in women and carcinoma of rectum is more common in men ... *CSDT 13/e 659*

16. Ans. is a, b, c, i.e. MC type adenocarcinoma; Surgery is the treatment of choice; Surgical treatment indicated inspite of hepatic metastasis *Ref. Devita 8/e p 1286-1290*

Treatment of Rectal Carcinoma	
Low anterior (sphincter saving) resection	***Combined abdominoperineal resection***
For tumor of upper 2/3 of rectum (more commonly done) Resection of tumor with at least 2 cm margin of normal bowel below lower edge of tumor with total mesorectal excision followed by stapled colorectal anastomosis	For extensive tumor of lower third of rectum Distal sigmoid, rectosigmoid, rectum and anus are removed followed by permanent end-sigmoid colostomy. *It is not performed in case of peritoneal Seeding or fixation to bony pelvis*

17. Ans. is a, c, d Low fiber diet; Low fiber, high fat intake; Smoked fish

Ref. Devita 8/e, p 1234

Already explained, see answer no. 4

18. Ans is a, b, c i.e. Polyps seen in other places such as nasopharynx, bladder, Polyps have no malignant potential as they are hamartomas in other sites, Polypectomy on colonoscopy is Rx of choice *Ref. Devita Stomach 8/e 1236; Sabiston 18/e p 1400*

In peutz Jegher's syndromes, polyps are found in small bowel; stomach, colon, sinus, lung, urinary bladder.

For details see answer No. 9

19. Ans. is a i.e. Juvenile polyp *Ref. Robbin's 8/e p 817*

Juvenile polyp itself are not malignant, but syndrome associated with it i.e. juvenil polyposis increase the risk of colorectal Ca

Refer ans. no 6 for details

20. Ans is d i.e. Jejunum *Ref. Maingott's 11/e p 633, Robbins 8/e p 817*

Most common location of Peutz-Jegher's polyp is in upper gastrointestinal tract, specially the upper Jejunum ..... Maingott

Refer ans. no 9 for details

21. Ans. is d i.e. Epidermal cyst and osteomas

Ref. Robbins 8/e p 816, Maingott's 11/e p 632

Osteomas are seen in Gardner syndrome, a variant of FAP

- In classic FAP adenomatous polyp begin to develop in the late teens and early twenties.

Refer ans. no 12

23 Tumour of Anal Region

What's Important ?
- Treatment
- Risk Factors

- Accounts for ***1.5%*** of malignancy of GIT.
- *Age :* 60 - 65 years.
- Sex : F > M (for anal canal), M = F (for tumors of anal margin).

Etiology and risk factor

- Factors associated with increased risk are :
  - HPV infection (particularly 16 and 18) } ***Especially for squamous cell carcinoma***
  - HIV infection
  - History of STD
  - Anogenital warts
  - History of cervical, vaginal, vulvar cancer
  - Long term steroid
  - Cigarette smoking.

Classification

AJCC divided anal region tumors into : *... CSDT 12/e p 720*

Cancer of Anal canal – *It includes the cancers arising from upper to the lower border of the internal anal sphincter* (from pelvic floor to anal verge). 70% of tumor arise here.

Cancer of Anal margin – *Includes the cancers arising outside the anal verge but presumably **within 5 - 6 cm** radius of skin.* 30% of tumor arise here.

Pathology

The current WHO classification used only two terms for anal tumors: *..... Devita 8/e p 1302*

1. *Anal intraepithelial neoplasia:* Precancerous changes in the squamous epithelium of the anal canal and perianal skin.

2. *Squamous cell carcinoma:* For invasive Ca, the generic term "**squamous cell ca**" is recommended. This term will replace various subtypes (basaloid, keratinizing) used in previous classification. Adenocarcinoma are also included in this term. Small cell carcinoma with mucinous microcysts are retained as separate entities.

Clinical features

- SCC of anal canal are usually preceded by highgrade AIN
- Main symptoms are ***rectal bleeding to mucous discharge,*** tenesmus, sensation of lump in anus.
- Some patients may come with a mass in inguinal region due to metastatic inguinal lymph node.
- *Tumors of anal margin* presents at an ***early stage*** than anal canal tumors.

Diagnosis and Staging

Mostly clinical and made by digital rectal examination, anoscopy, bilateral groin palpation, biopsy.
CT and MRI – For assesing the tumor size and establishing nodal and distant disease.

Staging is as follows :

Primary Tumor (T)	
TX	Primary tumor cannot be assessed
T0	No evidence of primary tumor
Tis	Carcinoma in situ
T1	Tumor 2 cm or less in greatest dimension
T2	Tumor more than 2 cm but not more than 5 cm in greatest dimension
T3	Tumor more than 5 cm in greatest dimension
T4	Tumor of any size invades adjacent organ(s), for example, vagina, urethra, bladder [involvement of the sphincter muscle(s) alone is not classified as T4].
Regional Lymph Nodes (N)	
NX	Regional lymph nodes cannot be assessed
N0	No regional lymph node metastasis
N1	Metastasis in perirectal lymph nodes(s)
N2	Metastasis in unilateral internal iliac and / or unilateral inguinal lymph node(s)
N3	Metastasis in perirectal and inguinal lymph nodes and / or bilateral internal iliac and / or bilateral inguinal lymph nodes.
Distant Metastases (M)	
MX	Distant metastasis cannot be assessed
M0	No distant metastasis
M1	Distant metastasis.

Prognostic factors

- Anatomic extent (Tumor size) is the most important prognostic factor. *...Devita 8/e, p 1305*
- Extrapelvic metastases carry worst prognosis.

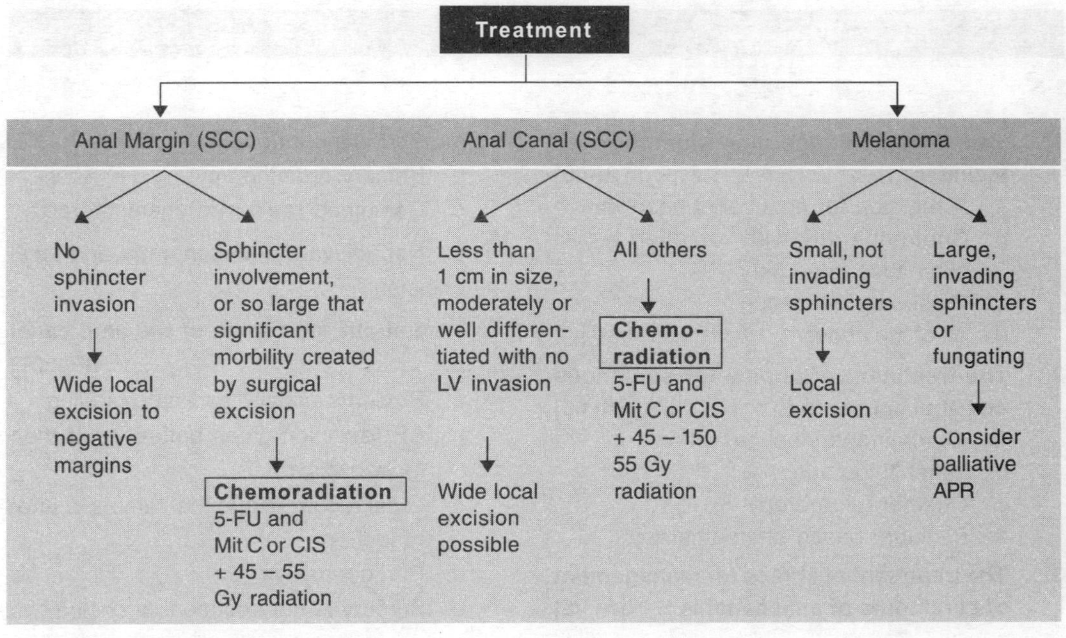

ANAL INTRAPEPITHELIAL NEOPLASIA

- ***Premalignant*** lesion of anal canal.
- Epithelium shows features of dysplasia as seen in cervical and vulvar epithelium.
- It is of three types :

AIN I	AIN II	AIN III = Ca in situ = Bowen's disease
Dysplasia limited to lower 1/3rd	Dysplasia limited to lower 2/3rd	Dysplasia in whole epithelium thickness

Etiology

- HPV 16, 18
- Immunosuppression.

Treatment :

– AINI, AINII - No treatment

– AIN III - Excision; excision with grafting; laser ablation cryoablation or cytotoxic creams (5 flurouracil).

QUESTIONS

1. **True statement regarding Nigro regimen includes: [AI-08]**
   a. A regimen for anal canal neoplasm
   b. Chemotherapy with radiation as an alternative to surgery
   c. Preserve continence
   d. All of the above
2. **The treatment of choice for squamous cell anal cancer is : [AI 06]**
   a. Abdominoperineal resection
   b. Laser fulgaration
   c. Chemoradiotherapy
   d. Platinum based chemotherapy
3. **The treatment of choice for management of carcinoma of anal canal is : [AI 06]**
   a. Abdominoperineal resection
   b. Primary radiotherapy
   c. Combined radio and chemotherapy
   d. Neoadjuvant chemotherapy and local excision
4. **True about melanoma of the anal canal is : [PGI 07]**
   a. Presents usually as anal bleeding
   b. AP resection gives better result than local excision
   c. Local recurrence at the same site after resection
   d. Radiosensitive
   e. Surgery is the treatment of choice

ANSWERS, REFERENCES, EXPLANATIONS WITH INFORMATIVE ILLUSTRATIONS

1. **Ans. is d i.e. All of the above**
   Ref. Sabiston 18/e, p 1459

   Combined chemotherapy for Anal Canal Epidermoid/squamous cell carcinoma
   - Introduced by Norman Nigro in 1974 called as Nigro Regimen
   - Initially used to shrink the tumor, so as to make them resectable, but surgical specimen showed no evidence of tumor in the patients who underwent surgery after this regimen

     Protocol: *Nigro protocol was neoadjuvant*
     – Radiation (30 Gy) was given in 15 sessions over a 3 week period
     – 5 FU wa administered at a dose of 1000 mg / m^2 / day in 2 cycles of 4 days each. 1st cycle starts on day 1 of radiation therapy, second cycle starts on day 29
     – Mitomycin C (15 mg / m^2) was administered as a single dose on day one of treatment
     – This was followed by APR, 6 weeks after completion of radiation therapy.
   - As surgical specimen of these patient showed no evidence of tumor, abdominoperineal resection had been excluded is later series of patient.
   - The introduction of this multimodal therapy preserves continence, avoid colostomy and offer similar survival advantage
   - Based on ongoing studies radiation (4500 – 5400 Gy), 5 FU and either cisplatin (preferrred), mitomycin C constitutes primary treatment of most anal squamous cell Ca.

   ... Maingot 11/e, p 737

2. **Ans. is c i.e. Chemoradiotherapy** *Ref. Bailey and Love 25/e, 1260*

"Primary treatment of anal canal cancer is combined modality treatment or CMT = Nigro regime" *... Bailey and Love 25/e, p 1269*

- Radical surgery (APR) is done in those with persistent or recurrent disease folloowing CMT
- Abdominoperineal resection with colostomy scarifies anal sphincter but the majority of adenocarcinoma are still treated with radical surgical approach.
- Defunctioning stoma may be indicated when treatment and disease regression is associated with radionecrosis, incontinence or fistula.

Remember: Treatment of choice for early cancer of anal verge or anal maragin is wide local excision including tumor free margin of 2.5 cm.

3. **Ans. is c i.e. Combined radio and chemotherapy** *Ref. Bailey & Love 25/e, p 1260*

Already explained, kindly see answer no. 1

4. **Ans. is a, e i.e. Presents usually as anal bleeding, surgery is treatment of choice** *Ref. Schwartz 9/e, p 1054*

Melanoma of anal canal usually presents with bleeding, pain or anal mass.

Melanoma :

- Rare, tumour comprise less than 1% of all anorectal malignancies.
- *Most patient have distant metastasis* or deeply invasive tumour at the time of diagnosis.
- For patient with resectable disease APR or wide local excision is treatment of choice.
- Since recurrence is common after both APR and wide local excision, because of morbidity associated with APR, local excision is recommended.
- Efficacy of adjuvant chemotherapy or radiotherapy remains unproven.

Hepatic Tumour

What's Important ?

- **Treatment Modalities**
- **Fibrolamellar Carcinoma**
- **Spread**

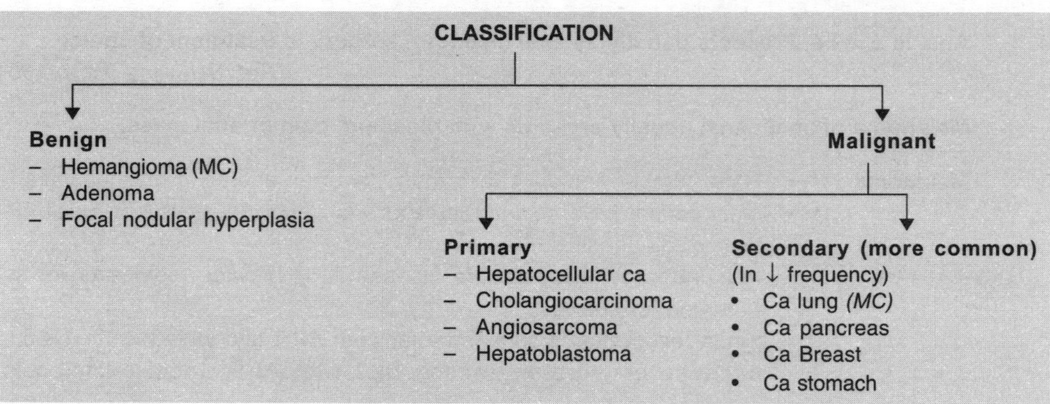

HEMANGIOMA

- ***Cavernous hemangioma*** is most common benign hepatic tumor. ... *CSDT 13/e p 524*
- After skin and mucous membrane, liver is most common site of hemangioma.
- Female > Male.
- Most are ***solitary subcapsular*** growth which remain asymptomatic but when large (> 4 cm) cause abdominal pain or palpable mass.

Diagnosis

- Scintography, contrast enhanced CT scan, MRI or angiograpy.
- FNAC is rarely indicated.

Treatment

a. *If asymptomatic* (even when found during laparotomy) : no treatment is necessary.
b. *If symtpomatic :* excision by lobectomy or enucleation.

Remember : Radiotherapy or embolization may be tried in patient who are poor condidates of surgery.

HEPATIC ADENOMA

- Benign neoplasm developing from hepatocyte.
- Occur almost ***exclusively in women*** in 3rd - 4th decade and is associated with oral contraceptive use.
- Tumor consist of well circumscribed mass of normal appearing hepatocytes without bile duct or central vein.

Clinical presentation

- Asymptomatic in 50%.
- 50% presents with right upper quadrant pain or acute intrabdominal hemorrhage and shock.
- There is strong association of acute bleeding episode and mensturation.
- Only physical finding is palpable liver in some cases.

Diagnosis

- Hepatic CT and US can reveal a mass lesion.
- Arterial phase helical CT and MRI with contrast **(best)** can distinguish adenoma from focal nodular hyperplasia.
- As most of these tumor are hypovascular hepatic *scintography reveals cold defect.*
- Aspiration biopsy is safe but ***core biopsy is contraindicated*** due to risk of bleeding.

Treatment

- Most important predictor of treatment is size.

  Size > 6cm : Whether symptomatic or asymptomatic tumor should be excised.

  Size < 6cm : In asymptomatic and with mild symptoms, conservative management by discontinuing OC's and periodic ultrasound is recommended.
  In symptomatic, complicated and those which fail to regress - excision is done.
- OC's are contraindication for whole life .

FOCAL NODULAR HYPERPLASIA

- Benign lesion with *no malignant potential,* found predominantly in women in 4th decade.
- Use of OCs may stimulate development or growth of the tumor.
- Grossly the tumor is well circumscribed, firm with pathognomic cut section showing central stellate scar with radiating fibrous septa that compartmentalize the lesion into lobules.
- Histologically these are nodular aggregation with normal appearing hepatocyte *without central vein or portal triad, but bile duct proliferation is seen.*

Clinical features

- Most patient are asymptomatic and few with symptoms present with right upper quadrant mass or discomfort.
- In contrast to hepatic adenoma these tumors rarely enlarge or bleed.
- Few patient with focal nodular hyperplasia may develop portal hypertension.

Diagnosis

- ***CT scan*** demonstrate the tumor and usually the central stellate scar.
- ***Arteriographic*** pattern is of hypervascular lesion.
- MRI best modality ... *CSDT 13/e p 526*

Treatment

- Symptomatic - Exicision
- Asymptomatic - No treatment
- Stop OCs.

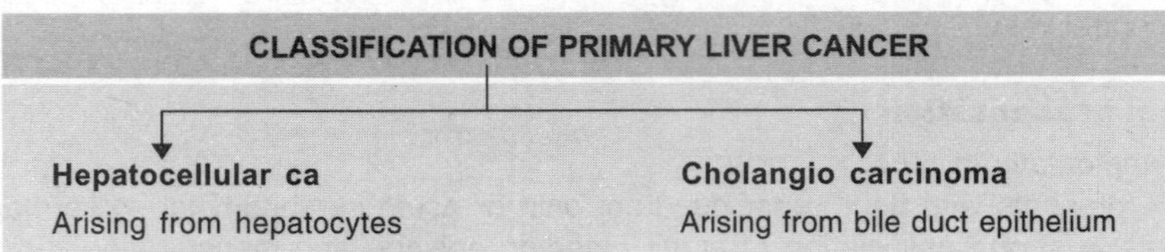

HEPATOCELLULAR CARCINOMA

- Most common abdominal tumor.
- Most common solid organ tumor world wide.
- Incidence ↑ with age (peak 40 – 60); M : F – 4 : 1

Etiology and risk factor

Condition	Risk	Condition	Risk
Cirrhosis		***Genetic diseases***	
Hepatitis B virus infection	High	Hemochromatosis	High
Hepatitis C virus infection	High	Hereditry tyrosinemia	High
Alcohol use	High	α1-Antitrypsin deficiency	Moderate
Autoimmune chronic active hepatitis	High	Ataxia telangiectasia	Moderate
Cryptogenic cirrhosis	Moderate	Types 1 and 3 glycogen-storage disease	Moderate
Primary biliary cirrhosis	Low	Galactosemia	Moderate
Environmental Agents		Hereditary hemorrhagic telangiectasia	Moderate
Thorotrast	Moderate	Prophyria cutanea tarda	Moderate
Androgenic steroids	Moderate	Wilson disease	Low
Smoking	Moderate	Alagille's syndrome (congenital cholestatic syndrome)	Moderate

Pathology

- Mostly arise from ***right lobe***
- Grossly hepatocellular Ca may be :
  a. Unifocal – Single
  b. Multi focal – Widely distributed nodules of variable size
  c. Diffusely infiltrative.
- Diffuse and multifocal form are usually associated with metastasis.
- Hepatocellular Ca are usually paler than the surrounding and if green hue present, it represent well differentiation and is due to bile secretion.
- Characteristic feature of HCC is *invasion of portal vein and to a lesser extent the hepatic vein,* leading to extensive intrahepatic metastases and tumor may reach even upto IVC and right side of heart.
- **On histology:**
  – It range from well differentiated to highly anaplastic undifferentiated lesion.

– ***Fibrolamellar hepatocellular carcinoma :***
  - It is a distinct form of HCC which tends to occur in young males and females (M:F = 1:1).
  - Mostly arise in left lobe.
  - Not associated with ***HBV or cirrhosis.***
  - Consist of well circumscribed schirrous mass which on microscopy show well differentiated cells.
  - It has better prognosis.
  - Grow slowly and are not associated with fibrolamellar carcinoma.

Spread

- HCC spreads extensively within liver by contagious growth and by development of satellite nodules.
- Metastases outside liver occur mostly by ***venous invasion.*** ***Hematogenous*** metastases occur specially to lung.
- **Lymphatic :**
  - ***More common*** in fibrolamellar variant.
  - Perihilar, peripancreatic and para-aortic nodes are involved in upto 1/2 of cases of HCC.

Clinical features

- Most common symptom is *abdominal pain.* ... *Devita 8/e, p 1136*
- Other symptoms are: *weakness, fullness, weightloss, anorexia, jaundice* and *vomiting.*
- Central necrosis and acute hemorrhage may lead to death.
- *Unexplained weight loss in a patient known to have cirrhosis suggest hepatocellular carcinoma.*
- ***Hepatomegaly*** is the most frequent physical sign. Other are : *hepatic bruit, ascites, splenomegaly.*

Paraneoplastic syndromes

- HCC cause variety of paraneoplastic syndromes. Important ones are :

– Hypoglycemia	– Erythrocytosis
– Hypercalcemia	– Hypercholestrolemia
– Dysfibrinogemia	– Carcinoid syndrome
– ↑TBG level	– Porphyria cutenia tarda
– VIP associated diarrhoea	– Cryofibrinogemia
– Sexual changes (testicular atrophy, gyanaecomastia).	

Staging ... *Devita 8/e, p 1134*

Americal joint committee on cancer staging system.	
Primary tumor (T)	
TX	Primar tumor cannot be assessed
T0	No evidence of primary tumor
T1	Solitary tumor without vascular invasion
T2	Solitary tumor with vascular invasion, or Multiple tumors $\leq$ 5 cm
T3	Multiple tumors > 5 cm or tumor involving a major branch of the portal or hepatic veins
T4	Tumors with direct invasion of adjacent organs other than the gallbladder or with perforation of visceral peritoneum.

Regional lymph nodes (N) (Regional lymph nodes are para-aortic and paracervical nodes)	
NX	Regional lymph nodes cannot be assessed;
N0	No regional regional lymph node metastasis
N1	Regional lymph node metastases.

Distant metastases (M)	
MX	Distant metastasis cannot be assessed
M0	No distant metastasis
M1	Distant metastasis.

Stage grouping			
I	T1	N0	M0
II	T2	N0	M0
IIIa	T3	N0	M0
IIIb	T4	N0	M0
IIIc	Any T	N1	M0
IV	Any T	Any N	M1

Diagnosis

a. ***Tumor markers :*** Tumor markers for HCC are :
   - AFP - Raised in 50-70% of cases (value>200ng/ml are suggestive) but not raised in fibrolamellar variant.
   - *Des carobxy prothrombin (DCP) protein induced by vitamin K abnormality (PIVKA-2) – ↑ in upto 80% cases.*
     Both AFP and PIVKA-2 are elevated in chronic hepatitis and cirrhosis.
   - Hep par 1– It has emerged as the most sensitive and specific immunohistochemical marker of HCC.

b. ***Imaging :***
   - USG is *initial investigation of choice and best method* for screening in high risk group.
   - Arterial phase CT and MRI with contrast enhancement are preferred imaging studies to characterize size and vascularity of tumor (HCC is mostly hypervascular).
   - FDG-PET is used for detection of metastatic disease.
   - MRI is best way to show hepatic vein extension. *... Devita 8/e, p 1138*

c. ***Biopsy :***
   - Liver biopsy is diagnostic but seeding of needle tract by tumor is a potential risk. So *biopsy is contraindicated if* imaging studies are diagnostic or if surgical resection is planned.

Treatment

Treatment options for Hepatocellular carcinoma.

Surgery :	– Partial hepatectomy
	– Liver transplantation.
Local ablative therapies :	– Cryosurgery
	– Microwave ablation
	– Ethanol injection
	– Acetic acid injection
	– Radiofrequency ablation.

Regional therapies : ***Hepatic artery transcatheter treatments***
- Transarterial chemotherapy
- Transarterial embolization
- Transarterial chemoembolization
- Transarterial radiotherpay : - Yttrium 90 microspheres
  - Iodine 131 Lipiodol.

Conformal external beam radiation therapy

Systemic therapies :
- Chemotherapy
- Immunotherapy
- Hormonal therapy+growth control.

Stage I and Stage II : Principal is to use the treatment option that allows maximum sparing of hepatic parenchyma.

a. ***Surgical exicision :***
- Goal is to obtain 1 cm margin of normal tissue around the tumor.
- For tumor < 5cm - A nonanatomic wedge exicision is done.
- For tumor > 5cm and for deep tumors - Anatomic resection is performed.
- Intraoperative ultrasonography is performed to screen rest of the liver.

Remember :
- *Child pugh classification* is most imporant prognostic factor for tolerance of hepatic surgery.
- Only patient with child A should be considered for resection.
- Patient with child B and C and stage I and II should be reffered for transplant.

b. ***Transplantation :*** Stage I and II tumour in the setting of cirrhosis and other chronic hepatic disease.

c. ***Local ablation strategies :*** Radiofrequency ablation is a technique that uses heat to ablate tumors :
- It is best suited to tumors < 3cm.
- Can not be used for tumor > 5m and tumour close to bile duct.
- Complete preservation of hepatic parenchyma is possible.

d. ***Local injection therapy :***
- Most commonly used agent is ethanol.
- The maximum size of tumor that can be treated is 3 cm.
- Acetic acid is another agent which has been reported to have lower chances of recurrence.

e. ***Adjuvant therapy :*** In stage I and II there is no role of adjuvant chemotherapy.

Stage III and IV :

a. ***Surgery :*** In Stage III patient without cirrhosis a major hepatectomy provides the best chance of long term survival. *For stage IV surgery is not recommended.*

b. ***Transplantation :*** Unless the tumor can be down staged with chemotherapy, these patients are *not candidate of liver transplant* due to high chance of recurrence.

c. ***Systemic chemotherapy :*** Not much effective.

d. ***Regional chemotherapy :*** This is ideal therapy in these patients.
   - *Most effective* drug are cisplatin and doxorubicin.
   - *Transcatheter chemoembolization (TAC)* : Uses some embolizing agent like suinase, lipoidol, gelatin in addition to chemotherapy.

Summary of treatment

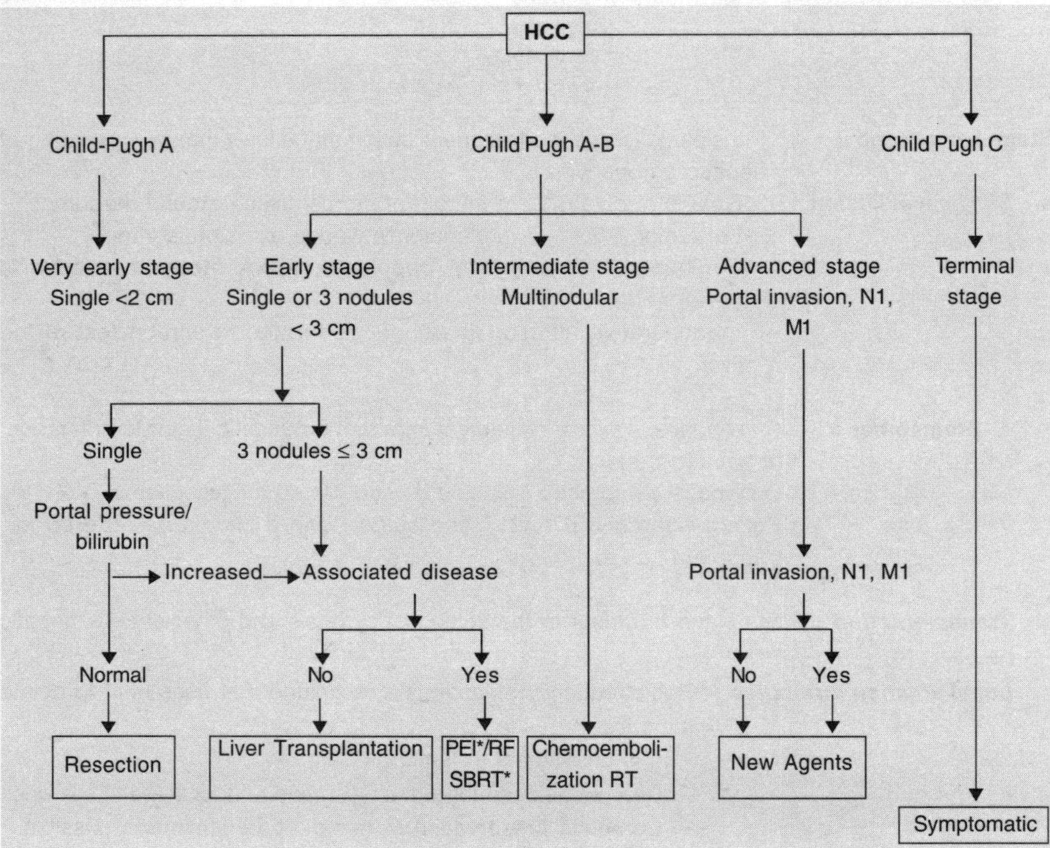

* *PEI-Percutaneous ethanol injection*
* *SBRT- Stereotactic body radiotherapy*

CHOLANGIOCARCINOMA

- Malignancy of biliary tree arising from bile duct within and outside of the liver.
- Age > 60 years; M > F

Etiology and risk factors	
• Primary sclerosing cholangitis	• Polycystic liver disease
• Choledochal cyst	• Cigarette smoking
• Caroli disease	• AIDS
• Liver fluke (clonorchis sinesis and opisthorchis viverrini)	• Chronic caliculi of bile duct
• Prior exposure to thorotrast (used in radiography of biliary tree)	

Pathology

Site : *Hilar cholangiocarcinoma* are most common followed by distal cholangiocarcinoma and intrahepatic cholangiocarcinoma.

Morphology : Grow along the intrahepatic portal system to form tree like pattern. Lymphatic and vascular invasion is prominent giving rise to extensive intrahepatic metastasis.

Histology : – Most cholangiocarcinoma are adenocarcinoma.

Divided in to 3 types :

1. ***Sclerosing :*** Most common, associated with marked *desmoplastic* and fibrous stroma
2. ***Nodular :*** Mass forming
3. Papillary

– Cholangiocarcinoma are ***not bile stained*** as the tumors cells are not capable of synthesizing bile.

Spread :
– Metastasize hematogenously to lung, bones (mainly vertebral), adrenals, brain.
– Lymphnode metastasis to nearby nodes.

Remember : *Klatskin tumor :* Tumour at the bifurcation of CBD.

Clinical features

- Most patient present in ***late stage.***
- Most common presentation is ***painless jaundice*** followed by pruritis, abdominal pain and weight loss.
- Jaundice occur early with distal and hilar cholangiocarcinoma, but very late with intrahepatic ones.

Remember : ***Most common*** cause of painless obstructive jaundice is Ca pancreas.

Staging : *Same as HCC*

Diagnosis

LFT:
– Reveals elevated markers of cholestasis (↑ ALK–PO_4tase, ↑ GGT)
– ↑ Bilurubin (Bilirubin is normal in case of intrahepatic tumors).

Tumor marker – CEA and CA-19-9 are most important tumor marker.

Radiology – US and CT are preferred imaging technique.

Choledochoscopy – Gold Standard for cholangiocarcinoma.

Treatment

– *Intrahepatic cholangiocarcinoma :* Resection if possible.

– *Hilar cholangiocarcinoma :* Enbloc resection of at least one lobe of the liver and the extrahepatic bile duct, and a complete periportal lymphadenectomy.

– *Distal cholangiocarcinoma :* Pancreaticoduodenectomy with resection of the extrahepatic bile duct.

SECONDARY (METASTATIC) TUMOR OF LIVER

- More common than primary.

- Most common site of primary are : *Ca lung > Ca colon > Ca pancreas> Ca Breast > Ca stomach.* *... Devita 7/e, p 991*
- **Clinical ciriteria of secondaries in liver :**
  - Both lobes are enlarge
  - Nodular growth with umblication (due to cental necrosis) is characteristic
  - Sharp border
  - Evidence of primary
  - Thrill or bruit never occur
  - *Raise in $ALKPO_4$ tase is most consistent abnormality. Tumor markers like CEA, CA 19-9, CA-125 are often elevated*
  - CT or USG guided biopsy is diagnostic
- **Imaging**
  - Contrast enhanced CT scan is the initial imaging modality to detect liver metastasis
  - FDG PET is the most sensitive diagnostic modality *... Devita 8/e p 2495*

QUESTIONS

1. **All of the following modalities can be used for in-situ ablation of liver secondaries except : [AI 06]**
   a. Ultrasonic waves
   b. Cryotherapy
   c. Alcohol
   d. Radiotherapy
2. **Marker of hepatocellular ca are all except: [AIIMS May 07]**
   a. Alfa feto protein
   b. PIVKA2
   c. Neurotensin
   d. Alfa2a globulin
3. **All of the following are modalities of therapy for hepatocellular carcinoma except : [AIIMS 05]**
   a. Radiofrequency ablaton
   b. Transarterial catheter embolization
   c. Percutaneous acetic acid
   d. Nd yag laser ablation
4. **Which one of the following hepatic lesion can be diagnosed with high accuracy by using nuclear maging ? [AIIMS 06]**
   a. Hepatocellular carcinoma
   b. Hepatic adenoma
   c. Focal nodular hyerplasia
   d. Cholangiocarcinoma
5. **Incorrect statement regarding secondaries of liver is: [PGI Dec 05]**
   a. Secondaries are more common than primary
   b. Raise in alkaline phosphate is seen in most cases
   c. Metastasis from colorectal carcinoma is associated with worse prognosis
   d. Surgery can be done for advanced metastatic disease

ANSWERS, REFERENCES, EXPLANATIONS WITH INFORMATIVE ILLUSTRATIONS

1. **Ans. is a i.e. Ultrasonic waves** *Ref. Devita 8/e, p 1140*

Ultrasonic waves are not used in situ ablation of liver secondaries.

Modalities for insitu ablation of liver secondaries :

- Hepatic arterial chemotherapy
- Chemoembolization
- Cryotherapy
- Radiofrequency ablation
- Percutaneous ethanol injection
- Whole liver irradiation ± chemotherapy.

2. **Ans. is c i.e. Neurotensin**

Ref. Devita 8/e, p 1137; Fletcher Histiopatholgy of Tumors 3/e, p 429 - 430

Neurotensin is increased in pancreatic endocrine tumor (not in HCC) and small cell Ca of lung.

Diagnosis of HCC

Tumor Marker :

- AFP – Raised in 50-70% of cases (not > 70%).
  - Level >200ng/ml are suggestive.
  - Level >1000ng/ml are diagnostic.
  - Level comes down after resection and raise again on recurrence.
- PIVKA-2 – Raised in 80-85% of cases.
- Hep Part1 – Most sensitive and specific immunohistochemical marker.
- Albumin ISH – Highly sensitive and specific.
- Both AFP and PIVKA-2 are ↑ in cirrhosis and chronic hepatitis.

Imaging :

- Ultrasonography is initial IOC and best method for screening.
- Arterial phase CT and MRI with contrast are best method for staging.
- FDG-PET : to detect metastatic disease.
- MRI is best way to show hepatic vein extension.

Biopsy :

- Percutaneous core or US guided aspiration biopsy are diagnostic but due to potential risk of seeding of needle tract, *biopsy is reserved only for cases in whom imaging is not diagnostic.*
- Biopsy is contraindicated if resection is planned.

Associated Lab findings :

- Anaemia with erythrocytosis and Leukocytosis.
- ↑ Alkaline PO_4tase.

3. Ans. is d i.e. Nd Yag laser ablation *Ref. Devita 8/e, p 1140*

No, it is not actetic acid surprised ! just see below.

Treatment options for Hepatocellular carcinoma

Surgery	**Local ablative therapies**
Partial hepatectomy Liver transplantation Ethanol injection Radiofrequency ablation	Cryosurgery Microwave ablation Acetic acid injection
Regional therapies : hepatic artery transcatheter treatments	**Systemic therapy**
Transarterial chemotherapy Transarterial embolization Transaterial chemoembolization Transarterial radiotherapy - Yttrium 90 microspheres - Iodine 131 lipiodol	Chemotherapy Immunotherapy Hormonal therapy + growth control

Treatment of HCC

HCC < 2 cm : Radiofrequency ablation, percutaneous ethanol injection or resection.

HCC > 2 cm no vascular invasion : Liver resection, Radiofrequency ablation, or liver transplantation.

Multiple unilobar disease *(Tumour with vascular invasion) :* Aggressive intrahepatic arterial chemoembolization followed by liver transplantation.

Bilobar disease : Same as multiple unilobar disease.

Extrahepatic HCC and bilobar disease with IVC invasion : No successfull treatment.

Remember :
- Percutaneous acetic acid is associated with lower rate of local recurrence in comparision to ethanol.
- Transarterial catheter embolization : It is a technique by which chemotherapy is given directly to liver and simultaneously embolisation is done by embolizing agent such as Lipoidal, gelatin, starch or PVC.

4. **Ans. is c i.e. Focal nodular hyperplasia**

Ref. Bailey & Love 25/e, p 1086; CSDT 11/e, p 578

To solve this question one, must known about nuclear imaging of liver.

Liver is made of two types of cell : ***1. Hepatocytes***
2. Kupffer cells

Based on this there are two types of radionucleide imaging :

1. ***Iodide imaging (Hepatocyte based imaging) :*** Iodide is Tc^{99m} labelled radionucleide that is administered intravenously which is taken by hepatocyte and then excreted in to bile.

   Thus, it is used for imaging of functional liver parenchyma and trace the flow of bile. Its clinical **uses** are :

   a. To asses functional liver mass, (only functional hepatocyte can process radionucleide)
   b. Demonstration of biliary leak
   c. Choledochal cyst
   d. To diagnose biliary obstruction
   e. Demonstration of gall bladder function
   f. Differentiation of hepatocellular tumor.

2. ***Sulphur colloid scintography (Kupffer cells based)***

   This is particulary used in hepatic mass lesion, to see whether they contain Kupffer cell or not.

   Interpretation is :

   Hot spot : Tumor contain Kupffer cell, Only example is *focal nodular hyperplasia.*

   Cold spot : Tumor mass lacking kupffer cell eg. *Hepatic angioma, adenoma, primary* or *metastatic cancer.*

Remember :

– Primary or metastatic ca	:	Field defect on both Iodide and colloid scintography.
– Hepatic angioma or adenoma	:	Normal iodide scan with defective colloid scintography.
– Focal nodular hyperplasia	:	Both iodide and colloid scintography are normal.

5. **Ans. are c and d i.e. Metastasis from colorectal carcinoma is associated with worse prognosis, surgery can be done for advanced metastatic disease**

Ref. Devita 7/e, p 2366

"Prognosis of liver metastases depend on primary site, metastasis of colorectal origin has best prognosis". *... Devita*

- Surgery is reserved only for patient with unilobar metastases with enough disease free hepatic parenchyma.

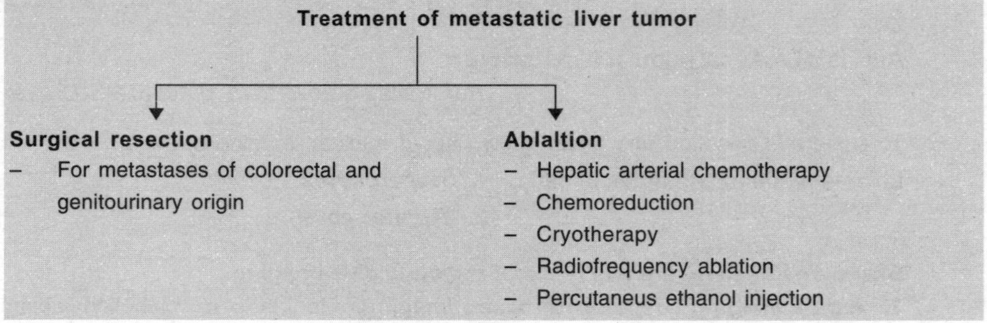

Clinical ciriteria of Secondaries in liver

- Both lobes are enlarge
- Nodular growth with ***umblication*** (due to cental necrosis) is characteristic
- Sharp border
- Evidence of primary
- Thrill or bruit never occur
- Raise in AlKPO4 is most consistent abnormality.

25 Carcinoma of Gall Bladder

What's Important ?

- Etiology
- Treatment

- Most common biliary tract malignancy, but rare in India.
- Age : 7th decade; F > M

Etiology and risk factor

- ***Gall stones :*** 70 - 80% of cases are associated with gall stones
- Calcification of gall bladder (porcelin gall bladder)
- Female sex
- Older age
- Typhoid carriers - Cholecystoenteric fistula
- Presence of anomalous pancreaticobiliary duct junction
- Obesity, inflammatory bowel disease, polyposis coli

Pathology

- Site : ***Fundus (60%)*** > **body** (30%) > **Neck** (10%) *... Devita 8/e p 1173*
- Type : MC type is ***adenocarcinoma.***
- Carcinoma of gall bladder exhibit two patterns of growth : a. ***Infiltrative*** MC
  b. Ulcerative
- Gall bladder cancer have a *remarkable propensity to seed and grow in peritoneal cavity as well as along needle biopsy sites and in laproscopic port site.*
- By the time these neoplasm are discovered most have invaded the liver centrifugally.
- ***Lung*** is *commonest* site of the hematogenous metastasis.

Clinical presentation

- Most patient present with biliary colic or chronic cholecystitis, jaundice is a late feature.
- *Persistent right upper quadrant pain with recent weight loss in old female is characteristic presentation.*

Diagnosis

- As most patient present with chronic cholecystitis, *most patient are diagnosed incidentally* at the time of surgery or pathologic review of resected gall bladder.
- Tumor marker CA 19 - 9 is *best serum* marker for gall bladder cancer. ... *Devita 8/e, p 1175*
- **Imaging :**
  - US - Demonstrate GB stone and wall thickening but these are not specific for carcinoma.
  - CT - Reveal mass in 80% of cases.
  - MRI - *Better than CT.*
- **Biopsy :**
  - Percutaneous fine needle aspiration or cone needle biopsy should be performed in cases that are not considered for resection.
  - When diagnosis is certain and resection is possible, intra-operative biopsy is done.

Treatment

- ***Prophylactic cholecystectomy :*** For cases of porcelain gall bladder.
- ***Extended cholecystectomy :*** For resectable disease and for gall bladder carcinoma recognised at laprotomy. In this cholecystectomy is performed along with wedge resection of adjacent 3 - 5cm of normal liver and dissection of lymphnode in the hepatoduodenal ligament.

Incidental gall bladder cancer after Simple cholecystectomy.

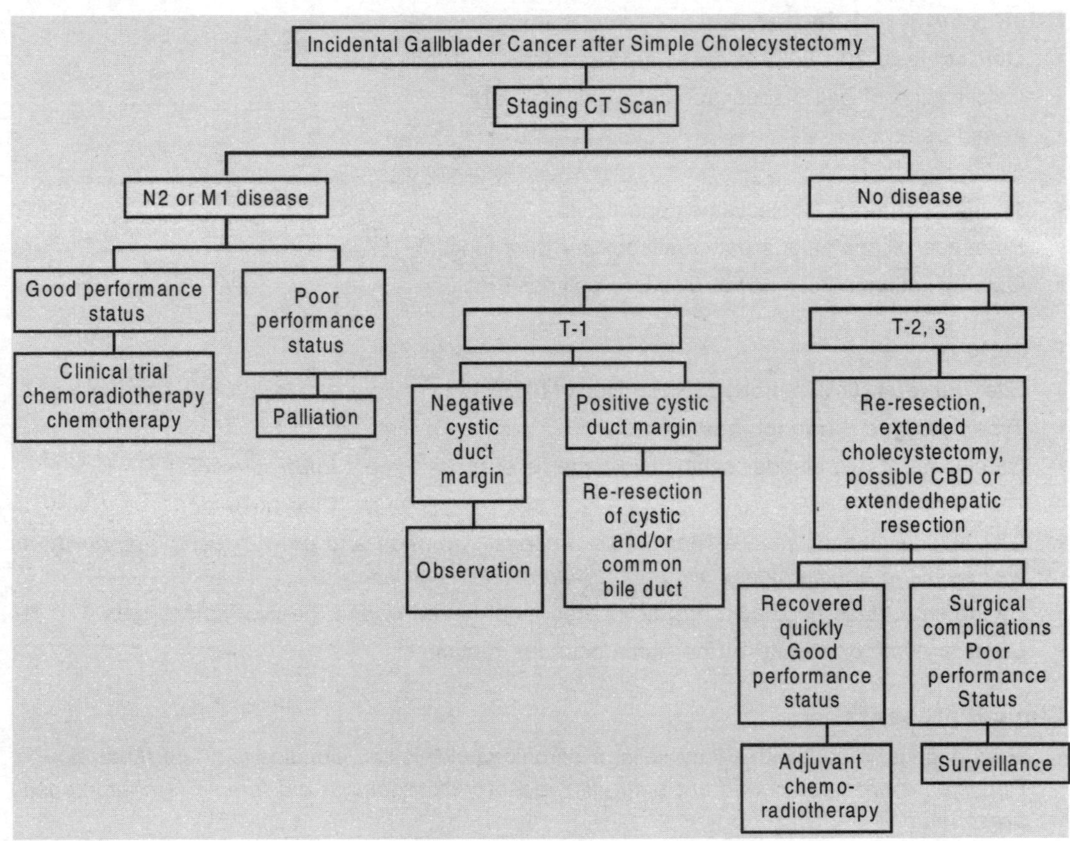

Remember : Asymptomatic gall stone is not an indication of cholecystectomy as the incidence of gall bladder cancer in patient of choledocholithiasis is very low (0.3%).

PORCELIN GALL BLADDER

- Calcification of gall bladder after long standing inflammation.
- Seen in plain radiograph.
- Associated with 10% – 15% of cases of gall bladder carcinoma.
- Due to high risk of developing carcinoma (20 times) ***prophylactic cholecystectomy*** is indicated.

QUESTIONS

1. **Risk factors for malignant change in an asymptomatic patient with a gall bladder polys on ultrasound include all of the following except: [AI 2009]**
   a. Age > 60 years
   b. Rapid increase in size of polyp
   c. Size of polyp > 5 mm
   d. Associated gall stones
2. **Factors associated with gallbladder Ca:**
   a. Chronic cholesterol stone **[PGI 05]**
   b. Hyperlipidemia
   c. Chronic gallbladder disease
   d. Hepatitis
   e. Porcelain gallbladder
3. **In a male after laparoscopic cholecystectomy, carcinoma gallbladder Stage I detected on histopathology. What is the next appropriate management :**
   a. Conservative and follow up **[AIIMS 08]**
   b. Radical portal lymphadenectomy
   c. Radiotherapy - Chemotherapy
   d. Excision of portal site

ANSWERS, REFERENCES, EXPLANATIONS WITH INFORMATIVE ILLUSTRATIONS

1. **Ans. is c i.e. Polyp > 5 mm in length** *Ref. Sabiston 18/e, p 1578*

Gallbladder polyps

• **Polyps of gallbladder are:**	– Cholesterol polyps (**MC benign mass of GB**) – Adenomyomatosis – Benign adenomas – Malignant adenocarcinomas
• **Factors signifying malignancy:**	– Old age (> 60 years) – Coexistence of gall stones – Size > 10 mm – Increasing size

Treatment

– Cholecystectomy is the treatment of choice for all patient with symptomatic polyp or those with any risk factor of malignancy
– Asymptomatic lesion < 10 mm without any risk factors can be managed by serial follow up with ultrasound

2. **Ans. is a, c and e i.e. Chronic cholesterol stone; Chronic gallbladder disease; Porcelain gallbladder** *Ref. Devita 8/e, p 1157*

Risk factor for carcinoma gallbladder:

- Gall stone (MC) (larger the size of stone, more is risk).
- Porcelain gallbladder (Calcified gallbladder).
- Cholecystoenteric fistula

Contd...

Contd...

- Chronic typhoid carriers
- Older age, female sex
- Anomalous pancreaticobiliary junction
- Adenomatous polyp > 1 cm in diameter
- Adenomyomatosis, gallbladder adenomas, and epithelial dysplasia
- Genetic factors include K ras and p53 mutations

Remember : – Limey bile is ***not a premalignant*** condition.

3. **Ans. is a i.e. Conservative and follow up**

Ref. Devita 8/e, p 1182; Blumgart surgery of Liver and Biliary tract 4/e p 778

"Incidentally discovered cancers after cholecystectomy is common and this is sufficient treatment for most T1 cancers, exception are patient with positive cystic duct margin who should undergo definitive complete resection and patient with T1b tumor who also should be considered for an extended repeat resection". ... *Blumgart 594*

26 Cancer of Kidney, Ureter and Bladder

What's Important ?

- Diagnosis and Treatment
- Histology and Cytogenetics for PGI

KIDNEY TUMORS

- Both benign and malignant tumors occur in kidney.
- With the exception of oncocytoma, benign tumors rarely cause clinical problem.
- Most common renal tumor is ***renal cell carcinoma*** followed by Wilms tumor which is found in children.

RENAL CELL CARCINOMA

Also called as ***hypernephroma = Adenocarcinoma of kidney.***

- Previously referred as *"Internist tumor"* owing to its common systemic manifestation, rather than local one. Now more appropriately it is called as "radiologist tumor" due to high frequency of incidental detection by radiologist.

Incidence and predisposing factors

- Accounts for **85%** of renal cancer in adults.
- Occurs usually in older individuals with male - female ratio of 2 to 3 :1.
- RCC occurs in both sporadic and hereditary forms (tends to affect young individuals).
  The **hereditary variant** of RCC are :
  - Von Hipple lindau syndrome (VHL) (Clear cell RCC)
  - Hereditary papillary carcinoma. (Papillary type RCC)
  - Hereditary leomyomatosis RCC (Papillary type 2 RCC)
  - Birt–Hogg–Dube (BHD) syndrome. (Chromophobe RCC)
- Tobacco is the ***most significant risk factor.***
- **Other risk factors are :**
  - Obesity
  - Hypertension
  - Exposure to Asbestos, Petroleum products
  - Chronic renal failure (specially due to analgesic nephropathy)
  - Long term dialysis, who develop renal cysts

Classification of RCC

A. **Clear cell carcinoma :**
   - Most common type of RCC.
   - Mainly sporadic.
   - Both sporadic and familial RCC are associated with loss of sequence on ***chromosome 3*** either by translocation (3:6; 3:8; 3:11) or deletion. This region harbours the VHL gene.

B. **Papillary carcinoma :**
   - Characterized by Papillary growth pattern.
   - Most common cytogenetic abnormalities are **trisomies 7**, 16 and 17. Loss of 18 in sporadic form. Trisomy 7 in familial form. This is due to mutated MET gene on chromosome 7.

C. **Chromophobe renal carcinoma**
   - Represent 5% of RCC.
   - Composed of cells with prominent cell membrane and eosinophilic cytoplasm with a halo around nucleus
   - These tumor exhibit multiple chromosome loss and extreme hypodiploidy.

D. **Collecting duct (Bellini duct) carcinoma :**
   - Rarest type of RCC.
   - Composed of malignant cells enmeshed with in a prominent fibrotic stroma typically in medullary location.

Pathology and Morphology

Clear cell carcinoma :

- Arise from *proximal tubular epithelial* cells particularly of cortex.
- Occurs as *solitary unilateral* lesion, often a *pseudocapsule* is formed around tumor by compression of surrounding tissue.
- Tumor cells are clear and contain glycogen and lipids.
- Most are well differentiated.

Papillary carcinoma :

- Arise from *DCT* can be multifocal and bilateral
- Has got highest propensity to invade IVC
- They are typically *hemorrhagic* and *cystic.*
- Papiilar ca is the MC type of RCC in patient with dialysis associated cystic disease.
- Composed of cuboidal and low columar cells.
- Psammoma bodies may be present.

Chromphobe renal carcinoma :

- Arise from intercalated cells of collecting duct.
- Composed of pale eosinophilic cells often with a perinuclear halo.
- Associated with best prognosis.
- Arranged in solid sheets with concentration of largest cell around blood vessel referred to as plant like structure

Collecting duct carcinoma :

- Arise from intercalated cells of collecting duct.
- Has got very aggressive course.
- Shows hobnail pattern of growth

Spread

- Tumour extends directly through the walls of collecting duct to renal pelvis and ureter.
- One of the characteristic of RCC is its tendency to ***invade the renal vein.*** Further extension produces a continuous cord of tumour in the inferior vena cava and even in right side of heart.
- Most common sites of distant metastases are lungs > soft tissue > bone > liver.

... Devita 8/e, p 1337

Clinical features

- Most common and consistent presentation is ***hematuria.***
- ***Classical triad*** of *gross hematuria, abnormal mass and pain* is seen ***only in 9%*** of patient.
- Other symptoms are : fever, weight loss, malaise. Approx 30% of patient have metastatic disease.
- ***Paraneoplastic syndromes*** associated with RCC are :

– Polycythemia	– Hypercalcemia
– Hypertension	– Hepatic dysfunction (Stauffer syndrome)
– Feminization and masculinization	
– Neuromyopathy	– Amyloidosis
– Eosinophillia	– Leukemoid reaction

- It may cause lower extremity oedema by occluding IVC.

Diagnosis

- **CT** is the diagnostic procedure of choice. CT is modality of choice for imaging a renal mass.

... Devita 8/e, p1338

- **IVU** is the initial *investigation of choice* for hematuria.
- **Diagnostic protocol** is IVU → US → CT.
- **MRI** less accurate than CT in evaluating renal mass.
  However, MRI is most accurate non invasive means of detecting tumor thrombi in renal vein or IVC.
- **Isotope bone scans:** For bone metastasis
- **Chest X-ray:** For pulmonary involvement

Remember : *Inferior venocavogram* is most specific and sensitive but ***invasive*** means to detect involvement of ***IVC.***

Staging

TNM classification						
Stage		***T***		***N***		***M***
I.	Tumour confined by renal capsule	T1	(< 7.0 cm tumour with minimal caliceal distortion)	N0 (nodes negative)		M0 (lack of distant metas-tases)
		T2	(> 7.0 cm tumour with caliceal deformity)			
II.	Tumour extension to perirenal fat or ipsilateral adrenal but confined by Gerota's fascia	T3a		N0		M0
IIIa.	Renal vein or inferior vena cava involvement	T3b	(renal vein involvement)	N0		M0
		T3c	(renal vein and caval involvement below the diaphragm)			
		T4b	(caval involvement above the diaphragm)			
IIIb.	Lymphatic involvement	T1-3		N1	(single homo-lateral regional node involved)	M0
				N2	(multiple regional, contralateral, or bilateral nodes involved)	
				N3	(fixed regional nodes)	
				N4	(juxtaregional nodes involved)	
IIIc.	Combination of IIIa and IIIb	T3-4		N1-4		M0
IVa.	Spread to contiguous organs except ipsilateral adrenal	T4a		N3-4		M0
IVb.	Distant metastases	T1-4		N0-4		M1

Treatment

Surgery :

- *For stage I, II, and IIIA : Open radical nephrectomy* which includes an enbloc removal of kidney and surrounding Gerota's fascia including ipsilateral adrenal, the renal hilar lymph nodes and proximal half of ureter. Paraaortic dissection has not been benefcial and is not recommended.
- *Patient with Stauffer's syndrome* are also candidate for *radical nephrectomy.*
- *Patient with solitary kidney those with Diabetes mellitus or renal insufficiency, those with tumor under 4 cm (even with normal opposite Kidney)* should be treated with *partial nephrectomy or renal insufficiency.* *... CSDT 13/e, p 942*

Radiotherapy : It is of little benefit except for *symptomatic bone metastasis.*

Chemotherapy :

- *No* effective chemotherapy is available for RCC.
- *Vinblastine* is single most effective agent.

Hormonal and therapy – *Medroxy progesterone* is used for metastatic RCC.
– Immunotherapy with *I FN* has 15 - 20 % response rate.

Biological therapy – Primary therapy *for wide spread metastatic RCC.*
– **Involves use of**
- IFNα and IL - 2
- *Combined IL - 2 and IFNα is the best treatment for widespread disease.*

Vascular endothelial growth factor targeted therapy:
– Sunitinib
– Sorafenib
– Temsirolimus

Radiotherapy: Indicated only for treatment of symptomatic bone metastasis

Remember : RCC is one of the tumor which may show *spontaneous regression.* Other are neuroblastoma, lymphoma.

Approaches to Nephrectomy for RCC

- ***Flank appraoch :*** Small tumor without venous involvement.
- ***Subcostal transperitoneal approach :*** When there is a large tumour in the middle on lower aspect of kidney or when vascular involvement is anticipated.
- ***Thoracoabdominal approach :*** When there is a large middle or upper pole tumour or there is extensive venacaval involvement.
- ***Laproscopic nephrectomy :*** This is a growing approach as it reduces postoperative hospital stay with equal survival rate.

BENIGN RENAL TUMORS

- Benign tumors are rare in kidney.
- Common benign tumors are :

Renal adenoma

– Most common *benign solid parenchyma lesion* of kidney. *... CSDT 12/e, p 1038*
– Histologically *indistinguishable from adenocarcinoma.*
– Treated as malignant tumor.

Oncocytoma

– Subtype of adenoma.
– Produce typical *spokewheel pattern on angiography.*
– Treatment is total removal.

Angiomyolipoma

– Seen in patient with *tuberous sclerosis.*
– Tumor > 5 cm should be surgically resected.

CARCINOMA OF RENAL PELVIS AND URETER

Features	Ca of Renal pelvis	Ca of Ureter
Incidence	Rare	Rare
Etiology	Smoking	Smoking
Histology	Transitional cell ca (MC); sq. cell ca (in cases of chronic inflammation and stone)	Transitional cell ca (MC)
Clinical feature	Hematuria (MC)	Hematuria (MC)
Diagnosis	IVU (showing hydronephrosis) *Confirmed by retrograde pyelography* (showing filling defect)	IVU (showing filling defect) Retrograde pyelograply shows filling defect in ureter "goblet sign'
Treatment	*Radical nephrectomy* with total removal of ipsilateral ureter and cuff of bladder	Nephroureterectromy Partial ureterectomy (for low grade, non invasive lesion)

BLADDER CANCER

Bladder cancer is fourth most common cancer in men and seventh most common carcinoma in women. In women bladder ca is the most common cancer of urinary tract (In males it is RCC).

Risk factors

Cigarette smoking	–	Most important risk factor.
Occupation	–	Work in dye, rubber and leather industry
Diet	–	Fried meat and high fat diet.
Infection	–	Schistosoma haematobium (↑ risk of both squamous and transitional cell carcinoma) but most cases of SCC are associated with it
Pelvic irradiation	–	increase risk of squamous cell ca.

Histology

- *95% of bladder tumor are of epithelial origin, rest being mesenchymal tumors.*
- Most epithelial tumors are *transitional tumors called as urothelial tumors.* Rest are squamous cell ca often seen on dome of bladder in patient with urachal remnant.

Pathology and Morphology

- The precursor lesion of invasive urothelial cancer are :
  - Non invasive papillary tumor ***(Kiss Ulcer)***
  - Flat urothelial ca called as carcinoma in situ = ***Malignant cystitis***
- **WHO/ISUP grading of urothelial tumor :**
  - Urothelial Papilloma
  - Papillary urothelial ca low malignant potential
  - Papillary urothelial ca low grade
  - Papillary urothelial ca high grade.
- Overall ***majority*** of tumor are of low grade.

- ***Most*** tumor develop at trigone and adjacent posterolateral wall and ureteral involvement is common.
- Tumor tends to be ***multifocal*** in bladder.

Clinical finding

- At presentation 75% of tumor are ***superficial,*** 20% are invasive.
- ***Hematuria*** is MC presenting feature, other are urgency, frequency.

Diagnosis

- **Cystoscopy :**
  - Cystoscopic evaluation forms the *main stay of diagnosis and staging.*
  - Superficial appearing tumor can be diagnosed and removed at the same time.
- **Urinary cytologic studies :**
  - Transitional cell tumors shed neoplastic cells in to the urine in large number which can be demonstrated by using flow cytometry. These studies are *most useful and gold standard for early diagnosis of recurrence* of transitional cell carcinoma.
  - Detection of biological markers such as NMP-22, fibrin degradation product basic feto protein in urine.
- **Imaging studies :**
  - US *can accurately demonstrate* moderately large tumor but miss small tumor.
  - CT and MRI both are equally effective for staging.

Note :
- Individual > 40 years who develop hematuria with normal IVU should have cystoscopy to exclude bladder carcinoma.
- Pelvic pain signifies extravesical spread.

Staging and Treatment

Stage	Involvement	Treatment
Ta	Mucosa only	Transuretheral resection ± intra vasical BCG (if high grade) followed by regular follow up.
T 1	Submucosal invasion (Lamina propria)	Transuretheral resection + intravesical chemoimmuno-therapy followed by regular follow up.
T 2a	Superficial muscle invasion	Total cystectomy and pelvic lymphadenectomy.
T 2b	Deep muscle invasion	Total cystectomy and pelvic lymphadenectomy.
T3	Perivesical fat invasion	Total cystectomy and pelvic lymphadenectomy.
T 3 - 4 N+	Regional Lymph invasion	Systemic chemotherapy (cisplatin based)
T 3 - 4 M1	Distant metastases	Systemic chemotherapy (cisplatin based)

Note :
- Open surgical excision (transabdominal) should be totally avoided. If by error a bladder containing a tumor is entered, then the tumor should be removed with post operative radiotherapy given to wound.
- BCG is most effective agent for intravesical chemotherapy.

IN SITU CARCINOMA (= MALIGNANT CYSTITIS)

- Replacement of normally well ordered epithelium by irregularly arranged cells with large nuclei and high mitotic index is called carcinoma in situ.
- **This may occur :**
  - Alone (primary CIS)
  - Association with a new tumor (concomitant CIS)
  - In patient who has previously had tumor (secondary CIS).
- **Symptoms :** It cause dysuria, suprapubic pain and frequency hence called malignant cystitis.

Prognosis : Treatment and prognosis depends on *degree of anaplasia (grade) and depth of penetration.*

QUESTIONS

1. **A 60 year old smoker came with history of one episode of painless and gross hemturia. The investigation of choice would be : [AIIMS 10, 06; AI 07]**
   a. Urine routine & microscopy
   b. Plain X-ray KUB
   c. USG KUB
   d. Urine microscopy for malignant cells

2. **In a case of bladder carcinoma all investigation can be done except : [AI 07]**
   a. Malignant cell in the urine
   b. Cystoscopy and biopsy
   c. Nmp - 22 test in urine
   d. CA - 125 in blood

3. **Paraneoplastic syndrome associated with RCC are all of the following except:**
   a Polycythemia **[AI 09]**
   b. Hypercalcemia
   c. Hypertension
   d. Cushing syndrome

4. **Most important prognostic factor for renal cell cancer is: [AIIMS Nov 09]**
   a. Size of tumor
   b. Pathological staging
   c. Nuclear grading
   d. Histologic type

5. **Which of the following is most effective intravesical therapy for superficial bladder cancer ? [AIIMS 05]**
   a. Mitomycin
   b. Adriamycin
   c. Thiotepa
   d. BCG

6. **The most common histologic variant of renal cell carcinoma is : [AIIMS 05]**
   a. Clear cell type
   b. Chromophobe type
   c. Papillary type
   d. Tubular type

7. **Robson's classification is used for :**
   a. Bladder ca **[PGI 05, 95]**
   b. Renal cell ca
   c. Testicular tumor
   d. Breast ca

8. **Chromophobe variety of RCC is associated with: [AI 10, AIIMS May 10]**
   a. Trisomy 7 and trisomy 17
   b. Loss of chromosome
   c. Gain of 5
   d. VHL gene mutation

ANSWERS, REFERENCES, EXPLANATIONS WITH INFORMATIVE ILLUSTRATIONS

1. **Ans. is d i.e. Urine microscopy by malignant cells**

Ref. CSDT 13/e 947; Devita 7/e, p 1169; Bailey & Love 25/e, p 1336

Painless gross hematuria in a smoker suggest bladder carcinoma.

Diagnosis of Bladder carcinoma

- **Cystoscopy :**
  - Cystoscopic evaluation forms the *main stay of diagnosis and staging.*
  - Superficial appearing tumor can be diagnosed and removed at the same time.
- **Urinary cytologic studies :**
  - Transitional cell tumors shed neoplastic cells in to the urine in large number which can be demonstrated by using flow cytometry. These studies are *most useful and gold standard for early diagnosis of recurrence* of transitional cell carcinoma.
  - Detection of biological markers such as NMP-22, fibrin degradation product basic feto protein in urine.
- **Imaging studies :**
  - US *can accurately demonstrate* moderately large tumor but miss small tumor.
  - CT and MRI both are equally effective for staging.

Clinical features of Bladder carcinoma

- Painless hematuria - Most common and most consistent.
- Acute retention of urine may occur due to pedunculated tumor.
- Constant *pain in pelvis* suggest extravesical spread.
- Late manifestation is nerve involvement causing pain referred to suprapubic region, groin, perinium and anus.

2. **Ans. is d i.e. CA - 125 in blood** *Ref. Devita 8/e, p 1359*

- NMP - 22 (Nuclear matrix protein) is seen in urine in about 40 - 60% cases of bladder ca.
- CA-125 is not elevated in bladder ca.

For more details, kindly see answer no. 1

3. **Answer is d i.e. Cushing's syndrome**

Ref. Harrison 17/e p 592; Robbins 8/e p 866

Guy's to be very frank some books have mentioned all options as paraneoplastic syndrome, but Cambell, Harrison has not mentioned Cushing syndrome. So it is taken as answer.

Paraneoplastic syndrome associated with RCC

Syndrome	Percent
Elevated ESR	55.6
Hypertension	37.5
Anemia	36.3
Cachexia, weight loss	34.5
Pyrexia	17.2
Abnormal liver function	14.4
Hypercalcemia	4.9
Polycythemia	3.5
Neuromyopathy	3.2
Amyloidosis	2

4. **Ans. is b i.e. Pathologic staging** *Ref. Campbell Urology 8/e p 2701*

Pathological staging is the single most important prognostic factor for RCC

... Campbell

Prognostic factors for RCC

a. **Tumor related**
   - Pathological stage
   - Tumor size
   - Histological subtype (Sarcomatoid or medullary cell histologic subtype denotes poor prognosis)
   - Nuclear grade

b. **Clinical factors:**
   - Performance status is the most consistently reported factor
   - Number of metastatic site

c. **Laboratory parameters:**
   - ↑ ESR, CRP (*bad prognosis*)
   - Anaemia, thrombocytosis (*bad prognosis*)
   - Biochemical markers: Serum LDH (>*1.5 time*), corrected calcium(> *10mg/dl*), carries high risk of mortality.

5. **Ans. is d i.e. BCG** *Ref. Devita 8/e, p 1362; CSDT 13/e, p 948*

"BCG is most effective agent currently used for intravesical chemotherapy."

... CSDT 12/e, p 1065

BCG induce T-cell recruitment and subsequent cytokine release at tumour site.

Indications of Intravesical therapy

- Multifocal CIS
- CIS associated with Ta or T_1 tumours
- Any grade III tumours
- Multifocal tumours
- Tumours that rapidly recur after TURBT of the initial tumour.

Complication of intravesical BCG

- Fever
- Joint pain
- Granulomatous prostatitis
- Sinus formation
- Disseminated TB.

6. **Ans. is a i.e. Clear cell type** *Ref. Robbin's 7/e, p 1016; 8/e p 965*

Relative frequency of histologic types of RCC

• Clear cell ca ***(MC)***	70 - 80%
• Papillary ca	10 - 15%
• Chromophobe carcinoma	5%
• Collecting duct (bellini duct) carcinoma	1%

Remember : Papillary ca is *most common* histologic type of RCC in patient of dialysis associated renal disease.

7. **Ans. b i.e. Renal cell Ca** *Ref. Devita 7/e, p 1147*

Robson classification was used in past for staging of RCC.

Robson's Classification

Stage I	Renal carcinoma is confined to kidney.
Stage II	Carcinoma extends through the renal capsule but is confined to Gerota's fascia.
Stage IIIA	Carcinoma involves the renal vein or IVC.
Stage IIIB	Carcinoma involving local hilar lymph nodes.
Stage IV	Tumour has spread to local, adjacent organs (other than adrenal glands) or distant sites.

The disadvantage of this system is that it combines stage with significantly different prognosis.

8. **Ans. is b i.e. Loss of chromosome** *Ref. Robbins 8/e, p 965*

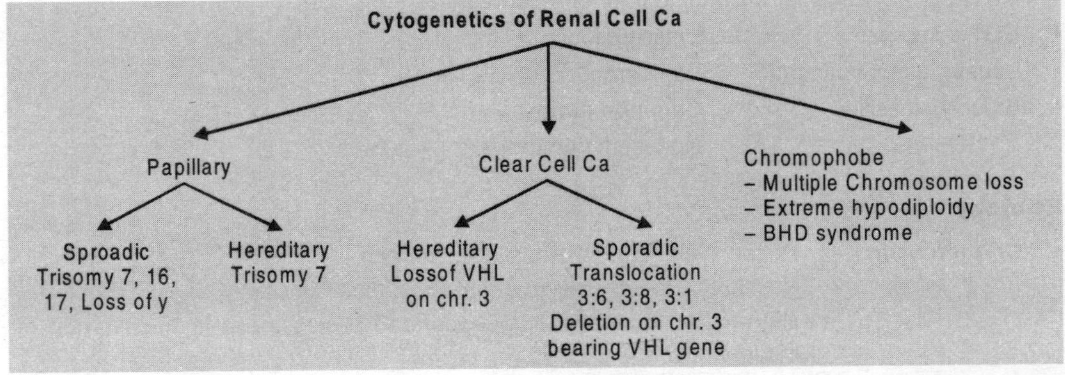

Cancer of Male Genital Tract

What's Important ?

- Diagnosis
- Treatment
- Etiology for PGI

TESTICULAR NEOPLASM

Testicular neoplasm are divided in to two major categories :

Germ cell Tumour	Sex cord stromal tumour
– Seminoma **(MC)**	– Leydig / interstitial cell tumour
– Teratocarcinoma	– Sertoli cell tumour (androblastoma)
– Choriocarcinoma	– Granulosa cell tumor
– Teratoma	– Yolk sac tumour
– Embryonal carcinoma	

- Gonadoblastoma has both germ cell & gonodal stromal elements. They almost always arise in gonads with some form of testicular dysgenesis
- *Germ cell tumour are mostly malignant and are more common than sex cord stromal tumor which are usually benign. Right testis is more commonly involved than left.*

GERM CELL TUMOR (GCT)

- GCT are MC testicular solid tumour in men between 20 - 35 years.
- GCT comprise > 91% of testicular tumours.
- Usually, affect young (25 - 35) age group.
- Broadly classified in to : – Seminomatous
  – Non seminomatous.

Etiology

- **Cryptorchism :**
  – Responsible for 5% of testicular tumour.
  – *Seminoma is* MC *testicular tumour in these patient.*
  – Higher the location of undescended testes more is the chance of malignancy.

– *Orchidopexy does not alter malignant potential* of cryptorchid testis but facilitates examination and tumor detection ... *CMDT' 10, p 1493*

- In utero DES exposure.
- Klinefelter's syndrome (increase risk of both testicular and mediastinal GCT) and testicular feminization syndrome.

Histogenesis and Cytogenetics

- Most GCT orginates from intratubular germ cell neoplasia (ITGCN) ...*Robbin's 8/e, p 988*
- *ITGCN is seen in all germcell tumor except spermatocytic seminoma, teratoma and pediatric Yolk cell tumor.*
- ITGCN progress to invasive GCT in approx 50% of cases.
- Histology of tumour depend on differentiation of germ cell.

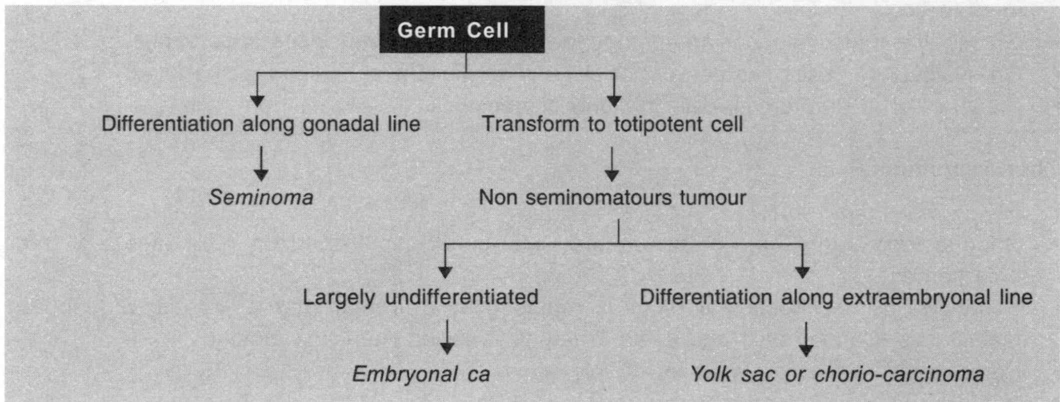

- Genomic change found in all germ cell tumour is an isochromosome of the short arm of **chromosome** ***12*** *(i12p).*

Morphology and Pathology

Seminoma :

- Affect age 25 - 35 years. *Never occur in infant.*
- Produce bulkymasses; cut surface is homogenous gray white and devoid of hemorrhage and necrosis.
- May extend to epididymis, spermatic cord but tunica albugenia is not penetrated.
- Classical seminoma don't contain AFP or HCG; but stain positive for *placental alkaline phosphate.*
- Mostly spread by *lymphatic route* to paraaortic LN.

Spermatocytic seminoma :

- It is different from seminoma both clinically and histologically. It is a slow growing tumor that does not produce metastasis
- Usually affect > 65 years age group and has good prognosis.
- It don't arise from ITGEN.

- Contains three types of cells:
  1. Medium sized cells (most numerous)
  2. Smaller cells resembling spermatocytes
  3. Scattered giant cells

Embryonal carcinoma

- Occurs mostly in *20 - 30 years* age group.
- More aggressive than seminoma.
- Histologically the cells grow as alveolar or tubular pattern.
- HCG or AFP or both may be detected in cells by immuno peroxidase.

Yolk Sac tumour

- Most common *testicular tumour in infants and children up to 3 years.* It has got best prognosis in all testicular tumor
- Grossly the tumour appear as homogenous, yellow white mucinous appearance.
- On microscopy - Lace like network of cell and schiller-Duval bodies may be found.
- Presence of AFP in tumour cells in highly characteristic.

Chorio carcinoma

- *Highly malignant.*
- Despite their aggressive behavior, they are usually small and do not cause testicular enlargement.
- Sometime primary testicular focus is replaced by a fibrous scar or leaving widespread metastases (Cannon ball) and death in few days called Hurricane tumour.
- Hemorrhage and necrosis are extremely common.
- HCG can be readily demonstrated.

Teratoma

- Affects age 20 - 30 years. Complex tumour having various cellular or organoid component.
- Usually large and composed of various tissues; gross appearance is heterogenous with solid and cystic areas.
- *In post pubertal male teratoma are regarded as malignant, regardless whether the elements are mature or immature.*
- Rarely non germ cell tumour (such as squamous cell ca) may arise in teratoma, these tumours are referred as teratoma with malignant transformation.
- Mostly spread by hematogenous route.

Mixed Tumour

- Most common of all testicular tumour (60%). ... *Robbin's 7/e, p 1045*
- Common mixtures are teratoma-embryonal ca; Seminoma with embryonal ca.

Note :
- Most common testicular tumour - Seminoma
- Most common histologic type - Mixed (If option is there, other wise seminoma).

Clinical features

- Most common symptom of testicular cancer is *painless enlargement of testis.*
- Occasionally hydrocoel (in 10%) may be presenting symptom.

Remember : In a young adult every testicular swelling should be considered malignant until proven otherwise.

Diagnosis

Serum markers

Tumour	Markers	
↓	*AFP*	*β HCG*
Seminoma	–	+
Teratoma	+/-	–
Embryonal Ca	+/-	+
Yolk cell tumour	+	–
Choriocarcinoma	–	+

- *LDH :* – Serum LDH reflects tumour burden, growth rate and cellular proliferation.
  - ↑ serum LDH has poor prognosis.
  - Elevated in both seminomatous and nonseminomatous type.
- *Placental alkaline phosphate :* elevated in seminoma.

Imaging Studies

- ***Scrotal ultrasound :*** It can readily determine whether the mass is intra or extratesticular in origin.
- ***Abdominal CT :*** Most effective technique for identifying metastatic disease.
- ***MRI:*** Not superior to CT.

Biopsy

- Biopsy is contraindicated through scrotal route because of spread to scrotal skin.

Treatment

Inguinal orchidectomy with high ligation of the cord at the internal ring is initial treatment for all testicular cancer.

a. **Non seminomatous tumour**
   - Following orchidectomy retroperitoneal lymphnode dissection is recommended.
   - *However, in patient with no evidence of retroperitoneal nodal enlargement on abdominal CT and with normal serum marker;* nodal dissection is not advised if patient can be followed. *... CSDT 13/e, p 954*
   - Patient with *extensive* retroperitoneal or chest metastases are best treated after orchidectomy by multiagents chemotherapy (etoposide and cisplatin + bleomycin) followed by removal of persistent mass.

b. Seminoma

- In absence of extensive distant spread, patient with pure seminoma should be treated with external beam radiotherapy to abdomen after orchidectomy.
- In presence of *metastases* multiagent chemotherapy is preferred.

SEX-CORD STROMAL TUMOUR

The two important tumours of this group are :

Leydig (interstitial) cells tumours	Sertoli cell tumours (andro blastoma)
• Derived from the stroma • May secrete androgens, estrogen or both • Present as testicular swelling, sexual precocity, gynecomastia	• Derived from sex cord • Composed entirely of sertoli cells • Secrete feminising hormone leading to gyanecomastia, loss of libido, aspermia.

TESTICULAR LYMPHOMA

- Most common form of testicular neoplasm in patient above 60 years. *... Robbin's 8/e, p 993*
- Most common secondary testicular tumour.
- Most common ***bilateral*** testicular tumour (MC *primary bilateral testicular tumour is seminoma).*
- Most common histologic type is diffuse large cell lymphoma.
- Prognosis is very poor.

PROSTATIC CANCER

- Most common form of cancer in men. *... Robbins 8/e p 996*
- 2nd MC cause of death due to cancer.
- ***Adenocarcinoma*** is the most common type of prostatic cancer.
- **Age :**
  - Affect man > 50, incidence ↑with ↑ in age.
  - Less common in Asians in comparison to Europeans.

Etiology and Cytogenetics

Risk is ↑ed by	Risk decreased by	
Advance age (most important risk factor). ↑ Fat intake	Lycopenes (found in tomato) Vitamin E Soy products	Vitamin D Selenium

The most common genetic alteration in ca prostate is hypermethylation of glutathione transferase (GSTP-1) gene promoter located on chromosome 11. *... Robbin's 8/e, p 996*

Pathogenesis and Morphology

• **Site**	– ***75%*** of prostatic cancer arise in ***peripheral zone*** (classically in posterior location). – ***15%*** occur in ***central zone.*** – ***10%*** (rarest) occur ***in transitional periurethral zone*** (MC site of BPH).
• **Spread**	– Spread occurs by direct local invasion and through blood stream and lymphatics.

	– ***Local invasion*** most commonly involves seminal vesicles and base of the bladder. – ***Hematogenous spread*** occurs chiefly to **bone** (MC axial skeleton) forming ***osteoblastic secondaries in lumbar spine > proximal femur > pelvis*** – ***Lymphatic spread*** occurs initially to obturator nodes followed by perivesical, hypogastric, iliac and paraaortic nodes.
• **Histology**	– Most 'e ***adenocarcinoma.*** – It is often accompanied by premalignant lesion, prostatic intraepithelial neoplasia which is characterized by large glands separated by moderate amount of stroma with normal appearing architecture. – Neoplastic tissue is gritty and firm which is difficult to visualize and easy to palpate. – Neoplastic glands are typically smaller than benign glands, but are more crowded and lack branching and papillary infoldings. *The outer basal layer of cells (typical of normal glands) is absent.* – ***Histologic finding specific for prostatic cancer is perineural invasion.***

Clinical features

- Incidental or stage A (T_1) Ca prostate is asymptomatic and not palpable and is diagnosed only by pathologist when prostate is removed as treatment of BPH.
- Stage B (T_2) or higher disease present as hard nodule on prostate felt during rectal examination.
- Metastatic disease present with bone pain (especially) pathologic fractures.
- Most common symptoms of prostatic Ca are bladder outlet distruction, sudden development of impotence, hematuria.

Screening

- It is recommended that screening for prostate cancer should *begin at 40 years for high risk and at 45 years for normal patient.* *... Robbin's 7/e, p 105*

• **Screening is done by :**	– DRE (Digital rectal examination) = Per rectal examination – Measurement of PSA – Transrectal ultrasound.
• **PSA measurement :**	– It is ***first line screening test*** – PSA is elevated in both *benign* and *malignant lesion* – Slight elevation is also seen after prostitis, endoscopic urethral manipulation – Levels > *4 ng/ml* are *abnormal* – PSA is most useful for *detecting recurrence* of tumour after treatment.

Diagnosis

Imaging :

- *Transrectal US* for staging of prostatic ca, most lesions are hypoechoic.
- *MRI* – For evaluation of the prostatic lesions as well as regional lymphnodes.
- *CT* – Plays little role.

- *Radionucleide scanning* :
  - For detecting bone metastases. Advised in patient with *PSA > 10mg / ml.*
  - A monoclonal antibody cyt - 356 (which identifies prostate specific antigens) has been couple with radio-isotopes for diagnoses of soft tissue metastases.

Biopsy :

- TRUS guided biopsy is better method than finger guided biopsy for detection of prostatic ca.
- Biopsy are taken from apex, mid portion and base of prostate.
- Differentiation of tumour is graded by a pathologist using *Gleason scale.* Tumour with Gleason sum of 7 or more is an aggressive cancer.

Treatment of prostate cancer related to tumor stage

Conventional Stage	TNM stage 1997	Clinical Findings	Treatment	15-Year-Recurrence-Free Survival (%)
A1	T1a	Nonpalpable tumor; incidental finding at transurethral prostatectomy (low-grade cancer seen in < 5% of of prostate).	Observation	100
A2	T1b	Same as above, except tumor is high grade, or > 5% of prostate is involved, or both.	Radical prostatectomy with pelvic lympha-denectomy Or	70-80
B1	T2a	Tumor involves 1 lobe or less	External beam radiation Or	85
B2	T2b	Tumor involves more than 1 lobe	Brachytherapy	60-70
C	T3a	Unilataeral extraprostatic extension		20-60
C2	T3b	Bilateral extraprostatic extension	Hormonal therapy (orchiec-tomy or LHRH/antiandrogen) plus external beam radiation	0-10
	T3c	Seminal vesicle invasion		
	T4a	Invades bladder neck or rectum		
	T4b	Invades levator mukscle and/or fixed to pelvic sidewall		
0	N^+ or M^+	Pelvic lymph node involvement or distant metastases	Hormonal therapy (orchiec-tomy or LHRH/antiandrogen) when symptomatic; irradia-tion for isolated bone pain	0-10

Curative therapy :

- *Radical prostectomy :*
  - Done for stage A_2 and B. Retropubic approach is used.
  - Involves removal of prostate, seminal vesicles and ampulla of vas deferens.
- In patient with *advanced local tumour (T_3, T_4) or stage C* androgen deprivation and external beam radiotherapy is procedure of choice.

Remember : Technique for Androgen ablation

- Surgical orchidectomy (Gold standard)
- Estramustine
- Megesterol acetate
- LHRH agonist
- DES
- Ketoconazole

Palliative therapy :

- For patient with metastatic disease.
- Consist of androgen deprivation therapy in the form of oral estrogen (DES) or B/L orchidectomy.
- The most important carcinogen smegma and HPV infection.

SARCOMA OF PROSTATE

- Occurs is children < 5 years
- Highly malignant
- Combination chemotherapy followed by surgery is the treatment.

CARCINOMA OF PENIS

- Rare disease occuring in 5th or 6th decade.
- Most penile cancer occur in uncircumcised males. Circumcision in neonatal period markedly ↓ chance of ca penis, however *circumcision performed during puberty or adult hood do not have same protective potential.*
- Most common histologic type is *squamous cell ca.*
- The most important carcinogen are smegma and HPV infection.
- ***Premalignant lesions :***
  - *Genital warts* (Buschke lowenstein tumour). Is a giant penile condyloma and may have foci of malignancy
  - *Erythroplasia of Queyrat or Paget's disease of penis*
  - *Bowens disease*
  - *Leukoplakia*
  - *Balanitis xerotica obliterans (Inflammatory condition of the glans and prepuce of unknown cause).*

Clinical features

- Majority of patient present with *non healing ulcer.*
- Foul smelling discharge, hematuria or phimosis may be presenting feature.
- *Urethra rarely involved* because it is protected by tough Buck's fascia.

Spread

- Direct to glans, prepucial skin and shaft.
- Lymphatic initially to inguinal nodes followed by internal iliac and paraortic nodes.

Diagnosis

- *Wedge biopsy* from edge of growth.

Staging and Treatment		
Stage	**Clinical finding**	**Treatment**
Stage I	• Tumour confined to prepuce • Tumour involving the glans	– Circumcision – Partial amputation with at least 2 cm margin from the palpable indurated edge of tumour
Stage II	• Tumour involving the penile shaft or corpora cavernosa	– Partial amputation / Total penectomy with perineal urethrostomy
Stage III	• Mobile regional nodal metastases with stage I or II	– Circumcision, partial amputation or total penectomy followed by ilioinguinal block dissection
Stage IV	• Tumour beyond penile shaft, fixed regional lymph node or distant metastases	– Radiotherapy + chemotherapy

Remember : Partial amputation is done only if adequate length of penile shaft ***(minimum 2.5 cm)*** for sexual function is left after macroscopic tumour free ***(with 2 cm margin proximally);*** otherwise total penectomy with perineal urethrostomy is done.

QUESTIONS

1. **A 50 years old man with h/o ca prostate wants to do screening. The most sensitive test is : [AIIMS May 10, AI 07]**
   a. Digital rectal examination
   b. PSA
   c. Digital rectal examination and PSA
   d. Endorectal coil MRI with T1, T2 weighted images
2. **Which of the following is true regarding testicular tumors ? [AI 06]**
   a. Are embryonal cell carcinomas in 95% of cases
   b. Bilateral in upto 10% cases
   c. Teratomas are more common than seminomas
   d. Usually present after 50 years of age
3. **Which one of the following is not used as a tumour marker in testicular tumours ?**
   a. AFP **[AI 05]**
   b. LDH
   c. HCG
   d. CEA
4. **Most common site of uretheral carcinoma in males: [AI 2010]**
   a. Bulbar
   b. Penile
   c. Prostatic
   d. Membranous urethra
5. **Hot flushes in prostate cancer are seen after treatment with: [PGI Dec 08]**
   a. Androgen receptor blocker
   b. Surgical castration
   c. Medical castration
   d. Radical prostatectomy
   e. Estrogen and cyproterone acetate
6. **Most common testicular tumor in prepubertal is: [AIIMS May 08]**
   a. Yolk sac tumor
   b. Embryonal cell Ca
   c. Seminoma
   d. Teratoma
7. **All are true about Gleason's staging except: [AIIMS Nov 08]**
   a. Score from 1-10
   b. High score is associated with bad prognosis
   c. Helps in grading of tumor
   d. Helps to decide about treatment modality
8. **All of the following clinicopathologic features are seen more often in seminomas as compared to nonseminomatous germ cell tumours of the testis except :**
   a. Tumors remain localized to testis for a long time **[AIIMS 05, 04]**
   b. They are radiosensitive
   c. They metastasize predominantly by lymphatics
   d. They are often associated with raised levels of serum AFP and HCG
9. **Which one of the following is the treatment of choice for a 4cm retroperitoneal lymph node mass in a patient with non seminomatous germ cell tumour of the testis :**
   a. Radical radiotherapy **[AIIMS 06]**
   b. High Orchidectomy + RPLND
   c. RPLND alone
   d. High Orchidectomy alone
10. **Which of the following is true about seminoma: [PGI Dec 05]**
    a. It is radiosensitive
    b. It arises only from cryptorchid testis
    c. AFP is not raised
    d. Surgical excision is treatment of choice
11. **Not true about carcinoma penis is :**
    a. Erythroplasia of Queret is a precancerous **[PGI Dec. 09]**
    b. 40% of patients are under 60 years of age
    c. Circumcision if done any time before puberty provides 100% protection against carcinoma penis
    d. More than 50% patients, have inguinal lymph node enlargement when they present

12. Intratubular germ cell tumour found adjacent to : [PGI 06]
a. Spermatocytic seminoma
b. Dysgerminoma
c. Yolk sac tumour
d. Embryonal carcinoma
e. Choriocarcinoma

13. All except used to detect carcinoma prostate gland : [PGI 06]
a. PSA
b. MRI
c. CT Scan
d. DSA
e. TRUS

14. Most useful screening method for screening of prostate ca : [PGI 06]
a. DRE
b. USG
c. MRI
d. PSA
e. CT Scan

ANSWERS, REFERENCES, EXPLANATIONS WITH INFORMATIVE ILLUSTRATIONS

1. Ans. is c i.e. Digital rectal examination and PSA

Ref. Devita 7/e, p 574; 8/e 1400, CSDT 13/e p 950

Screening tests for Prostate cancer

- ***Digital rectal examination :***
  - Most widely used and oldest technique.
  - Sensitivity 60 per cent.
  - Only one in three patient with positive DRE have prostatic carcinoma.
- ***PSA :***
  - Serine protease found in cytoplasm of prostatic cell.
  - PSA is abundant in seminal fluid. It has enzymatic activity which induces liquification of seminal fluid and the release of motile spermatozoa.
  - Serum level > 4 ng/ml is abnormal. Males with serum level > 4 ng/ml should undergo transrectal ultrasound
  - Sensitivity 80 - 90 per cent.
- ***Transrectal ultrasound :***
  - There was so much enthusiasm about the use of TRUS for screening but it is costly and has sensitivity of 41 - 79% only, when used alone.
  - Out of these screening test integration of DRE and PSA is the most suitable and best technique available.

Methods enhancing PSA specificity :
- ***Age specific PSA:*** [Age < 50 years. PSA should be < 2.5 ng / ml; Age > 70 years PAS < 6.5 ng / ml]
- ***PSA density:*** [PSA/Prostate volume] value < 0.15 ng/ml suggest cancer
- ***Percent free PSA*** (Total PSA – Complexed PSA). When less than 10% the risk of prostate cancer is 60%.

2. **Ans. is None or b i.e. Bilateral in upto 10% cases**

Ref. Bailey & Love 25/e, p 1384; CMDT '10, p 1493

Guys ! ***none of the given choice is totally correct.***

Let's see :

Option 'a'	***"Embryonal carcinoma forms less then 2% of testicular tumor."*** So, *option 'a'* is wrong.
Option 'b'	***"1 - 2% percent of primary testicular tumor is bilateral."*** *... CMDT '10, p 1493* ***"But bilaterality is seen in 15% of secondary testicular tumour."*** *... Devita 7/e, p 1290*
Option 'c'	***"Seminomas are most common testicular tumor and accounts for approximately 50% of GCT."*** *... Devita 8/e, p 1464* So, *option 'c'* is also wrong.
Option 'd'	***"Testicular tumor are most frequent in age group of 25 to 40 years."*** So, *option 'd'* is also wrong. **So, partial correct choice can be taken as answer.**

3. **Ans. is d i.e. CEA** *Ref. CMDT 10, p 1493; Devita 8/e p 1467*

"Several biochemical markers are important in the diagnosis of testicular carcinoma including HCG, α fetoprotein and LDH." *... CMDT 10, p 1493*

Testicular tumour markers

Testicular neoplasm	***AFP***	***β HCG***
Seminoma	–	+/–
Endodermal sinus tumor	+	–
Embryonal Ca	+/–	+
Chorio carcinoma	+	+
Teratoma	+/–	–

Immunohistochemical markers of testicular tumor

Seminoma	PLAP, OCT3/4, CD117 (Kit receptor)
Embryonal Ca	AE-1, CAM 5.2, CD 30
Yolk sac tumor	AE-1, CAM 5.2
Teratoma (Mature)	Vimentin
Cytokeratin is expressed in all epithelial tumor	

LDH :
- *Elevated in both seminomatous and non seminomatous type.*
- Reflects tumour burden.
- High value are associated with poor prognosis.

CEA :
- Elevated in carcinomas of colon, pancreas, lung, stomach and heart not in ca testis.

4. **Ans. is a i.e. Bulbarurethera** *Ref. Devita 8/e p 1453*

Site of uretheral cancer in ↓ order
- Bulbomembranous urethera (60%)
- Penile urethra (30%)
- Prostatic urethra (10%)

Cancer of male urethra
- Rare (Ca of female urethra is more common than Ca male urethra)
- Chronic irritation and infection are strongest risk factor. HPV-16 also has a causative role in the development of squamous cell carcinoma
- **Histology :** Squamous cell Ca > Transistional cell > Adenocarcinoma In prostatic urethra transistional cell Ca is more common
- ***Clinical presentation:*** Mostly present with obstructive symptoms (straining; diminished stream)
- **MRI** with contrast is *the ideal imaging modality*
- ***Treatment:*** Surgery is the main stay of treatment
- ***Prognosis:*** Most important prognostic factor for local control and survival is the anatomical location and extent of tumor. Anterior urethral (bulbar and penile) tumor are of low grade and more amenable to surgical exploration in comparison to posterior urethral (prostatic and membraneous) tumor

5. **Ans. is a, c, e i.e. Androgen receptor blocker, Medical castration, Estrogen and cyproterone acetate.** *Ref. CMDT 10, p 1487*

Androgen ablation therapy is given for stage C and stage D ca prostate.

Androgen ablation therapy		
Level	**Agent**	**Sequelae**
Pituitary	Estrogens	Gynecomastia, hot flushes, hypothalamus thromboembolic disease, erectile dysfunction
	LHRH agonists	Erectile dysfunction, hot flushes, gynecomastia, rarely anemia
Adrenal	Ketoconazole	Adrenal insufficiency, nausea, rash, ataxia
	Aminoglutethimide	
	Glucocorticoids	Gastrointestinal bleeding, fluid retention
Testis	Medical orchidectomy	Gynecomastia, hot flushes, erectile dysfunction
Prostate cell	Antiandrogens	No erectile dysfunction when used alone; nausea, diarrhea

6. **Ans. is a i.e. Yolk sac tumor** *Ref. Campbell urology 8/e p 2879; Robbin's 8/e, p 989*

Yolk sac tumor is the most common testicular tumor of infant and children

Testicular tumor	Age group
Seminoma	30-40
Yolk sac tumor	0-5
Lymphoma	After 60
Embryonal carcinoma	20-30
Choriocarcinoma	20-30

7. **Ans. is a i.e. Score 1-10** *Ref. CMDT 10, p 1486; Harrison 17/e, p 596*

Gleason staging system

- Most popular grading system for prostate carcinoma
- Based on architectural rather than histologic criteria
- **Grade 1** (well differentiated) - 5 (undifferentiated) are assigned which correlates with tumor volume, stage and prognosis
- Most poorly differentiated area determines biologic behavior. Perineural and extracapsular spread are also recorded
- Primary grade is applied to architectural pattern of cancerous gland occupying largest area of specimen while secondary pattern is assigned to next largest area of cancerous growth
- Adding the sure of primary and secondary pattern gives Gleason score (2-10) for each tumor

Remember: Other risk prediction tools after radical prostatectomy are Kattan nomogram (most widely used) and CAPRA nomogram (also uses Gleason grade)

8. **Ans. is d i.e. They are often associated with raised levels of serum AFP and HCG**

Ref. Bailey & Love 25/e, p 1385 -1387

Comparison of seminoma with teratoma

	Features	Seminoma	Teratoma
1.	Cell of origin	Seminiferous tubules in the mediastinum of the testis	Totipotential cells in the rete-testis
2.	Incidence	35 - 40%	20%
3.	Age group	30 - 40 years	20 - 30 years
4.	Shape of testis	Retained	Not retained
5.	Surface	Smooth	Irregular
6.	Cut surface	Smooth	ariegated – nodules, cysts
7.	Consistency	Firm	Firm or soft (cystic)
8.	Spread	Mainly lymphatic	Predominantly blood
9.	Tumour markers	Placental alkaline PO_4	HCG – malignant teratoma
10.	Radiation response	Excellent – melts like snow	Less sensitive

9. **Ans. is b i.e. High orchidectomy + RPLND** *Ref. Harrison 17/e, p 601*

Stage	Extent of Disease	Seminoma	Nonseminoma
IA	Testis only, no vascular / lymphatic invastion (T1)	Radiation therapy	RPLND or observation
IB	Testis only, with vascular / lymphatic invasion (T2), or extension through tunica albuginea (T2), or involvement of spermatic cord (T3) or scrotum (T4)	Radiation therapy	RPLND

Contd...

Contd...

Stage	Extent of Disease	Seminoma	Nonseminoma
IIA	Nodes < 2 cm	Radiation therapy	RPLND or chemotherapy often followed by RPLND
IIB	Nodes 2 - 5 cm	Radiation therapy	RPLND +/– adjuvant chemotherapy or chemotherapy followed by RPLND
IIC	Nodes > 5 cm	Chemotherapy	Chemotherapy, often followed by RPLND
III	Distant metastases	Chemotherapy	Chemotherapy, often followed by surgery (biopsy or resection)

Combination chemotherapy consist of Cisplatin + Etoposide + /-Bleomycin.

Remember : Transcrotal orchidectomy is contraindication as it permits the development of alternate lymphatic channel pathways to inguinal and pelvic lymph nodes.

10. Ans. is a, c and d i.e. It is radiosensitive; AFP is not raised; and Surgical excision is treatment of choice *Ref. Devita 8/e p 1464; CMDT 10/e, p 1493*

- Only 2% of GCT develops in inguinal cryptorchid testes and 5-20% of these patient develop tumor in normal descended testis. Both seminoma and teratoma are radiosensitive
- Treatment of both seminoma and teratoma is high inguinal orchidectomy
- AFP is never elevated in seminoma while hcg is occasionally elevated in seminoma (in 15-20%)

11. Ans. is c i.e. Circumcision if done any time before puberty provides 100% protection against carcinoma penis *Ref. Devita 8/e, p 1455*

Carcinoma of Penis

- Rare disease occuring in 5 or 6 decade.
- Most penile cancer occur in uncircumcised males. Circumcision in neonatal period markedly decrease chance of ca penis, however *circumcision performed during puberty or adulthood do not have same protective potential.*
- Most common histologic type is squamous cell ca.
- **Premalignant lesions :**
  - Genital warts (Buschke lowenstein tumour)
  - Erythroplasia of Queyrat or Paget's disease of penis
  - Bowens disease
  - Leukoplakia
  - Balanitis xerotica obliterans.
- Majority of patient present with non *healing ulcer.*
- Foul smelling discharge, hematuria or phimosis may be presenting feature.

Spread :

- Direct to glans, prepucial skin and shaft.
- Lymphatic initially to inguinal nodes followed by internal iliac and paraotic nodes.

Staging and Treatment

Stage	Clinical finding	Treatment
Stage I	• Tumour confined to prepuce • Tumour involving the glans	– Circumcision – Partial amputation with at least 2 cm margin from the edge of tumour
Stage II	• Tumour involving the penile shaft or corpora cavernosa	– Partial amputation / Total penectomy with perineal urethrostomy
Stage III	• Mobile regional nodal metastases with stage I or II	– Total penectomy followed by ilioinguinal block dissection
Stage IV	• Tumour beyond penile shaft, fixed regional lymph node or distant metastases	– Radiotherpy + Chemotherapy

12. **Ans. is b, d and e i.e. Dysgerminoma; Embryonal carcinoma; and Choriocarcinoma**
Ref. Robbin's 7/e, p 1041

Intratubular germ cell neoplasia is seen adjacent to all germ cell tumour except for spermatocyticf seminoma, epidermoid and dermoid cyst, pediatric teratoma, yolc sac tumour.

- Intratubular germ cell neoplasia is the presumed precurrer of all germ cell tumours.
- ***It is encountered with the high frequency in :***
  - Crypto-orchidism
  - Prio germ cell tumour
  - Androgen insensitivity syndrome
  - Gonadal dysgenesis syndrome.
- Untreated ITGCN progresses to invasive germ cell tumour in approx. 50 per cent of cases over 5 years of follow-up

13. **Ans. is c and d i.e. CT Scan; and DSA** *Ref. CSDT 13/e, p 950*

CT scan is not routinely recommended in CA prostate, as MRI is more accurate and informative

14. **Ans. is d i.e. PSA** *Ref. CSDT 13/e, p 950*

PSA estimation is single most useful screening test for screening of ca prostate.
PSA testing nearly doubles the detection rate possible with DRE alone.

According to Americian cancer society PSA testing should be offered to all men > 50 years and > 45 years in those with high risk (black race, family history).

Management of prostatic Nodule on Digital Rectal Examination

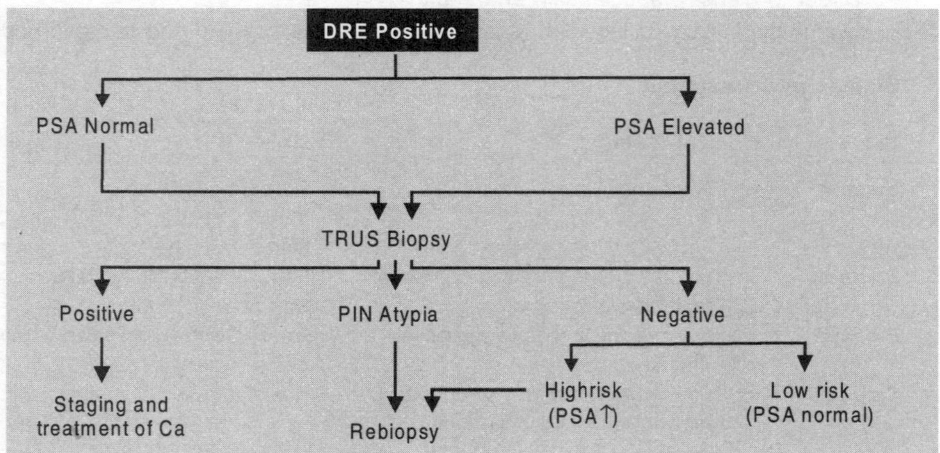

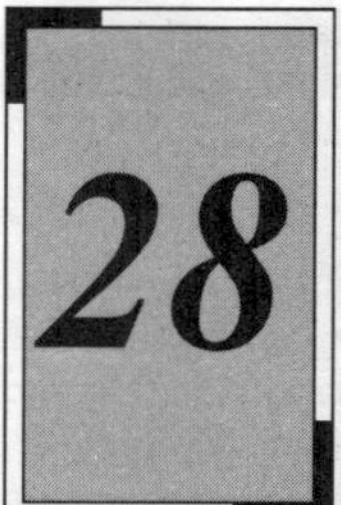

28 Myeloid Leukemia

What's Important ?

- Prognostic Factor
- Phildelphia Chromosome
- Diagnostic Criteria

Heterogenous group of neoplasm orginating from hematopoetic progenitor cells of myeloid series. Based on their course, the myeloid leukemias have been ***classified into:***

1. Acute myeloid leukemia
2. Myelodysplatic syndrome
3. Myeloproliferative disorders (which include CML)

ACUTE MYELOID LEUKEMIA

- Tumor of hematopoietic progenators caused by oncogenic mutations that impede differentiation leading to the accumulation of myeloid blast in the marrow.
- AML primarily affects middle age group and frequency increases as age advances

Etiopathogenesis

- AML are associated with acquired / genetic alterations that inhibit terminal myeloid differentiation as a result normal marrow elements are replaced by relatively undifferentiated blast cells.
- **Predisposing factors:**
  - *Hereditary :* Down's syndrome, Kline filter syndrome, Patau syndrome; Ataxia telangectasia, Fanconi anaemia, Blooms syndrome.
  - Radiation (For all leukemias except CLL).
  - Occupational exposure to benzene.
  - *Drugs :* Alkylating agents are MC drugs causing treatment associated AML (bad prognosis).

Classification

- The most widely used system in current use is revised FAB classification.
- **M2** is most common of all AML.
- ***Recently WHO classification*** has been proposed for AML.

Revised FAB Classification of Acute Myelogenous Leukemias

Class		Incidence (% of AML)	Features
M0	Minimally differentiated	2-3%	Blasts lack definitive cytologic and cytochemical markers of myeloblasts (e.g., myeloperoxidase negative) but express myeloid lineage antigens and resemble myeloblasts ultrastructurally.
M1	AML without differentiation	20%	Very immatrue, but ≥ 3% of blasts are peroxidase positive; few granules or Auer rods and little maturation beyond the myeloblast stage.
M2	AML with maturation	30-40%	Full range of myeloid maturation through granulocytes; Auer rods present in most cases; often associated with the t (8:21).
M3	Acute promyelocytic leukemia	5-10%	Most cell are hypergranular promyelocytes, often with many Auer rods per cell; patients are younger; high incidence of DIC; strong association with t (15 - 17).
M4	Acute myelomonocytic leukemia	15-20%	Myelocytic and monocytic defferentiation evident; monoblasts are positive for nonspecific esterases; subset associated with the inv.(16).
M5	Acute monocytic leukemia	10%	In M5a subtype, monoblasts (perioxidase-negative, nonspecific esterase-positive) and promonocytes predominate in marrow and blood; in M5b subtype, mature monocytes predominate in the peripheral blood; M5a and M5b occur in older patients; characterized by high incidence of organomegaly, lymphadeno-pathy, and tissue infiltration.
M6	Acute erythroleukemia	5%	Dysplastic erythroid precursors (some megaloblastoid, other with giant or multiple nuclei) predominate, and within the non-erythroid cells, >30% are myeloblasts; seen in advancecd age; makes up 1% of de novo AML and 20% of therapy-related AML.
M7	Acute megakaryocytic leukemia	1%	Blasts of megakaryocytic lineage predomiate; blasts react with platelet- specific antibodies directed against GPIIb/IIIa or vWF; myelofibrosis or increased marrow recticulin seen in most cases.

Clinical Presentation :

- Most patient present with in weeks or a few month due to symptoms related to anemia, neutropenia and thrombo-cytopenias.
- Most common ***initial symptom*** is fatigue and weakness.
- ***Bleeding diathesis*** present as cutaneous petechiae and ecchymoses, serosal hemorrage. This is particularly common with acute promyelocytic (M_3) Leukemia due to presence of procoagulants and fibrinolytic factors in auer rods.
- In tumors with monocytic differentiation (M_4 and M_5) infiltration of the skin ***(Leukemia cutis)*** and the gingiva is seen.
- Rarely AML may present with symptoms from a mass lesion located in the soft tissue, these mass lesion are called ***granulocytic sarcoma*** or ***choloroma*** which are usually associated with M_2.
- DIC is more common in AML than ALL; it is most commonly seen in ***M_3 variant***

Physical findings :

- Fever, splenomegaly lymphadenopathy, hepatomegaly, sternal tenderness.
- Significant GI ***bleeding,*** Intrapulmonary hemorrhage, Intracranial hemorrhage are seen particularly in M_3 .

Diagnosis :

- Based on presence of $\geq$ 20% myeloblast in blood and / or bone marrow.
- **Peripheral smear** *show Anaemia (Normocytic normochromic).*
  - Leucocyte count is variable (5000/μl – 1,00,000/μl). Occasionally peripheral smear have no detectable leukemic cells/blasts (Aleukemic); in these patient diagnosis can be made only by Bone marrow examination.
  - Platelet count - usually < 10, 0000 / μl.
- **Bone marrow examination** *show*
  - Myeloblast form > 20% of the cells of B.M.
  - Positive myeloperoxidase reaction in > 3% blast distinguish AML from ALL.
  - Auer rods and phi bodies are pathognomonic of AML. Phi bodies are fusiform or spindle shaped rods similar to auer rods, but require special strains for hydroperoxidases ... *Wintrobes 12/e, p 1848*
  - Myeloid blasts are identified by the presence of Auer rods, or by sudan black, myeloperoxidase, chloroacetate esterase, or nonspecific esterase positivity on cytochemical stains ... *Wintrobes 12/e, p 1843*
  - Blast exhibiting megakaryocytic differention (M_7) are usually accompanied by ***marrow fibrosis.***
  - **Monoblast** have folded or lobulated nuclei; *lack auer rods; peroxidase negative and nonspecific esterase positive.*
- **M0** and **M7** can only be diagnosed by multiparameter flow cytometry by detection of characteristic antigen.
  - M0 : Diagnosed by flow cytometeric demonstration of myeloid specific antigen CD - 13 or CD 33.
  - M7 : Diagnosed only by demonstration of platelet specific antigen CD 41, CD 42b or CD 61 or by electron microscopic demonstration of myeloperoxidase. ... *Wintrobes 12/e, p 1858*

Prognostic factor :

Clinical:

- ***Age at the time of diagnosis is most important*** prognostic factor *(Harrison 17/e, p 680).* Patient with age > 60 years signify poor prognosis.
- ***Secondary AML*** has extremely bad prognosis.

> Secondary AML is AML preceded by bone marrow disorder including MDS or myeloproliferative disorder, or a history of cytologic therapy for a prior malignancy.

- **Morphology:**
  - Favorable morphological features include presence of Auer rods (M_1–M_4) and of eosinophils (M_2)
  - Morphological dysplasias are unfavorable
  - M_0, M_6, M_7 generally have lower survival rate

- **Immunophenotype:**
  - CD34 + MDR expression is poor prognostic feature
  - Absence of CD7, CD33 is poor prognostic sign
  - *Secondary AML* has extremely *bad prognosis.* Secondary AML is AML preceded by bone marrow disorder including MDS or myeloproliferative disorder, or a history of cytotoxic theory for prior malignancy
- **Chromosomal abnormality :**
  - Patient with t (8:21) inv 16: t15:17 are associated with good prognosis.
  - Patient with complex karyotype, inv (3) or 7 has poor prognosis.
  - No cytogenetic abnormality has moderatility favourable outcome.
  - High TLC, CNS bleeding, relapse contributes to poor outcome.

Treatment :

Divided into two phase induction and post remission management. Initial goal is to acheive quick CR (complete remission).

- **CR** – CR is defined by examination of both blood and bone marrow.
  - **Criteria for CR includes :**
    - Blood neutrophill ≥ 1500/μl
    - Platelet ≥ 1 lakh / μL
    - Circulating blasts should be absent
    - In bone marrow : - Blast < 5%
      - Auer rods should be absent.
    - Extramedullary leukemia should be absent
    - The currently recommended criteria do not include requirements with regard to bone marrow cellularity or duration of response ... *Wintrobes 12/e, p 1858*

- **Induction chemotherapy**

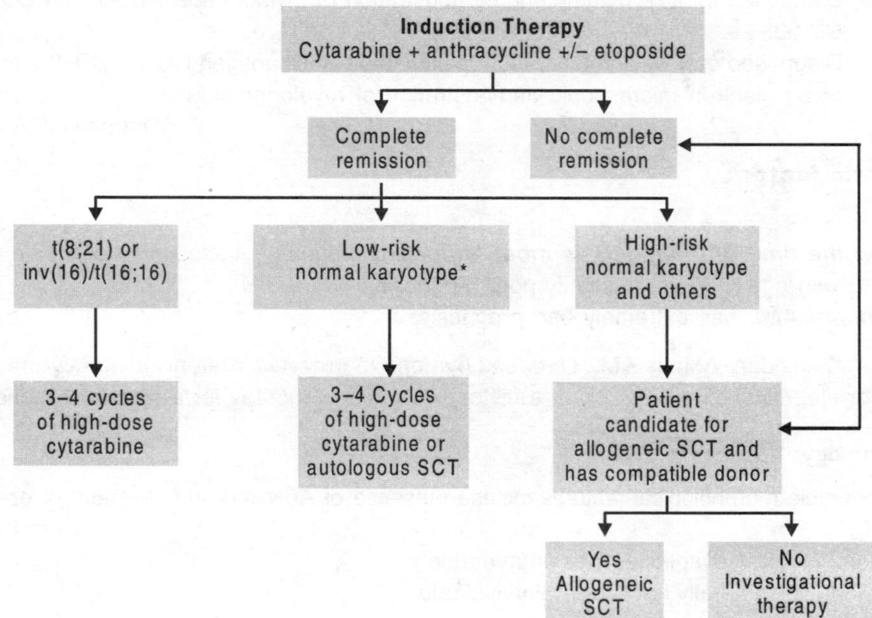

- **Treatment of Promyelocytic leukemia**
  - With cytorbine and daunorubin 10% patients of M_3 develop DIC, so these drugs are best avoided
  - *Tretinoin (ATRA)* is Drug of choice. It induces the differentiation of leukemic cells.
  - ATRA does not produce DIC but produces another complication called retinoic acid syndrome, which is characterized by fever, dyspnea, chest pain, pulmonary infiltrates, pleural and pericardial effusion. This is managed by steroids
  - ATRA is not effective in other forms of AML.
  - Arsenic trioxide given in cases refractory to ATRA.
- **Relapse**
  - Most important factor predicting response at relapse is the length of previous CR.
  - If patient is eligible allogenic SCT should be considered.
  - For elderly patient Gemtuzumab ozogamicin (antibody directed against CD – 33) is an alternative.

CHRONIC MYELOGENOUS LEUKEMIA

- CML is a clonal myeloproliferative disorder of pleuropotent hematopoietic progenitor cell characterized by excessive proliferation of marrow granulocytes, erythroid precursor, megakaryocytes and connective tissue forming cells.
- CML affects primarily middle years age group (25 - 60 years).
- Distinguished from other chronic myeloproliferative disease by presence of characteristic reciprocal translocation between chromosome 9 and 22, the resulting ***chr. 22 is called philadelphia chromosome.***

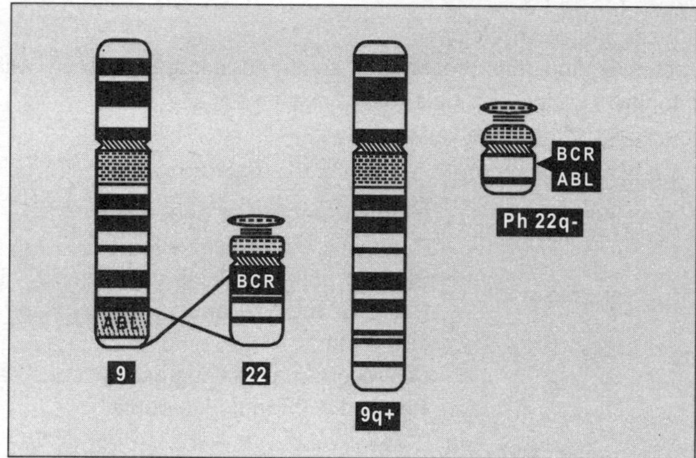

Mnemonic :

- A comes before B similarly 9 comes before 22.
- Now, they move forward so A goes over B or 9 over 22.The resulting phaldelphia chromosome codes for 210 kD fusion protein which has tyrosine kinase activity.

Remember :
- Philadelphia chromosome is also seen in acute leukemia in which 190 KD BCR - ABL fusion protein is formed.
- FISH and RT-PCR are most sensitive method to detect philedelphia chromosome.

Etiology :

- No clear etiolgic agent known.
- Cigarette smoking accelerate the progression to blast phase.
- Radiation.

Clinical Presentation :

- CML is a ***triphasic disease.*** At dignosis > 90% of patients are in chronic phase.
- Most patient complaint of lethargy, weakness, night sweats, weight loss, abdominal discomfort.
- Generalized lymphadenopathy and fever indicate accelerated disease progression.
- On physical examination – ***Splenomegaly*** is MC sign, mild hepatomegaly may also be found.

Diagnosis :

1. **Chronic phase**
   - Peripheral blood
     - ↑ TLC (> 10,000/μl) with various degrees of immaturity of granulocyte series
     - < 5% circulatory blast
     - Anaemia
     - Most important finding is neutrophilic leukocytosis and basophilia
     - Platelet count is usually elevated (other leukemias have thrombocytopenia)
     - *LAP score* (Leucocyte alkaline phosphate) is typically low in CML cells.
   - On BM examination
     - Hypercellularity i.e 100% cellular (normally 50% cellular 50% fat).
     - ME ratio 9 : 1 to 15 : 1
     - < 10% blast and promyelocyte
     - A characteristic finding is presence of scattered storage histiocyte with wrinkled green blue cytoplasm called sea blue histiocytes
     - Increased deposition of reticuline fibers.
2. **Accelerated phase**
   - Defined by development of :
     - Increase degree of anaemia
     - Cytogenic clonal evaluation
     - Blood or marrow blasts between 10 - 19%
     - Blood or marrow basophill ≥ 20% or platelet count < 100,000/μl
     - LAP score may be decreased or increased.
     - Persistant thrombocytopenia
3. **Blast crisis :**
   - Defined as acute Leukemia with blood or marrow blast > 20%.
   - Hyposegmented neutrophills may appear.
   - LAP score ↑ in Blast crisis. ... *Wintrobes 11/e, p 2243*

Philadelphia chromosome detection: This is must for diagnosis of CML. Three methods are available for pH chromosome detection.

1. Conventional cytogenetic analysis (gold standard)
2. Fluorescence in situ hybridization
3. RT PCR analysis

Prognostic factors :

Prognostic factor for CML		
	Sokal index	***Hasford system***
Basis	– *Based on chemotherapy treated patient*	– *Based on interferon α treated patient*
Factors	– Percentage of circulating blast – Spleen size – Platelet count – Cytogentic clonal evaluation – Age	– Age – Spleen size – Percentage of circulating blasts – Platelet count – Percentage of eosinophills and basophills

- Age, percentage of circulating blast, spleen size, platelet count, percentage of eosinophil and basophil are most important prognostic factor.

Treatment :

- Drugs of choice for CML is ***Imatinib mesylates*** (Gleavac) which inhibits tyrosine kinase activity of phildelphia chromosome. The most common toxicity of imatinib are periorbital swelling, rash, myalgia and myelosupression.
- The outcome is assesed by testing BM and blood after 6 months.

Response Criteria in CML	
Hematologic	
– Complete response	White blood cell count <10,000/μl, normal morphology Normal hemoglobin and platelet counts
– Incomplete response	WBC ≥ 10,000 / μl
Cytogenetic	*Percentage of bone marrow metaphases with t(9;22)*
– Complete response	0
– Partial response	≤ 35
– Minor response	36 - 85
– No response	85 - 100
Molecular	*Presence of BCR/ABL transcript by PCR*
– Complete response	None
– Incomplete	Any

- Patient with poor response should be considered for a allogenic SCT.
- Hydroxyurea and interfon α should be considered in patient who can not tolerate imatinib.
- Other drugs used were Busulphan and Hydroxyurea.

Remember : – The only available curative therapy for CML is allogenic BM transplantation.

... Harrison 16/e, p 638

Treatment of blast crisis :
- Generally ineffective, only imatinib is some what effective.
- If remission acheived patient should be considered for allogenic SCT.

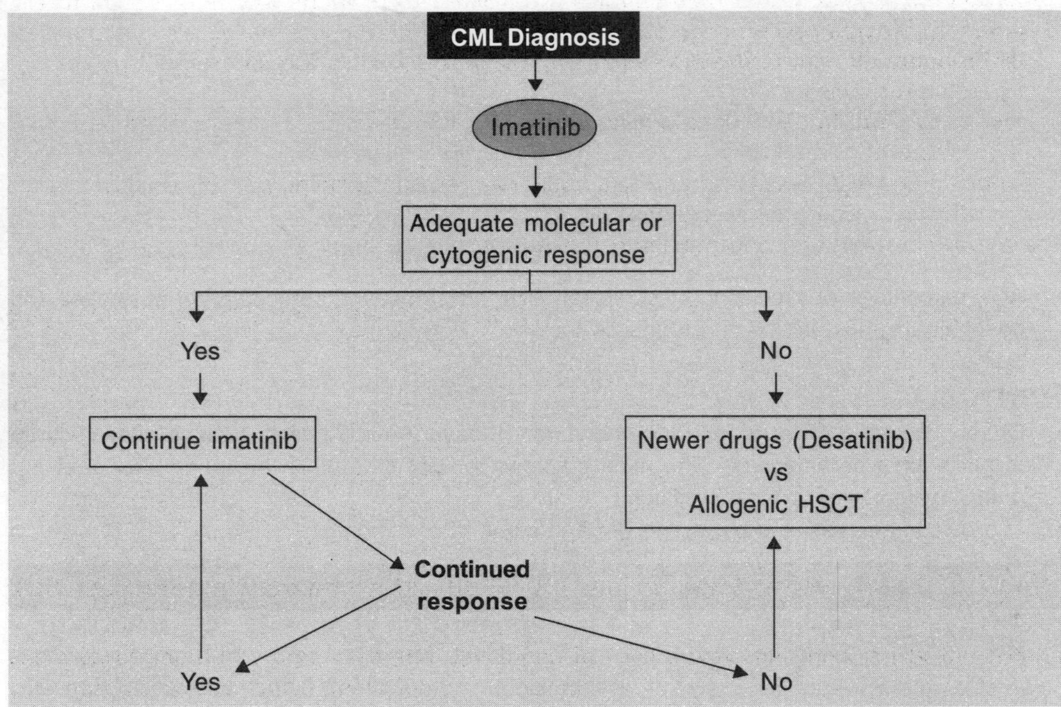

QUESTIONS

1. **The following are associated with AML except : [AI 07]**
   a. Turner's syndrome
   b. Down's syndrome
   c. Patau syndrome
   d. Klinefelter syndrome
2. **All of the following immunohistochemical markers are positive in neoplastic cells of granulocytic sarcoma, except : [AI 06]**
   a. CD 45 RO
   b. CD 43
   c. Myeloperoxidase
   d. Lysozyme
3. **Poor prognosis in AML is indicated by: [AI 08]**
   a. Inversion 16
   b. Translocation 15/17 (t15; 17)
   c. Normal cytogenecity
   d. Monosomy 7
4. **AML with gum infiltration, hepato-splenomegaly: [AIIMS 08]**
   a. ALL
   b. M3
   c. M2
   d. M4
5. **DIC is seen in which type of AML? [AI 08]**
   a. M1
   b. M3
   c. M4
   d. M6
6. **Marker for granulocytic sarcoma: [AIIMS 08]**
   a. CD33
   b. CD38
   c. CD117
   d. CD137
7. **All-trans-retinoic acid is used in the treatment for: [AI 08]**
   a. Acute promyelocytic leukemia (PML)
   b. Acute lymphoid leukemia (ALL)
   c. Chronic myeloid leukemia (CML)
   d. Chronic lymphoid leukemia (CLL)
8. **Drug of choice for chronic myeloid leukemia (CML) is: [AI 08]**
   a. Hydroxyurea
   b. Imatinib
   c. Infliximab
   d. IFN
9. **Which of the following signifies bad prognosis in AML: [AIIMS 06]**
   a. Monosomy 7
   b. t (:21)
   c. Inversion 16
   d. Cells with normal genotype
10. **A 15 year old boy presented with one day history of bleeding gums, subconjunctival bleed and purpuric rash. Investigations revealed the following results Hb-6.4 gm/dL; TLC-26,500/mm^3 Platelet 35,000 mm^3; prothrombin time 20 sec sec with a control of 13 sec; partial thromboplastin time 50 sec; and Fibrinogen 10mg/dL. Peripheral smear was suggestive of acute myeloblastic leukemia. Which of the following is the most likely ?**
    a. Myeloblastic leukemia without maturation
    b. Myeloblastic leukemia with maturation
    c. Promyelocytic leukemia [AIIMS 06]
    d. Myelomonocytic leukemia
11. **A peripheral smear with increased neutrophils, basophils, eosinophils, and platelets is highly suggestive of :**
    a. Acute myeloid leukemia [AIIMS 06]
    b. Acute lymphoblastic leukemia
    c. Chronic myelogenous leukemia
    d. Myelodysplastic syndrome
12. **Which of the folowing is not compatable with a diagnosis of juvenile myelomonocytic leukemia : [AIIMS 05]**
    a. Peripheral blood monocytosis more than 1x10^9/L
    b. Increased hemoglobin F level for age
    c. Presence of bcr/abl fusion gene
    d. GM-CSF hypersensitivity of myeloid progenitors in vitro

13. Which one the following is not a criterion for making a diagnosis of chronic myeloid leukemia in accelerated phase :
a. Blasts 10-19% of WBC's in peripheral blood **[AIIMS 08]**
b. Basophils 10-19% of WBC's peripheral blood
c. Increasing spleen size unresponsive to therapy
d. Persistent thrombocytosis ($>1000 \times 10^9$/L)

14. Laboratory evaluation for the differential diagnosis of chronic myeloproliferative disorders includes all the following except:
a. Chromosomal evaluation **[AIIMS 07]**
b. Bone marrow aspiration
c. Flow cytometric analysis
d. Determination of red blood cell mass

15. True about CML **[PGI 08]**
a. Myelofibrosis
b. 6 : 9 : 22 seen
c. Increased basophil in peripheral smear
d. Decreased LAP score

16. In CML, following pathological finding in blood is diagnostic **[PGI 06]**
a. Myelocytes, metamyelocytes, promyelocytes
b. Neutrophilia
c. Basophilia
d. Leukocytosis

ANSWERS, REFERENCES, EXPLANATIONS WITH INFORMATIVE ILLUSTRATIONS

1. Ans. is a i.e. Turner's syndrome *Ref. Wintrobes 12/e, p 1845*

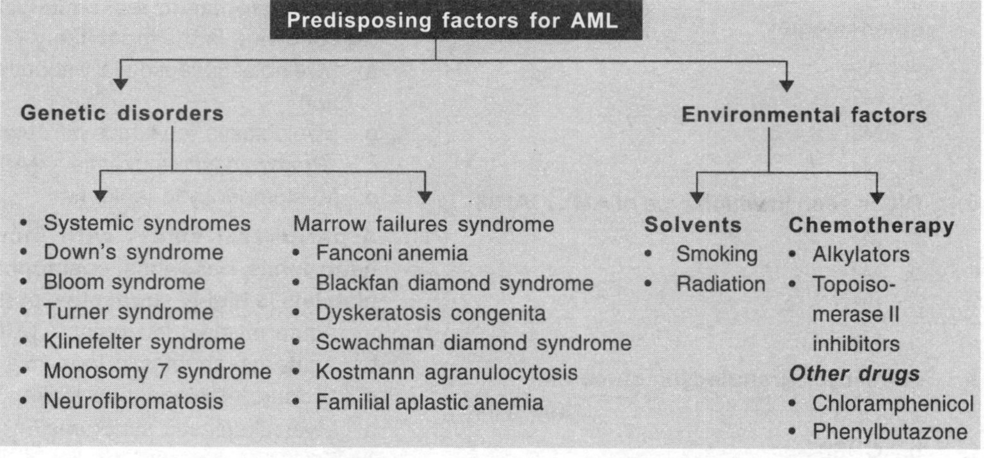

2. Ans. is a i.e. CD 45 RO *Ref. Wintrobe 12/e, p 1848, table 71.2; Devita 7/e, p 1943, 2114*

Granulocytic Sarcoma

- It is a type of extramedullary leukemia.
- It is a tumour mass of **myeloblast or immature myeloid** cells occurring in an extrameduillary site or in bone
- They were initially termed **chloromas** or myeloblastomas (tumor of leukemic cells)
- But now the name has changed to **granulocytic sarcoma or myeloid sarcomas.**

- Granulocytic sarcomas can occur in following conditions:
  i. In patients AML (particularly M_2)
  ii. In patients with chronic myeloproliferative disorder (CMPD) or a myelodysplastic syndrome
  iii. As relapse in patients previously treated for primary or secondary acute leukemia
  iv. De novo in healthy subjects
- It has predilection for CNS (brain or epidural space), bones and soft tissue of head and neck (especially the orbits).
- They have green hue due to myeloperoxidase.

Note:
- CD 43 is present in AML.
- *CD 45 RO is present in most T-cell lymphoma, some B-cell lymphoma* (not in AML).

Diagnosis

- The definitive diagnosis of Granulocytic sarcoma can be made only on ***immuno-histochemistry***
- Since it is a tumour of the myeloid origin the panel includes antibodies commonly used for diagnosis of meyloid neoplasm
- The best immunohistochemical stains used for this include ***MPO (myeloperoxidase) and lysozyme***

The immunoreactivity of various antibodies in a case of Granulocytic sarcoma includes:

• Myeloperoxidase	:	97%
• Lysozyme	:	93%
• CD 117	:	87%
• CD 34	:	47%
• CD 45	:	84%
• CD 43	:	97%
• CD 68	:	93%
• Bcl-2	:	68%
• TdT	:	37%
• CD 79a	:	20%
• CD 20	:	10%
• CD 3	:	10%

- **CD 33** is a sensitive marker for myeloid cells and gives a reactivity of > 95% but use is limited by non availability and non reliable result.

3. **Ans. is d i.e. Monosomy 7** *Ref. Harrison 17/e, p 680; Wintrobes 12/e, p 1860*

Prognostic factor of AML

- **Age** at the time of diagnosis is most important pretreatment risk factor ; Age>60 signify poor prognosis.

- **Chromosomal abnormality :**
  - Good prognostic - t(8:21); t(15:17); inv.(16)
  - Moderately favourable - no cytogenetic abnormality
  - Poor - Abnormality of chromosome 5 or 7, Complex karyotypes, Inv (3), 3q rearrangement
- High TLC, CNS bleeding, relapse are associated with poor prognosis.
- Prolong symptomatic interval with cytopenias of more than 1 month signify poor prognosis.
- **Attainment of CR** is most important treatment associated prognostic facror which also include rapidity with which CR is acheived and duration of CR.

4. Ans. is d i.e M4 *Ref. Robbin's 7/e, 693*

- Leukemia skin infiltration or ***leukemia cutis*** occur in upto 15% of patient with AML and is associated with involvement of other extramedullary sites including the CNS. The lesions are often violaceous and nodular and are more common in patients with monocytic component of AML ***(M_4 & M_5)****. Gum infiltration is also characteristic to monocytic leukemia* ***(M_5 > M_4)***. The skin lesions may preceede the diagnosis and are radiosensitive, but patients should usually be treated with chemotherapy

Class	Special feature
M0 (Minimally differentiated AML)	Blast are myeloperoxidase negative resemble myeloblast ultra-structurally. Requires immunophenotyping for diagnosis
M1 (AML without differentiation)	≥ 3 of blast are peroxidase positive
M2 (AML with maturation)	**MC** type of AML; Auer rods is present in most cases Affects children and young adults, associated with chloromas
M3 (Acute promyelocytic leukemia)	Affect younger age group (30–40) High incidence of bleeding diathesis and **DIC, $CD13^+$, $CD33^+$, HLA DR(–)** Faggot cells present
M4 (Acute myelo monocytic leukemia)	Monoblast are positive for non specific esterase Associated with *leukemia cutis*
M5 (Acute Monocytic)	Associated with *leukemia cutis* High incidence of *organomegally,* lymphadenopathy and tissue infiltration
M6 (Acute erythroleukemia)	Seen in advanced age Most common secondary AML
M7 (Acute megakaryocytic leukemia)	High incidence of marrow fibrosis ↑ marrow reticulin is seen in most cases

5. Ans. is c i.e. M_3 *Ref. Robbin's 8/e, p 622*

Incidence of DIC is highest in acute promyelocytic leukemia followed by acute monocytic leukemia

6. Ans. is c i.e. CD 117 *Ref. Wintrobes 12/e, p 1848*

Already explained

7. **Ans. is a i.e. Acute promyeloytic leukemia** *Ref. Harrison 17/e, p 682*

ATRA (All trans retinoic acid) = tretinoin is an oral drug that induce the differentiation of leukemic cells bearing the t(15 : 17)

Rational for ATRA use

- t (15 : 17) translocation in M_3 produces a fusion gene (PML-RAR) involving retinoic acid receptor gene (RAR) and promyelocytic leukemia gene (PML)
- This fusion gene tends to block the differentiation of cells
- ATRA tends to overcome this block and results in differentiation of cells

Toxicity

- Characteristic toxicity is retinoic acid syndrome occurring with in 3 weeks of treatment
- It is characterized by fever, dyspnea, chest pain pleural and pericardial effusion
- The syndrome is related to adhesions of differentiated cells to pulmonary vascular endothelium
- Treatment is strenoid and chemotherapy

Translocations asociated with AML		
• M2 (AML with maturation)	–	t(8:21)
• M3 (Acute promyelocytic leukemia)	–	t(15:17)
• M4 (Acute myelomonocytic leukemia)	–	Inv. (16)

8. **Ans. is b i.e. Imatinib** *Ref. Harrison 17/e, p 685*

Imatinib mesylate is a specific inhibitior of Bcr/Abl, PDGFR and Kit tyrosine kinases. ***It is the most effective drug for CML.*** Imatinib function through competitive inhibition at the ATP binding site of the Abl kinase, this leads to inhibition of tyrosine phosphorylation of proteins involved in Bcr/Abl signal transduction

Route : Oral

Mechanism of resistance : There are four mechanism :

1. Gene amplificaton
2. Mutations at the kinase site
3. Enhanced expression of multidrug exporter proteins
4. Alternative signaling pathway

Note: Desatinib is the other drug approved by FDA for CML including imatinib resistant CML.

9. **Ans. is a i.e. Monosomy 7** *Ref. Wintrobes 12/e, p 1860*

Already explained, kindly see answer no. 4

10. **Ans. is c i.e. Promyelocytic leukemia** *Ref. Robbin's 8/e, p 622*

- **This is a case of DIC which is suggested by :**
  - Acute onset of bleeding
  - Thrombocytopenia
  - Increase PT
  - Increase partial thromboplastin time
  - Decrease fibrinogen

- The most common leukemia associated with DIC is acute promyelocyle leukemia, hence answer.
- Leukemic cells of promyelocyle leukemia release procoagulant and fibrinolytic factors which leads to DIC.

Striking feature	Type of AML
– DIC	– Promyelocytic leukemia
– Infiltration of skin & gingiva	– M_4 & M_5

11. Ans. is c i.e. CML
See below

Let's consider peripheral blood picture of every option.

Option "a" :	**AML** • Neutropenia • Anemia (normocytic normochromic) • Throbocytopenia • Myeloblast constituting 10 - 100% of white cells.
Option "b" :	**ALL** • Increase TLC • Neutropenia • Thrombocytopenia • Increase blast cells (40 - 90%).
Option "c" :	**CML** • Increase TLC with various degree of immaturity. • DLC may show basophilia, eosinophilia, monocytosis in addition to neutrophilia. • Increase platelet count (in accelerated or blastic phase thrombocytopenia is seen).

12. Ans. is c i.e. Presence of bcr / abl fusion gene

Ref. Wintrobes 12/e, p 2001; CPDT 19/e, p 859

"Juvenile Myelomonocytic leukemia = Juvenile CML is Philadelphia negative and clinically aggressive, with course similar to, that of AML."

Criteria for Diagnosis of Juvenile Myelomonocytic Leukemia
Required criteria
• Peripheral blood monocytes > 1.0 × 10^9 / L • Blasts + Promonocytes < 20% in blood and marrow • Absence of philadelphia chromosome or BCR/ABL fusion gene
Optional criteria
• Increased hemoglobin F for age • Immature granulocytes in peripheral blood • WBC count > 10 × 10^9 / L • Clonal chromosomal abnormality (Monosomy 7)

Comparison of juvenile and adult chronic myelogenous leukemia		
Feature	**JMML / Juvenile CML**	**Adult CML**
Age at onset	< 2 years old	> 3 years old
Clinical presentation	Abrupt onset; eczematoid skin rash, marked lymphadenopathy, bleeding tendency	Nonspecific constitutional complaints, massive splenomegaly, variable hepatomegaly
Chromosomal alteration	Monosomy, or del(7q) in 20% of patients	t (9;22) present in 90% of patients
Laboratory features	Moderate leukocytosis (>10,000/ml), thrombocytopenia, monocytosis (>1000/ml), elevated fetal hemoglobin, normal to diminshed leukocyte alkaline phosphatase, elevated muramidase	Marked leukocytosis (>100,000/ml), normal to elevated platelet count, decreased to absent leukocyte alkaline phosphatase, usually normal muramidase

13. Ans. is d i.e. Persistent thrombocytosis *Ref. Wintrobes 12/e, p 2008*

Features of Accelerated Phase (AP) or Blast Phase (BP) of Chronic Myeloid Leukemia.

Symptoms of AP	**Signs and laboratory features of AP**
Fever	Inceasing peripheral basophilia to >20%
Weight loss	—
Refractory splenomegaly	Marrow blasts >19%
Bone pain	Cytogenetic clonal evaluation
	Difficult to control white blood cells with antiproliferative treatment
	Marrow reticullin or collagen fibrosis
	Thrombocytopenia (<100,000/ml) unrelated to treatment
Symptom of BP	**Signs and laboratory features of BP**
Similar to AP plus	Peripheral blood blasts >20%
-Lymphadenopathy	Marrow blasts >20%
-Extramedullary blastic chloromas	Clumps of blasts on marrow marrow examination
	Extramedullary blastic proliferation

14. Ans. is c i.e. Flow - Cytometric analysis *Ref. Harison 16/e, p 626; Robbins 8/e, p 626*

Myeloproliferative disorders includes :

– Typical CML : Morphologic variants
  - Chronic eosinophilic leukemia
  - Chronic basophillic leukemia
  - Chronic neutrophilic leukemia.

- – Essential thrombocytosis
- – Polycythemia vera
- – Idiopathic myelofibrosis
- – Chronic myelomonocytic leukemia proliferative type (CMML)
- – Atypical phildelphia negative chronic myeloid leukemia.

- These disorders are grouped together as *they involves the clonal expansion of a multipotent hematopoietic proginator cell* with over production of one or more of formed element of the blood.
- Differentiation among various types require bone marrow and blood examination and other specilized investigation as shown below :
  - – Red cell mass : Diagnostic for PCV in which it is ↑ed
  - – Chromosomal evaluation : Diagnostic for CML showing t9:22
  - – Bone marrow aspiration : Dry tap diagnostic for myelofibrosis.
- *Flow cytometric analysis used to assess the immunophenotype of the cell, it is of no use in myeloproliferative disorder.*

15. Ans. is a, b, c and d i.e. All options are correct

Ref. Harrison 17/e, p 684; Wintrobes 11/e, p 2241

Hematologic finding of CML

- Most important haematologic finding is *marked leukocytosis* and basophillia (often > 100,000/μl).
- The circulating cells are predominantly neutrophills, metamyelocyte and myelocytes with less than 10% myeloblasts.
- **DLC**
  - – Neutrophil ↑
  - – Basophil ↑
  - – Eosinophill ↑
  - – Monocyte ↓ (Absolute monocytosis with relative monocytopenia)
- Anaemia - Normocytic normochromic
- Platelet count - Increased
- Blasts < 5% (usually less than 3%)
- *LAP score* ↓ in chronic phase; ↑ in blast crisis

Bone marrow finding

- Cellularity ↑
- ME ratio ↑
- Significant degree of reticulin stained fibrosis (collagen fibrosis is rare)

Chromosomal finding

- Characteristic chromosomal finding is t9:22 leading to formation of philadelphia chromosome. *Philadelphia chromosome codes for 210kda protein which has tyrosine kinase activity.*

Remember :
- Philadelphia chromosome is not seen exclusively in CML as it is also found in ALL (10% cases); AML.
- Philadelphia negative CML are called *atypical CML.*

16. Ans. is a i.e. Myelocytes, metamyelocytes, promyelocytes

Ref. Robbin's 8/e, p 627; Harrison 17/e, p 683

- As diagnostic finding has been asked, there would be only one answer.
- Neutrophilia, basophilia or leukocytosis are not diagnostic for CML.

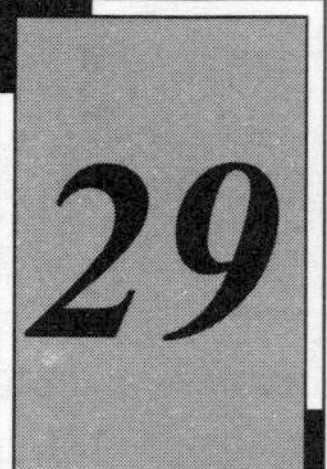

Lymphoid Leukemia

What's Important ?

- **Diagnosis and Treatment of ALL**
- **Diagnosis and Presentation of CLL**
- **Immunophenotype**

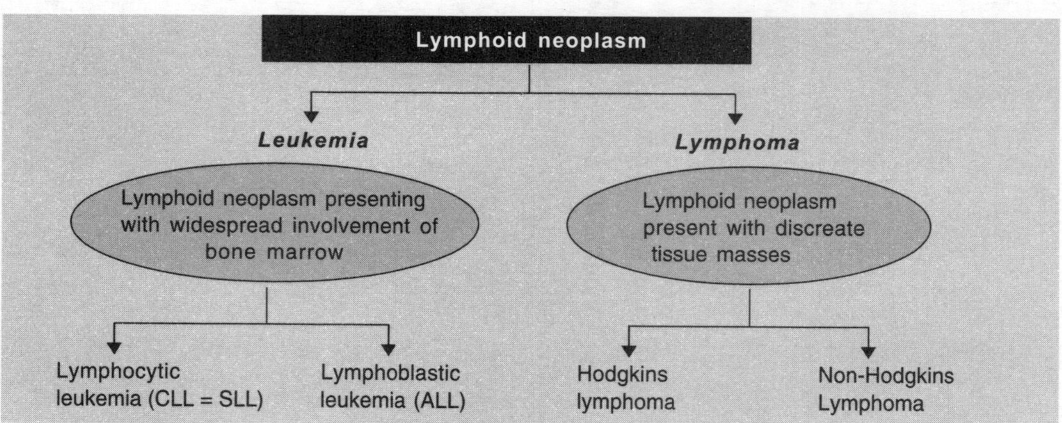

ACUTE LYMPHOBLASTIC LEUKEMIA / LYMPHOMA

- ALL includes a group of neoplasm composed of immature precursor B (pre B) or T (pre T) lymphocyte referred to as ***lymphoblast.***
- *ALL is the most common malignancy of childhood.*
- Peak age of onset is 4 years; M > F

Etiology and Risk factor :

- Cause is unknown but, risk is increased in :
  - **B**loom's syndrome
  - **A**taxia telangiectasia
  - **D**own's syndrome
  - **F**anconi Anaemia

Mnemonic : **BAD F**riend

- HTLV and EBV infection are associated in some cases.

Histopathology and Cytogenetics :

- *ALL is characterized by homogenous infiltration of bone marrow by leukemia blasts. ALL can be of B-cell origin or T-cell origin.*

	B-cell ALL	T - cell ALL
Incidence	More common	Less common
Age	<4 years	Adolescent age group
Presentation	Leukomatous presentation ↑TLC	Lymphomatous presentation often with thymic involvements Lymphadenopathy and spleenomegally are more common
Immunophenotype	Cell express TdT CD 19 & CD 10, lack surface Ig; with variable expression of CD-20	Cells express TdT and CD1, CD2, CD5, CD7 with variable expression of other T-cell marker (CD3, CD4, CD8)
Genotype	t (12:21) is most common chromosomal abnormally	Rearrangement of TALL gene is most common

- ***Note :*** TdT is expressed by all lymphoid blast and 20% - 25% myeloid blast.
- *Cells of ALL are differentiated from AML by presence of relatively condensed chromatin, absence of conspicuous nuclei and immunophenotyping.*

Cytochemical identification of acute leukemias

Type	Peroxidase	Suddan Black	Chloroacetate Esterase	Nonspecific Esterase	Periodic Acid-Schiff	Morphologic Features
Lymphoblastic (ALL)	–	–	–	–	+	Single nucleolus
Myeloblastic (AML)	+	+	+	–	–	Multiple nucleoli, Auer rods
Monocytic	–	–	–	+	–	–
Myelomonocytic	+	+	+	+	–	–

- Alpha-napthyl butyrate esterase staining is indicative of monocytic differentiation.
- *As rate of growth is very high starry sky pattern is seen in bone marrow examination.*
- *Chromosomal abnormalities include hyperdiploidy, t (12:21 '**MC** in childhood'), t (9:22 '**MC** in adulthood'); t (4:11); Hypodiploidy.*
- Acid phosphatase is most useful for T-cell ALL, where it stains as a block or patch.

Clinical finding :

- Similar to AML most patients present with complaint symptoms related to decrease production of hematopoetic cells.

In children:

- ↓MC symptom are fatigue, lethargy, fever, bleeding, bone and joint pain

...Wintrobes 12/e, p 1889

In adults fever is the most common symptom

- Most common physical signs are splenomegaly > lymphadenopathy > hepatomegaly.
- Testes may be enlarged secondary to leukemia infiltration.
- Leukemic infiltration of cranial nerve may cause cranial nerve palsy with marked nuchal rigidity.

Lab findings :

- **Peripheral smear :** At presentation most patient have a decrease in at least one cell type (single cytopenia) i.e. *neutropenia (MC)* or thrombocytopenia, anaemia.

a. **TLC** :	– WBC count is usually low or normal (≤10,000/µl). – In 20% of patient TLC is > 50,000/µl
b. **RBC** :	– Peripheral smear show anaemia and abnormalities in red cell such as tear drop cell.
c. **Thrombocyte** :	– Most patient of ALL have decreased platelet count.

- **Bone marrow examination :**
  - *Bone marrow aspiration is the standard method of establishing diagnosis.*
  - Marrow is hypercellular with replacement of fat spaces.
  - Myeloid and erythroid precursor are normal and megakaryocytes are decreased or absent.
  - Lymphoblast from bone marrow are confirmed by histochemical and cytogenetic analysis.
- **CSF examination :** About 5% of patient present with CNS leukemia which is defined as CSF WBC count ≥ 5/µl with blasts present on cytocentrifuged specimen or presence of cranial nerve palsy. *... Wintrobes 12/e, p 1823*
- **Serum chemistry** : ALL shows :
  - ↑ Uric acid
  - ↑ LDH
  - Hyperphosphatemia
  - Hypocalcemia

  ... Wintrobes 11/e, p 2145
- **Imaging :**
  - Plane X-ray of long bones and spine show demineralization, periosteal elevation, growth arrest lines, or compression of vertebral bodies.
  - Chest X-ray may shows mediastinal widening and tracheal compression.
  - Abdominal US may show kidney enlargement due to leukemic infiltration and intra-abdominal adenopathy.

Diagnostic criteria :

- Diagnosis of ALL is based on demonstration of lymphoblast in the bone marrow.
- Lymphoblast required for diagnosis is set at 25%. *... Wintrobes 12/e, p 1891*

Classification :

- According to FAB on the basis of cytological examination ALL is divided in to : L_1, L_2, L_3.
  - **L1** is MC type of ALL in children and has best prognosis.
  - **L2** is MC type of ALL in adults. *... Devita 7/e, p 2093*
  - **L3** has worst prognosis.

Prognostic factors :

Determinants	Favourable	Unfavourable
White blood cell count	<10x10⁹/L	>200x10⁹/L
Age	3-7 year	<1, >10 year
Gender	Female	Male
Node, liver, spleen enlargement	Absent	Present
Central nervous system leukemia	Absent	Present (blasts + pleocytosis)
FAB morphologic features	L1	L3
Ploidy	Hyperdiploidy	Hypodiploidy <45
Cytogenetic markers	Trisomies 4, 10, and/or 17 t (12; 21)	t (9;22) t (4, 11) [mll af4]
Time to remission	<14d	>28d
Minimal residual disease	$<10^{-4}$	$>10^{-3}$

Treatment :

- **Induction** : To achieve remmission most commonly used drugs are oral prednisone or dexamethasone, intravenous vincristine and daunorubicin, IM asparaginase, Intrathecal methotrexate.
  : Remission is conventionally defined by : <5% blast in cellular marrow, recovery of peripheral neutrophils, platelets, absence of detectable extramedullary leukemia
- **Consolidation** : By using cyclophosphamide, L asparginase.
- **Maintenance** : Drugs used are 6 mercaptopurine and methotrexate.
- CNS and testes are sanctuary sites of extramedullary leukemia. So, presymptomatic or prophylactic intrathecal chemotherapy using methotrexate is critical part of ALL treatment. *Testicular biopsy at the end of treatment are replaced by only physical examination.*
- Bone marrow transplant is not used as initial treatment for ALL as most patients gets cured by chemotherapy. But patient with t(9:22), t(4:11), may have better cure by early BMT.

... *CPDT 19/e, p 855*

Treatment of Relapse			
Site	*Bone marrow (MC)* ↓	*Isolated testes* ↓	*CNS* ↓
Treatment	Very difficult to cure BMT may be useful	B/L testicular irradiation and Chemotherapy	Cranial irradiation, triple intrathecal therapy and systemic therapy

Remember : Tumor lysis syndrome may complicate treatment of ALL, so alkalinization of urine in necessary.

CHRONIC LYMPHOCYTIC LEUKEMIA

- CLL and SLL (Small lymphocytic leukemia) are characterized by accumulation of non proliferating *(Wintrobes 11/e, p 2429)* mature appearing lymphocytes in the blood, bone marrow, or lymph node or spleen.
- CLL and SLL are morphologically phenotypically, genotypically indistinguishable, differing only in *degree of peripheral blood lymphocytosis* ***(for CLL absolute lymphocyte count > 5000 / mm³).***

Predisposing factors

- Unlike other leukemias it is not associated with any environmental or occupational exposure.
- Family history of CLL and Ataxia telangiectasia increase risk of CLL.

Cell of origin

- CLL cells are B lymphocytes and are unique in being CD5+; CD 19+; CD23+ and CD27+ (Marker of memory cell) with weak or no expression of surface immunoglobulin, CD 20, CD 79.
- Recent evidence suggest that these ***tumor cells are derived from memory B-cells*** *(Wintrobes 12/e, p 2215)* not from a naive B cell, or follicular center cell. Expression of CD5 and CD23 are due to malignancy induced gene activation.

Molecular genetics

- The most common chromosomal abnormalities are deletion of 13q 12-14, 17p, 17pq, trisomy 12q.

Pathology

- Lymphnode architecture is diffusely effaced by predominant population of small lymphocyte mixed with large cells called ***prolymphocyte.***
- Prolymphocyte may gather focally to form loose aggregates called ***proliferation centers.*** These proliferation centers are pathognomonic for CLL/SLL.
- Peripheral blood contain increased number of lymphocyte. These cells are fragile and get disrupted in process of making smear producing Smudge cells = Basket cells.
- BM infiltration of spleen and hepatic portal tract is also present.

Clinical features

- Most patient presents at age > 50.
- Mostly asymptomatic or only non specific symptoms such as weight loss, anorexia, easy fatigue are present.
- Generalized lymphadenopathy, hepatosplenomegaly are most frequent physical findings.
- With disease progression patient of CLL develop immunosuppression resulting in ***recurrent infection and septicemia;*** later being the major cause of death in CLL.
- Inspite of immunosuppression patient of CLL have an increased incidence of *autoimmune disorder particularly autoimmune hemolytic anaemia and autoimmune thrombocytopenia.*
- CLL/SLL may ***transform to aggressive lymphoma*** inform of :
  - *Prolymphocytic transformation (15-30% of patient)* - Characterized by worsening of cytopenias, increasing spleenomegaly, and increasing number of lymphocytes in peripheral blood.
  - *Diffuse large B-cell lymphoma transformation = Richter syndrome (10% of patient)* - Characterized by rapidly enlarging mass within lymph node and spleen.

Laboratory findings

- *Peripheral blood :* a. Absolute lymphocytosis
  b. Lymphocyte count > 500/μl for CLL
  c. Smudge cells and basket cells seen.
- In bone marrow and lymphnodes proliferation centres (pathognomonic) may be seen.
- Immunophenotyping : – Cells are positive for CD5, CD23, CD27, CD18, Cd20 (low).
  – There is low expression of surface immunoglobulin.

Differential diagnosis

Most common is ***prolymphocytic leukemia*** which is characterized by *marked leukocytosis, minimal lymphadenopathy with a median survival of less than 10 months.*

Criteria for Diagnosis

- According to **NCI-COG** diagnosis of CLL require. *... Devita 8/e, p 2281*
  1. A peripheral blood lymphocyte count of greater than $5 \times 10^9/L$, with less than 55% of cells being atypical. The cells should have :
     a. B-cell specific differentiation antigens (CD-19, CD-20 and CD-23) and be CD5+ without other pan - T-Cell markers.
     b. Either κ or γ chain surface Ig, confirming monoclonicity.
     c. Low density surface Ig.

2. Bone marrow aspirate showing > 30% lymphocytes.
3. *Lymphocyte counts less than 5 x 10^9 / L can be put under SLL.*

However recently, it lhas been suggested that diagnosis can be made with the presence of chronic absolute increase in blood lymphocytes (> 4 × 10^9/L) having the typical morphological and immunopathological features (CD5+, CD79 –, CD 103 –, CD19+) *... Wintrobes 12/e, p 2223*

Staging

Two staging system are used (RAI system Binet staging)

Stage	Clinical Features	Median Survival, Years
RAI SYSTEM		
0 : Low risk	Lymphocytosis only in blood and marrow	> 10
I : Intermediate risk	Lymphocytosis + lymphadenopathy + splenomegaly ± hepatomegaly	7
III : High risk	Lymphocytosis + anemia	1.5
IV	Lymphocytosis + thrombocytopenia	1.5

Treatment

- ***Chemotherapy*** is treatment of choice. ***Most effective*** drug are fludarbine and chlorambucil.
- Addition of steroid improve response.
- ***Monoclonal antibodies :*** Rituximab (directed against CD20) and Alemtuzumab (IgG-1 antibody directed against CD52) are used in resistant case.
- ***Splenectomy*** : For treatment of autoimmune anemia and thrombocytopenia.
- ***Radiotherapy*** : For local bulky lesion.
- ***Allogenic BMT*** : For younger patient.

Markers of poor prognosis in	
Confirmed	**Investigational**
– Advance stage – Male – Atypical morphology – Peripheral lymphocyte doubling time of < 12 month – CD 38 positivity – High β2-microglobulin level – Diffuse marrow histology – High lactate dephydrogenase – Fludarabine resistance	– Lack of IgVH gene mutation – Expression of ZAP-70 protein – del 11q22-q23 (loss of ATB gene); del 17p13, trisomy 12 – Increased serum levels of CD-23, TNFα, thymidine kinase

Cause of Death

- Most common cause of death is ***septicemia.***
- CLL increased the risk for development of ***second malignancy*** particularly Hodgkins disese, melanomas, CNS tumor and lung cancer.

... Devita 7/e, p 2141

QUESTIONS

1. **All are good prognostic factors in childhood ALL except : [AI 07]**
   a. Early pre B-cell subtype
   b. Precurser B-cell ALL
   c. Hyperdiploidy
   d. Female gender

2. **B-Cell prolymphocytic leukemia patients differs from those with B-Cell chronic lymphocytic leukemia in : [AI 06]**
   a. Presenting at younger age
   b. Having a lower total leukocyte count
   c. Having a prominent lymphadenopathy
   d. Having a shorter survival

3. **A four year old boy was admitted with a history of abdominal pain and fever for two months, maculopapular rash for ten days, and dry cough, dyspnea and wheezing for three days. On examination, liver and spleen were enlarged 4cm and 3cm respectively below the costal margins. His hemoglobin was 10.0g/dl, platelet count 37x10^9/L and total leukocyte count 70x10^9/L, which include 80% eosinophils. Bone marrow examination revealed a cellular marrow comprising 45% blasts and 34% eosinophils and eosinohilic precursors. The blasts stained negative for myeloperoxidase and non specific esterase and were positive for Cd19, Cd10, DC22 and Cd20.**
   Which one of the following statements in not true about this disease ? [AI 05]
   a. Eosinophils are not part of the neoplastic clone
   b. t (5:14) rearrangement maybe detected in blasts
   c. Peripheral blood eosinophilia may normalize with chemotherapy
   d. Inv (16) is often detected in the basts and the eosinophils

4. **A 48 year old man was admitted with a history of weakness for two months on examination cervical lymph nodes were found enlarged and spleen was palpable 2cm below costal margin hemoglobin was 10.5 g/dl platelet count 237 x 10^9/L and total leucocyte count 40x10^9/L, which include 80% mature lymphoid cells with coarse clumped chromatin Bone marrow revealed nodular lymphoid infiltrate. The peripheral blood lymphoid cells were positive for CD-19, CD-5, CD-20 and CD-23 and were negative for CD-79 B and FMC-7. The histopathological examination of lymph node in this patient will most likely exhibit effacement of lymph node architecture by : [AI 05]**
   a. A pseudofollicular pattern with proliferation centers
   b. A Monomorphic lymphoid proliferation centers
   c. Predominantly follicular pattern
   d. A diffuse proliferation of medium to large lymphoid cells with high mitotic rate

5. **Bad prognostic factor in ALL**
   a. Philadelphia syndrome [PGI 09]
   b. Male sex
   c. ↑ WBC count
   d. Hyperdiploidy
   e. Age < 1 year

6. **The poor prognostic factor associated with ALL in children is: [AIIMS 09]**
   a. Total leucocyte count 4000-100000
   b. Age less than 2 years
   c. Testicular involvement
   d. Blast in peripheral smear

7. **A 17 year old boy presented with TLC of 138 x 10^9 / L with 80% blasts on the peripheral smea. Chest X-ray demonstrated a large mediastinal mass. Immunophenotyping of this patient's blasts would most likely demonstrate :**
   a. No surface antigens (null kphenotype)
   b. An immature T cell phenotype (Tdt / D34 / CD7 positive) **[AIIMS 06]**
   c. Myeloid markers, such as CD13, CD33 and CD15
   d. B-cell markers, such as CD19, CD20 and CD22

8. **A 48 year old woman admitted with a history of weakness for two months. On examination, cervical lymph nodes were found enlarged and spleen was palpable 2 cm below the costal margin. Her hemoglobin was 10.5 g/dl, platelet count 237x109/L and total leukocyte count 40x10^9/L, which included 80% mature lymphoid cells with coarse clumped chromatin. Bone marrow revealed a nodular lymphoid infiltrate. The peripheral blood lymphoid cells were positive for CD19, CD5, CD20 and CD23 and were negative for CD79B and FMC-7.**
   What is the most likely diagnosis ?
   a. T-cell rich B-cell lymphoma with leukemic spill over in blood
   b. Chronic lymphocytic leukemia
   c. Mantle cell lymphoma **[AIIMS 05]**
   d. A definite diagnosis cannot be made in this patient without lymph node biopsy

9. **Congenital syndrome associated with lymphoproliferative malignancy includes:**
   a. Bloom syndrome **[PGI 05, 02]**
   b. Fanconi's anemia
   c. Turner syndrome
   d. Chediak Highashi syndrome
   e. Ataxia telangiectasia

ANSWERS, REFERENCES, EXPLANATIONS WITH INFORMATIVE ILLUSTRATIONS

1. **Ans. is b i.e. Precurser B-cell ALL** *Ref. Wintrobes 12/e, p 1892*

Pre B-cell ALL comprises approximately 20% of childhood ALL and has been associated with poorer outcomed compared to early pre B-cell ALL.

Depending on the developmental phase of B-cell involved. ALL can be:

- **Early pre B-cell ALL :** Comprises 2/3 of childhood ALL and is associated with good prognosis
- **Pre-B cell ALL:** Accounts for 20% of childhood ALL and is associated with a poor outcome compared to early pre-B cell ALL
- **Mature B-cell ALL :** Rarest, accounting for 1-2% childhood ALL. Children with B-cell ALL are older and have a poor response to standard ALL therapy. Thus poor prognosis

Determinants	Favourable	Unfavourable
White blood cell count	$<10x10^9/L$	$>200x10^9/L$
Age	3-7 year	<1, >10 year
Gender	Female	Male
Node, liver, spleen enlargement	Absent	Present
Central nervous system leukemia	Absent	Present (blasts + pleocytosis)
Testicular enlargement	Absent	Present
FAB morphologic features	L1	L3
Ploidy	Hyperdiploidy	Hypodiploidy <45
Cytogenetic markers	Trisomies 4, 10, and/or 17 t (12; 21)	t (9;22) t (4, 11)
Time to remission	<14d	>28d
Minimal residual disease	$<10^{-4}$	$>10^{-3}$

Total WBC count at the time of diagnosis is the single most important determinant of prognosis *...Wintrobes 12/e, p 1892*

2. **Ans. is d i.e. Having a shorter survival** *Ref. Wintrobes 12/e, p 2227; Devita 8/e, p 2289;*

Prolymphocytic leukemia is characterized by larger, less mature cells than CLL and the nucleus has condensed chromatin.

In prolymphocytic leukemia ≥ 55% of blood cells are prolymphocyte (In CLL it is < 55%).

Features	B - Cell Prolymphocytic leukemia	B-cell CLL
Cells	Larger, less mature	Comparatively mature
TLC	Marked leukocytosis	Leukocytosis is less marked
Prolymphocyte count	≥ 55% of TLC	< 55% of TLC
Immunophenotype	CD 5+/–, Sig/–, CD20+, CD79+	CD 5+, CD 23+, CD20+/–, CD79+/–
Clinical presentation	Usually symptomatic with fever, weight loss, splenomegaly	Usually asymptomatic
Lymphadenopathy	Minimal	Marked
Survival	Median survival < 3 years	Comparatively better prognosis

Guys ! I am unable to get any information about age; but as survival rate is cleary less that would be answer.

3. **Ans. is d i.e. Inv (16) is often detected in the basts and the eosinophils**

Ref. Wintrobes 12/e, p 1996; Journal of Hematology 2000; 79 (5), 272 - 274

This is a case of ALL with hypereosinophillic syndrome and Inv.(16) is not found in cases of ALL.

Why ALL ?

- Blasts are negative for myeloperoxidase and non specific esterase.

Type	*Myeloperoxidase*	*Sudan black*
AML	+	—
ALL	—	+

- ***Presence of positive immunological markers*** : CD 19, CD 20, CD 22 indicate a B - cell Lineage ALL.
  Immunological markers for B-cell lineage ALL : CD 19, CD 20, CD 22, CD 79a, cCD 22, cCD 79a.

Hypereosinophillic Syndrome (HES) :

- Idiopathic hypereosinophillic syndrome is a rare condition characterized by extremely high levels of peripheral blood eosinophil counts. These eosinophills are reactive and are not part of neoplastic clone.
- Clinical picture of dry cough, dyspnea, wheezing are further suggestive of HES. CNS damage is also common.
- This is differentiated from eosinophillic leukemia by the ***absence of eosinophilic blast cells.***
- There is no effective treatment. Cytokines such as IFNa and anti IL-5 have raised some hopes.

Other options :

- *'In contrast to myeloproliferative disorders where Eosinophils are part of the neoplastic clone, eosinophilia in patients with ALL is believed to be a reactive process.'*

... Journal

4. **Ans. is d i.e. A diffuse proliferation of medium to large lymphoid cells with high mitotic rate** *Ref. Wintrobes 11/e, p 2438; Robbin's 7/e, p 673*

The patient in question is a case of chronic lymphocytic leukemia *as indicated by the characteristic clinical picture and immunophenotypic characteristics.* (Typically, CLL cells express CD5, CD19, CD23 and show absence of CD79B, CD22 and FMC7).

Histopathological examination in a case of typical SLL/CLL shows

- Diffuse effacement of lymphocyte architecture by small to medium sized lymphocyes with clumped chromatin, indistinct or absent nucleoli and scanty cytoplasm.

- In many cases prolymphocyte gather together focally to form loose aggregates referred to as proliferation centre. These proliferation centres when presents are pathognomic for CLL.
- In CLL, the peripheral blood contains increased number of small, round lymphocytes with scant cytoplasm. These cells are fragile and frequently disrupted in the process of making smear producing so called *Smudge cells.*

Thus, a diffuse proliferation of medium to large lymphoid cells with high mitotic rate is consistent with a histo-pathological picture of CLL and hence is the single best answer here.

CLL	
Clinical picture and Laboratory parameters	***Immunophenotype (Same for both SLL / CLL)***
• Weakness together with cervical lymph node enlargement and splenomegaly • Increased total leucocyte count with 80% mature lymphoid cells • Anemia • TLC > 5 x 10^9 / L	• Positive for CD5, CD 19 and CD 23 and absence of CD 79 B, CD - 10

Thus, ***although an option stating*** *'diffuse proliferation of small to medium lymphoid cells with variable number of large cells with a high mitotic rate'* would have been more correct, but with the available options, *option 'd'* is the single best answer.

5. Ans. is a, b, c and e i.e. Philadelphia syndrome, Male sex, ↑ WBC count, Age < 1 year

Ref. Wintrobes 12/e, p 1892

Already explained

6. Ans. is c i.e. Testicular involvement *Ref. Wintrobes 12/e, p 1892*

Already explained

7. Ans. is b i.e. An immature T-cell phenotype *Ref. Robbin's 8/e, p 602*

This is a case of T-cell ALL.

Why ?	• Presence of 80% blast in peripheral smear clearly suggest ALL. • Adloscent age group and large mediastinal mass is suggestive of T-cell phenotype.

Immunophenotyping of ALL

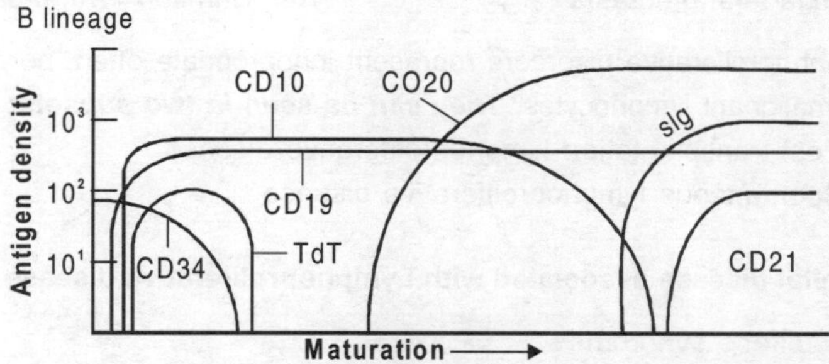

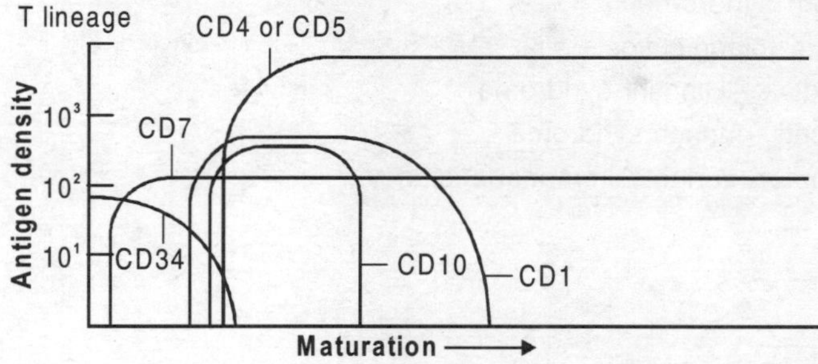

Note : CD 34 can be expressed by blasts of all lineges especially if the cells are primitive.

8. **Ans. is b i.e. Chronic lymphocytic leukemia** *See below*

Following table makes thing clear to you.

Immunophenotypes of Chronic lymphocytic leukemia and other Chronic B-cell disorders.

Condition	*smIg*	*CD5*	*CD10*	*CD11*	*CD19*	*CD20*	*CD22*	*CD23*	*CD25*	*CD43*	*Cd79b*	*CD103*	*FMC7*
Chronic lymphocytic leukemia	Dim	++	–	–/+	++	Dim	–/+	++	+/–	+	–	–	–/+
Prolymphocytic leukemia	+++	–/+	–/+	–/+	++	+++	+	++	–/+	+	++	–	+
Hairy cell leukemia	+++	–	–	++	+++	+++	+++	–	+++	+	+	+++	+++
HCL variant	+++	–	–	++	+++	+++	+++	–	–	+	+	+++	+++
Marginal zone B-cell lymphoma	++	–	–	+/–	++	++	+/–	+/–	–	–/+	++	–	+
Marginal cell lymphoma	++	++	–/+	–	++	++	++	–	–	+	++	–	++
Follicular lymphoma	++	–/+	++	–	++	++	++	–/+	–	–	++	–	++

9. **Ans. is a, b, d and e i.e. Bloom syndrome; Fanconi's anemia; Chediak Highashi syndrome; and Ataxia telangiectasia** *Ref. Harrison 17/e, p 689; CPDT 19/e, p 868*

- Lymphoprolierative disorders represent inappropriate often, polyclonal proliferation of nonmalignant lymphocytes. ***They can be seen in two subsets:***
  a. Post-transplantation lymphoproliferative disease
  b. Spontaneous lymphoproliferative disease

Congenital disease associated with Lymphoproliferative disease :

– Klinefelter's syndrome
– Downs syndrome
– Bloom syndrome
– Ataxia telangiectiosis
– Chediak - Higashi syndrome
– Wiscott - Aldrich syndrome
– Common variable immunodeficiency.

30 Hodgkins and Nonhodgkin Lymphoma

What's Important ?

- **Types of Hodgkin Lymphoma**
- **Hairy Cell Leukemia**
- **Mantle Cell Leukemia**

On the basis of site of origin and spread lymphomas are divided into Hodgkins lymphoma and Non-Hodgkins lymphoma.

Hodgkin lymphoma	Nonhodgkin lymphoma
– Localized to a single axial group of nodes (Cervical, mediastinal, para-aortic)	– More frequent involvement of multiple peripheral nodes
– Orderly spread by contiguity	– Noncontiguous spread
– Mesenteric nodes and Waldeyer ring rarely involved	Waldeyer ring and mesenteric nodes commonly involved
– Extranodal involvement uncommon	– Extranodal involvement common

HODGKINS LYMPHOMA (= HODGKINS DISEASE)

- Arise in single lymphnode or chain of node. Most commonly ***supra-clavicular*** and cervical nodes are involved.
- Age / sex - Show ***bimodal*** distribution. 1st peak (major) in the third decade of life and 2nd small peak occurs after age of 50 years. M > F.

Etiology

- Exact cause is not known, risk is increase in :
  - Primary relatives of patient of Hodgkin lymphoma
  - Previous EBV infection
  - AIDS patient.

Cell of Origin

- ***Reed Sternberg*** cells are considered malignant cells of HD; but they represent very small portion (0.1 - 1%) of tumor cells.
- RS cell induce accumulation of reactive lymphocyte; eosinophils; histiocyte by secreting cytokines such as IL-5, IL-6, IL-13, TNF) which makes the major portion of tumor.

- Till now exact origin of RS cell is not known.
- *RS cells are CD30+, CD15+ CD19+/–, CD20+/–.*
- RS cells of lymphocytic predominant HL are CD30⁻ and CD15⁻ and are CD45⁺
- **Cytogenetics**
  - RS cells are aneuploid and often possess diverse clonal aberration, chromosomal aberration
  - Gain of chromosome 2p is also common.

Classification

WHO has classified HD in to following types. ... *Devita 8/e, p 2174*

- ***Nodular sclerosis*** (Most common)
- Classical HL
- Lymphocyte predominant, nodular
- Lymphocyte rich classic HL
- Lymphocyte depleted
- Mixed cellularity
- Unclassified HL

Pathology

- **RS cell :** Diagnostic RS cell are large (15 to 14µm in diameter) and have either multiple nuclei or a single nucleus with multiple nuclear lobes, classical RS cells are binucleate and have inclusion like ***owl eyed nucleoli.***
- **Variants of RS cells are :**
  a. Mononuclear variant : Contain single round or oblong nucleus with a large inclusion like nucleolus.
  b. Lacunar cells : They have more folded or multilobate nuclei surrounded by pale cytoplasm.
     - They are predominant in the nodular sclerosis subtype.
  c. Lymphocytic and histiocytic variants (L+H cells) - They resemble popcorn kernels and are specific to lymphocytic predominant subtype.

Types

Subtype	Morphology and Immunophenotype	Typical Clinical Features
Nodular sclerosis (MC)	Frequent lacunar cells with diagnostic R-S cells, Characteristic fibrous bands dividing cellular areas into nodules are present. CD15+, CD30+, EBV-	Stage 1 or 2 disease. Frequent mediastinal involvement. F=M, most patient young adults. Good prognosis.
Mixed cellularity	Frequent mononuclear and diagnostic R-S cells 70% EBV+ CD 15+, CD30+, 70% EBV+	Mostly present at advance stage disease. M > F. Biphasic incidence, peaking in young adults and again in adults older than 55. Relatively poor prognosis
Lymphocyte-rich	Frequent mononuclear and diagnostic R-S cells 40% EBV+ CD15+, CD30+	Uncommon. M>F. Tends to be seen in older adults

Contd...

Contd...

Lymphocyte depletion	Reticular variant : Frequent diagnostic R-S and variants with a paucity of background reactive cells; Diffuse fibrosis variant; hypocellular fibrillar background with scattered diagnostic most EBV+, CD30+, CD15+	Uncommon, More common in older males, HIV-infected individuals, and in developing countries More likely to present with advanced disease. Worst prognosis
Lymphocyte predominance	Frequent L & H (popcorn cell) variants in a background of follicular dendritic cells and reactive B cells. R-S cells CD20+, CD15–, C30–; EBV–	Uncommon. Young males with cervical or axillary lymphadenopathy Excellent prognosis

Note : *Lymphocyte predominant Hodgkin's disease is now recognized as an entity distinct from classic Hodgkins disease as it does not express marker of RS cell i.e. CD30 and CD15 and express CD-45.*

Spread

- HD characteristically spread to anatomically contagious nodes.
- Nodal disease precedes splenic disease, splenic disease usually precedes hepatic disease and hepatic disease usually precedes marrow involvement and extranodal disease.

Clinical feature

- Patient characterstically presents with painless enlargement of lymph nodes (Most common left cervical and left supraclavicular nodes). Most common ***extra nodal sites are liver,*** bone marrow and lung.
- **Nodes** are discrete and freely movable.
- Mediastinal involvement is discovered on chest X-ray.
- Bone marrow infiltration is seen in advanced cases and is suggested by leukopenia, anaemia, thrombocytopenia and elevated alkaline phosphate.
- Occasionally HD present with fever of unknown origin particularly in mixed cellularity type.
- Rarely the fever persist for days to weeks followed by afebrile interval and then recurrence. This pattern is called Pel-Epstein fever.
- ***Cutaneous manifestation include :*** Erythema nodusum, icthyosiform atrophy.
- *Unusually HD may present with :*
  - Severe unexplained itching
  - Nephrotic syndrome
  - Immunohemolytic anaemia
  - Bleeding (due to thrombocytopenia is rare but characterstic symptom)
- Pain in lymphnode on alcohol ingestion.
- B symptoms : Weight loss, fever and night sweats signify advanced disease.

Diagnosis and staging

- Diagnosis of HD is made on biopsy by demonstration of RS cell. Although RS cell are prerequisite for diagnosis, they must be present in appropriate *background of non neoplastic inflammatory cells lymphocyte; plasma cells eosinophils.*

- In the past surgical (An Arbor staging) staging was done, but now it has been replaced by non invasive staging, Staging evaluation of patient include :
  - Complete blood count, ESR
  - Serum chemistry for LDH
  - Chest radiography
  - CT of chest, abdomen and pelvis
  - Bone marrow biopsy.
- **Costwolds staging for Hodgkin's lymphoma**

Stage I	Involvement of a single lymph node region or lymphoid structure (e.g., spleen, thymus, or involvement of a single extralymphatic site (IE).
Stage II	Involvement of two or more lymph node regions on the same side of the diaphragm (hilar nodes, when involved on both sides, constitute stage II disease); localized contiguous involvement of only one extranodal organ or site and lymph node region (s) on the same side of the diaphragm (IIE).
Stage III	Involvement of lymph node regions on both sides of the diaphragm which may also be accompanied by involvement of the spleen (III_S) or by localized contiguous involvement of only one extranodal organ site (IIE) or both (IIISE).
III1	With or without involvement of splenic, hilar, celiac, or portal nodes.
III2	With involvement of paraaortic, iliac, and mesenteric nodes.
Stage IV	Diffuse or disseminated involvement of one or more extranodal organs or tissues, with or without associated lymph node involvement.

Designations applicable to any disease stage

A	No symptoms.
B	Fever (temperature, >38ºC), drenching night sweats, unexplained loss of >10% body weight within the preceding 6 months.
X	Bulky disease (a widening of the mediastinum by more than one-third or presence of node ≥ 10cm.
E	Involvement of a single extranodal site that is contiguous or proximal to the known nodal site.

Bad prognostic factor for HL

- Serum **A**lbumin <4g/dl (most important)
- Hemoglobin <10.5g/dl (**A**naemia)
- **M**ale gender
- **S**tage IV disease
- **A**ge ≥ 45 year
- White blood cell count (**T**LC) ≥ 15,000/mm³
- **L**ymphocyte count < 600/mm³ or < 8% of white blood cell.

Mnemonic : Agra **T**ujhe **SALAM**

Treatment

Stage	Treatment
Early stage favourable (Stage 1A or IIA)	Extended field radiotherapy
Early stage unfavourable	4-6 cycles of chemotherapy + Involved field radiotherapy
Advanced stage	6-8 cycles chemotherapy + Radiotherapy to residual tumor and bulk.

- Most effective chemotherapeutic regimen is combination of :
  - **A**driamycin (Doxorubicin)
  - **B**leomycine - B
  - **V**incristine - V
  - **D**acarbazine - D

  Mnemonics : **ABVD** regimen
- Other commonly used regimen is MOPP (Mechlorethomine, Vincristine, Procarbazine, prednisone)

NON HODGKINS LYMPHOMA

Hematologic malignancies presenting as lymphoma with frequent extranodal involvement are included in this group.

Clinical characteristics of Patients with common types of Non-hodgkin's lymphomas (NHL)

Disease	Median Age, years	Frequency in children	Bone marrow involvement (%)	5 years survival (%)
Mantle cell lymphoma	63	Rare	64	27
Extranodal marginal zone B cell lymphoma of MALT type	60	Rare	14	74
Follicular lymphoma	59	Rare	42	72
Diffuse large B cell lymphoma	64	~25% of child hood NHL	16	46
Burkitt's lymphoma	31	~30% of Child hood NHL	33	45
Precursor T cell lymphoblastic lymphoma	28	~40% of child-hood NHL	50	26
Anaplastic large T/null lymphoma	34	Uncommon	13	77
Peripheral T cell non-Hodgkin's lymphoma	61	~5% of Childhood NHL	36	25

Follicular lymphoma

- Lymphoma of follicular B cells (Centrocytes and centroblasts) which has at least a partially follicular pattern.
- It is MC form of NHL in western countries but rare in India and other Asian countries.
- Immunophenotype / Cell of origin : Cell resemble normal germinal B-cell and express CD-19, CD-20, CD-10 (CALLA) and surface immunoglobulin, unlike CLL / SLL follicular lymphoma cells are CD5(-).
- Ki 67 fraction is lower than that of reactive follice.

- ***Cytogenetics :***
  - Hallmark of typical follicular lymphoma is a (14:18) translocation that juxtaposes *the IgH locus on chromosome 14 and the BCl-2 Locus on chormosome 18.*
  - Rearrangement of 3q27 is found in some case.
- ***Morphology :***
  - Follicular lymphoma is composed of a mixture of centrocytes (cleaved follicular centers cells) and centroblasts (large non cleaved follicle center cells) and by definition has at least a partially follicular pattern. Centrocytes are more in number.
  - Bone marrow involvement is common and characterstically takes the form of paratrabecular lymphoid aggregates.
  - *Splenic involvement* is limited typically to white pulp.
- ***Clinical features :***
  - Present as painless generalized lymphadenopathy.
  - Extranodal involvement to CNS and GIT is relatively uncommon.
  - Histological transformation occur in 30% to 50% cases, most commonly to diffuse large B-cell lymphoma or rarely to tumor resembling Burkitt lymphoma which is associated with acquisition of chromosome translocation involving C-Myc locus.
- ***Treatment :***
  - Follicular lymphoma is one of malignancies most responsive to chemotherapy and radiotherapy.
  - *Early stage* follicular lymphoma is best treated by *radiotherapy.*
  - *Advanced case :* Salvage *chemotherapy.*
  - *Transformed disease : CHOP* chemotherapy, however prognosis is very poor.
  - Monoclonal antibody against CD-20 is recommended in *advanced cases.*

Diffuse large B-cell lymphoma

- Most common type of NHL. ... *Harrison 17/e, p 696*
- DLBCL is a neoplasm of large transformed B-cells with nuclear size equal to or exceeding that of normal macrophage or more than twice the size of normal lymphocyte.
- ***Immunophenotype :*** Cell express B-cell marker CD-19 and CD-20 with variable expression of CD-5 or CD-10. Most have surface Ig and all are negative for TdT.
- ***Cytogenetics :*** Most frequent abnormality is dysregulation of BCL-6, located on 3q27.
- ***Morphology :***
  - Tumor composed of large cells.
  - Extranodal involvement to GIT and bone marrow is common.
- ***Clinical feature :*** DLBCL patient typically presents with a rapidly enlarging mass at a lymphnode or extranodal site.
- ***Treatment :***
  - Combination chemotherapy with CHOP. plus rituximab
  - Autologous bone marrow transplantation.
- ***Special subtypes :***

  A. *Immunodeficiency associated lymphoma :* Occurs in cases of severe T-cell deficiency eg. End stage HIV infection, SCID, solid organ and bone marrow transplantation. These neoplastic B-cells are often latently infected with EBV.

B. *Body cavity large cell lymphoma :* Arise as malignant pleural or ascitic effusion mostly in patient with HIV infection. All these tumor cells are infected with KSHV/HHV -. Tumor cells do not express surface B or T cell marker but often have clonal IgH rearrangements.

Burkitt Lymphoma

- Rare in adults but most common *type of NHL in children.*
- ***Immunophenotype :*** Tumor composed of relatively mature B cells expressing surface IgM, monotypic κ or α light chain. Cells are positive for CD-19, CD-20 and CD-10.
- ***Molecular genetics :*** Burkitt lymphoma are associated with t(8:14) involving Cmyc gene (on Chromosome 8) and IgH locus (on chromosome 14). Most cases of Burkitt lymphoma shows latent infection by EBV.
- Cells of Burkitt lymphoma are histologically and phenotypically similar to L3 ALL, *So, when Burkitt cells are found with features of leukemia, designation is Burkitt leukemia = L3 ALL.*
- ***Morphology***
  - Involved tissue shows diffuse infiltrate of intermediate sized lymphoid cells.
  - High mitotic rate and apoptotic tumor cell death with starry sky appreance is typical.
- ***Clinical course***
  - Mostly present at extranodal site.
  - Three distinct forms are found :
    a. *Sporadic Burkitts lymphoma :* Abdomen is the most common site of sporadic type, mostly presenting as right lower quadrant mass or with an acute abdomen secondary to an ileocaecal intususception.
    b. *Endemic Burkitts lymphoma :* Head and neck region is most common site of endemic type, presenting as mass involving the *mandible.*
    c. *Immunodeficiency associated lymphoma,* seen in patient of HIV.
  - Disease is rapidly progressive and has propensity to metastasize to CNS.
- ***Treatment :***
  - Combination chemotherapy incorporating high dose of cyclophosphamide.
  - Prophylactic therapy to the CNS is mandatory.
  - Radiation therapy is reserved for patient, who initially present with CNS involvement.

Mantle Cell Lymphoma

- MCL is a neoplasm of small to medium sized B-cell with irregular nuclei which resemble centrocytes and over express cyclin D-1.
- Mostly occur in ***elder*** age group.
- Tumor cell closely resemble mantle zone cells so, the name.
- ***Immunophenotype :***
  - MCL in thought to be malignant proliferation of naive B-cells.
  - Cells express CD-19, CD-20 and CD-5 but negative for CD23 (differentiating feature from CLL / SLL).
  - Cells express high level of surface Ig.
  - *Nuclear cyclin D1 protein is present in all cases and is gold standard for diagnosis.*

  ... Devita 8/e, p 2125
- ***Cytogenetics :*** Characteristic abnormality is t(11:14) involving IgH locus (on chromosome 14) and BCL1 (on chromosome 11).

- ***Morphology :*** Two pattern of nodal involvement is seen :

a. **Mantle zone pattern :** Tumor cell surround or efface B-cell producing nodular appearance.

b. **Diffuse pattern :** Tumor cells are distributed diffusely :
   - There is proliferation of small cells only and large cells resembling centroblasts are absent, (differentiating from CLL/SLL).
   - Bone marrow involvement is common and is typically nodular. ...*Devita 8/e, p 2125*
   - Splenic white, pulp may be involved.
   - Occasionally multifocal mucosal involvement of the small bowel and colon produces lymphomatoid polyposis.

- ***Clinical course :***
  - Most patient present in advanced cases with generalized lymphadenopathy, bone marrow and liver involvement.
  - Prognosis is poor.
- ***Treatment :***
  - Current therapies are unsatisfactory.
  - CHOP and CVP chemotherapy prolong survival in some cases.

Marginal Zone Lymphoma (MALToma) = Mucosa associated lymphoma

- Maltoma is an extranodal lymphoma consisting of heterogenous B-cells found at mucosal sites.
- They tends to arise in tissues involved by chronic inflammatory disorders such as *salivary gland in Sjogren disease, stomach in helicobacter gastritis.*
- Present as single ulcer or mass.
- They remain localized for prolong periods at sites of origin.
- Cell of origin is supposed to be post germinal center memory B cell. ... *Devita 7/e, p 1973*
- Most common site is stomach, but can occur in lung, thyroid, intestine, salivary gland.
- ***Treatment :***
  - Chemotherapy and H.pylori eradication is *treatment of choice* for gastric MALToma.
  - Local therapy such as surgery and radiotherapy is effective in other cases.

Hairy cell leukemia

- Rare lymphoproliferative disorder characterized by cytopenia and splenomegaly.
- Tends to occur in males.
- ***Immunophenotype / Cytochemistry :***
  - Tumor cells are CD 19+, CD 20+, CD 22+, CD 25+, CD 103+, CD 5–, CD 23 –
  - They stain strongly for surface immunoglobulin and FMC-7.
  - HCL cells are characterized by presence of tartate resistant acid phosphatase.
- ***Morphology :***
  - Leukemic cells have fine hair like projections that are best recognized under phase contrast microscope.
  - Bone marrow is always involved in focal or interstitial pattern showing fried egg appearance. BM aspiration may show dry tap.
  - HCL in contrast to other NHL tends to infiltrate red pulp of spleen. Other NHL infiltrate white pulp.

- ***Clinical features :***
  - Pancytopenia : Resulting from bone marrow failure
  - Splenomegaly : Often massive (MC sign)
  - Hepatomegally
- ***Treatment :***
  - Pentostatin (2 deoxycofromycin) and cladribine (DOC) are main stay of treatment.
  - Prognosis is excellent.

T-CELL AND N-K CELL NEOPLASM

Adult T-cell lymphoma/leukemia

- Adult T-cell lymphoma/leukemia is a neoplasm of CD-4 T cells seen in patient infected by HTLV-1 after a latency of approximately 50 years.
- Shapes of cell varies widely but most frequently cells with multilobed nuclei called clover leaf or flower cells are found.
- Tumor cells are CD2+, CD3+, CD5+, CD4+, CD7–.
- Most patient present with aggressive disease manifested by lymphadenopathy, hepatosplenomegaly, skin infiltration, hypercalcemia, lytic bone lesion and elevated LDH level.
- ***Treatment*** : No treatment is satisfactory and median survival is only 70 days.

Remember : – Other manifestation of HTLV-1 – Tropical spastic paraperisis and HTLV-1 associated myelopathy.

Peripheral T cell lymphoma, unspecified

- This entity includes predominantly nodal and occasionally extranodal T-cell lymphoma which do not have consistent immunophenotypic, genetic or clinical features.
- Although no morphological character is pathognomic, characteristic finding include :
  - Diffuse effacement of architecture of involved lymphnode.
  - Tumor composed of small intermediate and large malignant T-cell with infiltrate of reactive cells such as macrophage, and eosinophil.
- Diagnosis can be made only on immunophenotype and by definition lymphoma have a *mature T-cell phenotype lacking TdT and usually expressing CD-2, CD-5, surface CD-3.*
- Most patient present with generalized lymphadenopathy accompanied by eosinophilia, pruritis, fever and weight loss.
- ***Treatment :*** Combination chemotherapy is given, but prognosis is poor.

Cutaneous T-cell lymphoma

- CTCL is a neoplasm of mature CD4 + helper T-cells characterized by involvement of skin.
- *Mycosis fungoides and Sezary syndrome are two different manifestation of CTCL.*
- Associated with **HTLV-1** infection.
- **Hall mark** of CTCL of mycosis fungoides is :
  - *Sezary lutzner cells* (CD 4 cells)
  - *Pautrier microabscess.*
- Clinically patient present with scaly red brown patches. Over time nodal metastasis and visceral metastases occur.
- ***Sezary syndrome :*** Cuntaneous T-Cell lymphoma with circulating tumor cells and erythroderma is called sezary syndrome.

- ***Treatment :*** – Localized lesion - Radiotherapy
  – Advanced cutaneous lesion - Topical glucocortcoid, nitrogen mustard, phototherapy, psoralen.

Anaplastic large cell lymphoma (ALK positive)

- Rare, defined by the presence of rearrangements in the ALK gene on chromosome 2p33
- Tumor is composed of large anaplastic cells, some containing horseshoe shaped nuclei and voluminous cytoplasm *(so called hallmark cells)*
- This tumor typically affect young adults, frequently involve soft tissue and carries a very good prognosis

Remember :

Lymphoma	Characteristic translocation	Mnemonics
Burkitts lymphoma	t(8:14)	8≈**B**
Mantle cell lymphoma	t(11:14)	**M**≈IVI≈II
Follicular lymphoma	t(14:18)	Fourteen t18 (R is 18th letter)

QUESTIONS

1. **Mycosis fungoides which is not true :**
   a. It is the most common from of cutaneous lymphoma **[AI 07; AIIMS 06]**
   b. Pautriers microbacess are seen
   c. Indolent course and easily amenable to treatment
   d. Erythroderma seen and spreads to peripheral circulation
2. **Mantle cell lymphomas are positive for all of the following except : [AI 06]**
   a. CD-23
   b. CD-20
   c. CD-5
   d. CD-43
3. **All of the following statement regarding primary effusion lymphoma are true except : [AI 06]**
   a. It generally presents in elderly patient
   b. There is often an association with HHV-8
   c. The proliferating cells are NK cells
   d. Patients are commonly HIV positive
4. **The classification proposed by the international Lymphoma Study Group for non-Hodgkin's lymphoma is known as: [AI 05]**
   a. Kiel classification
   b. REAL classification
   c. WHO classification
   d. Rappaport classification
5. **The subtype of Hodgkin's disease, which is heterogenetically distinct from all the other subtypes, is : [AI 05]**
   a. Lymphocyte predominant
   b. Nodular sclerosis
   c. Mixed cellularity
   d. Lymphocyte depleted
6. **Which of the following statement pertaining to leukemia is correct : [AI 05]**
   a. Blasts of acute myeloid leukemia are typically sudan black negative
   b. Blast of acute lymphoblastic leukemia are typically myeloperoxidase positive
   c. Low leucocyte alkaline phosphate score is characteristically seen in blastic phase of chronic myeloid leukemia
   d. Tart rate resistant acid phosphatase positivity is typically seen in hairy cell leukemia
7. **About Burkitt's lymphoma – What is true?**
   a. CD34 +ve and surface Immuno Globulin +ve **[AIIMS 09]**
   b. CD34 +ve and surface Immuno Globulin –ve
   c. CD34 –ve and surface Immuno Globulin –ve
   d. CD34 –ve and surface Immuno Globulin +ve
8. **Post transplant lymphoma is?[AIIMS 08]**
   a. T cell
   b. B cell
   c. Null cell
   d. NK cell
9. **All are true about follicular lymphoma except: [PGI 09]**
   a. CD 20+
   b. CD 5+
   c. BCL-1 positive in follicular lymphoma whereas BCL-2 positive in mantle cell lymphoma
   d. Translocation of (14 : 18)
10. **Which of the following are characteristic markers for Hodgkin's lymphoma?**
    a. CD15 and CD30 **[AI 08]**
    b. CD15 and CD45

c. CD30 and CD68
d. CD15 and CD3

11. Most common primary lymphoma of spleen? [AIIMS 08

a. Hodgkin's lymphoma
b. Small lymphocytic lymphoma
c. Anaplastic lymphoma
d. Burkitt's lymphoma

12. Which of the following is not a B-cell neoplasm : [AIIMS 06]

a. Hairy cell leukemia
b. Angiocentric lymphoma
c. Mantle cell lymphoma
d. Burkitt's lymphoma

13. Which of the following statement on lymphoma is not True ? [AIIMS 06]

a. A single classification system for Hodgkin's disease (HD) is almost universally accepted
b. HD more often tends to remain localized to a single group of lymph nodes and spreads by contiguity
c. Several types of non Hodgkin's lymphoma (NHL) may have a leukemic phase
d. In general follicular (nodular) NHL has worse prognosis compared to diffuse NHL

14. Lymhocytic and histiocytic variant of cell is seen in : [AIIMS 05]

a. Follicular center lymphoma
b. Lymphocyte depleted Hodgkin's disease
c. Nodular sclerosis Hodgkin's disease
d. Lymphocyte predominant Hodgkins disease

15. Which of the following lymphomas is associated with HTLV-I virus infection :

a. Burkitt's lymphoma **[AIIMS 05]**
b. B-cell lymphoma
c. Adult T-cell leukemia and lymphoma
d. Hodgkin's disease

16. Treatment of Hodgkin's disease :

a. CHOP **[PGI 06]**
b. MOPP
c. ABVD

17. True statement regarding histological features of classical Hodgkins disease :

a. Mixed cellularity seen in background
b. Neoplastic cells more than non-neoplastic cells **[PGI 05]**
c. Both neoplastic and non neoplastic cells are seen
d. Cell are CD15 and CD30 positive
e. Reed-Sternberg cells are seen

18. All statement are false regarding mucosa associated lymphoma except :

a. Predisposed by H. pylori **[PGI 05]**
b. Chemotherapy sensitive
c. Surgical resection is treatment of choice
d. Associated with stromal polyp
e. Multiple lymphomas are seen

ANSWERS, REFERENCES, EXPLANATIONS WITH INFORMATIVE ILLUSTRATIONS

1. **Ans. is c i.e. Indolent course and easily amenable to treatment**

Ref. Harrison 17/e, p 697; Devita 8/e, p 2149

Though the course of mycosis fungoides is indolent prognosis is poor.

Mycosis fungoides (cutaneous T-cell lymphoma)

- Mycosis fungoides is the commonest cutaneous T-cell lymphoma.
- Disease is characterized by ***pauterier's microabscess*** (epidermotropic collections of CTCL cells and sezary lutzner cells) and ***sezary syndrome*** (generalized erythroderma and circulating tumor cells)
- **Clinical features :**
  - ***Prediagnostic phase :*** Asymptomatic scaling, erythematous macular eruption often in sun-shielded areas that lasts for month to years.
  - ***Patch phase :*** Thin barely palpable, erythematous and ectzematous lesions.
  - ***Plaque phase :*** More readily palpable erythomatous lesion.
  - ***Tumour phase :*** Neoplasm infiltrate extends below the dermis. In this phase erythroderma is seen.
- Tumor cells characterstically express ***CLA*** and chemokine receptor ***CCR-4*** and ***CCR-10***

Treatment

- Patient presenting in early stage *(which is rare)* are treated by radiotherapy.
- More advanced disease is treated with topical glucocorticoids, topical nitrogen mustard, phototherapy, psaralen with UVA, interferon, antibodies and systemic cytotoxic therapy, unfortunately these treatment are palliative.

2. **Ans. is a i.e. CD-23** *Ref. Wintrobes 12/e, p 2223; Robbin's 8/e, p 613*

"Mantle cell lymphoma is usually CD5 (+)ve and CD 23 - ve which can help to distinguish it from CLL/SLL."

Immunohistologic and Genetic Features of Common B-cell Neoplasms

Neoplasm	Serum Ig	CD 5	CD 10	CD 23	CD 43	CD 103	Cyclin D1	Genetic Abnormality
B-SLL/CLL	+	+	–	+	+	–	–	Trisomy 12;13q
Lymphoplasmacytic lymphoma	+	–	–	–	+/–	–	–	t(9;14); del 6(q23)
Hairy cell leukemia	+	–	–	–	+	++	+/–	None known
Splenic marginal zone lymphoma	–/+	–	–	–	+	+	–	None known
Follicular lymphoma	+/–	–	+/–	–/+	–	–	–	t(14;18); bcl-2
Mantle cell lymphoma	+/–	+	–	–	–	–	+	t(11;14); bcl-1
MALT lymphoma	+/–	–	–	–/+	–	–	–	trisomy 3; t(11;18)
Diffuse large B-cell lymphoma	+/–	–	–/+	NA	–	NA	–	t(14;18), t(8;14), 3q; bcl-2, myc, bcl-6
Burkitt's lymphoma	+	–	+	–	–	NA	–	t(8;14), t(2;8), t(8;22); c-myc; EBV –/+

CD19+,CD5+, CD23– immunophenotype is seen characterstically in mantle cell lymphoma.

Remember : Nuclear cyclin D1 protein is present in all cases of mantle cell lymphoma and is gold standard of diagnosis.

3. Ans. is c i.e. The proliferating cells are NK cells *Ref. Devita 8/e, p 2408 - 2410*

Lymphoma in AIDS patient	
Germinal B-cell orgin	***Post germinal B cell orgin***
– Burkitt lymphoma – Diffuse large B-cell lymphoma (centroblastic) – Primary Brain diffuse large B-cell lymphoma	– Diffuse large B-cell lymphoma (immunoblastic) – Primary effusion lymphoma – Plasmablastic lymphoma.

Primary effusion lymphoma "PEL" (= body cavity lymphoma).

- Orginates from ***post germinal B–cell (not NK cell).***
- Universally infected with *HHV-8 = KSHV.*
- Most cells are also infected with *EBV.*
- Develop in *pleural space* due to relative hypoxic environment.
- Present as pleural effusion.
- Poorly responsive to chemotherapy.

4. Ans. is b i.e. REAL classification

Ref. Devita 7/e, p 1967, 8/e, p 2107; Wintrobes 11/e, p 2071; Robbin's 7/e p 668; Journal of Clinical Oncology 1999, 17(12), 3835

"In 1994, the international lymphoma group developed a consensus on a list of disease that could be recognized by pathologist and that appear to be distinct clinical entity, Based on this they created the Revised European-American classification of lymphoid neoplasm (REAL)." ***... Devita 7/e, p 1967***

In 1997 members of European and American Hematopathology society published a new WHO classification of Hematologic malignancies. This uses an updated version of REAL classification and applies the principles of REAL classification to the classification of myeloid and histocytic neoplasm too. The project included a clinical advisory committee of international expert hematologist and oncologist.

Proponents of prior classification : Working formulation, KIEL, REAL and French-American. British are in agreement that the WHO consensus classification should replace existing classification. *...Text from Journal of clinical oncology 1999; 17(12) 3835*

Remember : WHO classification represents the first true international consensus on the classification of hematologic malignancies.

... Devita 7/e, p 1967

5. **Ans. is a i.e. Lymphocyte predominant** *Ref. Harrison 17/e, p 699*

"Nodular lymphocytic predominant Hodgkins disease is now recognized as distinct entity as RS cell of lymphocyte predominant Hodgkin lymphoma have a characteristic B-cell immunophenotype." *... Harrison 17/e, p 699*

Classification of Hodgkin's Lymphoma	
Classical	**Lymphocyte predominant**
– Nodular – Lymphocyte rich – Lymphocyte depleted – Mixed cellularity – Unclassifiable classic HL	
Immunophenotype of RS cell	
– CD30+, CD15+, CD25+, – CD71+, CD19+/–, CD20+/–	CD19+, CD20+, CD15– CD30–, CD45+, Tumor cells express J chain

6. **Ans. is d i.e. Tartarate resistant acid phosphatase positivity is typically seen in hair cell leukemia** *Ref. Wintrobes 12/e, p 1809; Harrison's 17/e, p 697*

Cells of Hairy cell leukemia contain an isoenzyme of acid phosphatase in the cytoplasm which in contrast to other isozymes is resistant to tartrate i.e. Tartarate resistant acid phosphatase (TRAP).

TRAP, was very important feature for diagnosis of hair cell leukemia, now it has been replaced by immunohistochemical staining.

Options 'a' and 'b'

Blast type	Myeloperoxidase	Sudan black	Non specific esterase	PAS	Morphologic features
ALL	–	+	–	+	Single nucleus
AML	+	–	+	–	Multiple nucleolus, Are rods absent

Option "c" : In blastic phase of CML, LAP score is increased ...*Wintrobes 11/e, p 2243*

Remember : Condition with ↓ LAP score : – Chronic phase of CML.
– Paroxysmal nocturnal hemoglobinuria.

Important features of Hairy cell leukemia

- Affect middle age group with male predominance.
- Cells are CD19+, CD20+, CD22+, CD 25 + CD103+, CD5–, CD23–.
- Cells stain strongly for *surface immunoglobulin and FMC-7.*
- HCL cells are characterized by *tartate resistant acid phosphatase.*
- Bone marrow is always involved showing ***fried egg appearance.***
- In contrast to others NHL, it tends to infiltrate red pulp of spleen.
- Clinically characterized by pancytopenia, splenomegaly, Hepatomegaly.
- ***Cladarabine*** is drug of choice.
- Prognosis is excellant.

Note : Other drugs used in HCL - Pentostatin, Interferon γ. Steroids have no role.

7. **Ans. is d i.e. CD34 –ve and surface Immuno Globulin positive**

Ref. Harrison 16/e, p 652; Robbin's 7/e, p 677

Burkitt's lymphoma

- Mature B-cell neoplasm found mostly in children.
- It is most common type of NHL in children.
- Cells characteristically shows **t(8:14).**
- **Occur in 3 ways :**
  1. Endemic form **(common)** – Always associated with **EBV** infection.
  2. Sporadic form – Rarely associated with EBV infection.
  3. Immunodeficiency associated lymphoma – Seen in patient of **HIV.**
- Immunophenotype – Cells are CD20+, CD10+, BCL6+ and express surface IgM, monotypic κ or α light chain, CD43– (*+ve in mantle cell lymphoma*), CD79 +ve
- ***Clinical presentation :***
  - Mostly present at extranodal site.
  - Endemic form present with involvement of jaw and other facial bones.
  - Abdomen is most site in sporadic form, mostly presenting as right lower quadrant mass or with an acute abdomen secondary to intusussception.
- ***Treatment :***
  - Combination chemotherapy incorporating high dose of cyclophosphamide is most effective.
  - Prophylactic therapy to CNS is mandatory.
  - Radiation therapy is to given only to those patient who initially present with CNS involvement.

Hairy cell leukemia is a rare B-cell neoplasm characterized by hair like projections on malignant cells when seen on phase contrast microscope.

8. **Ans. is b i.e. B cell** *Ref. Devita 8/e, p 2136*

Post transplant lymphoproliferative disorders

- Occur in 0.8-20.0% of transplanted patients
- Almost always EBV related
- The development of PTLD results from proliferation of EBV transformed B-cell clones when patient receive immunosuppressive therapy after transplantation. Occasional cases of Hodgkin lymphoma and T-cell NHL have also been reported
- **The WHO classified PTLD on the basis of histology**
  a. ***Early lesions:*** Reactive plasmacytic hyperplasia, infectious mononucleosis (IM) like lesions
  b. ***Polymorphic PTLD:*** IM like appearance with effacement of architecture and tissue destruction
  c. ***Monomorphic PTLD:*** Include DLBCL, burkit lymphoma, multiple myeloma, peripheral T-cell unspecified. Other types of T-cell lymphoma
  d. ***Hodgkin's and Hodgkin's*** like

- Two major risk factors for development of PTLD are pretreatment negative recepient EBV serology and the degree of post transplant immunosuppression

Clinical features

- Isolated extranodal disease is ***MC*** presentation. Though many cases present with lymphadenopathy or a mass. *The common site of extranodal disease are CNS, lung, GIT*

Treatment consist of reduction in immunosuppression, surgical excision. For PTLD after BM transplant, leukocyte infusion is the standard and highly effective therapy

9. **Ans. is b and c i.e. CD 5+, BCL-1 positive in follicular lymphoma whereas BCL-2 positive in mantle cell lymphoma** *Ref. Robbins 8/e, p 607*

- **Immunophenotype of follicular lymphoma**
  CD-19+, CD-20+, CD10+, Surface Ig+, BCL6+, CD5–
- The hallmark of typical follicular lymphoma is t (14: 18) translocation that juxtaposes IgH locus on chromosome 14 and the BCL-2 locus on chromosome 18

10. **Ans. is a i.e. CD-15, CD-30** *Ref. Robbins 8/e, p 618*

Already explained. See Answer No. 5

11. **Ans. is b i.e. Small lymphocytic lymphoma**
See below.

- ***Most common lymphoma of spleen is non Hodgkins lymphoma. Various subtypes in decreasing order of frequency are:***
  - Small lymphocytic lymphoma
  - Diffuse large B-celll lymphoma
  - Follicular lymphoma
  - Marginal zone lymphoma

Remember: Hemangioma is the most common primary tumor of spleen

12. **Ans. is b i.e. Angiocentric lymphoma**

Ref. Devita 8/e, p 2111; Robbin's 8/e, p 598;http://www.oncologychannel.com/nonhodgkins/types.html

Angiocentric lymphoma is a type of T-cell lymphoma that is associated with Epstein Barr virus (EBV) infection.

- It includes cancers that previously were labeled *"lethal midline granulomas," "nasal T-cell lymphoma,"* and *"lymphatoid granulomatosis."*
- Angiocentric lymphoma typically is characterized by a destructive nasal or midline facial tumor that is accompanied by invasive infiltrate.
- Other sites of involvement outside the lymph nodes (extranodal) are the skin, lungs, and central nervous system. This tumor often is very resistant to therapy and has a poor prognosis.

Precursor B-cell Neoplasms	Precursor T-cell Neoplasms
• Precursor-B lymphoblastic leukemia / lymphoma	• Precursor-T lymphoblastic leukemia / lymphoma
Peripheral B-cell Neoplasma	**Peripheral T-cell and NK-cell Neoplasm**
• Chronic lymphocytic leukemia / small lymphocytic lymphoma • B-cell prolymphocytic leukemia • Lymphoblastic lymphoma • Splenic and nodal marginal zone lymphoma • Extranodal marginal zone lymphoma • Mantle cell lymphoma • Follicular lymphoma • Marginal Zone lymphoma • Hairy cell leukemia • Plasmacytoma / Plasma cell myeloma • Diffuse large β-cell lymphoma • Burkitt lymphoma	• T-cell prolymphocytic leukemia • Large granular lymphocytic leukemia • Mycosis fungoides / sezary syndrome • Peripheral T-cell lymphoma, unspecified • Anaplastic large cell lymphoma • Angioimmunoblastic T-cell lymphoma • Enteropathy-associated T-cell lymphoma • Panniculitis like T-cell lymphoma • Hepatosplenic γδ T-cell lymphoma • Adult T-cell leukemia / lymphoma • NK / T cell lymphoma, Nasal type • NK-cell leukemia

13. Ans. is d i.e. In general follicular...
See below

Common NHL (in decreasing order of prognosis)	Five years survival rate
• Anaplastic large T / Null cell lymphoma	77%
• Extranodal marginal zone B-cell lymphoma of MALT type	74%
• Follicular lymphoma	72%
• Diffuse large B-cell lymphoma	46%
• Burkitt lymphoma	45%
• Mantle cell lymphoma	27%
Precurser T-cell lymphoblastic lymphoma	26%
• Peripheral T-cell NHL	25%

Thus follicular lymphoma have good prognosis in comparison to DLBCL

Other Options

Option "a"	Now, WHO classification is used for HD, and it is universally accepted.
Option "b"	I think there is no confusion in this option.
Option "c"	Leukemic transformation is though rare, but it may be seen in all lymphomas.

14. Ans. is d i.e. Lymphocyte predominant Hodgkins disease *Ref. Robbin's 8/e, p 618*

Variants of RS cell

- ***RS cells (Reed sternberg cell) :***
  - Quite large binucleate or bilobed cell with the two halves appearing as mirror images of each other. Cell contains inclusion like owl eyed nucleoli.
  - RS cells are pathognomic for Hodgkins disease.

- ***Lacunar cells :***
  - Cells with delicate folded or multilobed nuclei surrounded by abundant pale cytoplasm that is often disrupted during the cutting of sections. Leaving the nucleus sitting in an empty node.
  - Seen in nodular sclerosis type of HD.
- ***Lymphocytic and Histiocytic variants (L+H cells) = Popcorn cells***
  - Cells with polypoid nuclei resembling popcorn kernels.
  - These cells are specifically found in lymphocyte predominant subtype.

Classical RS cells are quite large, binucleate or bilobed, with the two halves appearing as mirror image of each other. Nucleus contains inclusion like owl eyed nucleoli.

For more details, kindly see answer no. 10

15. Ans. is c i.e. Adult T cell leukemia and lymphoma *Ref. Harrison 17/e, p 689*

Infectious Agents Associated with Lymphoid Malignancies

Infectious	Lymphoid Malignancy
• **Epstein-Barr virus**	• Burkitt's lymphoma
	• Post-organ transplant lymphoma
	• Primary CNS diffuse large B cell lymphoma
	• Primary effussion lymphoma
	• Hodgkin's disease
	• Extranodal NK/T cell lymphoma, nasal type
• **HTLV-I**	• Adult T cell leukemia/lymphoma
• **HIV**	• Diffuse large B cell lymphoma
	• Burkitt's Lymphoma
• **Hepatitis C virus**	• Lymphoplasmacytic lymphoma
• **Helicobacter pylori**	• Gastric MALT lymphoma
• **Human Herpes virus 8**	• Primry effusion lymphoma
	• Multicentric Castleman's disease

Factors increasing Risk of Malignant Lymphoma

- Inherited immunodeficiency disease
- Autoimmune disease
- Klinefelter's syndrome
- Sjogren's syndrome
- Chediak-Higashi syndrome
- Celiac sprue
- Ataxia telangiectasia syndrome
- Rheumatoid arthritis and systemic lupus erythematosus
- Wiscott-Aldrich syndrome
- Common variable immunodeficiency dis.
- Chemical or drug exposures
- Acquired immunodeficiency diseases
- Phenytoin
- Prior chemotherapy and radiation therapy
- Acquired hypogammaglobulinemia

Also remember :

Virus	Associated disease
• **HTLV1**	– Adult T cell lymphoma/leukemia – Tropical spastic parapersis – HTLV-1 associated Myelopathy
• **HTLV-II**	– T-cell variant of hair cell leukemia (not fully established) – Called as virus searching for disease.

16. Ans. is b and c i.e. MOPP; and ABVD *Ref. Harrison 16/e, p 654*

Regimen's for HD :
- **ABVD** – Adriamycin, bleomycin, vincristine, daunarubicin (best).
- **MOPP** – Mechlorethamine, vincristine, procarbazine, prednisone.

17. Ans. is are a, c, d and e i.e. Mixed cellularity seen in background; Both neoplastic and non neoplastic cells are seen; Cell are CD15, CD30 positive; and Reed-Sternberg cells are seen *Ref. Robbin's 8/e p 618*

In classical Hodgkins disease RS cells are present in the background of non neoplastic inflammatory cells (Lymphocytes, plasma cells, eosinophilics).
- **Major population** in the tumor belong to non neoplastic reactive cells with few neoplastic RS cells.
- **Popcorn cells** of lymphocyte predominant unlike RS cells of classical HD are CD30- and CD15-.

18. Ans. is a and b i.e. Predisposed by H. pylori; Chemotherapy sensitive

Ref. Harrison 17/e, p 694

Marginal Zone Lymphoma (MALToma) = Mucosa associated lymphoma
- Maltoma is an extranodal lymphoma consisting of heterogenous ***B-cells found at mucosal sites.***
- They tends to arise in tissues involved by chronic inflammatory disorders such as *salivary gland in Sjogren disease, stomach in helicobacter gastritis.*
- Present as single ulcer or mass.
- They remain localized for prolong periods at sites of origin.
- Cell of origin is supposed to be post germinal center memory Bcell.
- Most common site is stomach, but can occur in lung, thyroid, intestine, salivary gland.
- **Treatment :** – Chemotherapy and H. pylori eradication is treatment of choice for gastric MALToma.
  – Local therapy such as surgery and radiotherapy is effective in other cases.

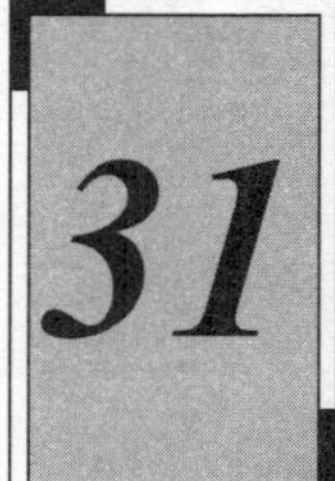

Plasma Cell Disorders

What's Important ?
- Diagnostic Criteria
- Clinical Features

Plasma cell disorder (also called as monoclonal gammopathies paraproteinemias = plasma cell dyscrasias) ***are monoclonal neoplasm which develop from common progenitors in the B lymphocyte lineage.***

It includes :
- Multiple myeloma
- Waldenstroms macroglobulenemia
- Heavy chain disease
- Primary amyloidosis.

Common Pathogenesis :

- Normally immunoglobulin is composed of two heavy chain (one of M,G,A,D,E) and 2 light chain (either K or λ).
- *Normally* ***light chains are synthesized in slight excess*** which are excreated by kidney.

... Harrison 17/e, p 700

- In *plasma cell disorder* there is excess synthesis of either light chains (Multiple myeloma) or heavy chain (heavy chain disease).
- Electrophoretic analysis of serum protein in these patient showns a broad peak in γ globulin (IgG) region. This sharp spike in this region called as M component (M for monoclonal). Less commonly M components may be seen in β_2 or α_2 globulin region.
- Antibody must be present at a conc. of > 0.5 g/dl to be detectable by electrophoresis.
- *M - component may be an intact antibody or isolated light or heavy chain.*
- **Confirmation** that such M component is truely monoclonal relies on immuno-electrophoresis.

MULTIPLE MYELOMA

Malignant proliferation of plasma cells derived from single clone with involvement of skeleton at multiple skeletal sites.

- Age > 50 years.
- Exact cause unknown.

- **Risk** is ↑ in *wood workers, farmers, those exposed to petroleum products, prior exposure to radiation.*
- **Proliferation** and survival of myeloma cells depend on IL - 6.
  – Most frequent **Karyotypic abnormality** are deletion of 13q and translocations involving in IgA heavy chain locus 14q. The most common translocations are t(11 : 14); ± (4 : 14)

Pathology and Clinical Feature

- **Bone**
  – Most common symptom is ***bone pain*** which usually involves back and ribs and is aggrevated by movement.
  – Most common bones involved are - verebral column > ribs > skull > pelvis.
  – Bone lesions are caused by ***proliferation of tumor cells*** and ***activation of osteoclast, suppression of osteoblast.*** These lesion appear as punched out defect consist of gelatinous, soft red tumor masses.
  – ***Micropscopic examination*** shows ↑ number of plasma cells which usually constitute > 30% of the marrow cellularity. Other cytlogic variant include flame cell (with fiery red cytoplasm), mott cell and cells containing inclusion bodies such as Russell bodies (cytoplasmic) Dutchner bodies (nuclear).

Remember : Multiple myeloma cause osteolytic lesion so, isotopic bone scan is less usefull than plain radiograph for diagnosis.

- **Infection**
  – 2nd MC symptom is susceptibility to bacterial infection.
  – Most common infection are pneumonias and pyelonephritis, MC ***pathogen*** are S.pneumoniae and S. aureus.
  – ***Susceptibility*** of infection is due to :
    - Hypogammaglobulinemia (after excluding M component)
    - ↓ in CD - 4 T cell
    - ↓ in granulocyte lysozyme concentration.
- **Renal abnormalities :**
  – Hypercalcemia is MC cause of renal failure in multiple myeloma. *...Harrison 17/e, p 703*
  – Renal damage is also contributed by : Bence Jones proteinuria, cast nephropathy and amyloidosis. Bence Jones protein are excess light chain that are excreted in urine they are ***directly toxic to tubular cells*** and also combine with urinary glycoprotein to form cast causing cast nephropathy.
  – ***Earliest manifestation*** of this tubular damage is adult Fanconi anaemia.
  – Patient with myeloma have ↓ anion gap.
- **Hematologic Abnormality :**
  – Normocytic normochromic anaemia due to replacement of normal marrow by malignant cell and also by inhibition of hematopoiesis.
  – Hyperviscosity - Normal relative serum viscosity is 1.8. Symptoms of hyperviscosity appear at level of 5 to 6. Chance of hyperviscosity is maximum with IgM myeloma.

Diagnosis

- ***Classical triad*** of myeloma is marrow plasmocytosis (> 10%), lytic bone lesions, and a serum or urinary M component. However diagnosis can be made in the absence of bone lesion if the plasmocytosis is associated with progressive ↑ in M component.
- Serum M component is most commonly IgG followed by IgA and IgD.
- Serum ***LAP score is usually normal*** due to absence of osteoblastic activity.

Diagnostic criteria of plasma cell Disorders
Monoclonal gammopathy of undetermined significance (MGUS)
• Protein in serum < 30 g/L • Bone marrow clonal plasma cells < 10% • No evidence of other B cell proliferative disorders • No myeloma-related organ or tissue impairment (no end organ damage, including bone lesions)
Asymptomatic myeloma (smouldering myeloma)
• M protein in serum ≥ 30 g/L and/or • Bone marrow clonal plasma cells ≥ 10% • No myeloma-related organ or tissue impairment (no end organ damage, including bone lesions) or symptoms
Symptomtic multiple myeloma
• M protein in serum and/or urine • Bone marrow (clonal) plasma cells or plsmacytoma • Myeloma-related organ or tissue impairment (end organ damage, including bone lesions)
Nonsecretory myeloma
• No M protein in serum and/or urine with immunofixation • Bone marrow clonal plasmacytosis ≥ 10% or plasmacytoma • Myeloma-related organ or tissue impairment (end organ damage, including bone lesions)
Solitary plasmacytoma of bone
• No M protein in serum and/or urine • Single area of bone destruction due to clonal plasma cells • Bone marrow not consistent with multiple myeloma • Normal skeletal survey (and MRI of spine and pelvis if done) • No related organ or tissue impairment (no end organ damage other than solitary bone lesion)[a]

Two important variant of myeloma are :

Solitary bone plasmacytoma	Extramedullary plasmacytoma
Single lytic lesion without plasmacytosis	Involves submucosal lymphoid tissue of nasopharynx with out plasmacytosis
Highly responsive to radiotherapy	Highly responsive to radiotherapy
Re-occur and progress to myeloma	Rarely re-occur

Remember : Staging system for Myeloma is functional system based on variety of clinical and laboratory test unlike anatomical staging for solid tumor.

Differential diagnosis

Most important differential diagnosis of myeloma is MUGS.

MUGS (Monoclonal gammopathy of uncertain significance)

- More common than myeloma
- Age > 50
- < 10% bone marrow plasma cells; < 3 g/dl M component; no urinary Bence Jones protein; no anaemia; no hypercalcemia.
- When bone marrow cells are exposed to radioactive thymidine. MUGs always have a labelling index < 1%, while myeloma always have a labelling index > 1%

Prognosis

- *Serum β2 microglubulin is single most powerful predictor of survival and can substitute for staging.*
- Patient secreting λ light chain have shorter survival than k secretors.
- *Cause of death in myeloma patient (in ↓ order of frequency) :* Progressive Myeloma > Sepsis > Renal Failure. *... Harrison 16/e, p 660*

Treatment

- *Patient with minimal disease should be observed without treatment in such patient chemotherapy should be given only when myeloma protein > 5g/dl. ... Harrison 17/e, p 705*
- *Patient with solitary plasmocytoma and extramedullary plasmocytoma* should be treated with radiotherapy.
- All patient with *stage II and stage III and symptomatic stage 1* are treated by chemotherapy.
- Formerly the combination chemotherapy (VAD) was used, but is being replaced by nonchemotherapy options.

  The combination of thalidomide + dexamethasome is as effective as VAD and is more convenient.
- Bortezomib - Proteosome inhibitor highly active in MM.
- Bisphosphnates reduce pathologic fracture.

WALDENSTROM'S MACROGLOBULINEMIA

- Malignant disease of **B - Cells** that appears to be ***hybrid of lymphocytes and plasma cells.***
- These cells characterstically secrete IgM paraprotein.

Pathogenesis and clinical features

- Disease develop between 60's and 70's.
- As there is hypersecretion of IgM, the major clinical manifestation is hyperviscosity syndrome.
- Disease is associated with lymphadenopathy and hepatosplenomegaly.
- Similar to myeloma it involves bone marrow, like myeloma serum M component is present in excess of 3g/dl but as the size of para protein (IgM) is large it is not excreated renally, so ***there is no renal damage,*** similarly there is no osteolytic lesions and hypercalcemia.

- ***Light chain subtype*** is k in most cases.
- Patient present with weakness, fatigue, recurrent infection and features of hyperviscosity syndrome i.e. epistaxis, visual disturbance, neurologic symptoms.

Diagnosis

- ↑ IgM praprotein (> 3 g/dl) ***without osteolytic lesion.***
- If there are osteolytic lesion diagnosis is multiple myeloma of IgM subtype.

Treatment

– Serious hyperviscosity syndrome should be treated with plasmapheresis.
– *Fludarabine and cladarabine* are ***highly effective*** single agent.

HEAVY CHAIN DISEASE

- Rare Lymphoblastic malignancy, in which patient secrete a defective heavy chain that usually have intact Fc fragment with deletion in the Fd region.
- The two main heavy chain disease are :
  – ***γ heavy chain disease (Franklin disease)***
    - It is characterized by *lymphadenopathy, fever, anaemia, hepatosplenom egaly.*
    - Most distinctive symptom is palatal edema which may progress to respiratory compromise.
    - Diagnosis depend on demonstration of serum Mcomponent (< 20g/l). The M component typically present in serum and urine.
  – ***α heavy chain disease (Seligmann's disease)***
    - Most common heavy disease.
    - Characterized by *infitration of lamina propria of the small intestine* with lymphoplasmocytoid cells.
    - Patient present with chronic diarrhoea, fever, weight loss.
    - *Diagnosis is difficult* as α heavy chains are difficult to demonstrate and appear as small inspite of sharp peak.

QUESTIONS

1. **Which of the following investigations is least useful in multiple myeloma: [AI 07]**
   a. Bone scan
   b. X-ray
   c. Bone marrow biopsy
   d. MRI
2. **Which of the following is not a major criteria for diagnosis of multiple myeloma: [AI 06]**
   a. Lytic bone lesion
   b. Plasmacytoma on tissue biopsy.
   c. Bone marrow plasmocytosis > 30%.
   d. M spike > 3g % for IgG, > 2 g% for IgA.
3. **A 58 year old woman, who had ache and recurrent chest infection for 6 months, develop sudden weakness of the legs and urinary retention. Her investigation showed a hemoglobin of 7.3 gm/dl, serum calcium – 12.6mg/dl, phosphate 2.5mg/dl, alkaline phosphate 100 m/l, serum albumin 3 gm/dl, globulin – 7.1 gm/dl. Urea 178 µg/dl. What is the most likely diagnosis : [AI 06]**
   a. Lung cancer
   b. Disseminated tuberculosis
   c. Multiple myeloma
   d. Osteoporosis
4. **Which of the following statement is not true:**
   a. Patient with IgD myeloma may present with no evident M-spike on serum electrophoresis [AI 05]
   b. A diagnosis of plasma cell leukemia can be made if circulating peripheral blood plasmoblasts comprise 14% of peripheral blood white cells in patient with white blood cell count of 11 x 10^9/L and platelet count of 88 x 10^9/L
   c. In smoldering myeloma plasma cells constitute 10-30% of total bone marrow cellularity
   d. In patient with multiple myeloma, a monoclonal light chain may be detected in both serum and urine
5. **Lympho Plasmacytoid lymphoma is associated with: [AI 10]**
   a. IgG
   b. IgM
   c. IgA
   d. IgE
6. **Hypercalcemia is associated with:**
   a. Multiple myeloma [AI '10]
   b. Ewings
   c. Osteosarcoma
   d. Chondrosarcoma
7. **An elderly male presents with headache, recurrent infections and multiple punched out lytic lesions on X-ray skull. The investigation that will best help in establishing a diagnosis is: [AI '09]**
   a. Protein electrophoresis
   b. Serum calcium
   c. Alkaline phosphatase levels
   d. Acid phosphatase levels
8. **Treatment of multiple myeloma A/E:**
   a. Bortezomib [PGI '09]
   b. Melphalan
   c. Hydroxyurea
   d. Ketoconazole
   e. Cyclophosphamide
9. **A 70 year old male has a patologic fracture of femur. The lesion appears a lytic on X-rays film with a circumscribed punched out appearance. The curetting from fracture site is most likely to show which of the following ? [AIIMS 06]**
   a. Diminished and thinned trabecular bone fragments secondary to osteopenia
   b. Sheets of atypical plasma cells
   c. Metastatic prostatic adenocarcinoma
   d. Malignant cells forming osteoid bone

10. In multiple myeloma a radionucleide bone scan will show : [AIIMS 06]
   a. Hot spots
   b. Cold spots
   c. Diffuse increased uptake of radio-nucleotide
   d. Diffuse decreased uptake of radio-nucleotide

11. Which one of the following is not a feature of multiple myeloma : [AIIMS 05]
   a. Hypercalemia
   b. Anemia
   c. Hyperviscosity
   d. Elevated alkaline phosphatase

12. True about smoldering myeloma is:
   a. Monoclonal gammopathy **[PGI 08]**
   b. Lytic bone lesion
   c. Hypercalcemia
   d. Bone marrow plasma cell > 10%

13. Best prognostic indictor of multiple myeloma at the time of diagnosis:
   a. Number of myeloma cells in the marrow **[AIIMS 08]**
   b. Beta microglobulin
   c. Alkaline phosphatase level
   d. Hypercalcemia

14. In multiple myeloma following are seen in: [PGI 05]
   a. Increased serum calcium
   b. Sclerotic bone lesion
   c. Bone fractures
   d. Renal failure
   e. Increased leucocyte alkaline phosphate

ANSWERS, REFERENCES, EXPLANATIONS WITH INFORMATIVE ILLUSTRATIONS

1. Ans. is a i.e. Bone scan *Ref. Harrison 17/e, p 704*

Bone lesions in multiple myeloma are lytic in nature and are rarely associated with osteoblastic new bone formation. Therefore isotopic bone scan is less useful in diagnosis than plain radiograph.

Lab Evaluation of Patient with Multiple myeloma

Presence and Characterization of Monoclonal Protein :

- Serum protein electrophoresis
- Quantitative immunoglobulin
- 24-H urine : total protein and Bence Jones protein immunofixation of urine and serum, serum-free light chains.

Radiologic Evaluation :

- Skeletal survey
- Magnetic resonance imaging with short time inversion recovery images
- Bone densitometry

Laboratory Evaluation :

- Complete blood cell count with reticulocyte and differential count
- Chemistry panel (renal, calcium, albumin, uric acid, lactate dehydrogenase) β2-Microglobulin, C-reactive protein.

Bone Marrow :

- Aspirate and biopsy : – Cytogenetics
  – Flow cytometry (DNA-clg)
  – Plasma cell labeling index

Specialized studies for Selected patients :

- Abdominal fat pad or rectal biopsy for amyloid
- Solitary lytic lesion biopsy
- Serum viscosity if IgM component or high IgA levels of serum M component > 7g/dL

2. **Ans. is a i.e. Lytic bone lesion** *Ref. Devita 7/e, p 2167*

The question is of 2006, at that time following criteria was followed.

Multiple Myeloma

Major criteria :

a Plasmacytoma on tissue biopsy.
b. Bone marrow plasmacocytosis with > 30% palsma cells.
c. Monoclonal globulin spike on serum electrophoresis exceeding 3.5 g/dL for IgG or 2g/dL for IgA, ≥ 1g/24h of K or λ light-chain excretion on urine electrophoresis in the presence of amyloidosis.

Minor criteria :

a. Bone marrow plasmacytosis 10% to 30%.
b. Monoclonal globulin spike present but less than the level defined above.
c. Lytic bone lesions.
d. Suppressed uninvolved immunoglobuins; IgM < 50 mg/dL, IgA < 100 mg/dL, or IgG < 600 mg/dL.

Diagnosis is confirmed when any of the following features are documented in symptomatic patients with clearly progressive disease.

For latest diagnostic criteria refer theory portion

Remember : **Classical triad of multiple myeloma -**
- Lytic bone lesion
- Bone marrow plasmacytosis
- Serum or urinary M component.

3. **Ans. is c i.e. Multiple Myeloma** *Ref. Harrison 17/e, 702*

Their is only one confusion in this question i.e. level of alkaline phosphate.

Now see,

Normal level of Alkaline PO_4 is 13 -100 μ/L or 0.2-1.6 ukat/L.

So, alkaline phosphate level is normal is patient. In multiple myeloma alkaline phosphate level is normal as there is no osteoblastic activity.

Clinical features of Multiple myeloma :

Symptoms	Common cause
– Bone pain	Pathologic fracture
– Easy fatigability	Anaemia
– Polyuria, Nausea, Vomiting	Hyper calcemia, Renal failure

Contd...

Contd...

Symptoms	Common cause
– Recurrent infection	Hypogammaglobulinemia (after excluding light chain) Low CD-4 count
– Bleeding tendency	Coagulopathy *(due to high level of paraprotein which interfere with factor VIII)*
– Paraplegia	Cord compression
– CNS symptoms, visual disturbance	Hyperviscosity
– Renal calculi	Hyper calcemia, Hyperurecemia.

Other options : In lung carcinoma chances of renal failure are rare. In TB hyperclacemia would not be there.

4. **Ans. is b i.e. A diagnosis of plasma cell leukemia can be made if circulating peripheral blood plasmoblasts comprise 14% of peripheral blood white cells in patient with white blood cell count of 11 x 10^9/L and platelet count of 88 x 10^9/L**

Ref. Wintrobes 12/e, 2414; Devita 7/e, p 2166

Plasma cell Leukemia contains more than 20% plasma cells in the peripheral blood with an absolute plasma cell count of more than 2x10^9/L.

Let us consider every option.

Option 'a': **IgD myeloma** ... *Wintrobes 12/e, p 2414*

- Accounts for 2% of all cases of multiple myeloma.
- Presence of monoclonal IgD in serum indicates myeloma.
- Generally presents with smal band or ***no evident M-spike*** on serum protein electrophoresis.
- Higher incidence of renal insufficiency, amyloidosis and proteinuria than IgG or IgA myeloma.
- Incidence of extra medullary involvement is higher and **survival is poor.**

Option 'b': **Plasma cell leukemia** ... *Wintrobes 12/e, p 2414*

- Plasma cell leukemia is ***rare*** form of plasma cell dyscrasias.
- By definition there are more than 20% plasma cells in the peripheral blood with an absolute plasma cell count of more than 2x10^9/L.
- Clinical presentation is more aggressive than that of multiple myeloma, with a higher presenting tumor mass and higher frequency of extramedullary involvement, anaemia, thrombocytopenia, hypercalcemia and renal impairement.
- Incidence of ***lytic bony lesion is slightly lower*** than that of multiple myeloma.
- Over all survival is poor.

Option 'c': **Smoldering (asymptomatic) Multiple myeloma (SMM)**

- It is ***intermediate stage*** between MUGS and multiple myeloma.
- *These is no anaemia, hypercalcemia and bone disease.*

Option 'd':

- Monoclonal light chain (Bence Jone protein) is detected in urine and serum.
- For detection by electrophoresis it must be present in excess of 0.5g/dl.

5. **Ans. is b i.e. IgM** *Ref. Wintrobes 12/e, p 2472; Harrison 17/e, p 706*

- **Lymphoplasmacytic lymphoma** (Walderstron Macroglobulinemia) in the Malignancy of mature B-cells characterized by monoclonal IgM in the serum

Cell of origin

- Postgerminal B-cells, posessing the characteristics of an IgM bearing memory B cells.

> **Note:** WHO and REAL group has classified Walderstron Macroglobulinemia as lymphoplasmacytic lymphoma because of its immunophenotypic and morphologic pattern.

6. **Ans. is a i.e. Multiple Myeloma** *Ref. Harison 17/e, p 703; Wintrobes 12/e, p 2377*

Hypercalcemia in Multiple myeloma

- Occurs in 18 - 30% of patient.
- Hypercalcemia occur due to ***activation of osteoclasts*** which mobilize calcium from bone.
- *Serum level correlates with symptoms*, i.e. ***severe*** symptoms when level >15 mg/dl, however in some patients even level of 12-13 mg/dl cauuse severe neurologic symptoms.
- **Treatment :**
  - *Vigorous hydration* followed by intravenous bisphosphate (eg. Pamidronate) is *treatment of choice.*
  - *Gluocorticoids* can also reduce serum Ca2+.
  - Calcium nitrate, mithramycin and calcitonin were used before advent of bisphosphonates and are rarely used now.
- **Prognostic importance :**
  - Ca2+ level above 15 mg/dl are associated wit poor prognosis and is independent risk factor for acute renal failure.

7. **Ans. is a i.e. Protein electrophoresis** *... Harrison 17/e, p 703-704*

*Headache **(d/t hyperviscosity)**, recurrent infections and multiple punched out lytic lesion suggest multiple myeloma*

- Protein electrophoresis (for measuring serum Ig and free light chain) supplemented by immunoelectrophoresis (sensitive for detecting low concentration of M component) is the most valuable investigation for diagnosis of multiple myeloma

8. **Ans. is c, d, e i.e. Hydroxyurea; Ketoconazole; Cyclophosphamide**

Ref. Harrison 17/e, p 705; CMDT 2010, p 471; Wintrobes 12/e, p 2380

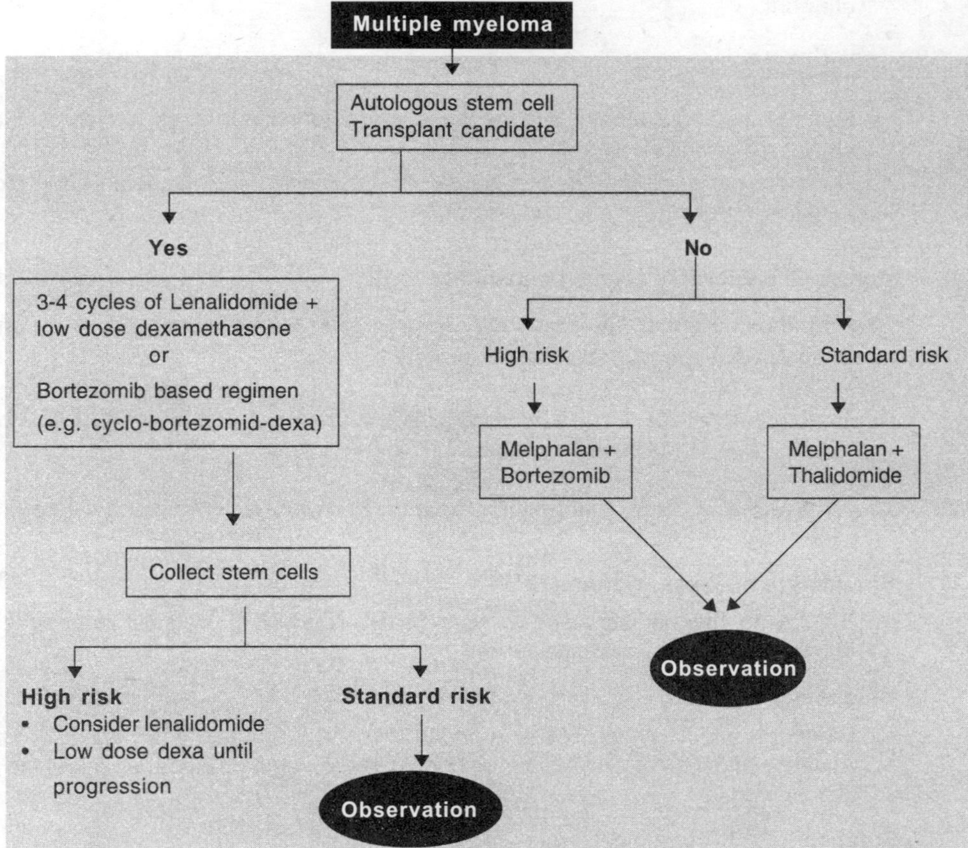

Note:
- Lenalidomide is more active and less toxic than thalidomide, so is preferred over it.
- Bortezomib is a proteosome inhibitor with neuropathy as major side effect
- Melphalan is not used in transplant candidates as it damages autologous stem cells

Other drugs effective in MM: Vincristine, doxorubicin, cyclophosphomide, cisplatin

9. **Ans. is b i.e. Sheets of atypical plasma cells** *Ref. Robbin's 7/e, p 679*

This is a case of pathologic fracture secondary to multiple myeloma as suggested by lytic punched out bone lesion in a patient of 70 years.

Bone lesions of Multiple Myeloma :
- ***Radiograph :*** Punched out defects of 1 to 4 cm.
- ***Macroscopy :*** Grossly multiple myeloma lesions consist of gelatinous soft red tumour mass.

- ***Microscopic examination :*** Reveals an increased number of plasma cells, which usually constitute more than 30% of marrow cellularity. The plasma cells infiltrate the marrow diffusely and present in sheet like masses that completely replace normal element.

10. Ans. is b i.e. Cold spots *Ref. Sutton Radiology 7/e, p 1339*

- Multiple myeloma lesions are negative on radionucleide scan and appear as cold spots.
- Normally radiographic skeletal survey is superior to radionucleide scan except in detecting rib lesion.

11. Ans. is d i.e. Elevated alkaline phosphate *Ref. Harrison 17/e, p 704*

"Serum alkaline phosphate is usually normal even with extensive bone involvement because of absence of osteoblastic activity" *... Harrison 17/e, p 704*

Remember : Plane X-ray is more sensitive than bone scanning for detection of bone abnormalities.

12. Ans. is a and d i.e. Monoclonal gammopathy; Bone marrow plasma cell > 10%

Ref. Wintrobes 12/e, p 2346

Smoldering multiple myeloma (SMM)

- SMM is an intermediate stage between MGUS and MM. It is almost identical to MGUS but represent more advance clone.

Diagnostic criteria

- Clonal plasmacytosis > 10% or a serum monoclonal protein of 30 g/L or more
- Absence of hypercalcemia, anemia, bone disease, renal insufficiency related to plasma cell neoplasm

Treatment: No treatment except close observation

Remember: ***Indolent myeloma:*** Nearly identical to SMM but with a small number of discrete bone lesion

Features	Multiple myeloma	Monoclonal gammopathy of undetermined significance
1. Age	> 50 years	> 50 years
2. Incidence	Less common	More common
3. Plasma cells	> 10 %	< 10%
4. M component	> 3 g/dl	< 3 g/dl
5. Bence Jones proteins	***Present :***	No urinary Bence Jones proteins
6. Clinical features	– Lytic bones lesion	No lytic bony lesion
	– Hypercalcemia	No hypercalcemia
	– Renal failure	No renal failure
	– Anemia	No anemia
7. Plasma cell : – acid phosphate	High	Low
– Glucuronidase	High	Low
8. Treatment	Required	No therapy required

Remember : ***Predictors of malignant transformation of MUGS***

- Size of M protein (most important predictior)
- Type of immunoglobulin (IgM or IgA MUGS have higher risk)
- Bone marrow plasma cells.

13. **Ans. is b i.e. Beta microglobulin** *Ref. Harrison 17/e, p 704; Devita 8/e, p 2322*

"Serum β-2 microglobulin is the single most powerfull predictor of survival and can substitute for staging."

Prognostic factors for multiple myeloma	
Tumour Burden - Related Factors	***Tumour Biology - Related Factors***
– β_2 - Microglobulin level	– Monosomy 13 or 13q
– Serum immunoglobulin level	– Plasma cell labeling index
– Number of lytic bone lesions	– Renal failure
– Hemoglobin level	– Miotic activity
– Serum calcium level	– Immunoglobulin A myeloma
– Percentage of bone marrow plasmacytosis	– C - reactive protein level
– Albumin level	– Lactate dehydrogenase level
	– Soluble interleukin - 6 receptor level

14. **Ans. is a, c and d i.e. Increased serum calcium; Bone fractures; and Renal failure**

Ref. Harrison 17/e, p 704

In multiple myeloma lytic bone lesions are seen (not sclerotic one).

Sclerotic bone lesions are seen in :
- Ca breast
- Ca prostate.

32

Pituitary Tumour

What's Important ?

- **Types**
- **Prolactinoma**

PITUITARY ADENOMA

- Most common cause of sellar mass. Most common cause of pituitary hypersecretion.
- It is responsible for 15% of intracranial tumors.
- Always *arise* from ***anterior pituitary or adeno hypophysis.***
- Two types : microadenoma (< 10mm)
macroadenoma (> 10mm)
- Tumor mass initially *compress pituitary gland* and, at a larger size, the *optic chiasma* and nerve superiorly further growth involves the cavernous sinus bilaterally, the third ventricle (some times producing hydrocephalus).
- **Associated** with *MEN, Carney syndrome, McCune albright syndrome.*

Classification

- Prolactinoma (MC) – 52%
- Hormone negative adenoma – 21%
- Growth hormone cell (somatotroph) adenoma – 27%
- Corticotropin secreting adenoma – 20%
- TSH secreting adenoma – 0.3%

Clinical features

- **Mass effect :**
  - Characteristically presents with ophthalmologic finding.
  - The classical ophthalmological finding are : Visual loss typically with *bitemporal hemianopsia* and loss of *colour discrimination* (specially red).
  - *Automated visual field testing* is ***more sensitive*** than simple confrontation.
- **Endocrinological effect :** Leads to characteristic symptom such as *hyperprolactinemia, cushing disease, acromegaly.*

Mass effect of pituitary tumour	
Impacted Structure	***Clinical Impact***
Pituitary	Hypogonadism Hypothyroidism Growth failure Hypoadrenalism
Optic tract	Loss of red perception Bitemporal hemianopia Superior or bitemporal field defect Scotoma Blindness
Hypothalamus	Temperature dysregulation Appetite and thirst disorders Obesity Diabetes insipidus Sleep disorders Behavioral dysfunction
Cavernous sinus	Ophthalmoplegia ± ptosis or diplopia Facial numbness
Frontal lobe	Personality disorder Anosmia
Brain	Headache Hydrocephalus Psychosis Dementia Laughing seizures

Diagnosis

- ***Imaging modality of choice is MRI.***
- Adenoma density is usually lower than that of surrounding normal tissue on T1 weighted imaging and signal intensity increases with T2 weighted images. The high phospholipid content of the posterior pituitary results in "Pituitary bright spot".
- Macroadenoma can be differentiated from other sellar mass as there is *sellar enlargement in macroadenoma, which is not seen in meningioma.*

Treatment

- **Medical :** Specially for hormone secreting tumors, e.g. Dopamine agonist (bromocriptine or carbergoline) are the *most effective* therapy for prolactinoma.
- **Surgery :**
  - *For macroadenoma :* Goal is to decompress visual pathway and reduce tumor bulk.
  - *For hypersecreting adenoma :* Goal is normalization of the hypersecretion with preservation of remaining normal pituitary function.
- Surgical approach of choice is transsphenoidal. *... Harrison 17/e, p 2203*

– **Radiation therapy :** Used either as primary therapy (steriotactic radio surgery) or more commonly as an adjunct to surgery or medical therapy.

PROLACTINOMA

- Most common pituitary adenoma.
- F : M - *20 : 1* (for microadenoma) *1 : 1* (for macro prolactinoma)
- Tumor size correlates with prolactin level.

Clinical features

- Amenorrhea
- Infertility
- Galactorrhea

} Women

- Mass effect in case of macroadenoma.
- Impotence
- Loss of libido
- Infertility

} Men

Diagnosis

- Prolactin > 100 μg/l in absence of medications which tends to ↑ prolactin; ↓ Estrogen; ↓ LH and FSH
- **MRI**

Treatment

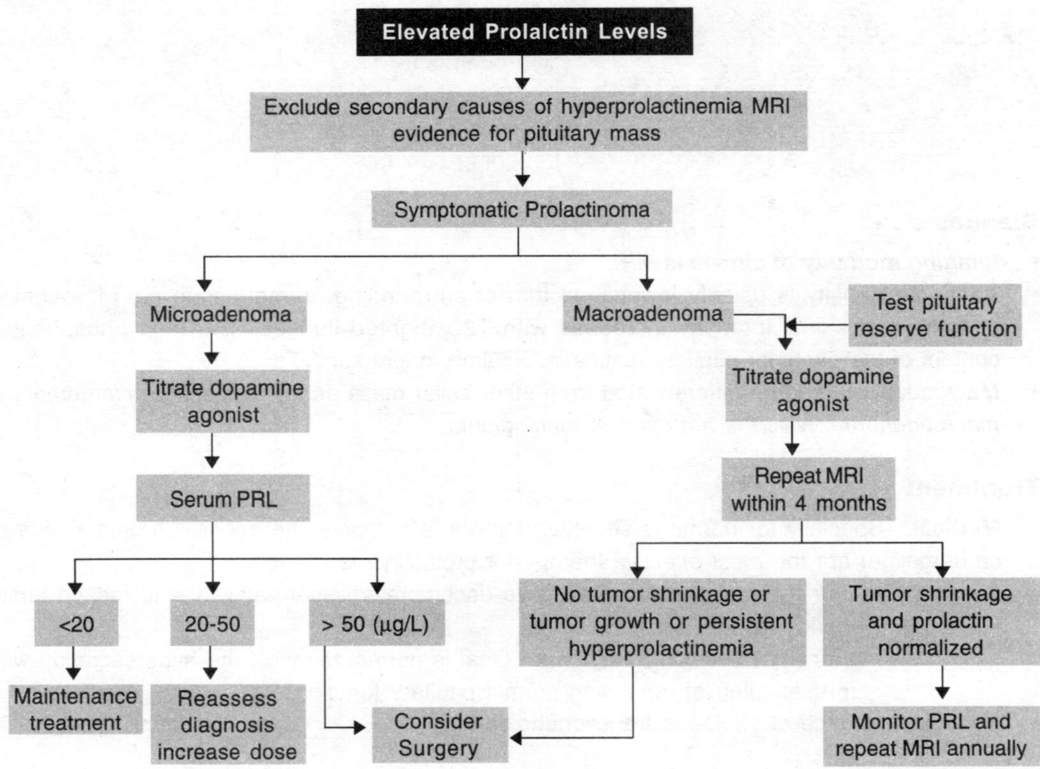

Dopamine agonist :

- Carberogline - *Long acting* dopamine agonist with high D_2 receptor affinity
- Bromocriptine - *Shorter acting*
- These drugs are TOC for prolactinoma (both micro and macro) and shrinks the size of about 70% tumor.

Surgery : Indicated when there is dopamine resistance or intolerance and Invasive macro-adenoma with compromised vision that fails to improve rapidly after drug treatment.

Remember : Hyperprolactenemia is ***most common*** pituitary hypersecretion in both males and females.

... Harrison 17/e, p 2204

QUESTIONS

1. **The most preferred approach for pituitary surgery at the present time is :** **[AI 06]**
   a. Transcranial
   b. Trans ethmoidal
   c. Transphenoidal
   d. Transcollasal
2. **In a lady with bilateral superior temporal quadrantopia and galactorrhea, the most probable cause is :** **[AI 09]**
   a. Pituitary macroadenoma
   b. Craniopharyngioma
   c. Sheehan's syndrome
   d. Pituitary hypophysitis
3. **Which of the following is the most common type of pituitary adenoma ?** **[AIIMS 05]**
   a. Thyrotropinoma
   b. Gonadotropinoma
   c. Prolactinoma
   d. Corticotropinoma

ANSWERS, REFERENCES, EXPLANATIONS WITH INFORMATIVE ILLUSTRATIONS

1. **Ans. is c i.e. Transphenoidal**
Ref. Devita 8/e, p 2014; Schwartz 8/e, p 1636

"The standard surgical approach for the majority of pituitary tumours is transphenoidal which is safer and better tolerated than the transcranial approach."

"Most pituitary adenoma are approached through the nose via transphenoidal approach."
... Schwartz

Transcranial approach is limited to the treatment of :
- Suprasellar tumour that are tough and fibrous.
- Tumours that extend laterally in the middle fossa.
- Tumours that extend anteriorly or beneath the frontal lobes.

Remember : ***Surgical treatment is indicated only in cases of :***
- **Macroadenoma compressing optic chiasma.**
- Growth hormone secreting tumour causing acromegally.
- ACTH tumour causing cushings disease.
- Prolactinomas not responding to surgical treatment.

2. **Ans. is a i.e. Pituitary macroadenoma**
Ref. Devita 8/e, p 2013

Galactorrhea along with visual field diffect suggest prolactinoma

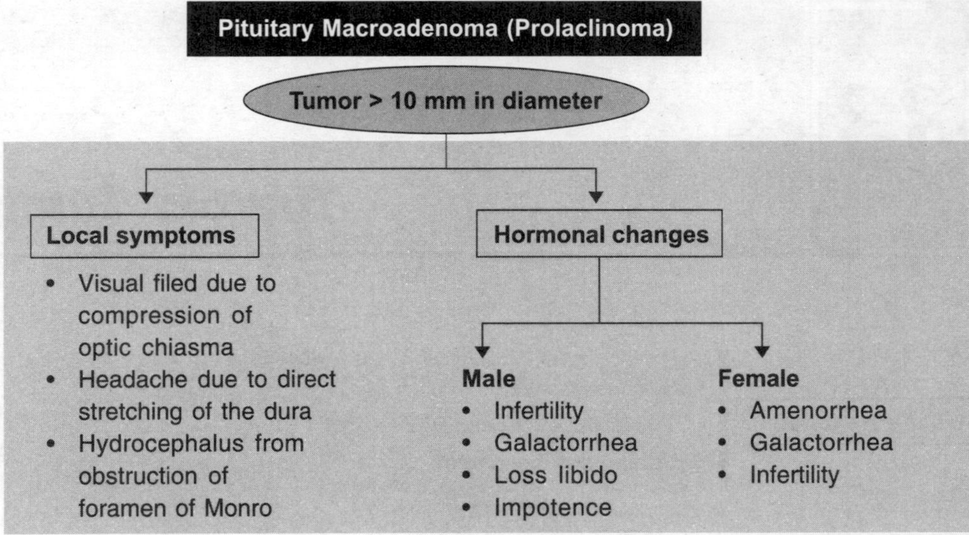

The classic ophthalmologic finding of pituitary microadenoma is visual loss typically starting with bitimporal hemianopsia and loss of colour discrimination.

5. Ans. is c i.e Prolactinoma *Ref. Devita 8/e, p 2013*

Types of Pituitary adenoma in Decreasing order :

Type		%
• Prolactinoma	–	52%
• Growth hormone cell adenoma	–	27%
• Hormone negative adenoma	–	21%
• Corticotropin secreting	–	20%
• TSH cell (Thyrotropin) adenoma	–	0.3%

33 Thyroid Tumour

What's Important ?

- Solitary nodule
- Types and Pathological Features
- Spread and Treatment

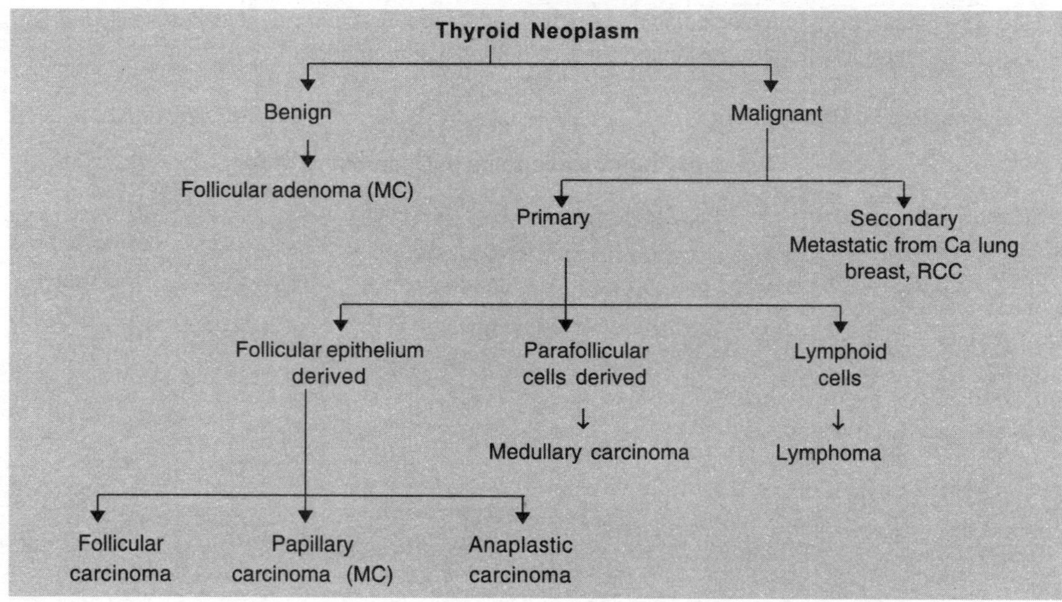

Epidemiology

Incidence of thyroid cancer is rapidly increasing and it is the most common endocrinal malignancy.

Etiology

- Radiation exposure to the thyroid gland
- Female sex and family history
- **Diet:** Iodine deficient, excessive intake of vegitable from crucifer family (which block iodine uptake)

FOLLICULAR ADENOMA

- Most common benign tumor of thyroid.
- Present as *solitary thyroid nodules.*
- On **histology** - The adenoma bulges from cut surface and compresses adjacent thyroid, this is ***surrounded by well defined capsule*** which *differentiate it from multinodular goitre in which there is no capsule.* *... Robbin's 7/e, p 1173*
- *Differentiation between follicular adenoma and carcinoma* can only be made by histological examination *(in carcinoma there is invasion of capsule or pericapsular blood vessels).*
- On ***radionucleide scanning*** it appear as cold nodules.
- **Treatment :** As they appear as cold nodules and 10% of cold nodules are malignant, treatment is lobectomy. *... Bailey and Love 25/e, p 792*

MALIGNANT TUMORS

Papillary carcinoma

- Most common malignant tumor of thyroid (75 - 85% of cases).
- **Radiation** exposure in < 5 years of age is **most important risk factor for** papillary carcinoma.
- Hashimoto thyroiditis and thyroglossal cyst are other risk factor.
- **Age :** 30 - 50, F > M.
- **Pathology :**
  - Solitary or multifocal lesion that are well differentiated. Papillary carcinoma < 1 cm are called as microcarcinoma
  - It may be capsulated and there may be cyst formation.
  - Characteristic hallmark of papillary neoplasm is ground glass or Orphan Annie eye nuclei.(clear or empty appeared nuclei).
  - Cytoplasmic invaginations in nuclei appear as intranuclear inclusions (pseudo inclusion).
  - Psammoma bodies often present. When ever psammoma bodies is found in thyroid specimen or perithyroidal tissue or lymphnode, a hidden papillary carcinoma must be considered.
- **Spread :**
  - Mostly lymphatic.
  - Hematogenous spread to bone and lung.
- **Clinical features :**
  - Mostly present as asymptomatic thyroid nodule.
  - May present as ***occult carcinoma*** i.e. *enlarged lymphnode with in jugular chain with impalpable thyroid.*
- **Diagnosis :**
  - On Radioactive iodine scan appear as ***cold nodule.***
  - Although FNAC is IOC for discrete thyroid nodule, *definitive diagnosis* can only be made by histology and microscopy
- **Treatment :**
  - Lobectomy + Isthemectomy is *treatment of choice* for < 1 cm tumor.
  - Near total or *Total thyroidectomy* for tumor > 2 cm in size.
  - *Treatment of secondaries* in lymphnode - Berry picking i.e. removal of enlarged LN only.
  - Functional modified radical neck dissection preserving the sterno-cleidomastoid muscle and spinal accessory nerve is performed if lymphnode in the lateral neck are clinically involved.
  - In patient with *unresectable disease, local recurrence* or metastatic disease, large dose of radio iodine is given.

- **Prognosis :** – Age at diagnosis (younger better) and presence of metastasis are most important prognostic factor
- **Follow up :** – Measurement of *serum thyroglobulin* is IOC. Residual disease is likely to be present when Tg >2 ng/ml.

Remember :
- Papillary carcinoma is thyroid carcinoma with best prognosis.
- ***Most common* occult carcinoma of thyroid is papillary carcinoma.**
- **Prognosis of occult carcinoma is *excellent.***

Follicular carcinoma

- **2nd** most common thyroid carcinoma.
- Affect older age group; F > M.
- **Risk factors :** – More prevalent in areas of *dietary iodine deficiency Nodular goiter.*
- **Pathology :**
  - Mostly solitary lesions showing capsular and vascular invasions
  - *Capsular and vascular invasions is the criteria to distinguish between follicular adenoma and follicular carcinoma.*
  - On microscopy, tumor composed of fairly uniform cells. In some cases *Hurthle cells* (bad prognostic sign) may be found.
  - Mostly *hematogenous* to *bone* (osteolytic); Lungs and CNS.
- **Clinical features :**
  - Mostly present as thyroid nodule.
  - Metastases in ***flatbones,*** presenting as pulsatile swelling.
- **Diagnosis :**
  - Cold nodule on isotope scan.
  - FNAC *can't distinguish* between follicular adenoma and follicular carcinoma so, histology is necessary.
- **Treatment :**
  - Near total thyroidectomy and total thyroidectomy.
  - Secondaries in bone :
    - Single : Radiotherapy
    - Multiple : Radio iodine
- **Prognosis :**
  - Poor prognostic factors are :
    - Age > 50
    - Primary tumor size > 4 cm.
    - Hurthle cell histology.
    - Presence of marked vascular invasion.

Anaplastic carcinoma

- Rarest and most aggressive.
- Most rapidly growing thyroid malignancy.
- Half patient have **history of multinodular goitre**; 20% have **history of** well differentiated **thyroid carcinoma**, 20% have **concurrent** well differentiated thyroid carcinoma.
- Most cases have mutation in **p53** which is rare in well differentiated tumors.

... Robbin's 7/e, p 1178

- Typically presents in older patient with dysphagia, cervical tenderness and a painful neck mass.
- There is infiltration of carotid sheath and carotid artery pulsation are not palpable which is called as *Berry sign positive.*

- Prognosis is very poor.
- **Treatment** is surgery for resectable disease (which is present in very few patient). Palliation in the form of surgery (tracheostomy) in rest cases.

Medullary carcinoma

- *Neuroendocrinal in origin* derived from ***parafollicular cells*** or ***C cells of thyroid***.
- Two types sporadic *(common)* or familial (associated with MEN II).
- **Pathology :**
  - Can arise as *solitary nodule* (***sporadic***) or as *multiple lesion* involving both lobes of thyroid ***(familial).*** Familial cases are associated with C-cell hyperplasia
  - Characteristic features is presence of *amyloid stroma* derived from altered calcitonin molecule.
- **Spread :**
  - Involvement of ***lymph node*** and ***blood borne metastases*** to liver, bone (osteoblastic) is common.
  - It has strong predilection to metastasize in ***central compartment*** LN (the space between two internal jugular veins)
- **Clinical features :**
  - Due to tumor :
    - Present as mass in neck.
  - Due to paraneoplastic syndromes :
    - Diarrhoea *(MC paraneoplastic syndrome)*.
    - Secretes VIP, calcitonin, somatostatin, serotonin.
- **Diagnosis :**
  - I^{131} *scan is of no use* as tumours are TSH independent.
  - Calcitonin is raised in almost all cases of Medullary carcinoma and is used as *tumor marker.*
- **Treatment :**
  - Total thyroidectomy with central lymphnode dissection

    ... *Schwartz 9/e, p 1368*
- **Follow up :**
  - Level of Calcitonin falls after resection and is raises again in cases of recurrence, hence used for follow up.

Lymphoma

- Mostly arise in cases of ***hashimoto thyroiditis.***
- *Rapidly expanding thyroid mass in patient of Hashimoto's thyroiditis suggests diagnosis.*
- Most common type is *diffuse large cell lymphoma* ... *Harrison 17/e 2246*
- Highly ***radiosensitive.***
- **Treatment :** External beam radiotherapy + Chemotherapy

SOLITARY THYROID NODULE

- Most common cause - ***Follicular adenoma.***
- Investigation of choice and first investigations - ***FNAC.***

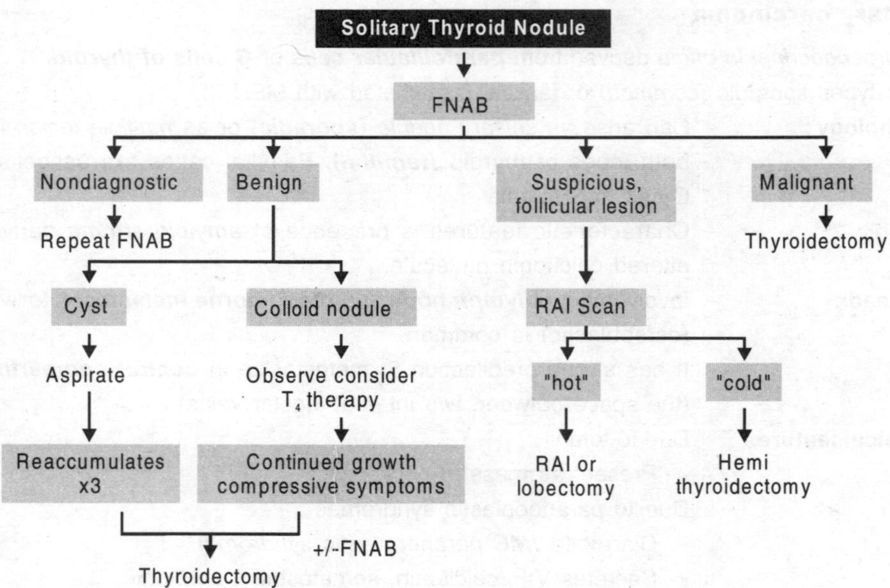

SECONDARY (METASTATIC TUMORS OF THYROID)

- **Rare,** most cases are found in autopsy.
- Most common site of primary are ***carcinoma breast***, carcinoma lung.

Remember : If thyroid metastases is detected **premortem** than **most common** site of primary are ***Renal cell carcinoma***, carcinoma breast, carcinoma lung.

... Devita 7/e, p 1518

Thyroid Operations

All thyroid operations can be assembled from three basic elements :

- *Total lobectomy*
- *Isthmusectomy*
- *Subtotal lobectomy :*
  - Total thyroidectomy = 2 x total lobectomy + isthmusectomy
  - Subtotal thyroidectomy = 2 x subtotal lobectomy + isthmusectomy
  - Near-total thryoidectomy = total lobectomy + isthmusectomy + subtotal lobectomy
  - Lobectomy = total lobectomy + isthmusectomy.

QUESTIONS

1. **Which is not a thyroid cancer : [AI 07]**
   a. Insular
   b. Markel cell
   c. Follicular
   d. Anaplastic

2. **Regarding thyroid lymphoma all are true except : [AI 07]**
   a. Thyroid lymphomas are more common in women than in men
   b. Respiratory difficulty cough, and dysphagia also can occur
   c. Slow growing
   d. Simulates anaplastic Ca

3. **Which of the following is used in treatment of differentiated thyroid cancer ? [AI 06]**
   a. ^{131}I
   b. 99 mTc
   c. 32 p
   d. ^{131}I NIBG

4. **Which of the following gene defect is associated with development of medullary carcinoma of thyroid? [AI 04]**
   a. Ret Proto Oncogene
   b. FAP gene
   c. Rb gene
   d. BRCA I gene

5. **The most common histologic type of thyroid cancer is : [AI 08; AI 04; AIIMS 05, 98]**
   a. Medullay type
   b. Follicular type
   c. Papillary type
   d. Lymphoma

6. **A well differentiated follicular carcinoma of thyroid can be best differentiated from a follicular adenoma by :**
   a. Hurthle cell damage
   b. Lining of tall columnar and cuboidal cells **[AIIMS May 10; AI 09]**
   c. Vascular invasion
   d. Nuclear features

7. **Which of the following would be the best treatment for a 2 cm thyroid nodule in a 50 year old man with FNAC revealing it to be a papillary carcinoma : [AI 09]**
   a. Hemithyroidectomy
   b. Subtotal thyrodectomy with modified neck dissection
   c. Near total thyrodectomy with modified neck dissection
   d. Hemithyroidectomy with modified neck dissection

8. **Which of the following feature of thyroid nodule on ultrasound is not suggestive of malignancy: [AIIMS May 10; AI 09]**
   a. Hyperechogenisity
   b. Hypoechogenisity
   c. Nonhomogenous
   d. Microcalcification

9. **Anaplastic carcinoma thyroid true are:**
   a. Well encapsulated **[PGI 08]**
   b. Will not invade surrounding structures
   c. Distant metastasis common
   d. Some degree of differentiation to papillary and follicular types seen

10. **Papillary carcinoma thyroid : [PGI 08]**
    a. Lymph node metastasis is common
    b. More common in female
    c. Can metastasize in lungs
    d. Multifocal in origin and invades to capsule
    e. Prognosis is bad

11. **One of the following is not correct in papillary carcinoma of thyroid :**
    a. Can be reliably diagnosed using fine needle aspiraton cytology
    b. Always unifocal **[AIIMS 06]**
    c. Typically spreads to the cervical lymph nodes
    d. Requires a total thyroidectory for large tumors

12. Ret proto oncogene mutation is a hallmark of which of the following tumors :
a. Medullary carcinoma thyroid
b. Astrocytoma **[AIIMS 06]**
c. Paraganglionoma
d. Hurthle cell tumor thyroid

13. Treatment of choice for medullary carcinoma of thyroid is : [AIIMS 05]
a. Total thyroidectomy
b. Partial thyroidectomy
c. I^{131} ablation
d. Hemithyroidectomy

14. Expression of following oncogene is associated with a high incidence of Medullary carcinoma of thyroid :
a. P-53 **[AIIMS 05]**
b. Her 2 neu
c. Ret protooncogene
d. Rb gene

15. In treatment of papillary carcinoma thyroid, Radio iodine destroys the neoplastic cells predominantly by : [AIIMS 05]
a. x-rays
b. β-rays
c. γ rays
d. α particles

16. A 45-year old male presents with 4x4 cm, mobile right solitary thyroid nodule of 5 months duration. The patient is euthyroid. The following statements about his management are true except :
a. Cold nodule on thyroid scan is diagnostic of malignancy **[AIIMS 05]**
b. FNAC is the investigation of choice
c. The patient should undergo hemithyroidectomy if FNAC report is inconclusive
d. Indirect laryngoscopy should be done in the preoperative period to assess mobility of vocal cords

17. The treatment of choice for Anaplastic carcinoma of thyroid infiltrating trachea and sternum will be:
a. Radical excision
b. Chemotherapy
c. Radiotherapy
d. Palliative/Symptomatic treatment

18. Thyroid Ca true about : [PGI 06]
a. Follicular Ca worst prognosis than Papillary
b. Papillary Ca spreads by hematogenous route frequently than follicular
c. Papillary Ca have increased mortality than follicular
d. Follicular Ca have more female incidence than papillary

19. In solitary thyroid nodule true are :
a. THR-Ab are always seen **[PGI 06]**
b. Lined by columnar epithelium
c. Diffuse hyperplasia of thyroid
d. Common in female
e. Thyroidectomy done in all cases

20. Low risk in Ca thyroid : [PGI 06]
a. Men < 50 yrs
b. Women < 40 yrs
c. Papillary Ca <5 cm
d. Metastasis
e. Follicular Ca >5 cm

21. Treatment of medullary carcinoma of thyroid with Lymphnode Metastases :
a. Subtotal thyroidectomy + Radioiodine
b. Subtotal thyroidectomy + Radiotherapy
c. Near total thyroidectomy + Radiotherapy
d. Near total thyroidectomy + Radioiodine **[PGI 05]**
e. Total thyroidectomy + Radiotherapy

ANSWERS, REFERENCES, EXPLANATIONS WITH INFORMATIVE ILLUSTRATIONS

1. **Ans. is b i.e. Merkel cell** *Ref. Harrison 17/e, p 2242*

Guy's I think there is confusion only between insular and merkel cell. Insular carcinoma is the variant of follicular carcinoma.

Classification of Thyroid Neoplasms
Benign
Follicular epithelial cell adenomas : • Macrofollicular (colloid) • Normofollicular (simple) • Microfollicular (fetal) • Trabecular (embryonal) • Hurtle cell variant (oncocytic)
Malignant
Follicular epithelial cell : Well-differentiated carcinomas • Papillary carcinomas : – Pure papillary – Follicular variant – Diffuse sclerosing variant – Tall cell, columnar cell variants • Follicular carcinomas : – Minimally invasive – Widely invasive – Hürthle cell carcinoma (oncocytic) • Insular carcinom[Q] • Undifferentiated (anaplastic) carcinomas • C cell (calcitonin-producing) : – Medullary thyroid cancer • Other malignancies : – Lymphomas – Sarcomas – Metastases – Other

2. **Ans. is c i.e. Slow growing** *Ref. Harrison 17/e, p 2246*

Thyroid lymphoma grows rapidly, infact a rapidly expending thyroid mass in a patient of Hashimoto's thyroiditis suggest thyroid lymphoma.

Important points about Thyroid lymphoma

- Rare tumor, F > M.

- Most cases arises in back ground of Hashimoto's thyroiditis.
- Diffuse large cell lymphoma is the most common type.
- Biopsy reveals sheets of lymphoid cells that can be difficult to distinguish from amaplastic thyroid Ca.
- It is highly radiosenstitive and surgical resection should be avoided as inital therapy.

3. **Ans. is a i.e. ^{131}I** *Ref. Schwartz 9/e, p 1365; William's Endocrinology 10/e, p 479*

^{131}I is an effective agent for delivering high radiation doses to the thyroid tissue with low spill over to other portions of the body.

Indication of I_{131} in thyroid cancer (Latest American thyroid association guidelines)

- All patients with Stage III or IV carcinoma
- All patients with Stage II younger than 45 years
- Most patients with Stage II older than 45 years
- Patients with Stage I disease who have aggressive histology, nodal metastasis, multifocal disease, extrathyroid or vascular invasion

Mechanism of Action :

- ^{131}I emits ***x-rays*** as well as **β *particles.***
- **X-rays** are useful for tracer studies.
- **b rays** are utilized for their destructive effects on thyroid cells.
- *Thyroid follicular cells undergo pyknosis and fibrosis.*

Complications of Radioactive Iodine Therapy (^{131}I)

Acute	Long-Term
Neck pain, swelling and tenderness	***Hemotologic***
Thyroiditis (if remnant present)	– Bone marrow suppression
Sialadenitis, taste dysfunction	– Leukemia
Hemorrhage (brain metastases)	***Fertility***
Cerebral edema (brain metastases)	– Ovarian/testicular damage, infertility
Vocal cord paralysis	– Increased spontaneous abortion rate
Nausea and vomiting	***Pulmonary fibrosis***
Bone marrow suppression	***Chronic sialadenitis, nodules, taste dysfunction***
	Increased risk of cancer
	– Anaplastic thyroid cancer
	– Gastric cancer
	– Hepatocellular cancer
	– Lung cancer
	– Breast cancer
	– Bladder cancer
	– Hypoparathyroidism

Remember: Screening with RAI is more sensitive than chest X-ray or CT scanning for delecting metastasis. However it is less sensitive than Tg measurement for same.

4. ***Ans. is a i.e. Ret proto oncogene*** *Ref. Robbin's 8/e, p 1125; Schwartz 9/e, p 1367-68*

"Medullary ca is associated with MEN II which is due to defect in RET protoncogene located on chromosome 10."

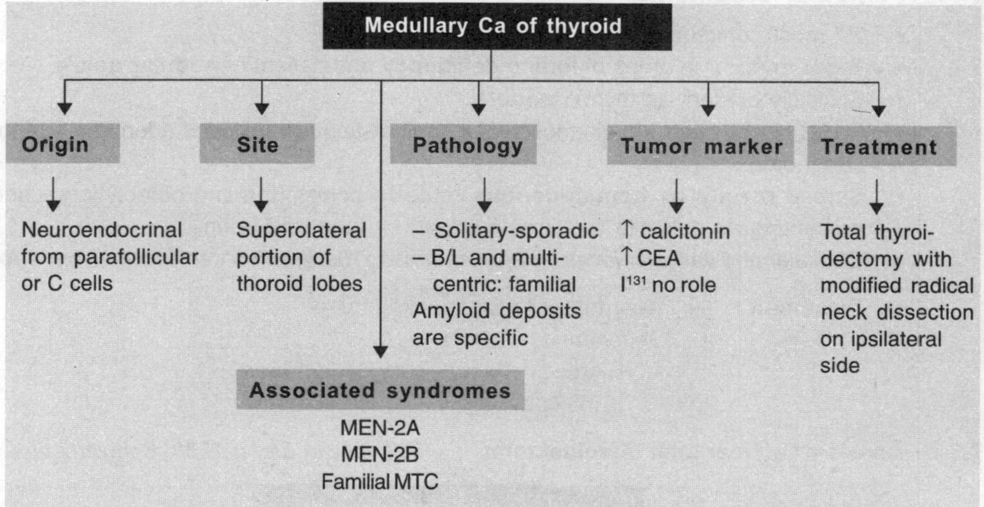

Remember:
- Calcitonin is a more sensitive tumor marker CEA is a better predictor of prognosis.
- Neck pain and aching is more common in Medullary Ca.

5. **Ans. is c i.e. Papillary type** *Ref. CMDT 10/e, p 1022*

Least malignant or Best prognosis is with Papillary Ca.

Characteristic features of Thyroid cancer

Features	*Papillary*	*Follicular*	*Medullary*	*Anaplastic*
Relative incidence	60%	20%	5%	1%
Average age	42	50	50	57
Females	70%	72%	56%	56%
Invasion				
Juxtanodal	+++++	+	+++++	+++
Blood vessels	+	+++	+++	+++++
Distant sites	+	+++	++	++++
Resemblance to normal thyroid	+	+++	+	±
^{123}I uptake	+	++++	0	0
Degree of malignancy	+	+++++	+++++	++++++++
5 year survival rate	85%	78%	62%	18%

Remember :

Features	Papillary (%)	Follicular (%)
• Recurrence rate	19	29
Location of Recurrence		
• Distant metastases	45	75
• Nodal metastases	34	12

6. **Ans. is c i.e. Vascular invasion** *Ref. Schwartz, 9/e, p 1364*

In follicular lesion malignancy is defined by capsular and vascular invasion

Follicular carcinoma

- 2nd most common thyroid carcinoma.
- Tends to occur in areas of **iodine deficiency** and patient of **nodular goitre.**
- Clinically present as thyroid **nodule.**
- FNAC is **not useful** in diagnosis as it can't distinguish follicular adenoma and follicular carcinoma.
- Spread **mainly by hematogenous** route to bones (forming osteolytic secondaries, presenting as pulsatile swelling) followed by lung and brain.
- *Capsular and vascular invasion* is the *criteria* to ***distinguish carcinoma from adenoma.***
- **Treatment :**
  - Near total or total thyroidectomy.
  - Secondaries in Bone :
    - Single → Radiotherapy
    - If multiple → Radioiodine

7. **Ans. is c i.e. Near total thyroidectomy** *Ref. Devita 8/e, p 1673; Schwartz 9/e, p 1363*

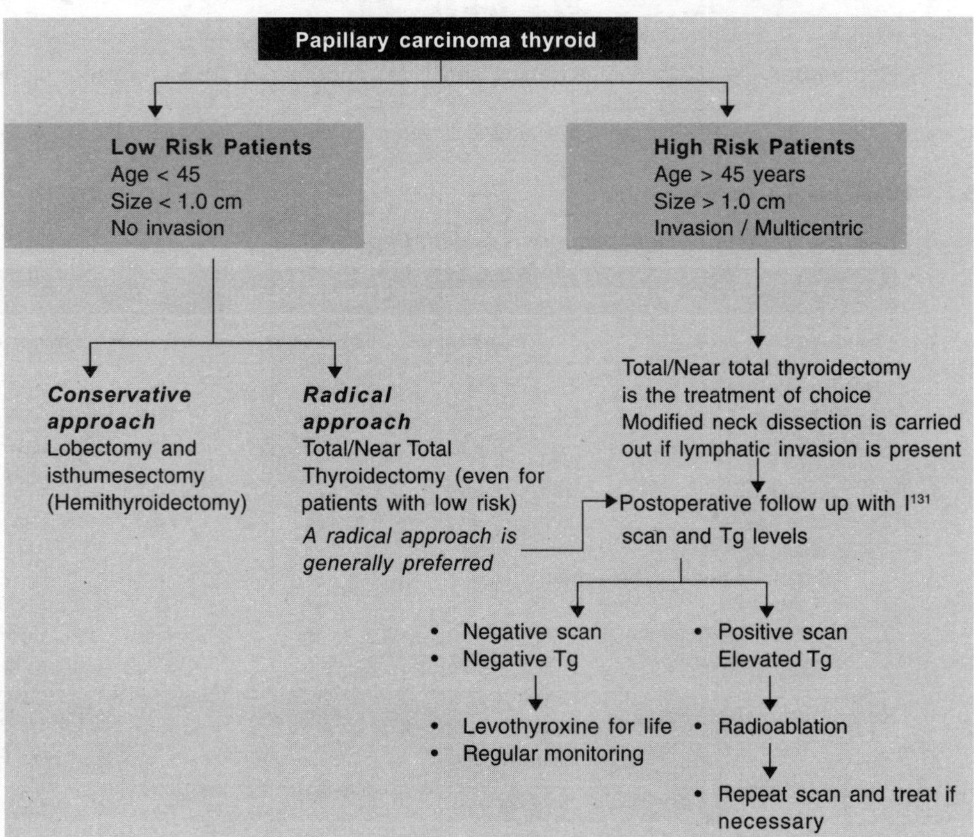

In low risk patients too radical surgery is preferred because of following reasons:

- Eliminates contralateral occult cancer

- Reduces risk of recurrence
- Enables the use of RAI to effectively detect and treat residual thyroid tissue or metastatic disease
- Increased sensitivity of serum Tg as tumor marker

8. Ans. is a i.e. Hyperechogenicity *Ref. Rumack 3/e, p 755*

Hyperechogenicity is suggestive of benign lesion

Feature	Benign	Malignant
Internal contents		
Purely cystic content	++++	+
Cystic with thin septa	++++	+
Mixed solid and cystic	+++	++
Comet-tail artifact	+++	+
Echogenicity		
Hyperechoic	++++	+
Isoechoic	+++	++
Hypoechoic	+++	+++
Halo		
Thin halo	++++	++
Thick incomplete halo	+	+++
Margin		
Well-defined	+++	++
Poorly defined	++	+++
Calcification		
Eggshell calcification	++++	+
Coarse calcification	+++	+
Microcalcification	++	++++
Doppler		
Peripheral flow pattern	+++	++
Internal flow pattern	++	+++

Differentiation of thyroid nodules according to echogenicity

Echogenecity of the Nodule	Most likely diagnosis
Hyperechoic, isoechoic	Adenomatous (colloid) noodule
Hypoechoic	Follicular adenoma Malignancy Metastasis
Mixed echogenicity	Large nodules (Folicular adenoma as well as colloid nodules) with regressive changes
Anechoic	Cyst

9. **Ans. is c and d Distant..., Some degree...** *Ref. Schwartz 9/e, p 1369; Robbins 8/e, p 1124*

Anaplastic Ca

- Accounts for 1% of all thyroid malignancy and is fastest, most aggressive thyroid neoplasm
- **Age:** 7th, 8th, decade, F > M
- **Pathology:** Most patients have preexisting goitre or thyroid cancer
  Gross: Tumor are firm, with invasion to surrounding structures
  Microscopy: Multinucleated giant cells, spindle cell, foci of papillary or follicular differentiation may be present which further suggest that anaplastic tumor arise from well differentiated tumor
- **Clinical presentation**
  - Typical patient has a long standing neck mass which rapidly enlarges and become painful due to invasion of nearby structures
  - Associated symptoms include dysphonia, dyspnea, dysphagia
- **Treatment**
  - At the time of diagnosis most patients have distant metastasis and only few patients survive beyond 6 months
  - All forms of treatment are disappointing Total thyroidectomy is most effective treatment, if possible
  - In other **cases tracheostomy may be needed to alleviate airway obstruction**

10. **Ans. is a, b, c and d Lymph node..., More common..., Can metastasize..., Multifocal in...** *Ref. CMDT 2/e, p 1022*

Already explained refer Ans. no. 5

11. **Ans. is b i.e. Always unifocal** *Ref. Robbin's 7/e, p 1178, 8/e, p 1121*

Papillary Ca can be solitary or multifocal lesion.

Papillary Carcinoma

- Most common, *least malignant, best prognostic* malignancy of thyroid.
- *Radiation exposure* is most important risk factor, other risk factor are Hashimoto thyroiditis, thyroglossal cyst.
- Age 20-40, F > M

12. **Ans. is a i.e. Medullary Ca thyroid** *Ref. Harrison 17/e, p 2244; Schwartz 9/e, p 1361*

RET mutation is hallmark of MEN-II Medullary Ca is the component of MEN-II.

Oncogenes and Tumor supression genes in Thyroid cancer	
Oncogenes	
RET	Sporadic and familial MTC, PTC
MET	Overexpressed in PTC
TRKI	Activated in some PTC
Ras	Follicular adenoma and carcinoma, PTC
PAX8/PPARγl	Follicular adenoma, follicular carcinoma
Tumor suppressors	
p53	Dedifferentiated PTC, FTC, anaplastic cancers
PTEN	Follicular adenoma and carcinoma

13. Ans. is a i.e. Total thyroidectomy *Ref. Bailey & Love 24/e, p 802*

Treatment of MCT is total thyroidectomy followed by modified radical neck dissection

14. Ans. is c i.e. Ret protooncogene *Ref. Schwartz 9/e, p 1361*

Already explained

15. Ans. is b i.e. β-rays *Ref. KDT 5/e, p 233*

Already explained, kindly see answer no. 3

16. Ans. is a i.e. Cold nodule on thyroid scan is diagnostic of malignancy *Ref. CSDT 12/e, p 281*

Only 20% of cold nodule and 1% of hot nodule are malignant. So, cold nodule on thyroid scan is not diagnostic of malignancy.

Indications of Surgical removal of Nodule :

- Suspicion of **c**ancer
- **Th**yrotoxicosis
- **C**osmetic deformity.
- Symptoms of **p**ressure
- Substernal **e**xtension

Mnemonic: Cancer Can Produce Extensive Thyrotoxicocis

17. Ans. is d i.e. Palliative / symptomatic treatment *Ref. Schwartz Surgery 9/e, p 1369*

Anaplastic carcinoma with distant metastasis or invasion in to locally unresectable structure such as trachea or vasculature of the anterior mediastinum should be treated by conservative and symptomatic surgery such as tracheostomy as radical treatment is not associated with increased survival.

18. Ans. is d i.e. Follicular Ca have more female incidence than papillary

Already explained, kindly see answer no. 5 *Ref. CMDT 10/e, p 1022*

19. Ans. is d i.e. Common in female *Ref. Schwartz 9/e, p 1358*

- **Solitary thyroid nodule (STN)** is a palpable discrete swelling within an otherwise apparently normal thyroid gland.
- **Incidence** : 1 - 10%.
- Male : Female = 1 : 4.
- The possiblility of neoplastic disease though rare, but is of major threat in STN.
- **Most represent non-neoplastic conditions like :**
  - Nodular hyperplasia
  - Simple cysts
  - Thyroiditis
  - Benign neoplasms-follicular adenoma
  - Carcinomas (uncommon).
- **Features of STN :**
  - They are more likely to be *neoplastic* than are multiple nodules.

- Nodules in *younger patients* are more likely to be neoplastic than are those in older patients.
- Nodules in *males* are more likely to be neoplastic than are those in females.
- History of radiation exposure is associated with an increased incidence of thyroid malignancy.
- Nodules that do not take radioactive iodine in imaging studies (cold nodules) are more likely to be malignant.

20. Ans. is b and c i.e. Women < 40 years; and Papillary Ca < 5cm

Ref. Bailey & Love 25/e, p 795

Risk group definitions in differentiated thyroid carcinoma are :

- **Low risk group :** 2% mortality in 25 years.
  - Male ≤ 40 years.] **Age**
  - Women ≤ 50 years.
  - Without distant metastasis
  - All older patients with intrathyroid papillary carcinoma or follicular carcinoma with minor capsular involvement, **tumors < 5 cm in diameter** and no distant metastases.
  - No extrathyroid extension
- **High risk group :** 46% mortality in 25 years.
  - All patients with distant metastases.
  - All older patients with extrathyroid papillary carcinoma or follicular carcinoma with major capsular involvement, tumors 5 cm or larger, regardless of extent of disease.

21. Ans. is e i.e. Total thyroidectomy + Radiotherapy

Ref. Devita 8/e, p 1678; Schwartz 9/e, p 1368

Treatment of choice for MCT : Total thyroidectomy + Radical or modified radical neck dissection.

"In patient with metastatic disease, outcome is poor as radiotherapy and chemotherapy are disappointing. Surgical resection still offer best chance of survival."

... Devita 8/e, p 1678

Remember : MCT do not take radioiodine, so radioiodine is not used rather contraindicated in MCT.

So, guys ! none of the choice is correct but *Schwartz 8/e, p 1424 puts radiotherapy above chemotherapy and surgery for all cases is total thyroidectomy,* so ***option 'e'*** can be taken as answer.

34 Parathyroid and Adrenal Tumour

What's Important ?

- Treatment of Parathyroid Adenoma
- Diagnosis of Pheochromocytoma

PARATHYROID NEOPLASM		
Hyperplasia	Adenoma ***(MC)***	Carcinoma

All cases present with primary hyperparathyroidism.

PARATHYROID HYPERPLASIA

- Responsible for 14% of cases of primary hyperparathyroidism.
- Usually effect ***all four*** parathyroid gland simultaneously but size may be different.
- Occur sporadically or component of MEN I and 2A syndrome.
- Microscopically there is ***chief cell hyperplasia*** in most cases.
- Combined weight of all glands is usually less than 1.0 gm.

PARATHYROID ADENOMA

- Most common ***cause of primary hyperparathyroidism.***
- Adenoma (weight 0.5 to 5.0 gm) is well circumscribed, soft and covered by capsule.
- In contrast to primary hyperplasia, glands beside adenoma are usually normal or shrunken.
- Adenoma most commonly involved ***inferior parathyroid.***
- Associated with MEN I and 2A syndrome.
- Usually asymptomatic.
- Symptoms are due to excess PTH.

Investigation

- Tc^{99m} isotope scan **(IOC).**
- Single photon emission computerised tomography (SPECT) *(Most accurate)* can detect abnormal parathyroid glands.

Treatment

- **Absolute indication of treatment are :**
  - Urinary tract calculi.
  - Markedly reduced bone density.
  - Serum calcium > 2.85 mol/lt.
- **In case of adenoma :** Only enlarged parathyroid is removed.
- **In case of hyperplasia :** When all parathyroid are enlarged subtotal parathyroidectomy is performed leaving a single vascularised gland (remnant equal to size of a normal parathyroid).
- **Patients with MEN syndrome :** As they have high risk of recurrent hyperparathyroidism, total parathyroidectomy is performed with auto transplantation of 50-100mg of parathyroid tissue in to brachioradialis muscle of forearm.

PARATHYROID CARCINOMA

- Rare
- Classical presentation is with symptomatic severe hypercalcemia, with very high PTH level.
- Gland usually weight > 10.0 gm.

Diagnosis

- It is based on invasion of surrounding tissue and metastases (cytology is unreliable).

Treatment

- Excision of tumor mass + Ipsilateral thyroidectomy + Node dissection if involved.

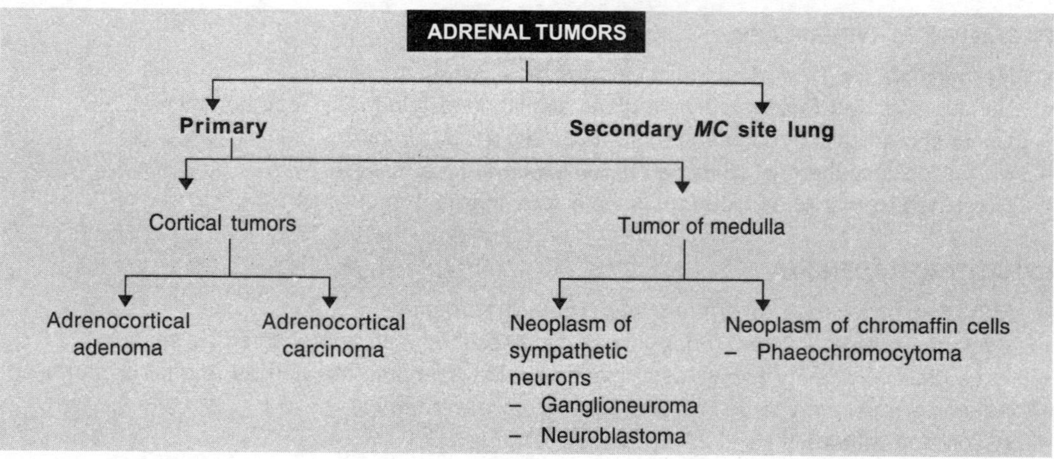

ADRENOCORTICAL ADENOMA

- Secrete either ***cortisol*** to cause cushing syndrome ***or aldosterone*** *(Conn's syndrome).*
- It is the most common cause of ***primary hyperaldosteronism.***

Morphologically

- Involve **left** side more frequently.
- *Adenoma secreting cortisol show cells of zona fasiculata while that secreting aldosterone also resemble fasiculata.*

... Robbins 7/e, p 1210

- In contrast to adenoma secreting cortisol, those associated with hyperaldosteronism don't suppress ACTH and there is no cortical atrophy of contralateral gland (which is found in cortisol secreting adenoma).

Features	Cortisol secreting adenoma	Aldosteron secreting adenoma
Clinical features	Present as Cushing syndrome	Hypertension, Hypokalemia, polyuria *without edema*
Diagnosis	Cushing syndrome in presence of *low ACTH*	Hypertension and Hypokalemia without edema in a patient not receiving potassium sparing diuretic
Treatment	Laparoscopic removal of adrenal with proper steroid replacement as contralateral gland is atrophied	Laproscopic removal

ADRENOCORTICAL CARCINOMA

- Rare neoplasm occur at ***any age group.***
- ***Inherited cause*** are Li-Fraumeni syndrome and Beckwith - Wiedmann syndrome.
- Morphologically large invasive lesion.
- Tendency to invade the adrenal vein, venacava and lymphatics.
- Distant metastases occur *mostly to lung and liver.*
- As tumor is mostly functional, patient presents with *cushing syndrome with virilization.*
- Radical resection is done when ever possible.
- **Principal drug** of treatment is mitotane an isomer of DDT.
- Prognosis is poor.

PHAEOCHROMOCYTOMA

- Tumors arise from **chromaffin cells in adrenal medulla and elsewhere.**
- Can be benign or malignant.
- Age : Can occur in all age group, familial tumor occur in younger.
- Sex : F > M

Etiology and Risk factor

- Pheochromocytoma can be familial or sporadic. Familial can be syndromic or nonsyndromic.
- Syndromes associated with pheochromocytoma are :
  - *MEN-2A and MEN-2B* - defect in RET protooncogene.
  - *Von hippel lindau* - Mutation is VHL gene.
  - *Von Recklinghausen syndrome* - Mutation in NF-1 gene.
  - *Sturge weber syndrome.*
  - *Paraganglionoma of neck*

Mnemonic: 2 MEN Hippel and Von Reckling present with sturge Weber syndromes

- Non syndromic familial pheochromocytoma - Most commonly associated with SDHB and SDHD mutation.

Pathology

- Most are unilateral and solitary.
- *Extra-adrenal pheochromocytoma* (10% cases) occur in organ of zuckerlandt in the periaortic region (most common **site**) and the carotid body. Extra adrenal pheochromocytoma more higher incidence of malignancy. *... Devita 8/e, p 1698*
- Adrenal tumor range from small lesion to large hemorrhagic mass.
- Histologically tumor composed of polygonal to spindle chromaffin cells clustered in to small nests or alveoli (Zelballen) by a rich vascular network. Nuclei are round with 'salt and pepper' chromatin.
- *Criteria for malignancy is based exclusively on presence of metastases, as even capsular or vascular invasion, can be present in benign tumors.*
- Pheochromocytoma synthesize and secrete catecholamine.
- Tumour are not innervated so catecholamine release does not result from neural stimulation.
- Also secrete other peptides including endogenous opoids, adrenomedullin, erythropoeten, parathyroid hormone related protein, neuropeptide.
- ***Most pheochromocytoma*** produce both NA and Adr, with NA > Adr.
- *Extra-adrenal pheochromocytoma/paraganglioma* secrete NA exclusively.
- Those associated with **MEN** may secrete Adr alone.
- *Increased production of dopamine and homovanillic acid is usually seen with malignant lesions.*

Pheochromocytoma usually follow *rule of 10.*

- 10% are familial.
- 10% are extradrenal
- 10% non familial adrenal pheochromocytoma are bilateral. Figure raises to 70% in case of familial.
- 10% arise in childhood.

Clinical feature

- Most common ***symptom*** are headache (due to hypertension) > sweating > palpitation.
- Most common ***manifestation*** is hypertension (hypertension is not a symptom).
- Cardiac manifestation are sinus tachycardia, sinus bradycardia, supraventricular arrhythmias and ventricular premature contraction.
- Carbohydrate intolerance.
- Increased hematocrit.

Diagnosis

- Demonstration of increased production of Catecholamine by following tests :
  a. ***Biochemical test***
     - *Plasma metanephrine is single most sensitive test* for secretory pheochromocytoma (both adrenal and extraadrenal)
     - Urinary VMA assay > 35 μmol (7.0mg) is significant.
     - Urinary assay for metanephrine.
     - Assay for unconjugated or free catecholamine.

b. ***Pharmacological test***

- Positive response to ***phentolamine*** (5mg bolus following a test dose of 0.5 mg) is a *reduction in B.P of at least 35/25mm Hg after 2 min.* But this is not diagnostic and biochemical confirmation is necessary.

- **Imaging :** – CT and MRI (Less sensitive).
  – Nuclear Imaging [123]Iodobenzylguanidine scan (MIBG scan) is highly specific and sensitive for both adrenal and extraadrenal pheochromocytoma.

... Bailey 25/e, p 813

Treatment

- ***Total laproscopic adrenalectomy*** is the treatment of choice.
- α ***Blockers (Prazocin or phenoxybenzamine):*** These are typically administered preoperatively to control BP. Optimal α blockade is achieved when supine arterial pressure is below 140/90 mm of Hg
- Calcium channel blockers (nifedipine or nicardipine) are very effective and may be used with or without α blockers. They are superior to phenoxybenzamine for long term use and for controlling hypertensive crisis
- **β blocker:** Only given after α blockade or calcium channel blockade. The use of β blocker without α blockade result in unopposed α action and worsening of hypertension
- Perioperative and post operative blood pressure monitoring should be done.
- **Malignant pheochromocytoma :**
  - Treated by surgical *resection followed by chemotherapy* consisting of cyclophosphamide, vincristine and dacarbazine.
  - Most common site of metastases is bone, liver and lymphnodes.

GANGLIONEUROMA

- ***Benign tumor*** consisting of mature sympathetic ganglion cells.
- Wide age group, F > M.
- Presents with pressure symptom and pain.
- Treatment is surgical excision.

QUESTIONS

1. **All of the following are features of pheochromocytoma except : [PGI 07]**
   a. Hypertensive paroxysm
   b. Palpitation
   c. Orthostatic hypotension
   d. Wheezing
2. **Which is not done in case of pheochromocytoma: [AIIMS May 07]**
   a. FNAC
   b. MRI
   c. CT
   d. MIBG
3. **Pheochromocytoma secretes, all except: [PGI 10]**
   a. Adrenaline
   b. Noradrenaline
   c. Parathyroid related protein
   d. Corticosterone
   e. Opoids
4. **Accidental finding of incidentaloma (Adrenal mass) on USG is detected. Following is/are to be ruled out : [PGI 06]**
   a. Cushing's disease
   b. Metastasis
   c. Adrenal adenoma
   d. Carcinoma
   e. Adrenal hyperplasia
5. **Which of the following is not a CT feature of adrenal adenoma: [AI 09, 10]**
   a. Low attenuation
   b. Homogenous density and well defined borders
   c. Calcification is rare
   d. Enhances rapidly, contrast stays in it for a relatively longer time and washes out late

ANSWERS, REFERENCES, EXPLANATIONS WITH INFORMATIVE ILLUSTRATIONS

1. **Ans. is d i.e. Wheezing** *Ref. Bailey & Love 25/e, p 813; Harrison 17/e, p 2270*

Symptoms in patient with Pheochromocytoma		
> 50% of patient	**20-40% of patient**	**< 20% of patient**
– **Headache** (**MC** symptom) – Sweating – Palpitation	– Pallor – Nausea – Fever – Tremor – Anxiety – Abdominal pain – Chest pain – Weakness – *Orthostatic hypotension* (due to ↓ plasma volume)	– Dyspnea – *Weight loss* – Flushing – Visual disturbance – ↑ Hematocrit – Carbohydrate intolerance – Hypercalcemia

Remember : Most common sign or most common manifestation of pheochromocytoma is paroxysmal or episodic hypertension

2. **Ans. is a i.e. FNAC** *Ref. Harrison 17/e, p 2257, 2270*

"Percutaneous fine needle aspiration of chromaffin tumors is contraindicated; indeed, pheochromocytoma should be considred before adrenal lesions are aspirated."

... Harrison

Biopsy of pin pheochromocytoma may result in excessive release of catecholamines and may cause hyptensive crisis.

Diagnosis of Pheochromocytoma		
Demonstration of ↑ catecholamines or catecholamine metabolite	Pharmacological test	*Demonstration of tumor*
– Urinary metanephrine (> 1.3 mg/day) – Urinary VMA (> 7.0mg/day) – Fractionated Plasma metanephrine **(best)**	– Phentolamine provocation test	– CT – MRI – MIBG scan **(Most sensitive) (Best for localization)**

3. **Ans. is d i.e. Corticosterone** *Ref. Harrison 16/e, p 2148 - 2149*

Beside catecholamines (Adr and NA) pheochromocytoma secretes

- Endogenous opoids
- Erythropoietin
- Neuropeptide γ
- ↑ production of dopamine and homovanillic acid (HVA) occur with ***malignant pheochromocytoma.***
- Adrenomodullin
- Parathyroid hormone related protein
- Chromagranin A

Remember :
- Most sensitive screening test for pheochromocytoma is urinary catecholamine and VMA level
- Best test for diagnosis : Fractionated plasma metanephrine.
- Best test for localization : MIBG scan

4. **Ans. is a, b, c, d and e i.e. All options are correct**

Ref. CT & MRI by Haga 4/e, p 1525; Robbin's 7/e, p 1218

Adrenal incidentiloma

- Incidental adrenal mass detected while imaging for any other reason.
- **Causes :**
  - Non secreting cortical adenomas *(MC)*
  - ACTH secreting adrenal adenoma (Cushing's disease)
  - Adrenocortical or Medullary malignancy
  - Pheochromocytoma
  - Adrenal hyperplasia
  - Metastatic Cancer
  - Abscess
  - Amyloidosis
  - Sarcoidosis, cysts.
- **Evaluation :**
  - Aim is to determine whether its is hyperfunctioning or malignant.
  - Features suggestive of malignancy are large size (> 4 to 6 cm), irregular margins, soft tissue calcifications, inhomogenicity.

- FNAC should be done only if pheochromocytoma has been ruled out.
- Hyperfunctioning is determined by measurement of 24h urine catecholamines.
- Serum electrolytes.
- Assesment of adrenal cortical functions by dexomethasone suppression testing.

Treatment : If tumor is hyperfunctional or malignant surgery is indicated. Rest cases are managed by following.

5. **Ans. is d i.e. Enhances rapidly, contrast ...** *Ref. Grainger Radiology 4/e, p 1388*

- Adrenal cortical adenomas are common benign tumor, They are usually asymptomatic and found incidently on abdominal CT
- Histologically they are composed of an admixture of clear, lipid rich cells arranged in small cord like patterns.

Etiology: Previous injury or vascular insult

Diagnosis: The goal is to differentiate adenoma from malignancy

- Most of them are detected incidently on CT abdomen

Features suggestive of benign nature include:

a. Well defined
b. < 3 cm size
c. Low attenuation due to presence of lipid cells (< 10 HU)

- If an adrenal mass with attenuation > 10 HU is found contrast enhance CT scan is indicated
- Benign lesions shows relatively rapid washout of contrast. The percent enhancement washout is calculated by the formula:

$$\frac{E-D}{E-U} \times 100$$

E = 70 second post contrast enhancement value

D = 15 min post contrast enhancement value

U = Unenhanced value

If percent enhancement is greater than 60% the lesion is benign

35 Carcinoid and Pancreatic Endocrinal Tumour

What's Important ?

- Site of Carcinoid Tumour
- Carcinoid Syndrome
- Gastrinoma
- Insulinoma

- These tumour comes under **neuroendocrine tumours (NETs).**
- These are *composed of sheets of small round cells with uniform nuclei* which synthesize and secrete various peptides and bioactive amines to produce specific clinical syndrome.
- These tumour were originally classified as **APUD omas** (Amine precursor uptake and decarboxylation) which also *include pheochromocytoma, Melanoma, medullary carcinoma of thyroid.*
- On histology they are *identified by their staining pattern.*
  - *Earlier silver staining* was used.
  - *Now* immunocytochemical localization of chromo-granin (A,B,C), neuron specific enolase or synaptophysin are used for identification.
- ***Conditions associated with NETs***
  - MEN type 1
  - VHL syndrome
  - Von Recklinghausen's disease (NF-1)
  - Tuberous sclerosis.

CARCINOID TUMOURS

- Occurs in **all age** group and at various sites.
- Classified on the basis of **site** of origin :
  - Foregut carcinoid (MC site ***bronchus).***
  - Midgut carcinoid (MC site ***ileum).***
  - Hindgut carcinoid (***Rectum)***.
- *Overall MC site are bronchus > rectum > colon.* ... *Devita 8/e, p 1723*
  (In some books appendix is given as MC site, guys ! be clear now bronchus and rectum are MC site).

Classification of Carcinoid Tumours

Origin

Histochemistry	Foregut	Midgut	Hindgut
Silver staining	Argentaffin-negative but argyrophilic	Argentaffin-positive	Argentaffin-negative (75%) often argyrophilic (55%)
Neuron-specific enolase	Positive	Positive	Positive
Chromogranin A	Positive	Positive	Positive (42%)
Cytoplasmic granules	Round, variable density	Pleomorphic, uniform	Round, variable density
Products	**Foregut**	**Midgut**	**Hindgut**
Tumour	Low 5-HT content, multihormonal	High HT content, multihormonal	Rarely 5-HT, multihormonal
Blood	ACTH		
Urine	5-HTP, 5-HT, 5-HIAA, histamine, and others	5-HT, 5-HIAA	Negative
Carcinoid syndrome	Occurs but may be atypical	Occurs frequently (with metastasis)	Rarely occurs
Metastasize to bone	Common	Rarely	Common

Pathology

- Carcinoid arising in stomach and ileum are frequently multicentric, rest arise as solitary lesion.
- Characteristic feature is solid yellow tan appearance with marked desmoplasia.
- *Malignancy* is most common in carcinoid arise in jejunum, ileum.
- *Risk of malignancy* is highest in pancreatic carcinoid tumour.
- Liver is the most common site of metastasis followed by bone and lung

Clinical features

- Depending on site and secreted products these tumour are classified into :
  a. **Carcinoid tumour without systemic features :**
     - Appendix carcinoid - mostly asymptomatic.
     - Small intestine carcinoid - MC presenting symptom are abdominal pain, intestinal obstruction, GI pain.
     - Rectal carcinoid - MC symptom are bleeding, constipation and diarrhea.
     - Bronchial carcinoid - MC symptom are pneumonia, hemoptysis and cough.

  Note : Guys ! *this does not means that these tumors does not produce systemic manifestation; but usually it is local symptom which predominates.*

  b. **Carcinoid tumour with systemic feature :**
  - ***Carcinoid tumour synthesize and secrete number of biologically active compounds :***
     - ACTH (More in foregut carcinoid)
     - Gastrin
     - Somatostatin (Duodenal carcinoid)
     - Insulin
     - Neurotensin
     - βMSH
     - Calcitonin
     - Glucagon

- Motilin
- Gastrin releasing peptide
- Serotonin
- Pancreatic polypeptide
- Vasoactive intestinal peptide
- Prostaglandins

- The most common systemic ***syndrome*** caused by carcinoid tumour is carcinoid syndrome.
- **Carcinoid syndrome :**
  - Most common symptom is diarrhoea.
  - M ≥ F
  - *Symptom/sign :*
    - Diarrhoea *(due to serotonin)*
    - Flushing *(due to histamine)* : Typically on upper part of body
    - Pain
    - Asthma/wheezing *(due to both Histamine and Serotonin)*
    - Pellagra *(as most tryptophan is used by tumour cells)*
    - Carcinoid heart disease *(due to both histamine and serotonin).*
  - In heart it causes *fibrosis of endocardium*. The dense fibrous deposits are MC on ventricular aspect of *tricuspid valve > pulmonary valve causing pulmonary stenosis and tricuspid regurgitation > Mitral valve > Aortic valve.*
  - **Site** of carcinoid causing carcinoid syndrome Midgut > Foregut > Hindgut > Unknown.
  - **Etiology :** Main secretory product of tumour cells of carcinoid syndrome is serotonin which is responsible for diarrhoea, wheezing, carcinoid heart disease.
  - **Pathology :** Patient may develop either typical or atypical carcinoid syndrome.
  - *Typical carcinoid syndrome* : Characteristically caused by midgut carcinoid.

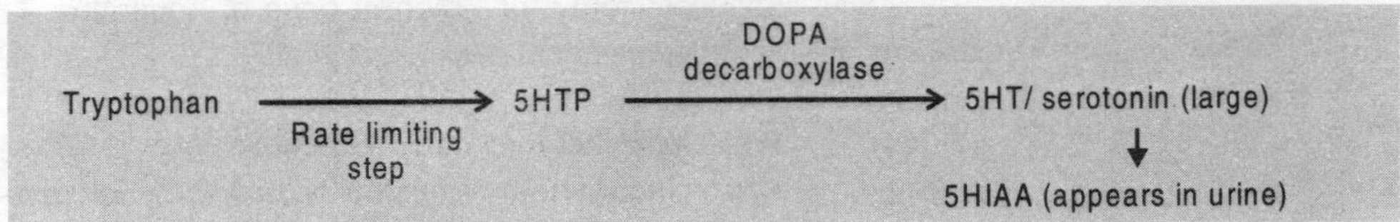

Thus there is increase in blood and platelet serotonin.

- *Atypical carcinoid syndrome* - caused by foregut carcinoid.
  - These are *deficient* in enzyme DOPA decarboxylase so *5HTP can't be converted to 5HT.*
  - In these patient plasma serotonin (5HT) levels are normal, but urinary 5HTP and 5HT are increase due to some conversion in kidney.
  - Urinary HIAA level is normal or only slightly increased.
- **Complication**
  - Most severe complication is carcinoid crisis which *particularly* occurs from foregut tumour or those with very high HIAA level.
  - It occur spontaneously or provided by stress, anaesthesia, chemotherapy or biopsy.
  - Patient develop intense flushing, diarrhoea, tachycardia and hypotension.
- **Diagnosis**
  - Diagnosis is based on measurement of urinary and plasma serotonin or its metabolite.
  - Urinary HIAA (>8mg/dl) is investigation of choice.
  - *Platelet serotonin :* Most sensitive investigation.
  - In case of atypical (Foregut) carcinoid - urinary 5HTP or 5HT should be measured.
  - *Localization* of tumour - Somatostatin receptor scintography (SRS) is best imaging technique. *... Devita 8/e 1728*

Prognosis

- Main determinants of survival is ***presence of liver metastasis.***
- Tumour mass is directly related to urinary HIAA level and is a marker of extent of disease.
- **Other poor prognostic factor are :**
  a. Male gender
  b. Older age
  c. Pancreatic or colorectal location (appendicular carcinoid has best prognosis)
  d. Presence of carcinoid crisis
  f. Depth of invasion.

Treatment

- ***Carcinoid syndrome*** **-** Octreotride and Lanreotide are most widely used agents.
- ***Carcinoid crisis*** **-** Octreotride is DOC.
- ***Tumour*** **-** Surgery is *treatment of choice.*

Site	Size	Treatment
Small intestine	Any size	Wide resection with enbloc resection of the adjacent lymphnode bearing mesentry.
Appendix	<1cm	Simple appendicectomy
	1-2cm	Simple appendicectomy/partial caecectomy or right hemicolectomy for lesion in base of appendix
	>2 cm	Right hemicolectomy
Rectum	<1cm	Local resection
	1-2cm	Wide local full thickness resection
	>2cm	Abdominoperineal resection or Low anterior resection
Gastric	<1cm	Endoscopic removal
	1-2cm	Total gastrectomy or antrectomy
	>2cm	Excision and regional lymhnode clearance.

- Isolated hepatic metastasis should be resected.
- Chemotherapy : Not effective
- Biotherapy : Using octreotide + interferon
- Hepatic artery embolization.
- *5 year survival rate* : Overall 50%.Highest for carcinoid of appendix and lowest for laryngeal carcinoid

PANCREATIC ENDOCRINE TUMOUR (PET)

- PET are ***vascular tumours*** with similar radiographic appearance and metastatic patterns of spread (i.e. primarily to regional lymphnode and liver).
- They can be functional (if associated with clinical syndrome due to hormone release) or Non functional (less common) which secrete pancreatic polypeptide which cause no specific symptom.
- *Except insulinoma most are malignant.*
- CgA is an acidic polypeptide which is elevated in about 60-100% PET *... Devita, 8/e, p 1707*

Gastrinoma (Zollinger - Ellison syndrome) :

- Most common ***malignant*** PET.

- It is tumour of delta islet cells.
- Most common **site** *duodenum* > *pancreas* (in pancreas MC site head).
- Most common symptom abdominal pain > Diarrhoea> reflux esophagitis.
- Associated with MEN - 1
- ***Diagnosis :*** Increased *fasting serum gastrin level (FSG) usually > 1000 pg/ml with gastric pH<2 suggest diagnosis of gastrinoma.* *... Devita 8/e, p 1712*

  Secretin stimulation test :
  - Most sensitive provocative test, provocative *test of choice.*
  - Rise in gastrin level by more than 200pg/ml diagnostic.

  Tumor localization :
  - Endoluminal US.
  - Somatostatin receptor scintigraphy (SRS) : Imaging modality of choice.
- **Treatment :**
  - *Proton pump inhibitor* are drug of choice.
  - Surgery is done for resectable tumour.
  - For unresectable disease - Streptozocin + 5fu is given.

Insulinoma :

- Endocrine tumour derived from beta cells.
- Most common **PET.**
- *Site* - Pancreas *(Head = Body = Tail).*
- *Characteristic feature* is WHIPPLE's TRIAD i.e. :
  a. H0ypoglycemic symptoms
  b. Blood glucose < 50mg/dl
  c. Immediate relief after ingestion of glucose.
- Most common ***symptom*** is *visual disturbance* (due to hypoglycemia).
- **Diagnosis :**
  - Increased insulin level (> 6 mU/ml) in presence of hypoglycemia (< 50 mg/dl).
  - Plasma peptide level is either increased or normal (distinguish from intake of excessive exogenous insulin in which it is decreased).
  - Localization by multidetector CT and endoscopic US
- **Treatment :**
  - As most are benign, they are usually treatable.
  - Octreotide and diazoxide are *most effective* agent to control hypoglycemia.
  - Other drugs used are phenytoin, verapamil, prednisone.
  - Non metastatic tumour should be surgically removed after controlling hypoglycemia.
  - For **malignant insulinoma,** Chemotherapeutic agent of choice is streptozocin and doxorubicin.

Glucagonoma, Vipoma, Somatostatinoma and Nonfunctional islet tumours are rare tumors for which refer table.

Pancreatic Endocrine Tumours				
Syndrome	***Hormone(s) Produced***	***Primary Hormone Effects***	***Pathologic Features***	***Clinical Features***
Zollinger-Ellison	Gastrin	Gastric acid hypersecretion	Delta cell islet tumours ; 60% malignant	Severe peptic ulcer disease often refractory to therapy; ectopic ulcers; diarrhoea;
Insulinoma	Insulin	Hypoglycemia with inappropriately increased serum insulin levels	Beta cell islet tumours; 80-90% benign	Hypoglycemic symptoms weight gain
Glucagonoma	Glucagon; pancreatic polypeptide	Hyperglucagonemia →glucose intolerance	Alpha cell islet tumours; 60% malignant	Slow-growing pancreatic tumour; hyperglycemia; eczematoid dermatitis, or necrolytic erythema; weight loss; anemia
Somatostatinoma	Somatostatin; pancreatic polypeptide	Somatostatin inhibits insulin, gastrin, and pancreatic enzyme secretion; decreased bile flow	Delta cell islet tumour	Pancreatic tumour; diarrhoea; steatorrhea; gallstones; diabetes mellitus; anemia
Pancreatic Cholera (MC cause is vipomas)	Vasoactive intestinal peptide, Pancreatic peptide	Net secretion of salt and water by gut	Delta cell tumour; >50% malignant	Pancreatic tumour with severe watery diarrhea; flushing; weight loss; *hypokalemia hypercalcemia; hypochlorhydria; hyperglycemia;* inoordinate fecal water and electrolyte loss.

QUESTIONS

1. In men -1 most common pancreatic islet tumour is : [AI 07]
a. Insulinoma
b. Gastrinoma
c. Glucagonoma
d. Somatostatinoma

2. DOC in zollinger-Ellison syndrome is :
a. Proton pump inhibitors **[AI 07]**
b. H2 blockers
c. Gestrectomy
d. Octreotide

3. In which of the following locations Carcinoid tumour is most common ?
a. Esophagus **[AI 05]**
b. Stomach
c. Small bowel
d. Appendix

4. Which of the following is true regarding carcinoids : [AIIMS 06]
a. Most common site is duodenum
b. Does not cause endocardial fibro-elastosis
c. Increases risk of Ca lung
d. Most common tumor of small intestine

5. A 45-year-old gentleman has undergone truncal vagotomy and pyloroplasty for bleeding duodenal ulcer seven years ago. Now he was intractable recurrent symptoms of peptic ulcer. All of the following suggest the diagnosis of zollinger ellison syndrome, except :
a. Basal acid output of 15 meq/hour
b. Serum gastrin value of 1000 pg/ml
c. Ulcers in proximal jejunum and lower end of esophagus **[AIIMS 06]**
d. Serum gastrin value of 200 pg/ml with secretin stimulation

6. Carcinoid syndrome produces valvular disease primarily involving :
a. Pulmonary valves **[AIIMS 05, 04]**
b. Tricuspid valves
c. Mitral valve
d. Arotic valve

7. For which of the following tumour gastrin is biochemical marker: [AIIMS 05; AI 02]
a. Medullary carcinoma of thyroid
b. Pancreatic neuroendocrine tumour
c. Pheochromocytoma
d. Gastrointestinal stromal tumour

8. Which of the following does'nt occur in patient with gastrinoma : [AIIMS 05]
a. Epigastric pain
b. Diarrhoea
c. Basal acid output (BAO) less than 15 meq/dl
d. Serum gastrin level > 200 pg/ml

9. All of the follwing are features of Zollinger Ellison symdrome except : [AIIMS 05]
a. Intractable peptic ulcers
b. Severe diarrhoea
c. Beta cell tumours of the pancreas
d. Very high acid out put

10. For differentiating between Insulinoma and Sulfonylurea related hypoglycemia, the test which is useful is? [AIIMS 08]
a. Antibody to Insulin
b. Plasma C-peptide level
c. Plasma Insulin level
d. Insulin: Glucose ratio

11. Which of the following can be seen in carcinoid syndrome? [AI '10]
a. Calcification of the ring of tricuspid
b. Intimal thickening
c. Fibrosis of tricuspid valve
d. Causes increased vascularization of tricuspid and pulmonary valves

12. Gold standard test for diagnosis of insulinoma is: [AI '09]
a. 72 hour fast test
b. Plasma glucose levels < 3 mmol/L
c. Plasma insulin level > 6μU/mL
d. Peptide level < 50 p mol/L

13. Gastrinoma leads to : [PGI 05]
a. Diarrhoea
b. Constipation
c. Achlororhydria
d. Multiple gastric ulcers
e. Gasric atrophy

ANSWERS, REFERENCES, EXPLANATIONS WITH INFORMATIVE ILLUSTRATIONS

1. Ans. is b i.e. Gastrinoma *Ref. Devita 8/e, p 1737*

- MEN-1 is an ***autosomal dominant*** trait characterized by hyperplasia or tumor of multiple endocrine organs, with ***hyperparathyroidism being the most common abnormality.***
- Patient with ZES in MEN-1 differ from sporadic cases as they frequently present at a younger age group. Their tumor are almost always multiple, small and usually located in duodenum, and surprisingly they have increased survival.

Pancreatic endocrine tumor associated with MEN

- Pancreatic polypeptide producing (80%)
- Gastrinoma (50%)
- Insulinoma (25%)

2. Ans. is a i.e. Proton pump inhibitors *Ref. Harrison 17/e, p 2354*

Gastrinoma (Zollinger Ellison Syndrome)

- ***Delta*** cell islet tumour.
- Most common ***malignant*** PET, associated with MEN-I.
- Most common ***site*** - ***Duodenum*** > Pancreas (*MC* site in pancreas - Head).
- Most common symptom - ***Abdominal pain.***
- Clinical feature - Abdominal pain > Diarrhoea > GERD.
- **Diagnosis :**
  - ↑ fasting gastrin level (> 1000pg/ml) with ↑ Basal acid output (> 15 meq/h).
  - Secretin stimulation test (Best): If gastrin level < 1000 pg/ml
    - Rise in gastrin level by 200 pg/ml is diagnostic
- **Treatment :** – Proton pump inhibitors (drug of choice) + surgery.
  – For unresectable disease - Streptozocin + 5fu is given.
- Recurrence rate is high after surgery.

3. Ans. is c i.e. Small bowel *Ref. Devita 8/e, p 1723: w.w.w.oncology.com*

Guys ! this was one of the most controversial question of AI-2005 as *except Harrison* all other books *(Bailey, Robbin, Schwartz)* **are going with appendix.**

But let me make you clear, be sure answer of this question is only and only small intestine. Why ?

- Until 1971 (1950-1971 study) – appendix was most common site.
- In study of 1973-1991 – Bronchus / lung becomes the most common site followed by ileum > rectum > appendix.
- ***In latest study 1992-1999 (2003)*** – MC site is :

Bronchus / lung >	Rectum >	ileum >	Colon>	Stomach>	Appendix
25% cases	18% cases	13% cases	7.6% cases	5.8% of cases	2.4% of cases

Mnemonic: BRICS.

Now, we do not think, any one wants to go with appendix.

Remember :
- Most common *site* of carcinoid : Bronchus > rectum > ileum > colon.
- **Site with *best* prognosis : Appendix.**
- **Site with *worst* prognosis or highest incidence of malignancy : pancreas.**
- *Overall* **MC** *site :* **Foregut > midgut > hindgut.**

4. Ans. is d i.e. Most common tumor of small intestine

Ref. Harrison 17/e, p 579; Robbin's 7/e, p 868

- In small intestine adenocarcinoma is the ***MC*** malignant tumor (35-50%) followed by carcinoid tumors (20-40%) but many books mention carcinoid tumor as ***MC*** tumor of SI.
- 50% of SI carcinoids are found in the distal ileum with most congregating close to ileocaecal valve
- **All other options are wrong as :**
  - *Most common* site of carcinoid tumor is bronchus.
  - Carcinoid tumor leads to dense fibrous deposit in endocardium.

5. Ans. is d i.e. Serum gastrin value of 200 pg/ml wil secretin stimulation

Ref. Harrison 17/e, p 2355; Devita 8/e, p 1713

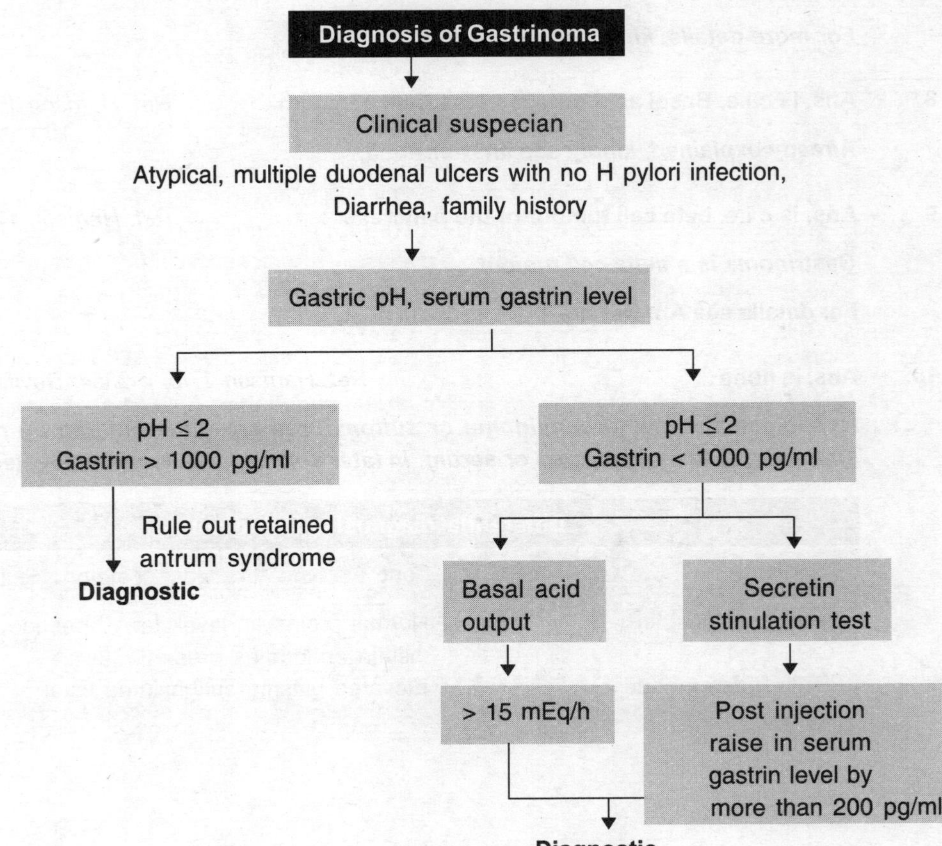

Remember: Other causes of hypergastrinemia with fasting gastrin <1000 pg/ml; Gastric pH ≤ 2:
- Antral G cell hyperplasia/hypergunction
- Gastric outlet obstruction
- Renal failure

6. **Ans. is b i.e. Tricuspid valve** *Ref. Harrison 17/e, p 2351*

"Carcinoid heart disease is due to fibrosis involving the endocardium primarily on the right side, these dense fibrous deposits are most commonly on the ventricular aspect of the tricuspid valve and less commonly on pulmonary valves cusps."

Carcinoid Heart disease :
- Only occur after hepatic metastasis.
- Mostly due to serotonin over production.
- Clinically present as triscupid regurgitation *(MC)*, Pulmonic stenosis or both.
- In left side mitral valve is involved predominantly

7. **Ans. is b i.e. Pancreatic neuroendocrine tumour** *Ref. Harrison 17/e, p 2354*

Gastrin is used as tumour marker for gastrinoma (=Zollinger Ellison syndrome) which is a type of PET.

For more details, kindly see answer no. 2

8. **Ans. is c i.e. Basal acid output < less than 15meq/h** *Ref. Harrison 17/e, p 2354*

Already explained, kindly see answer no. 5

9. **Ans. is c i.e. beta cell tumour of the pancreas** *Ref. Harrison 17/e, p 2354*

Gastrinoma is a delta cell tumour.

For details see Answer no. 2

10. **Ans. is none** *Ref. Harrison 17/e, p 2354; Devita 8/e, 1714*

Hypoglycemia due to insulinoma or sulfonylurea are differentiated by measuring sulfonylurea level in plasma or serum; in later sulfonylurea level is elevated

Differential diagnosis of insulinoma

Condition	Test
Exogenous insulin	Normal proinsulin level, low C-peptide level, insulin antibodies present
Insulin secretagoue (sulfonyl urea)	Elevated plasma sulfonylurea level

Diagnostics criteria of insulinoma

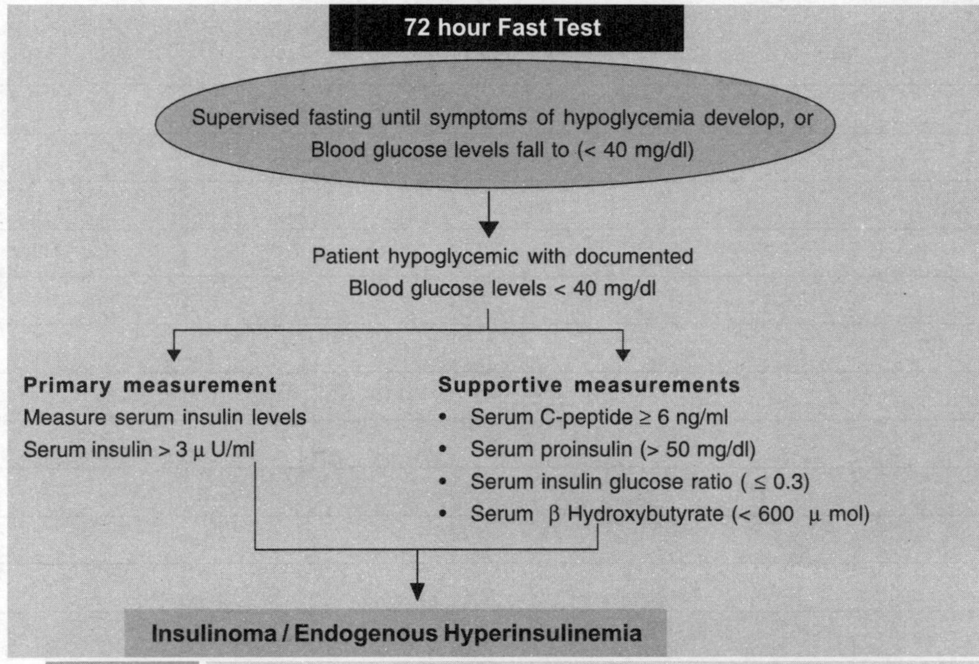

Note:
- Exogenous insulin do not contain C-peptide therefore an elevated insulin with no detectable C-peptide suggest exgenous insulin administration
- In patients taking sulfonylurea, it is endogenous insulin which is secreted. So these patient have an elevated C-peptide level and are most difficult to differentiate

11. Ans. is c i.e. Fibrosis of tricuspid value *Ref. Harrison 17/e, p 2351*

Already explained

12. Ans. is a i.e. 72 How fast test *Ref. Harrison 17/e, p 2354*

Already explained

Remember:

First 24 hours	:	70-80% of patients with insulinoma can be detected
Upto 48 hours	:	98% of patients with insulinoma can be detected
By 72 hours	:	100% of patients with insulinoma can be detected

13. Ans. is a and d i.e. Diarrhoea and Multiple gastric ulcer

Ref. Harrison 15/e, p 1803, 17/e, p 2355

Ulcers in gastrinoma

- Unusual location (***second part of duodenum*** and beyond) in addition to usual location (Stomach and 1st part of duodenum).
- Often ***multiple.***
- ***Refractory*** to standard medical therapy.
- ***Recurrence*** after acid reducing surgery.
- Associated with ***diarrhoea.***

Note : Gastrinoma leads to hypertrophy of acid secreting glands not, atrophy.

NOTES

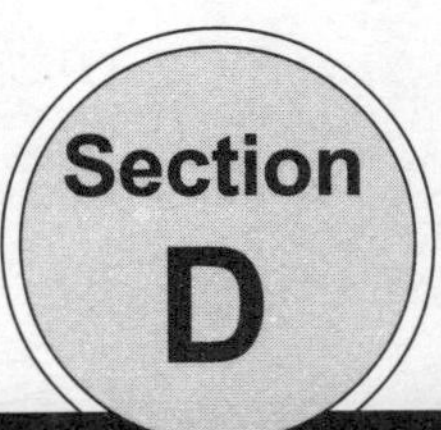

Miscellaneous Oncology

Unit XVIII	Gynaecological Oncology
Unit XIX	Pediatric Tumour
Unit XX	Ophthalmic Tumour
Unit XXI	Miscellaneous

Cervical, Vaginal and Vulval Tumour

What's Important ?

- Etiology and Risk Factors
- Management of CIN and CIS
- Staging and Spread of CA Cervix

CERVICAL INTRAEPITHELIAL NEOPLASIA (CIN)

- ***Disordered growth*** and development of epithelial lining of the cervix.
- *Precancerous lesion* of ca cervix.
- There are various degree of CIN :
  - **CIN I** : Disordered growth in lower third of epithelial lining (= Mild dysplasia).
  - **CIN II** : Abnormal maturation of two third of epithelial lining (= Moderate dysplasia).
  - **CIN III** : Involvement of more than two third of epithelial thickness (= Severe dysplasia).
  - **CIS** : Full thickness dysmaturity with *no basement membrane (stromal) invasion.*
- CIN II and CIN III are described as high grade squamous intraepithelial lesions (HSIL) according to latest *Bethseda classification.* They have propensity to progress and become inasive.

Age : – CIN is most commonly detected in women in their ***20 - 30 years (15 years younger than women with invasive carcinoma)***
– CIS (carcinoma in situ) in ***Age : 25 - 35 years***
– Ca cervix in ***Age : 45 - 55 years.***

Etiology

Risk factors for CIN and cervical cancer are similar and includes :

HPV
- Primary etiologic factor for development of CIN and ca cervix is HPV (Human papilloma virus).
- It is seen in *over 80%* of CIN and > 90% of ca cervix.
- *On basis* of strength of association they are divided in to :
  - ***Low risk group*** : (6, 11, 42, 43, 43) : Associated with condylomata and CIN I.
  - ***Intermediate risk group*** (33, 35, 51 and 52) : Associated high grade lesion (CIN II and CIN III) that tends to persist, but rarely progress.
  - ***High risk group :*** (16, 18, 31, 39, 45, 56, 58, 59, 68) : Associated with high grade lesion that progress to invasive carcinoma.

Remember : Condoms do not prevent transmission of HPV as it can also occur through labioscrotal contact. *... CGDT 10/e, p 834*

Smoking : Smoking and HPV has synergistic effects on development of CIN and invasive ca.

Other risk factor for CIN and ca cervix are :

- *Multiple* sexual partners
- *Early onset* of sexual activity
- *Delivery of first baby before 20 years*
- *Poor hygiene*
- *Immunosuppression*
- *High risk sexual partner* (i.e. ***sexual partner with a history of multiple sexual partner, HPV infection, low genital tract neoplasia, prior sexual exposure to some one with cervical neoplasia).***
- *History of STD (HIV, HSV, HPV)*
- *Multiparity with poor birth spacing*
- *Long term oral contraceptive pill use.*
- ***Note:*** *Women with circumcised sexual partner have lower incidence than uncircumcised partner. This is due to high incidence of HPV in uncircumcised male.*

Pathology

- **Most** CIN and cervical cancer *arise at junction* ***between the primary columnar epithelium of endocervix and the squamous epithelium of ectocervix.***
  - This junction is a site of continuous metaplastic change (Which is greatest in utero *and during 1st pregnancy and declines after menopause).* This junction is in *ectocervix* in 2/3rd of female and in *endocervical canal* in 1/3rd of female. ... *Devita 8/e p 1497*
- Histological changes ranges from nuclear enlargement and hyperchromasia in superficial epithelial layer (CIN) to total replacement of epithelium by immature atypical cells (CIS).

Clinical finding

- There are usually *no symptoms* and signs of CIN and the diagnosis is based on biopsy finding only.
- *Postcoital bleeding* may be the presenting feature in some patient.

Diagnosis

1. Pap Smear

- Pap smear is the *screening test* for diagnosis of ca cervix, CIN.
- Also helpful in detection of *endometrial polyps, endometrial hyperplasia*. It can also detect *actinomycosis* and *Trichomonas infection.*
- A speculum is introduced in vagina after lubricating with water only, it is applied to cervix and rotated 360° to abrade the surface slightly and to pick up cells from squamo columnar area of cervical os.
- A vaginal smear from lateral vaginal wall may be obtained for hormonal evaluation.
- Preservative (ethyl alcohol) is applied immediately to prevent air drying.
- Thin prep automates the preparation of pap smear and decrease the smears showing ASC US (abnormal squamous cells of uncertain significance). ... *CGDT 10/e, p 533*

- **Recommendation :** 2 consecutive smear after onset of sexual activity or > age 20.
  - If negative repeat every 3 years. ... *Harrison 16/e, 557*
- **Normal pap smear** shows *basophilic basal cells, acidophillic superficial cells, endometrial histiocytes, blood cells.*
- *Ascus is the most common finding on PAP smear* ... *Devita 8/e p 1500*

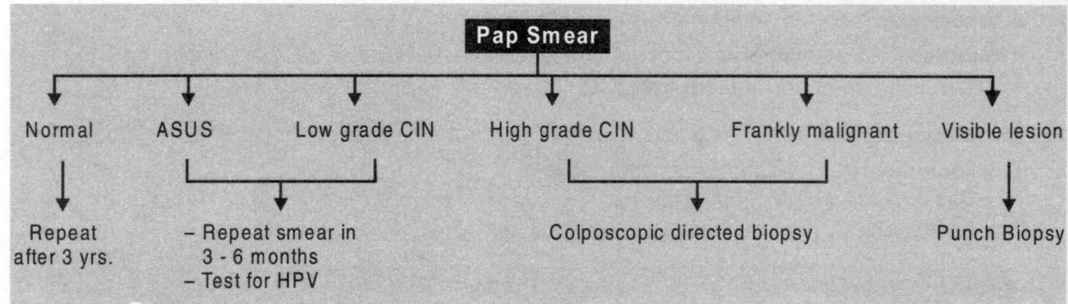

2. **HPV Testing** for detecting HPV infection.
3. **Schiller test :** Based on **principle** that normal mature squamous epithelium of the *cervix contains glycogen,* which combines with iodine to produce deep brown colour.
   - Non staining indicates abnormal squamous epithelium.
4. **Colposcopic examination**
   - Colposcopy is ***primary technique*** for evaluation of an abnormal cervical cytology smear.
   - Colposcope is ***binocular microscope*** which provide magnification of ***13.5***

   Indications for colposcopy are :
   - *Abnormal* cervical cytology *smear* or HPV testing.
   - Clinically abnormal or *suspicious* looking cervix.
   - Unexplained intermenstrual or *postcoital bleeding.*
   - Vulvar or vaginal neoplasia.
   - History of in utero *DES exposure.*

   Abnormal finding indicative of dysplasia are :
   - Leukoplakia or hyperkeratosis
   - Acetowhite epithelium
   - Mosaicism or punctation reflecting abnormal vascular pattern of the surface capillaries
   - Atypical vessels with bizarre capillaries with so called *corkscrew, comma shaped* or *spaghetti* like configuration suggest early stromal invasion.

- ***A colposcopic directed biopsy of severely abnormal areas should be done.***
- It is not indicated if growth is visible.

5. **Diagnostic cone biopsy**
   - **Indications :**
     - Unsatisfactory colposcopy
     - Lesion in cervical canal beyond the view afforded by colposcope
     - Disparency between histologic diagnosis of biopsy specimen and cytologic examination
     - If adenocarcinoma in situ or microinvasive Ca is suspected
   - Cone biopsy can cause bleeding, infection, cervical stenosis and incompetent os

6. **Molecular marker: Ag NOR:** New molecular marker for ca cervix. lesion with low molecular count regress, while those with high count progress

Treatment

Techniques for treatment of CIN are:

a. ***Ablative technique :*** This procedure includes *ablation of abnormal tissue* and *do not produce a tissue specimen* for additional histologic evaluation.

   It includes : – Cryotherapy (not require anaesthesia but a/w copious discharge)
   – Laser ablation with CO_2 laser

b. **Excisional procedure :** Involves *excision of abnormal area* and *allow further histology study.*

   This includes : – *Cold knife conization*
   – *Laser cone excision*
   – *LEEP (Loop electrosurgical, excision procedure)*

Situation	Ectocervical CIN	Endocervical CIN	CIN in Pregnancy	Adeno carcinoma in situ
Treatment	Cryotherapy Laser ablation /	*Deeper Leep /* cone biopsy	Even high grade CIN discovered during pregnancy regress. so *superficial LEEP conization during pregnancy is indicated only when micro-invasion is suspected.*	• Therapeutic conization in young women who wants to retain fertility • Hysterectomy in rest cases

CINI : Treat the infection and follow up Pap test every 3 - 6 months. If persist than ablative procedure done.

- ***LEEP*** is the ***procedure of choice*** for CIN II and CIN III. ... *CGDT 10/e, 840*
- ***CIN II in adolescent:*** *Follow up should be done as spontaneous regression is substantial*

CIS

- Depends on age and associated condition.
- *For age > 40 who have associated fibroid or DUB or patient who can not be followed,* simple vaginal or abdominal hystectomy is procedure of choice.
- For other cases LEEP conization or excisional conization is treatment of choice.

Progression of CIN

Majority of CINI regress, while ***majority of CIN III persist*** and ***progress.***

Fate of CIN

	CIN I	CIN II	CIN III
Regression	60%	40%	30%
Persistence	30%	35%	48%
Progression to cancer	< 1%	5%	22%

CANCER OF CERVIX

- Most common genital cancer in Indian women
- Average age of diagnosis 51 years.

Etiology

- Risk factor for cervical carcinoma are same as for CIN.

Pathogenesis

– HPV is *epitheliotropic*. After integration of HPV genome, their is upregulation of viral oncogene ***E6*** and ***E 7***

E6 and E7 → Forms complex with P53 and Rb
Immortalization→ Downregulation of p53 and Rb

- Carcinoma cervix is *slow developing process.* It takes ***approximately 15 years*** to develop ca cervix from CIN.

Pathology

- 70-75% of cervical carcinomas ***are squamous cell ca,*** rest are a *adenocarcinoma, adenosquamous ca, undifferentiated carcinoma.*

Squamous cell carcinoma

– Most cases *are associated* with ***HPV 16 infection.***
– Further classified into large cell non keratinized *(MC)* large cell Keratinized and small cell carcinoma (worst prognosis).

Verrucous carcinoma

– *Well differentiated* squamous cell ca.
– ***Associated*** with *HPV–6* infection.
– *Slow growing*, locally invasive, ***good prognosis.***

Adenocarcinoma

– Derived from glandular elements of cervix.
– Most cases are associated with ***HPV 18.***
– *Papillary variety* of adenocarcinoma, tends to occur in *younger women.*

Adenoma Malignum

– *Extremely well differentiated* adenocarcinoma.
– Associated with *Peutz jegher syndrome.*

Spread

Direct	Lymphatic	Hematogenous
To parametrium, Vagina, uterus, pelvic side walls	Lymphnodes involved (in order) are : Parametrial, hypogastric, obturator, external iliac and sacral	***Most common*** site of distant metastases is lung and liver *... Devita 8/e, p 1499*

Staging

FIGO staging is used :

FIGO Stage	Definition
Stage 0	Carcinoma in situ
Stage I	Cervical carcinoma confined to the cervix (extension to the corpus would be disregarded)
Stage IA	Invasive cervical cancer diagnosed by microscopy only
Stage IA1	Stromal invasion *no deeper than 3 mm,* no wider than *7 mm* in horizontal spread
Stage IA2	Stromal invasion greater than *3,* but less than *5 mm* & no wider than *7 mm* in horizontal spread
Stage IB	Clinically visible lesion confined to the cervix or microscopic disease greater than stage IA
Stage IB1	Lesion *not greater than 4 cm*
Stage IB2	Lesion *greater than 4 cm*
Stage II	Tumor extends beyond uterus but not to pelvic side wall or lower third of vagina
Stage IIA	Vaginal involvement without parametrial involvement
Stage IIB	Parametrial involvement
Stage III	Tumor extends to pelvic sidewall and/or causes hydronephrosis and/or extends to lower third of vagina
Stage IIIA	Involvement of lower third of vagina with no extension to sidewall
Stage IIIB	Extension to pelvic sidewall and/or hydronephrosis
Stage IV	Extension beyond the true pelvis or into mucosa of rectum or bladder
Stage IVA	Extension into adjacent organs
Stage IVB	Distant metastases

Stage IA is also called as microinvasive carcinoma

Clinical features

- ***Abnormal vaginal bleeding*** is earliest and most common symptom.
- ***Post coital bleeding*** is specific symptom.
- ***Pelvic*** pain, urinary abnormality are seen in advanced cases.

Diagnosis

Biopsy : Colposcopically guided biopsy or direct biopsy *(when tumor is visible).*

Conization : If cervical biopsy shows microinvasive cancer; cone biopsy is necessary to rule out deeper invasion.

Investigations advised in a case of ca cervix are : Complete blood count, Chest X-ray, IVP, MRI, PET *(to demonstrate involvement of pelvic or para aortic lymph nodes).*

Treatment

Stage	Treatment	
	Young women wants to retain fertility	*Rest cases*
1A1 *1A2,* *1B1(small)*	Conization Radical trachelectomy F/b therapeutic lympnadenectomy	Vaginal or abdominal hysterectomy ... *Devita 8/e p 1506* Radical Hysterectomy = Werthims hysterectomy or primary radiation with concomitant chemotherapy
1B2, IIA	Primary radiation therapy with concomitant chemotherapy or Neoadjuvant chemotherapy followed by radical hysterectomy and lymphadenectomy & subsequent chemoradiation (TOC).	Werthims hysterectomy with pelvic lymphadenectomy
II B to IVA	Primary radiation therapy (external beam + brachytherapy) with concomitant chemotherapy	
IV B and Recurrence	Combination chemotherapy (but discouraging)	

Note: – ***In chemotherapy - Cisplatin and 5 Fluorouracil are given in special situation.***
– ***Surgery is preferred in younger women as ovaries can be spared and radiotherapy can cause vaginal stenosis, atrophy***

Indications of adjuvant postoperative radiation in stage IA2 to IIA

- Positive lymph nodes
- Positive or close resection margin
- Microscopic parametrial involvement

Special situation

1. **Ca cervix during pregnancy**
   - Pregnancy do not affect the prognosis of cervical cancer.
   - ***For stage I to IIA -*** Cesarean radical hysterectomy and therapeutic lymphadenectomy as soon as adequate fetal maturity is achieved.
   - ***For higher stage*** treatment same as non pregnant with removal of product of conception.
2. **Carcinoma of cervical stump**
   - Radical trachelectomy and therapeutic lymphadenectomy in the medically fit patient.
   - Upper 2/3rd vaginal cancer show metastasis similar to Ca cervix while lower 1/3 metastasize to inguinal LN like vulvar cancer
3. **Cervical ca incidently diagnosed after simple hysterectomy**
   - ***Microinvasive disease :*** No additional treatment.
   - ***Invasive disease with no gross parametrial involvement :*** Radical parametrectomy, upper vaginectomy and lymphadnectomy.

Prognosis

- The major prognostic factors are : **Stage,** lymphnode status (most important single factor), tumor volume, depth of invasion and to a lesser extent histologic type and grade.
- Most common cause of death are uremia, pulmonary embolism or hemmorhage.

CANCER OF VAGINA

- Very rare, most common ***histologic*** type is ***epidermoid cancer*** (squamous cell ca).
- Most common ***site*** is posterior wall of ***upper third of vagina.***
- Upper 2/3rd vaginal cancer show metastasis similar to Ca cervix, lower 1/rd metastasize to inguinal LN like vulvar cancer.

Treatment : Invasive cancer is primarily treated by external beam and internal radiotherapy. In patient whom coitus is important surgery is considered.

Remember : A tumor should be considered primary vaginal ca only when cervix is uninvolved, otherwise It is classified as cervical ca with vaginal metastasis.

CANCER OF VULVA

- Most common **histologic type** is ***epidermoid (squamous cell ca).***
- Occurs mostly in post menopausal women with poor hygiene.
- ***HPV is strongly associated*** with vulvar ca in younger age group.
- ***Associated disorders*** are vulvar dystrophies, granulomatous veneral disease, diabetes.
- ***Paget's disease*** of vulva is an *intraepithelial lesion* and accounts for *5% of vulvar neoplasm.*
- Main route of **spread** of vulvar ca is direct extension. Primary route of lymphatic spread (which is rare) is to superficial inguinal, deep femoral and external iliac lymph node.
- Primary ***treatment*** is surgical removal of whole of the tumor.

QUESTIONS

1. **A 35 year old female comes with post coital bleeding, next step is: [AIIMS 08, 09]**
   a. A clinical examination and pap smear
   b. Vaginal inspection with acetowhite
   c. Visual inspection with Leyol's iodine
   d. Colposcopy directed biopsy
2. **Virus associated with cancer cervix is:**
   a. HPV b. HIV **[AI 08]**
   c. EBV d. HTLV
3. **Which of the following statements about squamous cell carcinoma of cervix is False: [AI 08]**
   a. Common at squamocolumnar junction
   b. CT scan is mandatory for staging
   c. Post coital bleeding is a early symptom
   d. HPV 16 and 18 are associated with high risk of carcinogenesis
4. **A 35 year old female $P_3 + O$ was found to have CIN grade III on colposcopic biopsy. Which of the following would be best initial management:**
   a. Cryosurgery **[AI 09, AIIMS May 10]**
   b. Conization
   c. LEEP
   d. Hysterectomy
5. **Patient diagnosed as squamous cell intraepithelial lesion which of the following has the highest risk for progression to carcinoma: [AIIMS 07]**
   a. Low grade squamous intraepithelial neoplasia
   b. High grade squamous intraepithelial neoplasia
   c. Squamous intraepithelial Ineoplasia associated with HPV 16
   d. Squamous intraepithelial neoplasia associated with HIV
6. **Papsmear shows Ca in situ. What is the best next logical procedure ? [AIIMS 06]**
   a. Conisation
   b. Colposcopy and Biopsy
   c. Hysterectomy
   d. HPV viral DNA testing
7. **True about Ca Cervix risk factors:**
   a > 90% associated with HPV **[PGI 06]**
   b. Nulliparity
   c. OCP
   d. Immunocompromised patients
8. **True about CIN : [PGI 06]**
   a. Premalignant lesion
   b. HPV predisposes
   c. Pap smear can detect it
   d. Chlamydia infection can predisposes
   e. Occurs at squamo-columnar junction
9. **HPV associated with adenocarcinoma of cervix : [PGI 05]**
   a. Type 6 b. Type 18
   c. Type 11 d. Type 42
10. **In Ca cervix lymphatic spread involves which of the following lymph node/ nodes: [PGI 09]**
    a. Obturator
    b. External iliac
    c. Inguinal lymphnode
    d. Femoral lymphnode
    e. Hypogastric lymphnode
11. **Most common agent associated with Ca. cervix: [AI 10]**
    a. HPV 16 b. HPV 18
    c. HPV 33 d. HPV 35
12. **A 40-year-old woman presenting with CIN III on pap smear treatment of choice?**
    a. Hysterectomy **[AI 10]**
    b. Colposcopy with leep
    c. Trachelectomy
    d. Conization
13. **Presposing Factors for Ca. Cervix:**
    a. Multiple sex partners **[PGI 10]**
    b. Genital wart
    c. HPV 16, 18
    d. Late menarche
14. **Lady undergoes total radical hysterectomy for Stage Ib Ca Cervix. It is found that Ca extends to lower part of body of uterus and upper part of cervix. Next step of management: [AIIMS May 10]**
    a. Chemotherapy
    b. Radiotherapy
    c. Chemoradiotherapy
    d. Follow-up

ANSWERS, REFERENCES, EXPLANATIONS WITH INFORMATIVE ILLUSTRATIONS

1. **Ans. is a i.e. a clinical examination and pap smear**

Ref. Shaw's 14/e, p 364; CGDT 10/e, p 841

Post coital bleeding is one of the specific symptom of cervical carcinoma

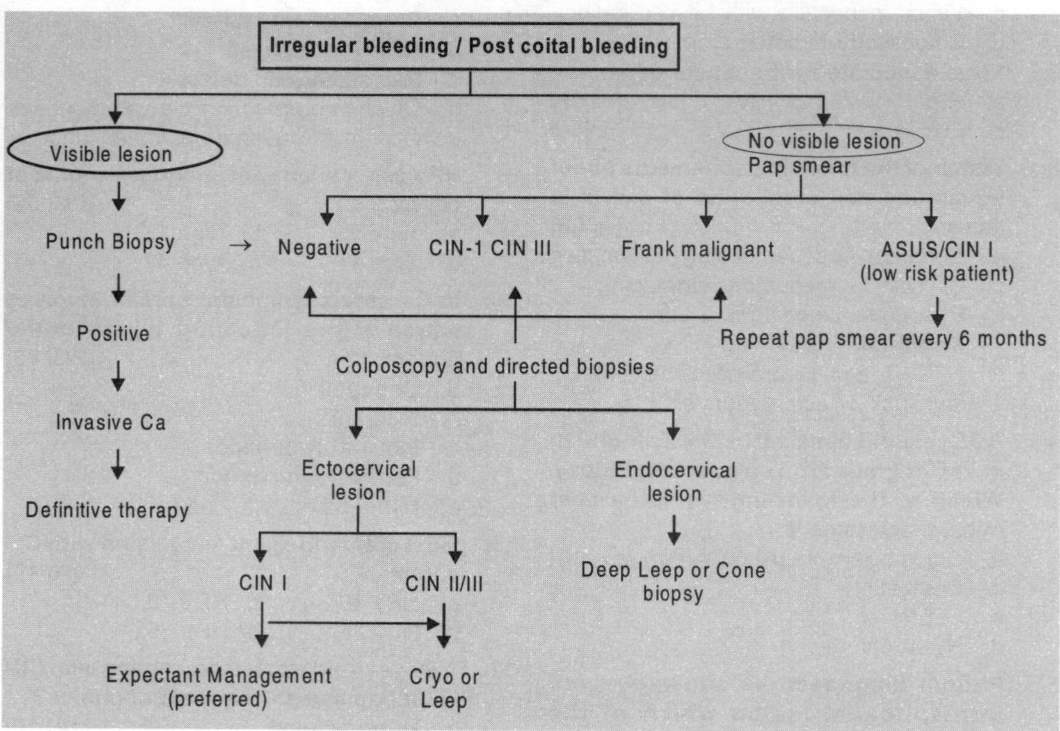

Note: In cases of postmenopausal women with post coital bleeding, pap smear is usually negative. So in these cases colposcopy and biopsy in IOC

2. **Ans. is a i.e. HPV** *Ref. CGDT 10/e, p 843*

HPV is associated with *80% of CIN and over 90% of invasive ca.*

HPV 18 is most common HPV in adenocarcinoma of cervix.

HPV 16 is most common HPV in squamous cell ca.

- On the basis of strength of association to ca cervix HPV has been classified in to :

Low risk type	Intermediate risk	Highrisk
6, 11, 42, 43 Cause CIN I and Condyloma accuminata	33, 35, 55 and 52 Cause CIN II and CIN III that don't progress	16, 18, 31, 39, 45, 56, 48, 59 Cause high grade CIN that progress to invasive Ca

3. **Ans. is b i.e. CT scan is mandatory for staging** *Ref. Devita 8/e, p 1504*

"FIGO specifically states that finding on examinations such as laparoscopy, CT and MRI are of value for planning therapy but as they are not always available and the interpretation of results are variable, So they should not be the basis for clinical stage".

Test required for FIGO staging

Examination	Radiological investigations	Endoscopic procedures	Others
• Detailed gynecological examination including: – Lymph node palpation – Bimanual rectovaginal examination	• Chest X-ray • Skeletal X-ray • IVP	• Colposcopy • Hysteroscopy • Cystoscopy • Proctoscopy	• Biopsy • Endocervical curretage • Rectal or bladder biopsy if proctoscopy or cystoscopy yield positive result

4. **Ans. is c i.e. LEEP** *Ref. Novak's 14/e 582; CGDT 10/e p 840*

"LEEP is the procedure for choice for treating CIN II, CIN III and CIS."

Current recommendation for hysterectomy in CIN
- Recurrency
- Positive margins
- Associated fibroid, DUB or prolapse
- If microinvasion is suspected
- Adnocarcinoma in situ who have completed their families
- For older women and women who can not be followed represent relative indication for hysterectomy

Note: For squamous carcinoma in situ (CIS) treatment of choice is LEEP conization or excisional conization. Hysterectomy is recommended only for above indications

5. **Ans. is b i.e. High grade squamous intraepithelial neoplasia**
Ref. CGDT 10/e, p 833

High grade squamous intraepithelial lesion (HSIL) is a term used in latest Bethseda classification. HSIL include CIN II and CIN III which have propensity to progress and become invasive.

In *Bethseda system* the cytological smear are evaluated histologically

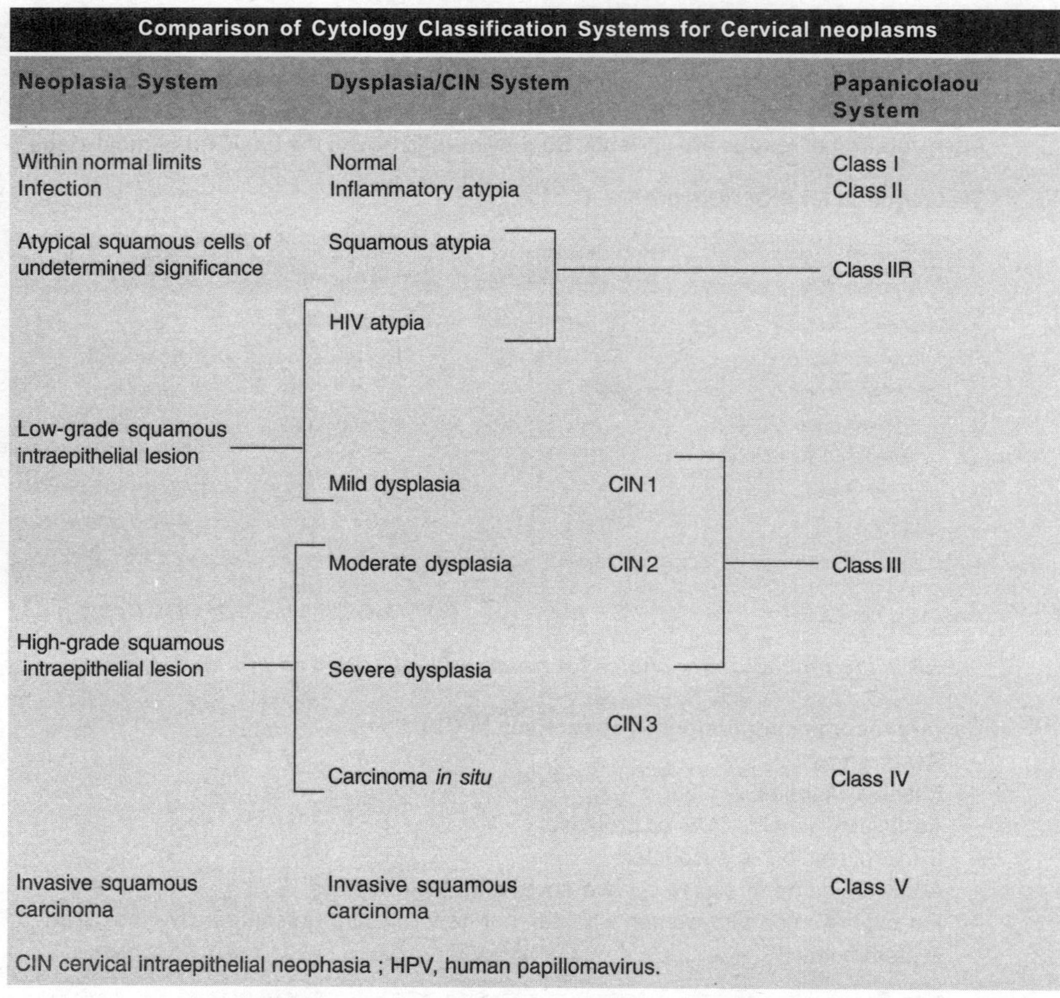

Comparison of Cytology Classification Systems for Cervical neoplasms

Neoplasia System	Dysplasia/CIN System		Papanicolaou System
Within normal limits	Normal		Class I
Infection	Inflammatory atypia		Class II
Atypical squamous cells of undetermined significance	Squamous atypia		Class IIR
	HIV atypia		Class IIR
Low-grade squamous intraepithelial lesion	HIV atypia; Mild dysplasia	CIN 1	Class III
High-grade squamous intraepithelial lesion	Moderate dysplasia	CIN 2	Class III
	Severe dysplasia	CIN 3	Class III
	Carcinoma *in situ*	CIN 3	Class IV
Invasive squamous carcinoma	Invasive squamous carcinoma		Class V

CIN cervical intraepithelial neophasia ; HPV, human papillomavirus.

6. **Ans. is b i.e. Colposcopy and Biopsy** *Ref. Shaw's 14/e, p 362*

Colposcopy and biopsy is indicated whenever pap smear shows abnormal area

Indication for Colposcopy

- Abnormal pap smear cytology
- To locate the abnormal areas
- To obtain biopsy
- Conservative therapy under colposcopic guidance
- Follow up of cases treated conservatively.

Indications of Cone biopsy

- If there is significant ***disparency*** between Colposcopic biopsy and the cytologic examination.
- If colposcopy is ***unsatisfactory.***
- If lesion extends to cervical canal beyond the view afforded by the colposcope i.e. ***endocervical*** lesion.

- As ***treatment*** of high grade CIN (CIN III)
- If an adenocarcinoma in ***situ*** or microinvasive ca is suspected.

***Mnemonic :* DUET S**inger

Contraindication : Gross visible lesion suggestive of invasive cancer as it predisposes the patient to serious pelvic infections and bleeding.

7. **Ans. is a, c and d i.e. > 90% associated with HPV; OCP; and Immunocompromised patients** *Ref. Shaws 14/e, p 359*

HPV DNA is found in 99.7% of all cervical carcinoma. ... COGDT 10/e p 843

Etiology and Risk factors for CIN and Ca-cervix

– HPV infection	– Smoking	– Delivery of first baby before age of 20 years
– Early onset of sexual activity	– Multiple sexual partners	
– History of STD	– High risk sexual partner	– Poor personal hygeine
– Multi parity	– Long term OCP use	– Poor socioeconomic status
– HSV-2 infection	– Immunodefciency (HIV)	

8. **Ans. is a, b, c and e i.e. Premalignant lesion; HPV predisposes; Pap smear can detect it; and Occurs at squamo-columnar junction** *Ref. Shaw's 14/e, p 359*

CIN (Cervical Intraepithelial Neoplasia)

- CIN refers to the histopathological entity in which a part or the full thickness of the stratified squamous epithelium is replaced by the cells showing various degree of dysplasia, however the basement membrane is intact.
- Most CIN arise at squamocolumnar junctions.
- Risk factors are same as for Ca cervix.
- **Diagnosis :**

– PAP smear	– Schiller test
– HPV testing	– Colopscopy
– Cone biopsy	

9. **Ans. is b i.e. Type 18** *Ref. CGDT 10/e, p 843*

Already explained.

10. **Ans. is a, b and e i.e. Obturator; External iliac; and Hypogastric lymphnode** *Ref. Devita 8/e 1498*

Lymphatic spread of Ca cervix.

Cervix has rich supply of lymphatics that drain the mucosal, mucularis and serosal layers. The lymphatic trunks exit laterally from uterine isthmus in ***three group :***

- Upper branch – Originates in anterior and lateral cervix, terminates in the uppermost hypogastric nodes.
- Middle branch – Drain to deeper hypogastric and obturator nodes.
- Lowest branch – Drain to external iliac and sacral nodes.

Additional posterio lymphatic channels arising from posterior cervical wall *drain to superior rectal nodes or may continue upward in to the subaortic nodes.*

Ca cervix follow orderly progression i.e. involve initially primary nodes in pelvis then to paraaortic nodes.

Other modes of Spread :

Direct	–	To parametrium, vagina, uterus, pelvic side walls.
Hematogenous	–	*Most common* site are lung and liver.

11. Ans. is a i.e. HPV 16 *....Ref. Robbins 8/e, p 1024*

HPV 16 is the most common HPV seen in cervical cancer.

Refer answer no. 2 for details

12. Ans. is b i.e. Colposcopy with LEEP *....Ref. Novak's 14/e, p 582; COGDT 10e/ p 840*

Already explained see answer no. 4

13. Ans. is a, b, c Multiple sex partners, Genital wart, HPV 16, 18

....Ref. Shaws 14/e, p 359

Already explained

14. Ans. is c i.e. Chemoradiotherapy *..... COGDT 10/e p 848*

Postoperative adjuvant radiation therapy with concomitant chemotherapy is indicated in women with localized cervical cancer at high risk for recurrent disease, such as

- Positive lymph node
- Positive or close resection margin
- Microscopic parametrial involvement
- ***In this setting adjuvant radiation with platinum based chemotherapy is superior to radiation alone.***

37 Uterine Tumour

What's Important ?

- Predisposing Factor
- Spread
- Staging
- Treatment

ENDOMETRIAL CARCINOMA

- Endometrial Ca is the most common *pelvic genital cancer in woman in world*
- Peak incidence is 6th and 7th decade.
- Most common type Adenocarcinoma. *... CGDT 10/e, p 855*

Etiology and Risk factors

Chronic estrogenic stimulation (Endometrial hyperplasia)	Associated illness	Personal factors	Drugs
– Estrogen replacement (no progestin) – Early menarche / late menopause – Nulliparity – Anovulation – Estrogen secreting tumors	– Diabetes mellitus – PCOD – Obesity – Hypertension – Hypertension – Prior pelvic radiotherapy – HNPCC syndrome	– Increasing age (Postmenopausal women) – White > Blacks – High Socioeconomic status – Family history	– Tamoxifen

Thus, ***Endometrial Ca classically affect obese, nulliparous, infertile, hypertensive and diabetic white woman.***

Remember :
- Combined oral contraceptive pills protect against endometrial carcinoma.
- Progesterone has an antiproliferative effect on endometrium and can induce apoptosis of endometrial cells.

Pathology

On the basis of pathogenesis endometrial carcinoma **can be of two type:**

Type 1: Characterized by exposure to unopposed estrogen. Usually arise after endometrial hyperplasia and are slow growing with well differentiation and good prognosis.

Type 2: Unrelated to hormonal exposure and commonly arise in setting of atrophic endometrium. Tumor show rapid progression and has poor prognosis

Endometrial hyperplasia

This occur mostly in association with hyperestrogenic state.

This is classified into :

1. ***Simple hyperplasia with out atypia.*** There is only crowding of cell without nuclear atypia. Also called as cystic hyperplasia, glands are cystically dilated and gives swiss cheese appearance.
   - Only 1% of cases progress to cancer.
2. ***Complex hyperplasia without atypia*** (Adenomatous hyperplasia).
   - Complex crowded appearance of glands with very little intervening stroma.
   - Progression to cancer is seen in 3–5% of cases.
3. ***Hyperplasia with atypia :*** Characterized by endometrial glands lined by enlarged cells with increased N : C ratio. It can be complex or simple.

   Progression to cancer occur in 8% & 29% of simple atypical and complex atypical hyperplasia respectively.

Histological types

• *Adenocarcinoma*	– *Most common* type of endometrial ca.
• *Squamous differentiation*	– Very well differentiated ***least malignant.***
• *Serous carcinoma*	– Occur in older women and with other risk factors. – Have propensity for ***lymphatic invasion.*** – Prognosis is unfavorable and patient should be treated similar to that of patient with ovarian tumor.
• *Clear cell carcinoma*	– Occurs in older women or younger women with history of in ***utero DES exposure.*** – Aggressive highly malignant and have ***worst prognosis.***
• *Miscellaneous types*	– Include mucinous carcinoma; squamous cell Ca (occur in association with cervical stenosis; pyometra and chronic inflammation).

Spread

Endometrial cancer can spread by four possible routes :

- **Direct extension :** Tumour extends to involve whole endometrial surface and extends to lower uterine segment and cervix. Invasion of myometrium with involvement of bladder, colon, adnexa.
- **Lymphatics :**
  - Uterus has rich lymphatic network.
  - Lymphatics from ***superior portion*** of fundus drain to paraaortic lymph nodes.
  - Lymphatics from ***middle and lower portion*** pass to external iliac nodes.
  - Lymphatics from ***lower uterine segment*** pass to external iliac, internal iliac and sacral nodes.
  - Few lymphatics from ***fundus*** pass through round ligament to superficial inguinal nodes.
- **Peritoneal implants :** Occurs due to transtubal spread.
- **Hematogenous :** Lung, liver and brain.

Clinical presentation

- ***Abnormal vaginal bleeding*** is most common presenting symptom.
- *Lower abdominal pain* secondary to uterine contractions.
- Severe cramps from hematometra or pyometra.

Remember :
- Endometrial Ca is associated with 12-15% cases of postmenopausal bleeding in 50-60 age group and 50%-60% of cases after the age of 80.
- Diagnosis of endometrial carcinoma should be considered in postmenopausal woman with any vaginal bleeding and premenopausal women with abnormal bleeding pattern who are obese and oligoovulatory.

Dignosis

1. ***Fractional curettage :***
   Dilation and fractional curettage is the definitive procedure for diagnosis of endometrial carcinoma.
   - *Should be performed in all cases with post menopausal bleeding.*
   - Perforation of uterus followed by intraperitoneal contamination with malignant cell is a common compliction and can be avoided by gentle surgical technique.
2. ***Endometrial biopsy :***
   - Can be performed in out patient settings by giving paracervical block.
     a. Aspiration biopsy
     b. Aspiration curettage – Most accurate out patient method for *evaluating endometrial ca*.
3. ***Pelvic Ultrasonography :***
   - To evaluate the size and thickness of uterus.
   - Post menopausal endometrium thickness > 5 mm is abnormal.
4. ***Estrogen and progestrone receptor assay :***
   - For planning adjuvant hormonal therapy.
   - Receptor content are inversely proportional to histologic grade.
5. ***Tumour marker :***
   - CA - 125 tumor marker of epithelial ovarian Ca can also be used for endometrial ca.
6. ***Other:***
   - CT for bowel and omental metastasis. MRI for myometrial and nodal involvement, Chest X-ray

Staging

Staging of endometrial Ca is done ***after surgical exploration***, ***grading*** is done by ***histopathology*** of tissue specimen.

FIGO Staging	
Stage I	Stage Ia G123 Tumour ***limited*** *to endometrium* Stage Ib 123 Invasion to ***less than*** *one-half the myometrium* Stage Ic G123 Invasion to ***more than*** *one-half the myometrium.*
Stage II	Stage IIa G123 *Endocervical glandular involvement only.* Stage IIb G123 *Cervical stromal invasion*

Stage III	Stage IIIa G 123 Tumour ***invades serosa*** and/or adenexa, and/or positive peritoneal cytology. Stage IIIb G123 Vaginal metastases Stage IIIc G123 Metastasis to pelvic and / or paraaortic lymph nodes
Stage IV	Stage IVa G 123 Tumour i***nvades bladder and/or bowel mucosa*** Stage IVb ***Distant metastases*** including intra-abdominal and/or inguinal lymph nodes.
FIGO Grading	
Grade I ***Grade II*** ***Grade III***	Tumors have less than ***5%*** of non squamous solid growth pattern. Tumor contain ***6-50%*** of non squamous solid growth pattern. Tumor with more than ***50%*** of solid growth pattern.

Treatment

TAH + BSO, peritoneal washing, omental biopsy and node sampling is the basic treatment, if possible.

Stage O *(Ca in situ)*	– Hysterectomy with or without B/ L salpingoopherectomy (BSO) for older women. – ***Progestin therapy / Mirena IUCD for Younger women***
Stage 1 A Grade I / II	– Total abdominal hysterectomy with or without B/L salpingo-oophorectomy.
Stage IB / IC / IA Grade III	– Same treatment as in grade I and Grade II followed by post-operative pelvic irradiation.
Stage II	– Pelvic *irradiation* (Brachytherapy) followed by TAH + BSO. External radiotherapy if nodes are positive. Wertheim's Hysterectomy is alternative.
Stage III	– Chemotherapy and Radio therapy.
Stage IV	– *Palliative* radiotherapy, chemotherapy and progesterone.

- **Progesterone therapy :** Medroxyprogesterone acetate (oral) and hydroxy progesterone caproate (parenteral) are used.
- **Chemotherapy :** Doxorubicin and cisplatin are most active agents.

Vaginal recurrence : *Excision followed by progesterone therapy if receptor assay is positive.*

- **Emergency measuores**

  Patient with endometrial Ca may present in emergency with :

  – Bleeding : ***Treatment is high dose radiation*** or ***embolization.***

  – Pyometra : High dose of broad spectrum antibiotic followed by gentle fraction curettage.

Prognostic factors

Major prognostic factors associated are : grade or cell type, depth of myometrial invasion and tumour extension to the cervix.

UTERINE SARCOMA

Accounts for 10% of uterine neoplasm.

Types

- ***Leiomyosarcoma*** – Most common
- ***Malignant mixed mullerian tumor (MMT)*** = Carcinosarcomas – *Mixture of carcinoma and sarcoma.* Serous carcinoma mixed with endometrial sarcoma is the most common histologic type.
- ***Adenosarcoma***
- ***Endometrial stromal sarcoma.***

Spread

Lymphatic permeation and ***contiguous*** spread are most common method.

Clinical features

Occur at any age but ***most prevalent*** after 40.

Abnormal bleeding is most common manifestation.

Chest X-ray may show coin lesion characteristic of uterine sarcoma. ... *CGDT 9/e, p 929*

Treatment

- ***Surgery*** is the primary modality of treatment.
- ***Radiation*** is used for emergency measures such as hemorrhage.
- ***Prognosis*** is very poor.

QUESTIONS

1. **Investigation of choice in a 55 years old post menopausal woman who has presented with postmenopausal bleeding : [AI 06, 98]**
   a. Pap smear
   b. Fractional Curettage
   c. Transvaginal ultrasound
   d. CA - 125 estimation

2. **The risk of endometrial carcinoma is the highest with the following histological pattern of endometrial hyperplasia: [AIIMS 06]**
   a. Simple hyperplasia without atypia
   b. Simple hyperplasia with atypia
   c. Complex hyperplasia without atypia
   d. Complex hyperplasia with atypia

3. **The following are indications for post operative radiotherapy in a case of carcinoma endometrium except :**
   a. Myometrial invasion of more tha half thickness **[AIIMS 05, 04]**
   b. Positive lymph nodes
   c. Endocervical involvement
   d. Tumor positive for estrogen receptors

4. **The risk of complex hyperplasia of endometrium with atypia progressing to malignancy in a postmenopausal woman is : [AIIMS 05, 04]**
   a. 3%
   b. 8%
   c. 15%
   d. 28%

5. **Stage III B endometrial Ca shows :**
   a. Vaginal metastasis **[PGI 06]**
   b. Lymph nodal metastasis
   c. Bowel involvement
   d. Lung metastasis

6. **Indication of adjuvant radiotherapy in Ca endometrium is/ are : [PGI 05]**
   a. Cervical involvement
   b. Lymph node involvement
   c. Carcinoma in situ
   d. Papillary serous tumor
   e. Estrogen receptor positive

7. **Indication for radiotherapy in carcinoma endometrium include all except :**
   a. Pelvic node involvement **[AIIMS 07]**
   b. Deep myometrial involvement
   c. Enlarged uterine cavity
   d. Poor differentiation

8. **Stage-IIIB endometrial carcinoma true is/ are: [PGI 09]**
   a. Vaginal metastasis
   b. Lymph node metastatis (paraaortic)
   c. Pelvic lymph node involvement
   d. Positive peritoneal cytology
   e. Rectal invasion

9. **True about endometrial carcinoma in clinical stage III:**
   a. Vaginal metastatis **[PGI 10, 09]**
   b. Para aortic lymph node involvement
   c. Pelvic lymph node invlvement
   d. Peritoneal lymph node involvement
   e. Inguinal lymph node involvement

10. **All are the risk factor for endometrial carcinoma except: [PGI 09]**
    a. Multiparity
    b. Obesity
    c. Early menopause
    d. Unopposed estrogen therapy
    e. Hypertension

ANSWERS, REFERENCES, EXPLANATIONS WITH INFORMATIVE ILLUSTRATIONS

1. **Ans. is b i.e. Fractional curettage** *Ref. Shaw's 14/e, p 874; COGDT 10/e p 860*

Diagnosis of endometrial carcinoma should be considered in postmenopausal woman with any vaginal bleeding and premenopausal women with abnormal bleeding pattern who are obese and oligoovulatory.

Fractional curettage

Dilation and fractional curettage is the definitive procedure for diagnosis of endometrial ca.

- *Should be performed in all cases with post menopausal bleeding.*
- *Separate samples from uterine body and endocervix should be taken.*

Endometrial biopsy

Can be performed in out patient settings :

a. Aspiration biopsy
b. Aspriation curretage – Most accurate out patient method for *evaluating endometrial ca.*

... COGDT 9/e, p 921

Remember : Endometrial carcinoma is one of the common cause of post menopausal bleeding.

2. **Ans. is d i.e. Complex hyperplasia with atypia** *Ref. COGDT 10/e, p 855 - 857*

Edometrial Hyperplasia

- It is a benign condition which may produce symptoms indistinguishable from endometrial Ca.
- Usually associated to hyperestrogenic state.
- Though reversible they are considered premalignant.

Types : They are classified as simple or complex and with or with out atypia.

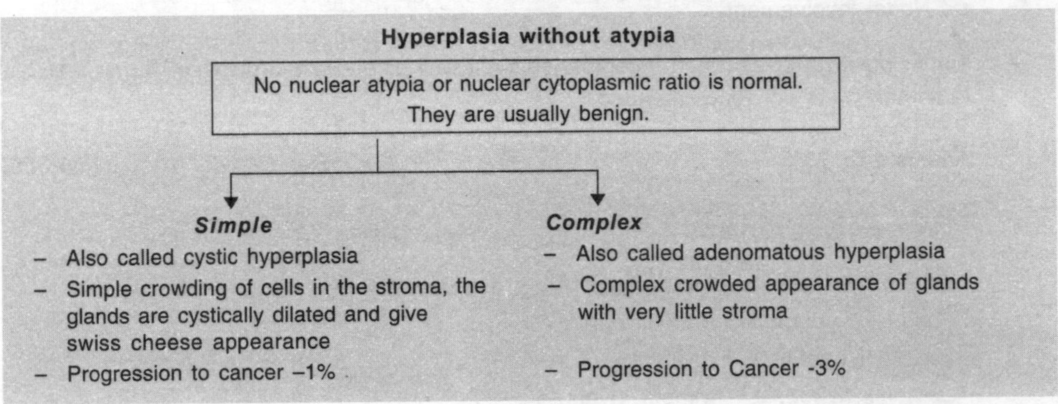

Contd...

Contd...

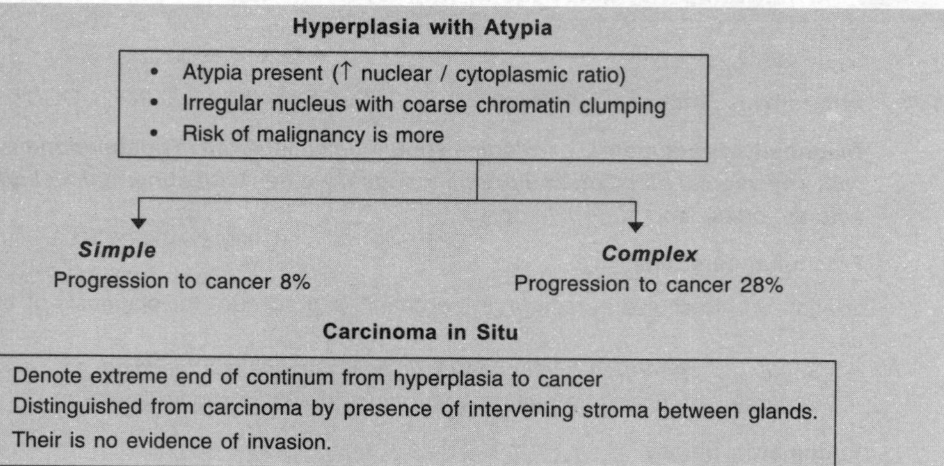

Carcinoma in Situ

- Denote extreme end of continum from hyperplasia to cancer
- Distinguished from carcinoma by presence of intervening stroma between glands. Their is no evidence of invasion.

Clinical feature : Present as abnormal bleeding, so endometrial sampling and fractional curretage are always necessary to rule out co-existing carcinoma.

Treatment :

- Treatment initially with progestin therapy.
- In peri and postmenopausal women who relapse after progestin therapy or who can not tolerate its side effect, hysterectomy is recommended.

3. **Ans. is d i.e. Tumor positive for estrogen receptors** *Ref. COGDT 9/e, p 924*

Indication of Adjuvant radiotherapy

- Extrauterine extension.
- Lower uterine or cervical involvement.
- Papillary serous or clear cell histology.
- Poor histologic differentiation (Grade III).
- Myometrial penetration greater than 1/3rd of thickness.
- Nodal involvement.

Tumor positive for estrogen receptors suggest well differentiated disease, So no adjuvant radiotherapy is not recommended.

4. **Ans. is d i.e. 28%** *Ref. COGDT 10/e, p 855 - 857*

Endometrial hyperplasia	Risk of progression
Simple hyperplasia without atypia	1%
Complex hyperplasia without atypia	3%
Simple hyperplasia with atypia	8%
Complex hyperplasia without atypia	28%

5. **Ans. is a i.e. Vaginal Metastasis** *Ref. COGDT 10/e, p 856*

Stage IIIb includes vaginal metastasis while metastasis to pelvic or paraaortic lymph nodes comes in stage IIIc.

6. **Ans. is a, b and d i.e. Cervical involvement; Lymphnode involvement; and Papillary serous tumor** *Ref. COGDT 9/e, p 924*

Already explained

7. **Ans. is c i.e. Enlarged uterine cavity** *Ref. COGDT 10/e p 862*

Already explained

8. **Ans. is a, d i.e. Vaginal metastasis, Positive peritoneal cytology**
Ref. COGDT 10/e p 856

Stage IIIb include vaginal metastasis, positive peritoneal cytology is seen is stage IIIa

Other Options

- Invasion of bowel mucosa : stage IV a.
- Lymphatic involvement (both pelvic and intra-abdominal) : Stage IV b

9. **Ans. is a i.e. Vaginal metastasis** *Ref. COGDT 10/e p 856*

Already explained

10. **Ans. is a, c, e i.e. Multiparity, Early menopause**

Ref. Shaws 14/e p 373, 374

Etiology and risk factors of endometrial carcinoma			
Chronic estrogenic stimulation (Endometrial hyperplasia)	**Associated illness**	**Personal factors**	**Drugs**
– Estrogen replacement (no progestin) – Early menarche / late menopause – Nulliparity – Anovulation – Estrogen secreting tumors	– Diabetes mellitus – PCOD – Obesity – Hypertension – Hypertension – Prior pelvic radiotherapy – HNPCC syndrome	– Increasing age (Postmenopausal women) – White > Blacks – High Socioeconomic status – Family history	– Tamoxifen

Ovarian Tumour

What's Important ?

- Classification
- Staging
- Tumour Markers
- Germ Cell Tumour and Sex Cord Stromal Tumours

- Tumors of ovary are common forms of neoplasia in women.
- Ovary is the site of both benign and malignant tumour, benign tumour tends to arise in middle age group and malignant tumours affect older women or children.

CLASSIFICATION

A. Surface Epithelial-Stromal Tumors	***B. Sex Cord-Stromal Tumors***	***C. Germ Cell Tumors***
Serous tumours Benign (cystadenoma) Cystadenoma of borderline malignancy Malignant (serous cystadeno-carcinoma) *Mucinous tumours* Benign Of borderline malignancy Malignant *Epithelial-stromal* Adenosarcoma Mesodermal (mullerian) mixed tumour *Clear cell tumours* Benign Of borderline malignancy Malignant *Transitional cell tumours* Brenner tumour Brenner tumour of borderline malignancy Malignant Brenner tumour Transitional cell carcinoma (non-Brenner type) *Endometroid (benign, borderline, malignant)*	*Granulosa-stromal cell tumours* Granulosa cell tumours Tumors of the thecoma-fibroma group *Sertoli-stromal cell tumours*; androblastomas *Sex cord tumour with annular tubules* *Gynandroblastoma* *Steroid (lipid) cell tumours*	*Teratoma* Immature Mature (adult) Solid Cystic (dermoid cyst) Monodermal (e.g., struma ovarii, carcinoid) *Dysgerminoma* *Yolk sac tumour* (endodermal sinus tumour) *Mixed germ cell tumours*

D. Malignant, Not Otherwise Specified

E. Metastatic Nonovarian Cancer (from Nonovarian Primary)

ETIOLOGY AND RISK FACTORS

Exact cause unknown, but risk is increased by :

- ***Repeated ovulation*** : Chronic anovulation, multiparity and history of breast feeding are protective (pregnancy is associated with a risk reduction of 13-19% per pregnancy).
- ***Polycystic ovarian syndrome*** : Increase risk by 2.5 times.
- ***Unopposed estrogen therapy*** – Increase risk of endometriod and epithelial tumours of ovary.
- Increased ***intake of saturated animal fats and alcohol.***
- ***Turner syndrome*** (increase risk of dysgerminoma and gonadoblastoma).
- ***Breast ovarian cancer syndrome*** (due to mutation of BRCA1 or BRCA2).
- ***HNPCC syndrome***.
- *Talc application on external genitalia*

Remember : Use of oral contraceptive decrease the risk of ovarian cancer by 50% for users of 5 years and longer.

Cytogenetics

Cytogenetic abnormality associated with *ovarian cancer are :*

- BRCA 1 and BRCA 2 mutation
- P - 53 mutation (Most common)
- HER 2 / neu mutation

PATHOLOGY

Epithelial neoplasms

Epithelial neoplasms are ***derived from the ovarian surface mesothelial cells*** and include 6 cell types :

– Serous	– Mucinous	– Endometroid
– Clear cell	– Transistional cell	– Undifferentiated

1. **Serous tumour :**
   - Present as cystic lesion; can be *either benign or malignant.*
   - They are MC epithelial tumour of ovary.
   - ***Serous cystadenocarcinoma*** are MC ***malignant tumour of ovary.*** ... *CGDT 10/e, p 872*
   - 60% of serous tumours are ***benign*** (cystadenoma); 15% ***borderline*** and 25% are ***malignant.***
   - *Benign cystadenoma is reported in younger age group. While serous cystadenocarcinoma occur more frequently with advancing age.* But they are associated with good prognosis.
   - *10-15%* of *cystadenoma* and *40-60%* of *cystadenocarcinoma* are bilateral.
   - ***Morphologically*** cystadenoma *present with a smooth glistening cyst* wall *with no epithelial thickening* or with small papillary projections.
   - Large amount of solid or papillary irregularity in the tumour mass and fixation or nodularity of the capsule are indicators of malignancy.
   - Histological examination show Psammoma bodies and lamellar calcification.
   - Serous tumour is ***classified as malignant*** only when nuclear atypia exceeds 4 cell layer thickness or stromal invasion occurs. *... Shaw's 14/e, p 334*

2. **Mucinous tumour :**
   - Mucinous tumours are multiloculated cyst lined by epithelium resembling the endocervix.

- Accounts for *20-25%* of all ovarian tumours and are the second most common type of epithelial tumours.
- Occur principally in ***middle age*** (30-50 years) and are notable for large size that they may attain.
- 85% of mucinous tumour are ***benign*** and 15% are ***malignant*** (mucinous cystadeno-carcinoma), ***bilaterality*** is observed in 10-15% of cases.
- Cut surface show multiloculi and honey combed ***appearance.***
- Pseudomyxoma peritonei may occur in ***associated with mucinous neoplasms*** of the ovary. Usually in lesions of low malignant potential.

3. **Endometriod tumour :**
   - Account for 10% of all ovarian cancer.
   - ***Most*** endometroid tumours are ***malignant*** and are *lined by glandular epithelium resembling the endometrium.*
   - Tumour is ***bilateral*** in 30-50% of cases and in 30% of patients coexisting endometriosis is also found.

4. **Clear cell carcinoma = Mesonephroid tumour :**
   - ***Aggressive*** tumour accounting for 1% of epithelial ovarian cancer.
   - Associated with ***hyperpyrexia*** and ***hypercalcemia*** (due to aggressive growth).
   - Histologically two cells are found - clear cells and hobnail cells.
   - Differentiated from mucinous neoplasm by periodic acid Schiff reaction.

5. **Brenner tumour =Transitional cell tumour**
   - Brenner tumour are uncommon solid fibroepithelial tumour accounting for < 1% of all ovarian neoplasms.
   - Mostly ***unilateral.***
   - Histologically tumour shows Walthard cell nest of transitional cells, cells have coffee bean nuclei.
   - Prognosis is poor.

6. **Undifferentiated Carcinoma :**
   - Account for < 10% of epithelial neoplasm.

Germ cell tumour

- Arise from germ cell element of the ovary.
- In contrast to other tumours of body, benign germ cell tumour tends to occur in middle and elder age group, while malignant ones have predilection for younger age group.It includes :

1. **Teratoma - Dermoid (Mature cystic teratoma) :**
   - Most common germ cell neoplasm.
   - On the basis of maturity they are divided into :
     a. ***Mature (Benign) teratoma = dermoid cyst***
        – Most common *benign tumour of ovary* in reproductive age group.
        – Most common neoplasm diagnosed during pregnancy.

- *Bilateral* in 10% to 15% of cases.
- Characteristically they are unilocular cyst containing hair and cheesy sebaceous material, teeth, bones, thyroid cartilage.
- About *1% of the dermoids undergoes malignant transformation* of one of the component element (e.g., thyroid carcinoma, melanoma, but most commonly squamous cell ca).

b. *Immature (Malignant) teratoma*

- Rare, mostly solid, differ from benign teratomas in the component tissue which resembles that observed in the fetus or embryo rather than mature adult tissue.
- Tumour occur *chiefly in prepubertal adolescents* and young women.
- Tumour grade is correlated with prognosis and extraovarian spread.

c. *Monodermal or specialized teratomas = (Struma ovarii and carcinoid)*

- Rare group of tumour, struma ovarii composed entirely of mature thyroid tissue which is hyperfunctional.
- Patients usually present with hyperthyroidism.
- Most of the tumours are innocent, but *malignant thyroid tumour* have been recorded.

2. Dysgerminoma :

- Most common ***malignant germ cell tumour***.
- Ovarian counter part of the seminoma of testis.
- Usually arise in ***young women or in childhood,*** with an average age 20 years.
- Risk is more in patient with *gonadal dysgenesis*.
- All dysgerminomas are ***malignant*** and develop as ***unilateral*** (in 80 to 90%) solid lesion of variable size.
- Histologically, dysgerminoma, mimics the pattern of primitive gonad, lymphocytic invasion may be seen which is a good prognostic indicator.

3. Endodermal sinus tumour = Yolk sac tumour :

- 3rd most common malignant tumour of germ cell origin. It is always bilateral.
- Mostly affect ***children or young adults***.
- ***Grows rapidly*** and aggressively, patient commonly presents with acute abdomen.
- Pathognomonic histologic finding is schiller - Duval bodies, which is single papilla lined by tumour cells.

Remember : Endodermal sinus tumour is most rapidly growing neoplasm that occurs at any site. ... *CGDT 10/e p 875*

4. Embryonal carcinoma :

- Very rare, but ***highly malignant*** tumour.
- Histologically, tumour consist of solid sheets of large polygonal cells that appear to merge together as syntcitium as plasmamembrane is poorly defined.

5. Choriocarcinoma :

- Very rare, unlike gestational choriocarcinoma, there is little elevation of HCG.

6. Gonadblastoma :

- More common in right ovary. Seen in patients with abnormal gonadal development.

7. Mixed germ cell tumour :

- These tumour contain two or more germ cell element.
- Dysgerminoma and endodermal sinus tumour occur together most frequently.

Sex Cord Stromal Tumors (= Mesenchyoma)

Originates either from the sex cord of the embryonic gonad or from the stroma of ovary (thecoma or fibroma).

1. Feminizing tumours :

- They are :

	Granulosa cell tumour	Theca cell tumour
	Incidence	*Common Rare*
Age	Occur at any age but more common after age of 40 years.	Occur after menopause.
Presentation	In prepubertal girl lead to precocious puberty, hypertrophy of breast. In adults suprathreshold level of blood oestrogen, may lead to amenorrhoea followed by prolonged bleeding. In post menopausal women, the most remarkable feature is post menopausal bleeding. ***Metastases*** is interesting *as opposite ovary first* become involved.	Usually present as postmenopausal – Bleeding – Associated with Meig syndrome (ovarian fibroma, ascites and right sided pleural effusion)
Microscopy	Granulosa cells exhibit – Coffee bean nuclei – *Call exner bodies*	Tumour consist of spindle shaped cell together with fat laden cells
Tumor marker	Inhibin	

Remember : In both of these tumour endometrium is hyperplastic and risk of carcinoma of endometrium is increased.

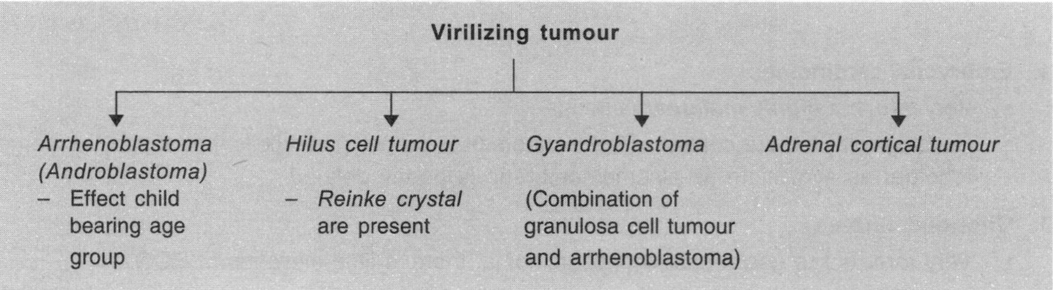

Spread

Ovarian carcinoma can spread in following ways :

- **Transcoelomic** – Most common and earliest mode of dissemination. Tumor cells are implanted over peritoneal cavity. Omentum represent the common site
- **Lymphatic** – To ***pelvic and para-aortic lymph*** nodes.
- **Hematogenous** – Rare, sites are lung and liver.
- **Direct** – To peritoneal surface of bladder rectosigmoid.

CLINICAL FEATURES

- Ovarian neoplasm typically develop as an *insidious disease* with few warning signs and symptom.
- In general, post menopausal women and prepubescent child are at greatest risk for developing a malignant adnexal mass.
- Menstrual abnormalities may be noted in reproductive age group, common in feminizing tumors.
- ***Virilizing tumour*** usually present with ***loss of secondary sexual characters,*** excess developments of hairs and deepening of voice.
- ***Early satiety and abdominal distension*** as a result of ascites are generally signs of advanced disease.
- ***Epithelial cancers*** of ovary are described as silent killers because, *they produce symptom only in advanced cases (70% of patient present with Stage II or Stage III)*. ***Abdominal discomfort and distension*** are most common symptom.
- ***Germ cell*** malignancies tends to stretch and twist the infundibulopelvic ligament causing severe pain while the disease is still confined to ovary; so most patients ***present in early stage.***
- ***Complications :***
  - Torsion (common in benign), rupture, infection, pseudomyxoma peritonei.
  - Intestinal obstruction - Most common ***cause of death*** in ovarian carcinoma.

DIAGNOSIS

- Whenever an adenexal mass is diagnosed it is necessary to distinguished between benign and malignant .

Pelvic Mass		
Physical examination		
	Benign	***Malignant***
Mobility	Mobile	Fixed
Consistency	Cystic	Solid or firm
Bilateral or unilateral	Unilateral	Bilateral
Cul-de-sac	Smooth	Nodular
Radiographic characteristics		
Size	Usually < 10 cm size	Any size
Septations	< 2 mm thickness	Multiple septalions > 3 mm in size
Calcification	Seen in teratoma	Usually absent
Omental caking	Absent	Seen
Ascitis	Absent	Present
Intra operative	Unilateral cyst with no adhesion Capsule intact	Solid areas with adhesion, rupture may occur Capsule is not intact

Intraoperative differentiation	
Benign	***Malignant***
Simple cyst	Adhesions
Unilalteral	Rupture
No adhesion	Ascites
Smooth surfaces	Solid areas
Intact capsule	Areas of hemorrhage or necrosis
Papillary excrescences	Multioculated mass
Bilateral	

Tumour marker

- Epithelial cancer : – One of the best characterized tumour marker in epithelial ovarian cancer is CA - 125.
  – It is the gold standard for tumour marker in the evaluation of pelvic mass.

Germ cell neoplasm	
• Dysgerminoma	PLAP +, LDH+, HCG + / –, AFP –
• Endodermal sinus tumour	AFP +, HCG –
• Immature teratoma	AFP ±, HCG –
• Mixed germ cell tumour	AFP + / –, HCG + / –
• Choriocarcinoma	AFP –, HCG +
• Embryonal carcinoma	AFP + / –, HCG +
• Epithelial cell neoplasm	CA - 125 +, Lysophosphatidic acid

... Novak's 13/e, p 1283

Radiography

- ***US*** is the most useful and most common ***radiographic test*** to evaluate adnexal masses. Transvaginal US has higher sensitivity then transabdominal US.
- Cyst that appear by US may be functional or neoplastic, functional cyst disappear after course of oral contraceptives, while neoplastic cyst do not.
- CT and MRI – To detect extraovarian spread, nodal status.

Diagnostic laparoscopy : For evaluating adenexal masses of uncertain pathology.

Frozen section : Definitive diagnosis can only be made by for frozen section.

STAGING

Given by FIGO. Surgical staging is used i.e. stage can not be determined prior to operation.

Procedures for surgical staging

- Sample of ascites or peritoneal washing from the paracolic gutters and pelvic and subdiaphragmatic surface for cytology.
- Complete abdominal exploration
- Intact removal of tumor
- Hysterectomy

- Infracolic omentectomy
- Biopsies of abdominal peritoneal implants; if none present, random biopsies from the paracolic gutter peritoneum, pelvic peritoneum and right subdiaphragmatic peritoneal surface.
- Pelvic and paraaortic lymph node biopsies
- Cytoreductive surgery to remove all visible disease.

Stage		
Stage I		***Growth limited to the ovaries***
Ia	–	one ovary involved.
Ib	–	both ovaries involved.
Ic	–	Ia or Ib and ovarian surface tumour, ruptured capsule, malignant ascites, or peritoneal cytology positive for malignant cells.
Stage II		***Extension of the neoplasm from the ovary to the pelvis***
IIa	–	extension to the uterus or fallopian tube.
IIb	–	extension to other pelvic tissues.
IIc	–	IIa or b and ovarian surface tumour, ruptured capsule, malignant ascites, or peritoneal cytology positive for malignant cells.
Stage III		***Disease extension to the abdominal cavity***
IIIa	–	Abdominal peritoneal surfaces with microscopic metastases.
IIIb	–	tumour metastases < 2 cm in size.
IIIc	–	tumour metastases > 2 cm in size or metastatic disease in the pelvic, para-aortic, or inguinal lymph nodes.
Stage IV		***Distant metastatic disease***
	–	Malignant pleural effusion
	–	Pulmonary parenchymal metastases
	–	Liver or splenic parenchymal metastases (not surface implants)
	–	Metastases to the supraclavicular lymph nodes or skin.

Prognostic factors

- ***Tumour stage*** is most important prognostic factor.

  Other are : – Histological grade, age, histologic type.
  – Mucinous and endometroid ca has better prognosis than serous and clear cell carcinoma of ovary.

TREATMENT

Surgery is the cornerstone of therapy for ovarian cancer regardless of cell type or stage of disease.

Epithelial neoplasm

A. Surgery

- Operation involves removal of primary tumour as well as associated metastatic disease (referred as debulking or cytoreductive surgery). The goal of cytoreductive surgery is to reduce tumor to less than 1cm in max diameter.
- In general ***contralateral adenexa should also be removed*** even when they are grossly normal *(CGDT10/e).* because of high risk of bilateral involvement. Exception to this generalization are made for ***young women with an apparent stage 1 tumour and when future fertility is an issue.***

- ***Hysterectomy and infracolic omentectomy is recommended*** as they are common site of metastasis.
- Any fluid in the peritoneal cavity should be aspirated.

B. Chemotherapy

- ***Excluding*** patient of Stage I a disease and grade I tumour ***chemotherapy is recommended in all*** other cases.
- Agent active against epithelial neoplasm are cisplatin, carboplatin, cyclophosphamide and pacletaxel.
- ***Most effective*** regimen is ***combination of pacletaxel and carboplatin***.

... CGDT 10/e, p 882

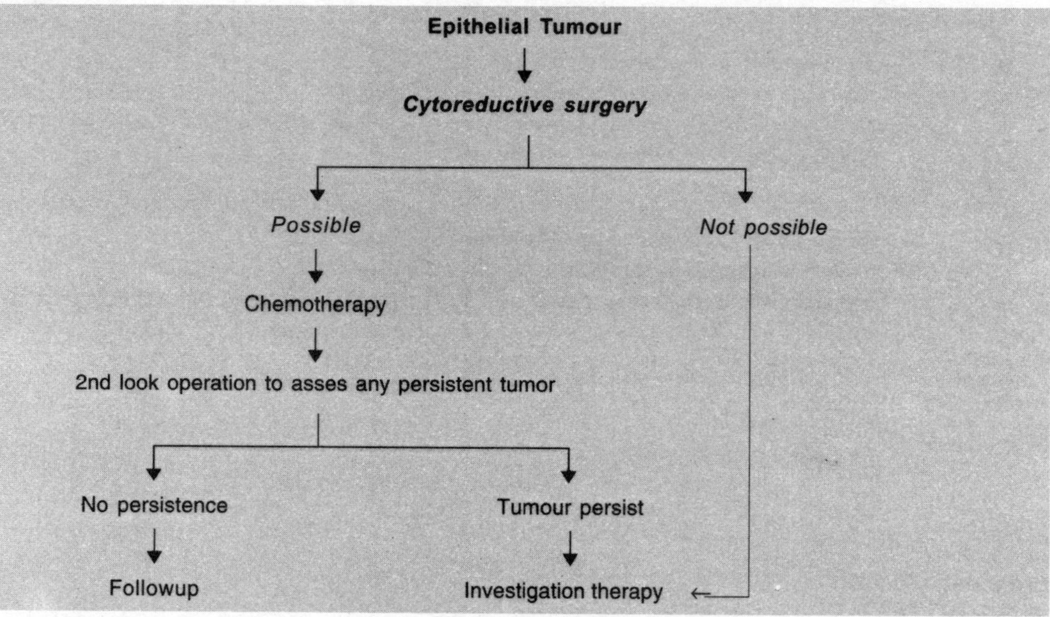

- **Radiotherapy** plays a very ***limited role*** in treatment of epithelial ovarian cancer.

Germ cell neoplasm

A. Surgery :

- As germ cell tumour are diagnosed at an early stage and affects young women, ***removal of the involved adenexa with preservation of contralateral adenexa*** and uterus is advocated.
- Dysgerminoma of the ovary has propensity to metastasize to ***pelvic and paraaortic nodes***, so biopsies of these structure is important.

B. Chemotherapy :

- Although dysgerminoma is most radiosensitive tumour identified it is ***treated with cisplatin containing chemotherapy*** *due to its potential for preserving fertility compared with radiotherapy.*
- Best is BEP ***(Bleomycin, Etoposide, Cisplatin).***

SPECIAL SITUATION

Treatment of Ovarian tumor in Pregnancy

- ***Elective operation*** of ovarian tumour in pregnancy is done in 2nd trimester between 14 to 18 weeks, as the chance of abortion is less and access to the pedicle is easy.
- ***Cesarian section*** is indicated for ovarian tumour diagnosed in late pregnancy when tumour is impacted in the pelvis. ***Tumour should be removed in the same setting.***

In case of ***complication*** tumour should be removed irrespective of gestational age.

Complication of ovarian neoplasm during pregnancy

- Torsion of pedicle : Usually occur during 8 - 10 weeks gestation of gestation.
- Intracystic hemmorhage
- Rupture
- Infection.

SECONDARY TUMOURS

(Tumours metastatic to ovary)

- Accounts for 25% of all ovarian malignancy.
- Most common primary site are breast, stomach, colon, endometrium. Highest risk of ovarian metastasis is seen in carcinoma of fallopian tube.
- ***Krukenburg tumour*** is by definition represent carcinomas of stomach metastatic to ovary.
- Secondary tumours are almost always bilateral.

FALLOPIAN TUBE CANCER

- Least common cancer of female genital tract
- Biological behaviour and pattern of spread are similar to epithelial ovarian cancer with papillary serous cystadenocarcinoma being most common
- Clinically present with triad of hydrops tubal profluens (watery vaginal discharge), pelvic pain and a palpable adenexal mass
- Treatment is same as that of ovarian epithelial cancer

QUESTIONS

1. Most common ovarian tumour to undergo torsion: [AI 07]

a. Serous cystadenoma
b. Mucinous cystadenoma
c. Brenner tumour
d. Benign cystic teratoma

2. Which of the following ovarian tumor is most prone to undergo torsion during pregnancy : [AI 06]

a. Serous cystadenoma
b. Mucinous cystadenoma
c. Dermoid cyst
d. Thecaleutin cyst

3. In which of the following genital tract malignancy, the risk of metastasis to ovary is the least ? [AI 06]

a. Carcinoma cervix
b. Carcinoma endometrium
c. Carcinoma fallopian tube
d. Uterine sarcoma

4. In a suspected case of ovarian cancer, imaging work up is required for all of the following except: [AI 06]

a. Detection of adnexal lesion
b. Characterization of lesion
c. Staging
d. Asses resectability

5. The most common pure germ cell tumor of the ovary : [AI 05; AIIMS 05, 04]

a. Choriocarcinoma
b. Dysgerminoma
c. Embryonal cell tumor
d. Malignant Teratoma

6. In a case of Dysgerminoma of ovary one of the following tumor markers is likely to be raised : [AI 05]

a. Serum HCG
b. Serum alphafetoprotein
c. Serum lactic dehydrogenase
d. Serum inhibin

7. A patient is diagnosed with ovarian cancer and planned for staging laparotomy. Surgical staging would involve all of the following except: [AI 09]

a. Peritoneal washings
b. Peritoneal biopsy
c. Omental resesction
d. Palpation of organs

8. Which of the following tumor markers is most likely to be raised in a case of dysgerminoma of the ovary: [AI 09]

a. Serum HCG
b. Serum Alphafetoprotein (AFP)
c. Serum Lactate Dehydrogenase (LDH)
d. Serum CA 19-9

9. A lady with treated CA ovary present in follow up with raised CA 125 level, next step: [AIIMS 08]

a. CT
b. PET
c. MRI
d. Clinical exam and serial follow up of CA125

10. Call-Exner bodies are seen in: [AIIMS 09, 08]

a. Granulosa cell tumor
b. Yolk sac tumor
c. Choriocarcinoma
d. Dysgerminoma

11. Call exner bodies seen in : [AIIMS 09]

a. Granulosa cell tumour
b. Endodermal sinus cell tumour
c. Ovarian fibroma
d. Teratoma

12. A female of 29 years underwent ovarian cystectomy. On biopsy it was found to be serous cyst adenocarcinoma. Further line of management is : [AIIMS 08]

a. Chemotherapy
b. Hysterectomy with diagnostic peritoneal wash
c. Salpingo-oophorectomy with diagnostic peritoneal wash
d. Follow up with serial CA 125 level

13. Which of the following is histological finding of endodermal sinus tumor :

a. Schiller-duval bodies
b. RS cell [AIIMS May 07]
c. Multinucleated giant cell
d. Plasma cells

14. Bilateral ovarian tumor is :

a. Endodermal sinus tumor
b. Embryonal cell ca
c. Dermoid [AIIMS May 07]
d. Dysgerminoma

15. CA-125 is a marker antigen for the diagnosis of : [AIIMS 06]

a. Colon cancer
b. Breast cancer
c. Brain cancer
d. Ovarian cancer

16. The pseudomyxoma peritonei occurs as a complication of the following ovarian tumor : [AIIMS 06]

a. Serous cystadenoma
b. Mucinous cystadenoma
c. Dysgerminoma
d. Gonadoblastoma

17. Sections from a solid-cystic uniliateral ovarian tumor in a 30-year old female show a tumor composed of diffuse sheets of small cells with doubtful nuclear grooving and scanty cytoplasm. No Call -Exner bodies are seen. The ideal immunohistochemistry panel would include : [AIIMS 06]

a. Vimentin, epithelial membrane antigen, inhibin, CD 99
b. Desmin, S-100 protein, smooth muscle antigen, cytokeratin
c. Chromogranin, CD45, CD99, CD20
d. CD3, chromagranin, CD 45, synaptophysin

18. All of the following are the markers for malignant germ cell tumors of ovary except: [AIIMS 05]

a. Ca - 125
b. Alpha feto protein
c. B HCG
d. LDH

19. Which of the following strategy has been recommended to reduce the heredity risk for ovarian cancer in women with BRCA - 1 and BRCA - 2 mutations : [AIIMS 05]

a. Use of oral contraceptive pills
b. Screening with transvaginal ultra-sound
c. Screening with Ca - 125
d. Prophylactic oopherectomy

20. Reinke's crystals are found in :

a. Arrhenoblastoma [PGI May 07]
b. Granulosa cell tumor
c. Dysgerminoma
d. Hilus cell tumor

21. What is the stage of Ovarian Ca with superficial liver metastasis with B/L ovarian mass : [PGI 06]

a. Stage I
b. Stage II
c. Stage III
d. Stage IV
e. Ca in situ

22. Tumor marker in dysgerminoma :

a. LDH [PGI 06]
b. AFP
c. β-HCG
d. CA-125

23. True about dygerminoma:

a. Radiosensitive [PGI 09]
b. MC malignant germ cell tumor
c. Bilateral usually
d. ↑ AFP
e. Common in prostmenopause

ANSWERS, REFERENCES, EXPLANATIONS WITH INFORMATIVE ILLUSTRATIONS

1. **Ans. is d i.e. Benign cystic teratoma**

Ref. Jeffcoate's Gynecology 6/e, p 529; Ultrasonography in Obstetric and Gynecology by Callen 4/e, p 878

Confused ! Dermoid cyst is the common name of benign cystic teratoma.

"Torsion is seen in 16% of dermoid and risk is increased during pregnancy and pueperium."

Dermoid cyst is the most common ovarian neoplasm **to show torsion.**

Remember :
- Most common ovarian tumour in pregnancy is mucinous cyst adenoma but mostly remains undiagnosed.
- Incidence of dermoid cyst is increased two fold during pregnancy and it is the most common neoplasm diagnosed during pregnancy.
- ***Hingorani sign :***
  - In ovariantumor during pregnancy.
  - Trendelenburg position can elicit the groove between two separate swelling.
  - Used to distinguish between ovarian tumour and fibroid. ... Callen

2. **Ans. is c i.e. Dermoid Cyst** *Ref. Jeffcoate's Gynecology 6/e, p 529; Dutta 6/e, p 310*

Complications of Ovarian tumours

- Torsion :
  - Most common complication
  - Most common in benign as they are mobile
  - ***Most frequent in dermoid cyst.*** *... Jaffecoat's 6/e, p 529*
- Rupture : – Can be traumatic or spontaneous.
- Pseudomyxoma of peritonium :
  - Peritoneal cavity is filled with coagulated mucinous material.
  - ***Mostly seen in cases of mucinous cystadenoma.***
- Infection: – Rare, most cases follow salpingitis.

Remember : Pseudomyxoma peritonei also seen in mucocele of appendix and carcinoma of large intestine.

3. **Ans. is a i.e. Carcinoma cervix** *Ref. Novak's Gynecology 13/e, p 1301*

Cervical cancer spread to ovary only in rare cases (<1%). Ovarian spread is more common with cervical adeno Ca in comparison to squamous cell Ca.

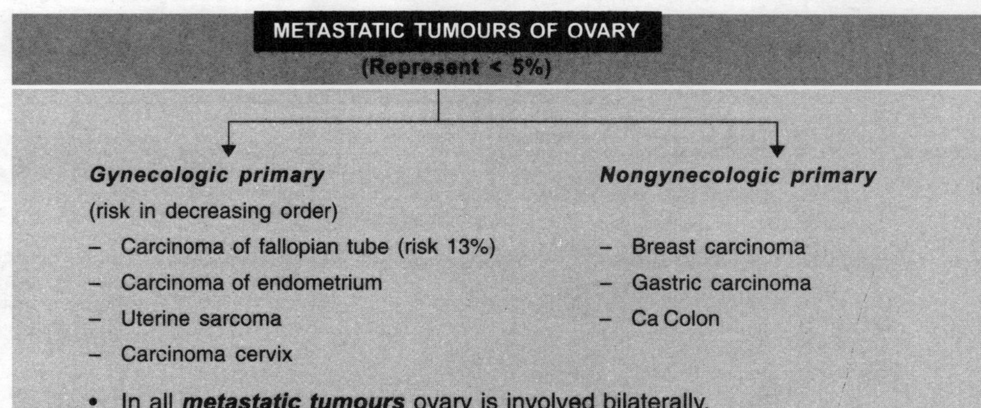

METASTATIC TUMOURS OF OVARY
(Represent < 5%)

Gynecologic primary (risk in decreasing order)	Nongynecologic primary
– Carcinoma of fallopian tube (risk 13%)	– Breast carcinoma
– Carcinoma of endometrium	– Gastric carcinoma
– Uterine sarcoma	– Ca Colon
– Carcinoma cervix	

- In all ***metastatic tumours*** ovary is involved bilaterally.

4. **Ans. is c i.e. Staging** *Ref. Novak's Gynecology 13/e, p 1261*

"FIGO staging is based on finding at surgical exploration."

... Novak's Gynecology

Role of Imaging in Ovarian tumour

- Imaging ***modality of choice*** - ***US.***
- Used to ***characterization of lesion*** into benign or malignant.
- To ***asses resectability.***
- To ***exclude*** extraperitoneal ***metastasis.***

5. **Ans. is b i.e. Dysgerminoma**

Ref. CGDT 10/e, p 875; Devita 8/e, p 1589; Novak's Gynecology 13/e, p 1284

"Dysgerminomas are the most common malignant germ cell tumours of the ovary and have been considered the female - equivalent of seminoma."

Dysgerminoma

- Most common *malignant germ cell tumour* of ovary.
- Primarily affect ***young women.***
- Mostly ***unilateral.***
- Pathologically it is a solid neoplasm with areas of softening due to degeneration.

... CGDT 10/e, p 875

- ***Histologically*** as in seminoma, it *mimics the pattern of primitive gonad*, lymphocytic infiltration may be seen (good prognostic sign).
- Clinically as with all germ cell tumour most dysgerminoma are diagnosed at an early stage.
- Unlike other germ cell tumour it ***does not secrete AFP*** and HCG is only rarely secreted, however it ***secretes LDH and placental alkaline phosphate***, which are used as tumour marker of dysgerminoma.
- Although dysgerminoma is most radio sensitive tumour, treatment of choice is ***surgery followed by cisplatin based chemotherapy*** as fertility can be preserved.

Treatment

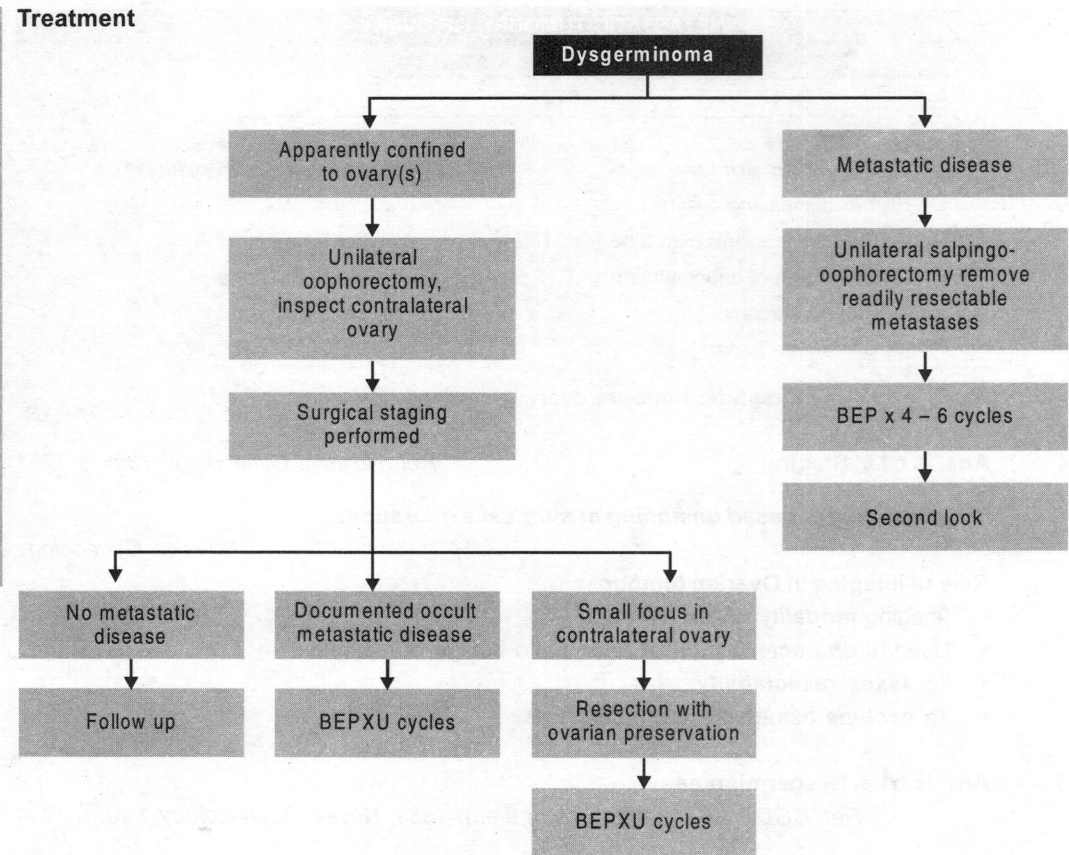

Remember :
- Most common germ cell tumour is mature teratoma = Dermoid cyst (which is benign).
- Most common malignant tumour of ovary is serous cyst adenocarcinoma.
- Most common tumor of ovary - Serous cystadenoma.

6. Ans. is c i.e. Serum lactic dehydrogenase *Ref. Novak's Gynecology 13/e, p 1282*

"Unlike other germ cell tumour dysgerminoma is not associated with raise in AFP and rarely increase HCG; however placental alkaline phosphate and lactate dehydrogenase are commonly produced by dysgerminomas and may be useful in monitoring the disease."

7. Ans. is d i.e. Palpation of organs *Ref. CGDT 13/e, p 880*

Palpation of organs is not a part of surgical staging.

Procedure for surgical staging of ovarian cancers

Surgical staging of Ovarian carcinoma includes following steps :

1. Any free fluid in pelvic cul-de-sac should be submitted for cytologic examination.
2. If no free fluid is present, peritoneal washing should be performed.

3. A systemic exploration of all the intrabdominal surfaces and **v**iscera is performed.
4. The **o**mentum should be resected from the transverse colon a procedure called as infracolic omentectomy.
5. The **r**etroperitoneal spaces should be explored to evaluate the pelvic and paraortic nodes.
6. Any **s**uspicious area or adhesions on the peritoneal surface should be sampled for biopsy.
7. The **d**iaphragm should be sampled by biopsy or scraping for cytological assessment.

Mnemonic : **F**luid washing of **V**iscera **OR** **S**uspicious area **D**one.

8. Ans. is c i.e. Serum LDH *Ref. Novak's 14/e p 1505*

Tumor marker	AFP	HCG	LDH	PLAP
Dysgerminoma	–	+/–	+	+

9. Ans. is a i.e. CT Scan *Ref. Devita 8/e p 1572*

"PET scan has no role in the diagnosis on subsequent follow up of the patient with ovarian Ca." ...Devita.

Surveillance after Ovarian Ca

– CA 125 is the most sensitive method for detection of relapse. CT is reserved for further evaluation of sign, symptoms, or serological evidence of relapse.

10. Ans. is a i.e. Granulosa cell tumor *Ref. Shaws 14/e, p 26; Robbins 7/e p 1102*

Cell Exner bodies are seen in Granulosa cell Itumor. They are small distinctive, gland like structures filled with on acidophillic material.

Note: Not all cases of granulosa cell tumor contain Cell Exner bodies, however if they are present diagnosis is definitely Granulosa cell tumor.

11. Ans. is a i.e. Granulosa cell tumor *Ref. Shaws 14/e, p 26; Robbins 7/e, p 1102*

Already explained

12. Ans. is d i.e. Follow up with serial CA 125 level *Ref. COGDT 10/e p 880*

Features are suggestive of stage Ia disease (higher stage is supposed to be identified intra-operatively)

For stage Ia disease it is only follow up with CA 125 level that is necessary.

13. Ans. is a i.e. Schiller-Duval bodies *Ref. CGDT 10/e, p 875*

Schiller : Duval bodiy which is a single papilla lined by tumour cells with a central blood vessel, is the pathognomic finding of endodermal sinus tumor (yolksac tumor).

Also remember :

• Granulosa cell tumor	• Call-Exner bodies
• Hilus cell tumor	• Reinke crystals
• Serous epithelial tumors	• Psammoma bodies
• Brenner tumor	• Walthard cell nest
• Polyembryonoma	• Embryoid bodies

14. Ans. is a i.e. Endodermal sinus tumor *Ref. CGDT 10/e, p 875*

Endodermal sinus tumor is bilateral in nearly 100% of cases.

Ovarian tumor	Bilalerality
Epithelial cell	
– Serous cystadenocarcinoma	40-60%
– Mucinous tumor	5–10%
– Endometroid tumor	30–50%
Germ cell	
– Dysgerminoma	10%
– Endodermal sinus tumor	100%
– Malignant sinus tumor	5%
– Dermoid cyst	10–15%
Sex cord stromal tumor	**Rare**
– Metastatic tumor	100%

Remember : Over all *most common* bilateral ovarian tumor is serous cyst adenocarcinoma.

15. Ans. is d i.e. Ovarian Cancer *Ref. Shaw's 14/e, p 383; Davita 8/e, p 1572*

CA–125 is the gold standard tumor marker for epithelial ovarian cancer.

- CA-125 is a glycoprotein and surface cell antigen which is secreted by malignant epithelial cells. CA 125>35u/ml suggest malignancy.
- It is also used to follow the response of adjuvant chemotherapy.
- However there are many other conditions in which CA 125 may be raised.
- Recently **lysophosphatidic acid** has also emerged as tumor marker for epithelial neoplasm.

Note : Other conditions associated with raised CA–125.

Neoplastic	Nonneoplastic
– Ca cervix	– Abdominal tuberculosis
– Endometrial carcinoma	– Pregnancy
– Ca breast	– Endometriosis
– Ca breast	– PID
– Ca lung	– Uterine fibroid
– Gastric Ca	– Ca fallopian tube

16. **Ans. is b i.e. Mucinous cyst adenoma** *Ref. Shaw's 13/e, p 367*

Pseudomyxoma peritonei

- Peritoneal cavity is filled with coagulated mucinous material adherant to the omentum and intestines.
- Usually ocurs with mucinous cystadenoma of ovary, but it has also been reported with mucocele of appendix and carcinoma of large intestine.
- The mesothelium of the peritoneum is converted in to high columnar cells similar to the cells lining mucinous cystodenoma. Laparotomy finding exactly resemble boiled sago pudding.
- Prognosis is poor even after removal of ovaries and appendix.

17. **Ans. is a i.e. Vimentin, epithelial membrane antigen, inhibin, CD 99**

Ref. Ackermann's Pathology 9/e, p 1692 - 1693

Guys! be clear that this is a case of granulosa cell tumour as Call-exner bodies may not be seen in few cases.

Granulosa cell tumour

- It is an feminizing ovarian neoplasm arising from granulosa cells in pre-existing follicles.
- *It is of two types :* – Adult granulosa cell tumour *(seen in child bearing age group).*
  – Juvenile granulosa cell tumour *(seen in first two decades).*

Pathological features

Gross : They are usually encapsulated with a smooth lobulated outline and have predominantly solid cut surface. Cysts filled with straw coloured or mucoid fluid may be seen.

Microscopy : Microscopic features of granulosa cell tumour are extremely variable, with different patterns of growth viz microfollicular (with Call-exner bodies), microfollicular, trabecular, insular and diffuse (sarcomatoid).

An important features is the presence of folds or grooves in the nuclei, resulting in coffee-bean appearance. Occasionally bizarre nuclei and multinucleated giant cells may be seen, they represent ***degenerative*** change *(not malignancy).*

Immunohistochemical marker : Vimentin, desmoplakin (desmosomal plaque protein), inhibin, follicle regulatory protein, CD99 (O13, MIC2), and A-103.

Now just learn the immunohistochemical marker of some important ovarian tumour.

Tumour	Immunohistochemical marker
• Serous tumour	CK7 +, CK8, CK9, CK90, EMA, B72.3, S-100 protein, WT-1 (in serous carcinoma), CK20 –
• Mucinous tumour	CEA, Keratin, EMA (particularly if malignant), MUC5AC (a gastric mucin gene), Dpc4, CK7, CK20 (in 50% of cases)
• Degerminoma	PLAP, CD117, GFAP, Desmin, Keratin +/–
• Teratoma	GFAP, Longchain polysialic acid

18. Ans. is a i.e. CA - 125 *Ref. Novak's Gynaecology 13/e, p 1282*

Carcinoma 125 is tumour marker of epithelial cell neoplasm (not for germ cell tumour).

19. Ans. is a i.e. Use of oral contraceptive pills

Ref. Devita 8/e, p 1574; Novak's 13/e, p 1257

Guys, *in this question age of patient is not given.* ***Prophylactic oopherectomy is recommended only in women > 35 years who have completed their family.***

Oral contraceptives are recommonded in all women.

"Surgery with prophylactic bilateral salpingo-oopherectomy (PBSO) is the most effective preventive strategy for patient with BRCA mutations to reduce cancer risk, but it can be accomplished only in women who have completed their family."

... Devita 8/e, p 1574

Chemoprophylaxis with OCP for 5 year decreases ovarian cancer risk by 50% in both the general population and women with hereditary ovarian carcinoma syndrome.

Recommendations

Current recommendations for management of women at high risk for ovarian cancer are as follows :

1. Women who appear to be at high risk for ovarian or breast cancer should undergo genetic counseling and, if the risk appears to be substantial, may be offered genetic testing for BRCA 1 and BRCA 2.
2. Women who wish to preserve their reproductive capacity can undergo screening by transvaginal ultrasonography every 6 months, although the efficacy of this approach is not clearly established.
3. Oral contraceptives should be recommended to young women before they embark on an attempt to have a family.
4. Women who do not wish to maintain their fertility or who have completed their families may undergo prophylactic bilateral salpingo-oophorectomy. The risk should be clearly documented, preferably established by BRCA 1 and BRCA 2 testing, before oophorectomy is performed.
5. In women who also have a strong family history of breast cancer, annual mammographic screening should be performed beginning at age 30 years.
6. Women with a documented HNPCC syndrome should undergo periodic screening mammography, colonoscopy and endometrial biopsy.

- Recommendation ***1, 2, 5 and 6*** are for early diagnosis. ***3, 4*** are for decreasing risk.

Remember: **Genetic syndromes associated with Ovarian Ca :**

- Turner syndrome (increase risk of dysgerminoma and gonadoblastoma).
- Breast ovarian cancer syndrome (due to mutation of BRCA - 1 or BRCA - 2).
  - Average age of diagnosis of BRCA-1 associated Ca is 48 years and that of BRCA-2 is 61 years
  - Risk is more with BRCA - 2
  - Prognosis is better than sporadic cancer.
- HNPCC syndrome - increase risk of colorectal cancer, ovarian cancer, endometrial cancer.

20. Ans. is d i.e. Hilus cell tumour *Ref. Shaw's 14/e, p 341*

Already explained

21. Ans. is c i.e. Stage III *Ref. Shaws 14/e, p 382*

Stage III ovarian tumor include tumor involving one/both ovaries, with microscopic implants outside the pelvis, and / or positive nodes (inguinal, retroperitoneal). Tumor limited to pelvis but with histological evidence of spread to bowel, omentum, presence of superficial metastases on the liver.

22. Ans. is a, c i.e. LDH, β-HCG *Ref. Novak's 14/e, p 1505*

Already explained see answer. no. 8

22. Ans. is a, b i.e. Radiosensitive, MC malignant germ cell tumor *Ref. COGDT 10/e, p 875*

Already explained see answer no. 5

39 Gestational Trophoblastic Tumour

What's Important ?
- Treatment
- Prognostic Factor

Definition : ***GTT are group of neoplasm arising from fetal tissue with in the maternal host.***

Components : Composed of ***both*** *syncytiotrophoblastic* and *cytotrophoblastic* cell except **PSTT** which is derived from intermediate trophoblastic cells.

It includes :

- Hydatidiform mole (complete and partial) (MC GTT).
- Invasive mole (Chorioadenoma destruens).
- Placental site trophoblastic tumour (PSTT).
- Choriocarcinoma.

Incidence and Risk factors

- Incidence is maximum ***in Asia*** and ***South America*** and least in US.
- Risk is more in women too elder (> *40*) or too younger (< *18 years*).
- Low ***socioeconomic status.***
- ***History*** of molar pregnancy.
- ***Diet*** deficient in protein, folic acid and carotene.
- ***Blood group A*** *women* married to group *O men*.

Categorization of Gestational trophoblastic neoplasia

a. Non metastatic disease : No evidence of disease outside uterus.
b. Metastatic disease : Any outside uterus.
   - *Good prognosis in metastatic disease if :*
     - Disease is present for short duration (< 4 months)
     - Serum β-hCG < 40,000 mIU/mL.
     - No metastasis to brain or liver
     - No significant prior chemotherapy
     - Not preceding term delivery
     - Metastasis limited to lung and vagina.

- *Poor prognosis in metastatic disease if :*
  - Long duration (> 4 months)
  - Serum β-hCG > 40,000 mIU/mL
  - Metastasis to brain or liver
  - Unsuccessful prior chemotherapy
  - Gestational trophoblastic neoplasia following term pregnancy.

FIGO Staging of Gestational trophoblastic disease :

I. Disease confined to uterus

II. Disease extending outside of the uterus, but limited to the genital structures (adnexa, vagina, broad ligaments)

III. Disease extending to the lung, with or without known genital tract involvement

IV. **Disease at other metastatic sites :**

A. No risk factors

B. One risk factors

C. Two risk factors.

Risk factors are :
- β-hCG > 100,000mIU/mL.
- Duration from termination of the antecedent pregnancy to diagnosis > 6 months.

HYDATIDIFORM MOLE

- It is ***benign*** neoplasia of chorion with malignant potential.
- In this chorionic villi is partly degenerated and partly hyperplastic, usually in the absence of fetus

Cytogenetics

- **Complete or true mole** are always *euploid* (have *a 46 XX* (***MC***) or *46 XY* karyotype) and chromosomes are entirely derived from the father.
  - They result from fertilization of empty or inactivated ovum with haploid sperm which then duplicates its own chromosome.
  - Phenomenon is known as ***androgenesis.***
- **Partial moles** are usually ***triploid.***

Pathology

- Hydatidiform mole are derived from ***extraembryonic trophoblast.***
- Cyst begin to develop from ***3rd to 5th*** week, the vesicle fluid is interstitial fluid rich in HCG.
- ***Ovary show bilateral*** theca lutein cyst *due to excessive HCG.*
- Tumor secrete thyrotropin and lead to ***hyperthyroidism.***

Clinical feature

- ***Bleeding*** : Vaginal bleeding is ***MC*** symptom. Blood may be mixed with fluid from ruptured cyst giving the appearance of *white* currants *in red currant juice.*
- Expulsion of grape like vesicles per vaginum ***(Diagnostic of vesicular mole).***
- Abdominal pain, eclampsia in first trimester of pregnancy.

- **On physical examination :** Size of uterus is more than expected *(MC sign)* and is doughy (soft) in feel, fetal parts are not palpable.

Remember : Hydatidiform mole should be suspected in any women with bleeding in 1st half of pregnancy, passage of vesicles, hyperemesis gravidarum, or preeclampsia / eclampsia with onset before 24 weeks.

Investigations

Sonography : **IOC**, show characteristic "snow storm" appearance.

HCG estimation : Most important characteristic of GTD is their capacity to produce HCG. HCG titre in urine (> 1 in 200) is significant.

X-ray: X-ray of both abdomen (if uterine size is more than 16 weeks) and chest (to rule out pulmonary embolisation of mole) should be done.

Treatment

Surgery

- ***Evacuation :*** Suction curretage is method of choice.
- ***Hysterectomy :*** Is an option for good surgical candidates not desirous of future pregnancy and older women (>35).
  - Hysterectomy only decrease the risk of malignancy and does not eliminate the necessity of follows up.
- ***Chemotherapy :***
  - **Prophylactic chemotherapy** is indicated in cases of :
    - Age > 35 years.
    - History of prior molar pregnancy, trophoblastic hyperplasia.
    - If patient can not be followed.
  - ***Drugs given are methotrexate or dactinomycin.***

Follow up : *Regardless of method of termination close follow up for **atleast 1 year** is essential.*

- ***It includes :***
  - History and clinical examination
  - HCG assay
  - Chest X-ray
  - Contraceptive advice : OC's are best.
- **Chemotherapy in follow up period.** Indications are :

a. β HCG level rising for 2 successive weeks or constant for 3 successive weeks.

b. β HCG level elevated at 15 weeks post evaluation.

c. Rising βHCG titer after reaching normal.

d. Post evacuation hemorrhage.

INVASIVE MOLE = CHORIOADENOMA DESTRUENS

- *Hydatidiform mole that invades the myometrium or adjacent structures.*
- Microscopic finding and treatment is same as hydatidiform mole.

MALIGNANT GESTATIONAL TROPHOBLASTIC NEOPLASIA

It includes choriocarcinoma and placental site trophoblastic disease.

CHORIOCARCINOMA

- Pure epithelial cell tumour composed of **syncytotrophoblast** and **cytotrophoblast** cells.
- Accompany or follow any type of pregnancy.
- Majority of growth arise in the ***body*** of uterus.
- Metastases occurs early mostly hematogenously. ***Lung*** is *MC* site of distant metastases.
- Metastases over vulva and lower third of vagina form ***purple hemorrhagic projections in or around vaginal orifice***, this appearance is pathognomic of choriocarcinoma.
- ***Symptom*** : Most common symptom is persistent or irregular uterine haemorrhage following an abortion, molar pregnancy or normal delivery.
- ***Investigation*** :
  - IOC is CT
  - Chest X-ray : Cannon ball appearance.

PLACENTAL SITE TROPHOBLASTIC DISEASE (PSTD)

- ***PSTD*** is derived from intermediate trophoblasts of the placental bed with minimal or absent syncytotrophablastic tissue.
- ***PSTD*** is resistant to chemotherapy, so hysterectomy is the recommanded treatment.

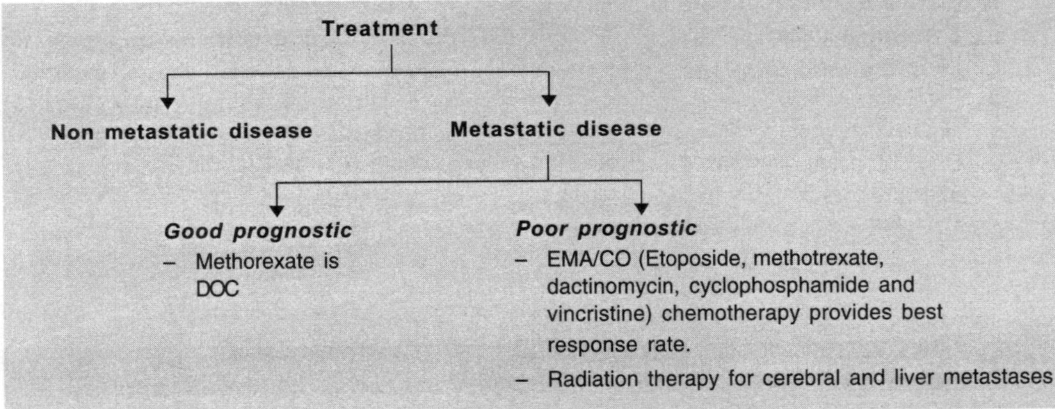

- Metotrexate is contraindicated in presence of renal failure and hepatocellular disease. In such case dactinomycin is recommanded.

QUESTIONS

1. **Most common site of metastasis from choriocarcinoma : [AI 07]**
   a. Lung
   b. Vagina
   c. Cervix
   d. Bone

2. **This highest incidence of Gestational Trophoblastic Disease is in : [AI 05]**
   a. Australia
   b. Asia
   c. North America
   d. Western Europe

3. **Bad prognostic markers of choriocarcinoma for treatment are : [PGI 06]**
   a. Liver metastasis
   b. Lung metastasis
   c. Previous H.mole
   d. High H.C.G titre
   e. Chemotherapy started 12 months after pregnancy

4. **False about partial mole: [AI 10]**
   a. Caused by triploidy
   b. Can be diagnosed early by USG when compared with complete mole.
   c. Can present as missed abortion
   d. Rarely causes persistent GTD

5. **True about H. mole: [PGI 10]**
   a. Always a/w raised uterine size for gestational age
   b. Raised HCG
   c. Hysterectomy in selected cases
   d. Chemotherapy is the freatment of choice
   e. Thyrotoxicosis

6. **Persistance of gestational trophoblastic tumor can be assesed with all except?**
   a. Enlarged uterus **[AIIMS May 10]**
   b. Persistence leutin cyst in ovaries
   c. Plateau of HCG
   d. Sub urethral nodule

ANSWERS, REFERENCES, EXPLANATIONS WITH INFORMATIVE ILLUSTRATIONS

1. **Ans. is a i.e. Lungs** *Ref. Shaw's 14/e, p 233; CGDT 10/e, p 887*

Most common sites of metastases in choriocarcinoma are : Lung > Brain > Liver.

Lung metastases of choriocarcinoma shows characteristic cannon ball appearance.

Choriocarcinoma

- Most malignant tumor of uterus.
- Mostly occur after evacuation of a hydatidiform Mole > Abortion > full term labour > ectopic pregnancy.
- Spread mostly ***hematogenously*** to lung.
- Metastases over vulva and lower third of vagina present as purple hemorrhagic projection around vaginal orifice.
- ***Symptoms :*** Most present as irregular or uterine hemorrhage following an abortion, molar pregnancy or normal delivery.

- ***Treatment :*** Most effective treatment is chemotherapy incorporating methotrexate or actinomycin D.

Hysterectomy is indicated in following conditions:

- High risk cases above 40 years, multiparous
- When chemotherapy is ineffective
- Haemorrhage due to uterine perforation
- Large sized growth in the uterus

2. **Ans. is b i.e. Asia** *Ref. Shaw's 14/e, p 226; Devita 7/e, p 1360*

"Incidence of gestational trophoblastic disease varies widely with figures as high as 1 in 120 in some areas of Asia and South America, compared to 1 in 1200 in the United States." *... Devita 7/e, p 1360*

In India incidence of gestational trophoblastic disease is 1 in 160.

Factors predisposing GTD :
- Low socioeconomic status
- History of molar pregnancy
- Diet deficient in protein, folic acid and carotene
- Blood group A women married to group O.

Remember : Risk of developing choriocarcinoma is highest after hydatidiform mole.

3. **Ans. is a, d and e i.e. Liver metastasis; High H.C.G. titre; and Chemotherapy started 12 months after pregnancy** *Ref. COGDT 10/e, p 893*

Treatment of malignant trophoblastic disease	
Good prognosis factor	***Poor prognostic factor***
– Serum βHCG <40,000 mIU/ml – Metastases confined to pelvis and lung – Therapy started with in 4 month	– Serum β HCG >40,000 mIU/ml – Brain or liver metastases – Prior unsuccessful chemotherapy of onset of disease – Onset following term gestation – Disease diagnosed more than 4 month after molar pregnancy.
Single agent chemotherapy	***Combination chemotherapy***
– Methotrexate is drug of choice – Actinomycin D is used in patient with hepatic dysfunction or intolerance to methotrexate	EMA/CO (Etoposide, Methotrexate, dactinomycin, cyclophsophamide and vincristine) is most effective. *... COGDT 10/e*

4. **Ans. is b i.e. can be diagnosed early by USG when compared with complete mole**

Ref. Shaws 14/e, p 227

The average age when a partial mole is diagnosed is at a later date than complete mole, around 24-26 weeks of pregnancy.

Comparison of Complete and partial hydatidiform moles:

Features	Complete	Partial
Karyotype	Diploid 46, XX or 46, XY	Triploid (69, XXY)
Embryo	Absent	Present
Villi	Hydropic	New hydropic
Trophoblasts	Diffuse hyperplasia	Mild focal hyperplasia
Implantation-site trophoblast	Diffuse atypia	Focal atypia
Fetal RBCs	Absent	Present
β-hCG	High (> 50,000)	Slight elevation (<50,000)
Frequency of classic clinical symptoms	Common	Rare
Risk for presistent GTD	20-30%	< 5%
Risk of developing choriocarcinoma	2-10%	< 1%
Uterine size	Always increased	Normal or small for gestational age
Scalloping of chronic villi	Diffuse	Focal
Trophoblastic stromal inclusions	Absent	Present

5. **Ans. is b, c, e Raised HCG, Hysterectomy in selected cases, Thyrotoxicosis**

Ref. Shaws 14/e p 227; Noveks 14/e, p 1585

Let's consider each option

Option 'a'

- Excessive uterine enlargement relative to gestational age is one of the classic sign of complete mole, although it was present in only about one half of patients.
- In partial mole uterine size is usually normal or small for gestational age on account of intrauterine fetal growth retordation.

Option 'b'

- Raised βhCG is seen in serum or urine of virtually all patients of hyadatiform mole or malignant trophoblastic disease and furthermore its level corelates closely with the number of viable tumor cells.
- The rate of decline in βHCG titre after successful evacuation is also important, In most cases βHCG values exhibit a progressive decline to undetectable levels with in 14 weeks. If hCG titer rises or plateu, it must be concluded that viable tumor continues to persist.

Option 'c, d'

Treatment of hyadatidiform mole

- Suction curretage is the treatment of choice, while hysterectomy remains an option for good surgical candidates not desirous of future pregnancy. Current recommendations restrict hysterotomy only to cases complicated by hemorrhage.

Option 'e'

- Hyperthyroidism in hyadatiform mole results from stimulation of thyrotropin receptors by β–hCG. It is seen in up to 10% of patients.

6. Ans. is d i.e. Suburetheral nodule *Ref. Shaws 14/e, p 231; Novaks 14/e 1591*

Persistant trophobastic disease is diagnosed when follow-up shows persistance of 'beta hCG level'. These patients usually present with:
- Irregular vaginal bleeding
- Theca leutin cyst
- Uterine subinvolution or assymetric enlargement
- Presistently elevated or plateau serum hCG levels.

40 Breast Tumour

What's Important ?

- Predisposing Factors
- Staging
- Mammography
- Treatment
- Causes of Discharge

Breast is a Modified sweat gland

Important Points :

- Most common ***disorder*** of breast
  - Fibroadenosis
- Most common ***tumor*** of breast
  - Fibroadenoma
- Most common ***carcinoma*** of breast
  - Scirrhous (ductal) carcinoma
- Most common cause of ***breast tenderness***
  - Fibroadenosis
- Most common cause of ***breast discharge***
  - Duct ectasia *(Paste like discharge)*
- Most common cause of ***bloody discharge*** from breast
  - Large duct papilloma
- Most common cause of ***death*** in breast Ca
  - Malignant pleural effusion
- Most common site of ***metastasis*** in breast Ca
  - Bone
- Most common ***site*** of breast Ca
  - Upper outer quadrant

    (*left more common than right 110:100*)

CLASSIFICATION OF BREAST NEOPLASM

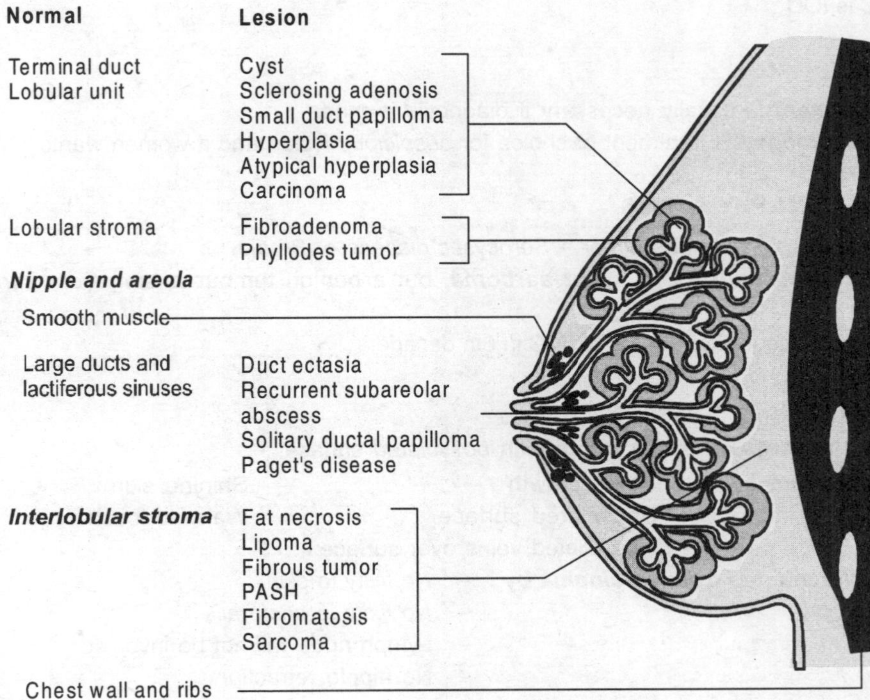

FIBROADENOMA

- Most common benign tumor of female breast.
- Most common age group ***15-30 years.***

Pathology

- Encapsulated spherical lesion.
- Composed of both fibrous and glandular tissue.
- Arise from interlobular stroma.

Etiology

- Increase sensitivity of focal area of breast to estrogen.

Types

- **Pericanalicular variety** *(Hard fibroadenoma)* due to proliferation of *connective tissue inside the elastic lamina.*
- **Intra canalicular variety** *(Soft fibroadenoma)* due to proliferation of *connective tissue outside the elastic lamina.*
- Giant fibroadenoma is the team applied for fibroadenoma > 5 cm.

Clinical presentation

- As *painless slowly growing solitary mobile lump* in breast.

Investigation

- Characteristic ***popcorn calcification*** is found in *mammography.*
- *FNAC* is IOC

Treatment

- ***No treatment*** is usually necessary if diagnosis is made.
- ***Excision biopsy*** is treatment of choice for *suspicious lesion* and if women wants.

CYSTOSARCOMA PHYLLOIDES

- Also called as *Phylloides tumor = Serocystic disease of Brodie.*
- Name is misnomer as ***it is not sarcoma,*** but a benign tumour *arising from intralobular stroma.*
- *Age* : Most occur after age of 40, MC in 6th decade.

Clinical features

- Present as ***large, massive tumor*** with *bosselated* surface.
- ***Characterized by :***
  - Rapid growth
  - Bosselated surface
  - Red dilated veins over surface
  - Shining skin
  - Warm to touch
- It is ***differentiated from carcinoma by :***
  - *No fixity* to *skin*
  - *No fixity* to *pectoralis*
  - Lymph node will not be involved
  - No nipple retraction

Spread

- Only *sarcomatous portion* **metastasize** through blood to lung.
- Lymphnode are not involved, so ***LN dissection is not performed.***

Treatment

- *Small* : ***Excision*** of lump or even subcutaneous mastectomy.
- *Giant or Recurrence* : ***Simple mastectomy.***
- *Malignant phylloides tumor* : ***Complete removal*** of tissue with rim of normal tissue.

Complication

- Recurrence.
- Turn into sarcoma or carcinoma.

CARCINOMA OF BREAST

- Most common ***cancer in women in world*** (*In India it is Ca cervix*).
- Most common ***cancer in urban women in India.***
- 2nd MC cause of cancer related death in women (1st being lung cancer). *... Robbins 7/e, p 282*
- Most common ***type*** is Adenocarcinoma.
- Almost all *carcinoma arise from* ***terminal duct lobular unit.*** *... Robbin's 7/e, p 1079*

Etiology and Risk factor

- ***Age*** – Incidence ↑ with age, *Mean age* is 60 years.
- ***Breast diseases*** increasing risk are ***:***
  - Mammary dysplasia *(fibrocystic disease of breast)*
  - *Proliferative* breast disease *without atypia* :
    - Moderate hyperplasia
    - Sclerosing adenosis
    - Papilloma
    - Complex sclerosing lesion
    - *Fibroadenoma with complex features.*
  - *Proliferative* disease *with atypia* :
    - Atypical ductal hyperplasia
    - Atypical lobular hyperplasia
  - Carcinoma in situ :
    - Lobular Ca in situ
    - Ductal Ca in situ
  - Cancer in one breast ↑ risk of Ca in other breast
- ***Chromosomal abnormality*** : BRCA-1, BRCA 2, p 53 mutation are most common abnormality in Ca breast in *both sporadic and familial.*
- ***Diet :***
  - ↑ Risk in post menopausal, obese women.
  - Vitamin C has protective role.
- ***Endocrinal***
  - Higher the exposure to femine hormone (estrogen & progesterone) higher the risk of developing Ca
  - Early menarche
  - Late menopause
  - Late first pregnancy
  - Combined OCS
  - Hormone secreting ovarian tumors

  } Increase the risk of carcinoma breast
- ***Family history***
- ***Geographical*** – Ca breast is a disease of white, western women.
- ***Radiation exposure and endometrial ca*** ↑ risk of ca breast.

Remember :
- Apocrine metaplasia is not associated with ↑ risk of cancer.
- More the children women has, less is the chance of developing breast Ca as breast feeding ↓ chance of Ca breast.

WHO Classification :

Most widely used, based on growth pattern and cytologic features.

... Devita 8/e, 1617

Although the classification uses the term invasive "ductal" and "lobular" carcinoma, ***this is not meant to indicate that former originates in duct and latter in the lobules of breast.***

The point must be noted that diagnosis of ***invasive ductal carcinoma is a diagnosis*** of exclusion i.e. subtype not classified into any other category like mucinous, tubular, etc. In practice the terms invasive ductal carcinoma, infiltrating ductal carcinoma, and infiltrating or invasive carcinoma of no special type are used interchangeably.

Breast Cancer			
Ductal	**Lobular**	**Nipple**	**Other**
– Invasive, NOS (MC) – Invasive with predominant intraductal component – Intraductal – Comedo – Inflammataory – Medullary with lymphocytic infiltrate – Mucinous – Papillary – Scirrhous – Tubular – Other	– In situ – Invasive	– Paget's disese – Paget's disese with intraductal Ca – Paget's disese with invasive ductal Ca	– Undifferentiated

Pathology

Ductal Ca in situ (DIS) = Intraductal carcinoma

- Malignant cells ***limited to ducts*** and ***lobules*** by basement membrane.
- *Most frequently* present as mammographic calcification and less as mass or nipple discharge.
- Divided in to ***5 subtypes*** - *Comedo Ca, solid, cribiform, papillary* and *micropapillary.*
- ***Comedo carcinoma*** is a *peripheral carcinoma in which the tumor cells block the ductules* by forming a case or plug producing a small cystic lesion and palpable lump
- DCIS Most commonly detected as an abnormality on screening mammography.
- ***Among cancer detected mammographically half are DCIS***
- DCIS is considered to be a *precursor of invasive ductal carcinoma* and thereby warrants treatment.

Lobular carcinoma in situ (LCIS)

- Always an incidental finding in a biopsy performed for another reason.
- LCIS is ***mostly multicentric*** and bilateral and *risk of invasive carcinoma* is *equal in both breast.*
- *Not detected on mammography* as there is no calcification.
- Tumor cells lack adhesin protein E cadherin, resulting in rounded cells without attachment to adjacent cells

Remember :

- LCIS is considered to be a marker of ↑ ed risk for development of breast cancer.
- DCIS is considered to be a non obligate precursor of invasive ductal carcinoma.

... Devita 7/e, p 1420

Invasive Carcinoma

- In women not undergoing mammography invasive Ca almost always present as mass and over half have lymphatic metastasis.
- In women undergoing mammography invasive Ca mostly present as density and 20% have lymphatic metastasis.

A. **Invasive ductal carcinoma = No special type carcinoma (NST) = Infiltrating ductal Ca**

- Most common ***type of breast Ca.***
- Most lesions are firm to hard which produce characteristic grating sound when cut.
- Well differentiated tumor express hormone receptor and do not over express *Her/neu* which is *over expressed in undifferentiated tumor.*
- ***Atrophic schirrious*** is a NST seen in elder patient, *when there is atrophy* of breast.
  - Recently developed technique that examined DNA, RNA and protein have provided a new molecular classification for NST group. Through gene expression profiling 5 major pattern have been identified.
    1. **Luminal A (50% of NST):** ER + ve and HER2 / neu negative. These cancers are slow growing and respond well to hormonal treatment.
    2. **Luminal B (20% of NST):** ER + ve, often over express HER-2 / neu. These cancers are of high grade and have a higher proliferation rate. They are more likely to show lymphatic metastasis. Response to conventional chemotherapy is good.
    3. **Normal breast like (8% of NST):** ER +ve, HER 2 / neu negative.
    4. **Basal like : (15% of NST) :** ER (–)ve, PR (–), HER-2 / neu (–)ve. They express markers typical of myoepithelial cells (basal keratin, P cadherin, P63 or laminin), progenitor cells (eg cytokeratins 5 and 6). They are also called **triple negative carcinoma**. Members of this grouip include medullary carcinoma, metaplastic carcinoma. They are of high grade, have a high prolieration rate and show aggressive course with frequent metastasis.
    5. **HER-2 positive:** This group comprises ER (–)ve carcinoma that overexpress HER-2 / neu protein. These cancers are usually poorly differentiated, have a high proliferation rate and are associated with a high frequency of brain metastasis.

B. **Invasive lobular carcinoma (ILC)**

- Comprise 5-10% of all invasive Ca.
- These tumors are detected as a mass on examination and density on mammography (no calcification).
- ***Histologic hallmark*** of ILC is the *tendency of tumor cells to invade the stroma in linear strands* (Indian file pattern).
- Tumor cells are *arranged in concentric ring* surrounding normal ducts.
- Most tumor show a loss of region on chromosome 16.
- They show *different pattern of metastasis* as they have *propensity to involve peritoneal and retroperitoneal surface, meninges (carcinomatous meningitis), GIT and ovaries and are less likely to metastasize to lungs.* This is due to loss of E-cadherin.

... Devita 7/e, p 1420

C. **Medullary carcinoma**

- 3rd Most common invasive Ca (5%). *... Devita 7/e, p 1421*
- Tends to occur in *younger* women *or reproductive* age group.
- Presents as well circumscribed mass *similar to fibroadenoma.*

- Histologically characterized by- solid syncytia like sheets.
- There is moderate to marked lymphatic infiltrate in tumor.
- Non infiltrative border.
- Most are *poorly differentiated,* despite this fact they have *better prognosis* (younger age group) than NST.

D. Mucinous (colloid) carcinoma

- Tends to occur in older women and grow slowly during the course of many years.
- *Extremely soft tumor* with grey blue gelatin appearance on microscopy.
- Slightly better prognosis.

E Tubular carcinoma (Cribiform carcinoma)

- ***Best differentiated*** form of invasive Ca. Bilaterality is seen in 9-30% of cases.
- Lesion are usually small and have favorable prognosis with less chance of nodal metastasis.
- Typically detected as small irregular mammographic densities in women with age > 40

F. Inflammatory carcinoma

- Breast Ca with *worst prognosis.*
- Aggressive and virulent form of carcinoma characterized by sudden enlargement, inflammation and infiltration of skin (always staged as T4d in stage III) with ***peaude orange appearance.***
- Tends to occur *during pregnancy and lactation.*
- *Differentiated* from breast abscess by ***absence of fever.***

G Metaplastic carcinoma

- Includes a variety of rare types of breast cancer (<1% of cell cases) such as matrix producing carcinomas, squamous cell carcinomas and carcinomas with prominent spindle cell component.
- They are ER-PR-HER-2/neu triple negative, often express myoepithelial proteins.

Paget's disease of Nipple

- Intraductal carcinoma involving *excretory duct* which infiltrate nipple and areola.
- Pathologically Paget's disease represent in situ carcinoma in the nipple epidermis
- Histologically characterized by presence of paget cells (large hyperchromatic cells with clear cytoplasm) in epidermis.
- Presents as ***eczema like condition*** of nipple and areola which persists after local treatment, so eczema of nipple should always be biopsied.

Spread

- Local : To involve remaining portion of breast, skin, pectoral muscle and even chest wall.
- Lymphatic : Axillary lymph node, Internal mammary chain of LN. Involvement of lymph node is not in chronological order.
- Hematogenous : Most common site is ***bone*** producing predominantly osteoblastic secondaries. ... *Campbell Orthopaedics 10/e, p 848*

Remember : – The site of tumor within the breast does not tell which node will be involved ... *Bailey 24/e, p 837*

– Supraclavicular LN or any contralateral LN represents advanced disease.

Clinical features

- Most common presentation is ***lump*** in breast.
- Bleeding per nipple.
- Fixation to skin, ulceration, peaud' orange, fixation to pectoralis and chest wall occur in advanced cases.
- ***Cancer-en- cursisse*** - skin of chest is ***infiltrated*** with carcinoma.
- Most common cause of death is ***malignant pleural effusion.***

Diagnosis and Staging

- **Clinical**

  Characteristic of malignant breast lump are :
  - Bloody discharge.
  - Puckering and dimpling of skin over breast.
  - Retracted nipple.
  - Presence of peau'd orange.
  - Nipple may be elevated.
  - Associated enlargement of axillary lymph node.

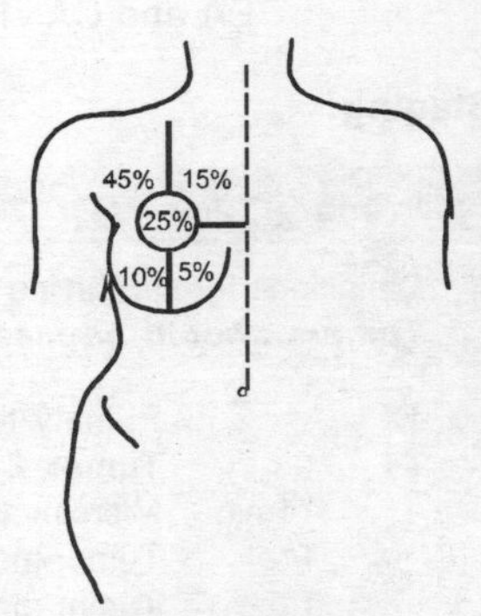

Frequency of breast ca at various sites

- **Investigation**

  a. ***Mammography :***
  - Used for both screening and evaluation of breast lump.
  - *Dose* of radiation - 0.1cGY.
  - Breast is exposed to low voltage high ampere X-ray, views are:
    - MLO (Meidolateral oblique) - Images greatest volume including axillary tail
    - CC (Craniocaudal). For medial aspect and provides better compression
    - 90° Lateral view – To determine exact location
    - Spot compression view
  - *Mammographic pattern* of Ca breast are :
    - Loss of architectural pattern
    - Calcification (*MC* finding)
    - Mass density *(spiculated density)*
    - Dilatation of duct
  - *Sensitivity* : 60 - 90%
  - *Specificity* : 30 - 40% for *non palpable*

    85 - 90% for palpable

Note: – The probability of cancer on screening mammography is determined by BIRAD (Breast imaging and reporting data system) assessment.

– When clinical diagnosis is already made, mammography is not done.

  b. ***Biopsy :***
  - *Most reliable* diagnostic test for Ca breast is open excisional biopsy, however it is recommended only in cases where diagnosis can not be made by simple means.
  - FNAB is most commonly empolyed biopsy method. Core needle biopsy is the most effective biopsy technique in OPD.

c. ***Imaging :***
- X-ray - For pleural effusion and bone metastases.
- US - To differentiate between cystic and solid lesion.
- MRI - Imaging of choice for breast with implant.
- CT - For detecting metastasis in liver and Brain.
- PET - Effective single scan for bone and soft tissue or visceral metastases.

d. ***Receptor assay*** :
- For progestin and estrogen to determine the senstivity to hormonal therapy.

e. ***Tumor marker :***
- CEA and CA -15-3 or CA 27-29 may be used as marker for *recurrent breast cancer.*

Staging

Primary Tumor (T)		
Definitions for classifying the primary tumor (T) are the same for clinical and for pathologic classification. ***Tumors should be measured to the nearest 0.1-cm increment.***		
TX		Primary tumor cannot be assessed.
T1		**Tumor *2 cm or less* in greatest dimension**.
	T1mic	Microinvasion 0.1 cm or less in greatest dimension.
	T1a	Tumor more than 0.1 cm but not more than 0.5 cm in greatest dimension.
	T1b	Tumor more than 0.5 cm but not more than 1 cm in greatest dimension.
	T1c	Tumor more than 1 cm but not more than 2 cm in greatest dimension.
T2		Tumor **more than 2 cm but not more than 5 cm** in greatest dimension.
T3		Tumor **more than 5 cm** in greatest dimension.
T4		**Tumor of any size with direct extension to (a) chest wall or (b) skin,** only as described below.
	T4a	Extension to chest wall not including pectoralis muscle.
	T4b	Edema (including peau d'orange) or ulceration of the skin of the breast or satellite skin nodules confined to the same breast.
	T4c	Both T4a and T4b.
	T4d	Inflammatory carcinoma.

Regional Lymph Nodes (N)		
NX		Regional lymph nodes *cannot be assessed* (e.g., previously removed).
N0		*No regional lymph node metastasis*.
N1		Metastasis to **movable ipsilateral a**xillary lymph node(s).
N2		**Metastases in ipsilateral axillary lymph nodes fixed or matted,** or in *clinically apparent* ipsilateral internal mammary nodes in the *absence* of clinically evident axillary lymph node metastasis.
	N2a	Metastases in ipsilateral axillary lymph nodes fixed to one another (matted) or to other structures.
	N2b	Metastasis only in *clinically apparent* ipsilateral internal mammary nodes and in the *absence* of clinically evident axillary lymph node metastasis.
N3		Metastasis in **ipsilateral infraclavicular lymph node**(s) with or without axillary lymph node involvement, or in *clinically apparent* ipsilateral internal mammary lymph node(s) and in the *presence* of clinically evident axillary lymph node metastasis; or metastasis in ipsilateral supraclavicular lymph node(s) with or without axillary or internal mammary lymph node involvement.
	N3a	Metastasis in ipsilateral infraclavicular lymph node(s).
	N3b	Metastasis in ipsilateral internal mammary lymph node(s) and axillary lymph node(s).
	N3c	Metastasis in ipsilateral supraclavicular lymph node(s).

Stage Grouping

Stage	Tumor (T)	Node (N)	Metastasis (M)
0	Tis	N0	M0
I	T1[a]	N0	M0
IIA	T0	N1	M0
	T1[a]	N1	M0
	T2	N0	M0
IIB	T2	N1	M0
	T3	N0	M0
IIIA	T0	N2	M0
	T1[a]	N2	M0
	T2	N2	M0
	T3	N1	M0
	T3	N2	M0
IIIB	T4	N0	M0
	T4	N1	M0
	T4	N2	M0
IIIC	Any T	N3	M0
IV	Any T	Any N	M1

Remember : Previously Manchester staging was used.

Prognostic factors

- **Axillary LN** status is the *most important* prognostic factor.
- Size of tumor.
- *Grading* (Bloom and Richardson grading) includes :
  1. Nuclear **p**olymorphism
  2. *Tubule formation* **Mnemonic** = **PMT**
  3. ***M**itotic rate*
- *Patient age* - very young and very old women have poor prognosis.
- Estrogen and progestin receptor expression - Good prognosis.
- *HER-2 over expression* - Poor prognosis.
- Proliferation rate (S phase fraction).
- **Histological type:** Tubular, mucinous, medullary, lobular and papillary type have good prognosis in comparison to NST.

Treatment

- **In situ carcinoma :**

A Ductal Ca in situ
- Excision (also referred to as lumpectomy or breast conserving surgery) plus definitive breast irradiation is the treatment of choice.
- Excision alone with out definitive breast irradiation (also referred as observation).
- Mastectomy in cases of diffuse lesion

B Lobular Ca in situ
- LCIS is best managed by careful observation.
- For patient who are unwilling to accept increased risk of breast cancer may be offered bilateral total mastectomy.

Remember : *Tamoxifen is effective is preventing invasive breast cancer in patient with lobular or ductal carcinoma.*

- **Invasive cancer**

Curative

– ***Surgery*** : For stage I and stage II disease and some patient of stage III

A. **Breast conserving therapy:**

BCT involves lumpectomy, sentinel lymphnode (SLN) biopsy, axillary dissection (if SLN is positive) followed by radiotherapy, systemic chemotherapy and hormonal therapy (in receptor positive)

Absolute contraindications:

- History of prior therapeutic irradiation
- Women with collagen vascular disease
- Pregnant women
- Multiple tumour focci
- Persistant positive margin after repeated surgical attempts

Senitel node biopsy has replaced axillary node dissection. In patient with no nodal involvement axillary dissection is avoided

B. ***Modified radical mastectomy***
- Standard therapy for most patient with breast Ca.
- Post operative *radiotherapy* is not usually necessary. ... *CSDT 12/e, p 314*

C. ***Radical mastectomy***
- Performed rarely.

– ***Radiotherapy*** : It is given after partial mastectomy or in QUART in total dose of 5000 - 6000 CGy in 5-6 week duration.

– ***Adjuvant therapy***

Palliative treatment

Given for disseminated stage III and stage IV cancer.

It includes :

1. ***Radiotherapy*** : Irradiation of the breast, chestwall, axillary and internal mammary and supraclavicular nodes,
   - To control *inoperable* lesions
   - To treat isolated *bone metastasis*
   - Chest wall *recurrence*
   - Brain *metastasis*
   - Acute spinal cord *compression.*
2. ***Hormone therapy*** - Agents used are :

Drug	Action
Tamoxifen	Antiestrogen
Diethylstilbestrol	Estrogen
Megestrol acetate	Progestin
Anastrozole	Aromatase inhibitor

- Hormonal therapy should be given in patient with receptor positive tumor i.e. in 90% cases.
- The *initial choice* of therapy is called primary therapy while *subsequent* endocrine treatment is called *secondary or tertiary hormonal therapy.*

Premenopausal patient	
Primary hormonal therapy	**Secondary or tertiary hormonal therapy**
– Tamoxifen (DOC) – B/L oophorectomy	– Tamoxifen (if not given in primary therapy). – If failed : Aminoglutethimide, megesterol or surgical adrenalectomy.
Postmenopausal patient	
Primary hormone therapy	**Secondary or tertiary hormone therapy**
– Tamoxifen **DOC**	– Who don't respond to initial tamoxifen should be given cytotoxic drugs such as CMF i.e. oydophosphamide, methotrexate 5 fluorouracil. – Who respond initially should be given diet hylstibesterol or megestrol acetate.

3. ***Chemotherapy :*** Indication are:
   - Presence of visceral metastases (specially brain or pulmonary).
   - If hormone treatment is failed.
   - If tumor is ER negative.

- Most useful single agent is **doxorubicin.**
- ErbB-2 (trastuzumab) (Herceptin) - Humanized antibody to erb B-2 combined with paclitaxel specially effective in tumor over expressing HER/neu.

Follow up

1. ***Local recurrence :***
   - Treated by irradiation and complete excision.
2. ***Edema of arm :***
   - Treated by mild diuretic Benzopyrone.
3. ***Breast reconstruction :***
   - Most commonly by implantation of silicone gel prosthesis in the *subpectoral plane* between the pectoralis minor and pectoralis major muscle.

Other are :
- *Saline filled prosthesis* - less chance of post prosthetic autoimmune disorder.
- *TRAM (Transrectus abdominous muscle) flap* - Most popular autologous technique.
- *Latissimus dorsiflap* - Provide less fullness.

Prevention

- Screening by mammography.
- **Self examination of breast :**
  - Monthly in all women > 20 years.
  - Should be performed 7-8 days after the menstural period.
  - Should be initially inspected while standing before a mirror, next in supine postion.
  - Each breast should be palpated.

MUST BE REMEMBERED

Cause of Breast discharge :

Ductectasia > Intraductal papilloma > Carcinoma are *most common* cause of breast discharge.

Breast discharge	
Discharge	**Lesion**
• Serous	Intraductal papilloma, fibroadenosis
• Greenish	Fibroadenosis
• Yellowish (pus)	Breast abscess
• Bloody	Duct papilloma *(Most common),* Duct carcinoma
• Milky	Galactocoele
• Paste like material	Duct ectasia *(also blackish or greenish)*

Breast surgery

- **QUART :** Quadrentectomy (***the entire segment of breast containing tumor)*** + Axillary block dissection + Radiotherapy.
- **Lumpectomy :** For tumor < 4 cm. ***Removal of tumor + a rim of at least 2 cm*** of normal breast tissue.
- **Simple mastectomy :** Removal of ***breast + small amount of skin.***
- **Modified radical mastectomy (Patey operation) :** Removal of ***entire breast with axillary block dissection*** with removal up to level III nodes.

  Structure Preserved are : - Pectoralis major
  - Nerve and blood supply of lattismus dorsi (thoracodorsal nerve)
  - Nerve to serratus anterior (Bells nerve)
  - Axillary vein
- **Radical mastectomy :** *MRM + removal of pectoralis major and minor, thoracodorsal nerve, artery to latissimus dorsi.*

  Structure preserved are : A – **A**xillary vein
  B – **B**ells nerve (Nerve to serratus anterior)
  C – **C**ephalic vein
- **Extended radical mastectomy :** Radical mastectomy + Removal of internal mammary lymphnodes.

CARCINOMA OF MALE BREAST :

- Rare
- Age > 60, ↑ ***incidence in men with prostate cancer gynecomastia***
- Invasion is more common
- Prognosis is worse
- Mostly present as painless lump
- Staging and treatment is same as breast ca in female.

QUESTIONS

1. **Which of this is a immunohistochemical marker for Pagets disease of the nipple of breast ? [AI 07]**
   a. S1000 b. Hmb 45
   c. CAM 5.2 d. CEA
2. **The most important prognostic factor in breast carcinoma is : [AI 06]**
   a. Histological grade of tumor
   b. Stage of the tumor at the of diagnosis
   c. Status of estrogen and progesterone receptors
   d. Over-expression of p-53 tumor suppressor gene
3. **The tumor which may occur in the residual breast or over lying skin following wide local excision and radiotherapy for mammary carcinoma is:**
   a. Leiomyosarcoma **[AI 06]**
   b. Squamous carcinoma
   c. Basal cell carcinoma
   d. Angiosarcoma
4. **The type of mammary ductal carcimoma in situ (DCIS) most likely to result in a palpable abnormality in the breast is :**
   a. Apocrine DCIS **[AI 06]**
   b. Neuroendocrine DCIS
   c. Well differentiated DCIS
   d. Comedo DCIS
5. **In which of the following types of breast carcinoma would you consider biopsy of opposite breast : [AI 06]**
   a. Adenocarcinoma - poorly differentiated
   b. Medullary carcinoma
   c. Lobular carcinoma
   d. Comedo carcinoma
6. **A blood stained discharge from the nipple indicates one of the following :**
   [AI 05; PGI 09, 10]
   a. Breast abscess
   b. Fibroadenoma
   c. Duct Papilloma
   d. Fat Necrosis of Breast
7. **All of the following hormonal agent used against breast cancer except : [AI 05, 04]**
   a. Letrazole b. Exemestane
   c. Taxol d. Tamoxifien
8. **A 25 year old female complaints of discharge of blood from single duct of breast. The most appropriate treatment is:**
   a. Radical duct excision **[AI 08]**
   b. Microdochectomy
   c. Radical mastectomy
   d. Biopsy to rule out carcinoma
9. **According to TNM classification in breast carcinoma, involvement of supraclavicular lymphnode indicates:**
   a. IIIa **[AIIMS Nov 08]**
   b. IIIb
   c. IIIc
   d. IV
10. **True about treatment of early breast carcinoma? [AIIMS May 08]**
    a. Aromatase inhibitors are replacing tamoxifen in premenopausal women
    b. Postmastectomy radiation therapy is given when 4 or more lymph nodes are positive
    c. Tamoxifen is not useful in postmenopausal women
    d. In pemenopausal women, multidrug chemotherapy is given in selected patient
11. **A 38 year old female presented with unilateral breast cancer associated with axillary lymphnode enlargement. Modified radical mastectomy was done, further treatment plan would be:**
    a. Observation and follow up
    b. Adriamycim based chemotherapy followed by tamoxifen depending on estrogen / progesterone receptor status **[AIIMS May 07]**
    c. Adriamycin based chemotherapy only
    d. Tamoxifen only

12. Triple assessment for CA breast includes:
a. History, clinical examination and mammogram **[AI 09]**
b. History, clinical examination and FNAC
c. USG mammogram and FNAC
d. Clinical examination, mammogram and FNAC

13. Moderately increased risk of invasive breast carcinoma is associated with which of the following benign lesions of breast: [AI 09]
a. Sclerosing adenosis
b. Atypical lobular hyperplasia
c. Apocrine metaplasia
d. Squamous metaplasia

14. Most sensitive investigation for DCIS (Ductal carcinoma in situ) of breast?
a. Mammography **[AI 09]**
b. Ultrasound
c. MRI
d. PET scan

15. True about male breast cancer: [PGI 09]
a. Does not follow gynecomastica
b. Lobular variety common
c. Estrogen recepter negative
d. Old age
e. Surgery is the treatment of choice

16. Aromatic inhibitor used in CA breast:
a. Letrozole **[PGI 09]**
b. Anastrozole
c. Exemestene
d. Tamoxifen

17. Which of the following is least likely to be associated with Ca breast in woman ?
a. BRCA - 1 **[AIIMS 06]**
b. BRCA - 2
c. Li Fraumenii syndrome
d. Ataxia telangiectasia

18. Which of the following features on mammogram would suggest malignancy? [AIIMS 06]
a. Well defined lesion
b. A mass of decreased density
c. Areas of spiculated microcalcifications
d. Smooth borders

19. Features that are evaluated for histological grading of breast carcinoma includes all except : [AIIMS 05]
a. Tumor necrosis
b. Mitotic count
c. Tubule formation
d. Nuclear polymorphism

20. In patient with breast cancer, chest wall involvement means involvement of any of the following structures except :
a. Serratus anterior **[AIIMS 05]**
b. Pectoralis major
c. Intercostal muscles
d. Ribs

21. Increased susceptibility to breast cancer is likely to be associated with a mutation in the following gene: [AIIMS 06]
a. p53 b. BRCA
c. Retinoblastoma [Rb] d. H-Ras

22. Blood stained nipple discharge is seen in: [PGI 09]
a. Breast abscess
b. Fibroadenoma
c. Duct papilloma
d. Fat necrosis

23. All of the following are used for reconstruction of breast except : [PGI 07]
a. Transverse rectus abdominus myocutaneous flap
b. Latissimus dorsi myocutaneous flap
c. Pectoralis major myocutaneous flap
d. Transverse rectus abdominus free flap

24. Contraindication for modified radical mastectomy in carcinoma breast :
a. Distant metatasis **[PGI 06]**
b. Fixity to chestwall
c. Axillary LN involvement
d. Supraclavicular LN involvement

25. B/L Breast Ca : [PGI 06, 05]
a. Lobular Ca
b. Ductal Ca
c. Comedo Ca
d. Cystosarcoma phylloids
e. Schirrous Ca

26. Breast Ca good prognosis markers : **[PGI 06]**
a. ER +ve [receptor]
b. Progesterone [receptors] +ve
c. HER - 2/neu [receptors] +ve
d. CD44 receptor +ve
e. P53 gene +ve

27. Conservative surgery for breast ca is not done in: **[PGI 06, 01]**
a. Low socioeconomic status
b. Age > 40 years
c. Multicentricity
d. LN Palpable in axilla
e. Family history of breast ca

28. About lymphatic spread of Ca breast, correct statement is : **[PGI 05]**
a. Axillary nodes are most commonly involved
b. Internal mammary nodes are also involved
c. If supraclavicular LN is involved then it is N_3
d. Axillary nodes are surgically resected in treatment

29. True about screening mammography :
a. Indicated in 50-70 years of age
b. Mortality reduced by 30% **[PGI 08]**
c. Radiation due to mammography can cause carcinoma
d. MRI is better than mammography
e. USG is better than mammography

30. Use of Tamoxifen for Breast cancer can cause all of the following adverse effects, Except. **[AI 09]**
a. Thromboembolism
b. Endometrial carcinoma
c. Carcinoma in contralateral breast
d. Cataract

ANSWERS, REFERENCES, EXPLANATIONS WITH INFORMATIVE ILLUSTRATIONS

1. s. is c i.e. CAM 5.2 *Fletcher Histopathology of Tumour 3/e, p 928*

severly inflammed nipple it is difficult to differentiate between paget's disease and e ma as the neoplastic cells also resemble keratinocytes. In such cases im ɔcytochemistry using antibodies to low molecular weight cytokeratins CK 8, 18, 19 (eg 1 5.2) which are not expressed in normal keratinocytes and found in over 90% of man. paget's disease, are invaluable.

Paget ease of Nipple

- Man tion of high grade DCIS involving excretory duct which infiltrate nipple and areola
- Presen eczema like condition of nipple and areola.
- Histolo characterized by presence of paget cells (large hyperchromatic cells with clea ɔlasm). Tumour cell may show positive staining for PAS-Positive disastase resistan s. Immunohistochemistry is diagnostic.

2. Ans. is b i.e. the tumour at the time of diagnosis *Ref. CSDT 13/e, p 301*

"Stage of the b r is overall most reliable indicator of prognosis as it include both tumor size a us."

Remember : Axillary e most important prognostic factor.

Prognostic factor in node negative breast cancer

Factor	Increased recurrence	Decreased recurrence
• Size	T_3, T_2	$T1, T_0$
• Hormone receptors	–	+
• DNA flow cytometry	Aneuploid	Diploid
• Histologic grade	High	Low
• S phase fraction	> 5%	< 5%
• Lymphatic or vascular invasion	Present	Absent
• Cathepsin D	High	Low
• HER-2/neu oncogene	High	Low
• Epidermal growth factor receptor	High	Low

3. **Ans. is d i.e. Angiosarcoma** *Ref. Sabiston 18/e, p 872; Bailey 25/e,p 845*

"Angiosarcoma and lymphangiosarcoma may develop as a complication of chronic lymphedema specially in patients of breast cancer." ... Bailey & Love

Angiosarcoma

- Vascular tumor arising in dermis after breast irradiation or in the lymphedematous upper extremity. Rarely it occur denovo too.
- Present as postirradiation vascular proliferation. The differential diagnosis is atypical vascular proliferation.
- Histologically tumor composed of anastmosing tangle of blood vessels in the dermis and subcutaneous fat.
- Clinically present as reddish brown to purpole raised rash within the radiation portals and on the skin of breast.
- Treatment includes surgery to ensure negative margins followed by split skin graft or myocutaneous flap.
- Lymphatic metastasis is very rare and lymphataic resection is not required.

Remember : Lymphoedema is *MC* and most worrisome complication of mastectomy.

Treatment of Lymphoedema :
- *Manual* lymphatic drainage.
- *Compression* garments / Bandaging.
- *Pneumatic* compression devices.

4. **Ans. is d i.e. Comedo DCIS**

Ref. Anderson Pathology 10/e, p 2368 - 2369; Ackerman 9/e, p 1795

"Majority of comedo DCIS present as palpable masses averaging 2-3cm in diameter."

...Anderson

DCIS	
Comedo DCIS	**Non comedo DCIS**
• 35-50%% of DCIS • Aggressive cytological features • Associated with invasive Ca in contralateral breast • Higher recurrence rate	• 50-65% • Relatively non aggressive • Not associated • Lower recurrence rate

5. **Ans. is c i.e. Lobular carcinoma**

Ref. CSDT 12/e, p 312; Robbins 7/e, p 1144, 8/e, p 1083

"Bilaterality occurs more often in women under age 50 and is more frequent when the tumor in the primary breast cancer is lobular."

Lobular carcinoma:

- Responsible for **5–10%** of all invasive Ca.
- Incidence is more among postmenopausal woman.
- Mostly present as a mass on examination **or density** on mammography i.e. no calcification.
- Most tumor show a loss of region on **chr. 16.**
- ***Histological hallmark*** of ILC is tendency of tumor cells to *invade in linear strands* (Indian file pattern) with minimal desmoplastic response
- Show ***different pattern of metastases*** and have propensity to involve peritoneal surface, meninges and git, OVARIES are *less likely to metastasize to lungs or bone.*

6. **Ans. is c i.e. Duct Papilloma** *Ref. Sabiston 18/e, p 867; Bailey 25/e p 831*

"Blood discharge is suggestive of cancer but is more often cause by benign papilloma in the duct."

Nipple discharge :

Most common cause are - *Duct ectasia > Intraductal papilloma > carcinoma.*

"In case of bloody discharge excision of the bloody duct system is indicated regardless the finding of ductography or cytology."

7. **Ans. is c i.e. Taxol** *Ref. Devita 8/e, p 1636-1638*

Taxol is trade name of Paclitaxel which is not a hormone.

Drugs used in Hormone therapy of Breast cancer		
SERM	**LHRH agonist (for ovarian ablation)**	**Progestin**
– Tamoxifen (Nolvodex) – Toremifen (Fareston)	– Goserelin (Zoladex) – Leuprolide (Lupron)	– Megesterol acetate (Megace) – Medroxyprogesterone acetate (provera)
Androgens	**Aromatase inhibitor**	**Pure anti estrogen**
– Fluoxymestrone (Halostesin)	– Aminoglutethimide – Letrozole (Femara) – Exemestane (Aromasin) – Anastrozole (Arimidex) – Exemestane (Aromasin)	– Fulvestrant (Faslodex) – High dose estrogen – Diethyl stibesterol

Contd...

Contd...

Drugs used in breast chemotherapy				
Anthracyclins	**Alkylating agent and related drug**	**Vinca alkaloids**	**Taxanes**	**Antimetabolites**
– Doxorubicin – Epirubicin – Mitoxantrone	– Cyclophosphamide – Melphalan	– Vinblastine – Vinorelbine – Etoposide – Gemcitabine	– Paclitaxel – Docetaxel – Methotrexate	– 5 Fluorouracil – Capecitabine

Remember :

Agents for targeted therapy in breast Ca

HER-2 neu overexpression:

- Trastuzumab (Herceptin): Antibody that binds HER-2/neu receptor

Vascular endothelial growth factor (VEGF)

- Bevacizumab (Avastin): Monoclonal antibody directed against VEGF

8. **Ans. is b i.e. Microdochectomy** *Ref. Bailey & Love 25/e, p 831; Sabiston 18/e p 867*

Bloody discharge from breast	
Single duct	**Multiple duct**
– Intraduct papilloma (MC) – Intraduct carcinoma – Duct ectasia	– Carcinoma – Ectasia – Fibrocystic disease

Duct Pappiloma

- **Benign lesion** of breast affecting middle aged women.
- Presents with ***small swelling just beneath the areola,*** palpation of which results in discharge of blood from nipple.
- Tumor is situated in one of the **large lactiferous duct.**
- It is premalignant lesion **(relative risk 1.5–2.0)**
- **Treatment:**
  - Microdochectomy – **Treatment of coice.**
  - Cone excision of major duct **(Head field operation).** When duct of origin of nipple bleeding is uncertain or when there is bleeding from multiple ducts.

Remember : – Dict papilloma is most common cause of bleeding discharge from nipple

Investigation in Case of Bloody discharge

- **Mammography**
- **Cytology**

} To detect cancer (but negative finding does not rule out cancer).

- **Ductography** : To localize the extent and site of bleeding duct.
- **Ultrasound** : To ***identify duct ectasia*** which has *characteristics tubular and echoic or hypoechoic appearance.*

9. **Ans. is c i.e. IIIc** *Ref. CSDT 13/e, p 291-292*

Metastasis to ipsilateral supraclavicular lymph node signifies N3. Minimum Stage with N3 is IIIc. ***Kindly see theroy portion for complete stage***

10. **Ans. is b i.e. Postmastectomy radiation therapy is given when 4 or more lymph nodes are positive** *... Ref. Devita 8/e, p 1635*

Lets consider each option

Option 'a' and 'c' *... Devita 7/e p 1635*

- Aromatase inhibitor (AI) are more beneficial than tamoxifen in postmenopausal women and are now becoming agent of choice
- In premenopausal women agent of choice still is tomoxifen
  Reason: In postmenopausal women, the main source of estrogen is aromatization of androgens as there is no estrogen from ovary. Aromatase inhibitors stop this aromatization
- This does not mean that tamoxifen is not effective in postmenopausal women. It is effective in both pre and postmenopausal women
- In premenopausal patients AI are not beneficial as residual ovarian function can lead to enhanced production of aromatase and thus overcome the effect of AI

Option 'b'

- Postmastectomy radiation therapy is defined *as the delivery of adjuvant radiation treatment to the chest wal and usually to the one or more regional lymph node*
- According to ASCO (American society of clinical oncology) post mastectomy radiation treatment is indicated *when there are four or more pathologically positive axillary lymph nodes and when the tumor is > stage II*

Option 'd'

- Adjuvant therapy is given in all cases of early breast Ca managed by breast conservation therapy
- Multidrug chemotherapy is the integral part of adjuvant therapy

11. **Ans. is b, i.e. Adriamycim based chemotherapy followed...**

Ref. Harrison 17/e, p 567; Schrawtz 8/e, p 492

Suggested approaches to adjuvant therapy

Age Group	Lymph Node Status	Endocrine Receptor (ER) Status	Tumor	Recommendation
Premenopausal	Positive	Any	Any	MDC + tamoxifen if ER-positive + trastuzumab in HER-2/neu positive tumors
Premenopausal	Negative	Any	>2 cm, or 1-2 cm with other poor prognostic variables	MDC+ tamoxifen if ER-positive + trastuzumab in HER-2/neu positive tumors
Postmenopausal	Positive	Negative	Any	MDC + trastuzumab in HER-2/neu positive tumors
Postmenopausal	Positive	Positive	Any	Aromatase inhibitors and tamoxifen with or without chemotherapy +

Contd...

Contd...

Age Group	Lymph Node Status	Endocrine Receptor (ER) Status	Tumor	Recommendation
				trastuzumab in HER-2/neu positive tumors
Postmenopausal	Negative	Positive	>2 cm, or 1-2 cm with other poor prognostic variables	Aromatase inhibitors and tamoxifen + trastuzumab in HER-2/neu positive tumors
Postmenopausal	Negative	Negative	>2cm, or 1-2 cm with other poor prognostic variables	Consider MDC + trastuzumab in HER-2/neu positive tumors

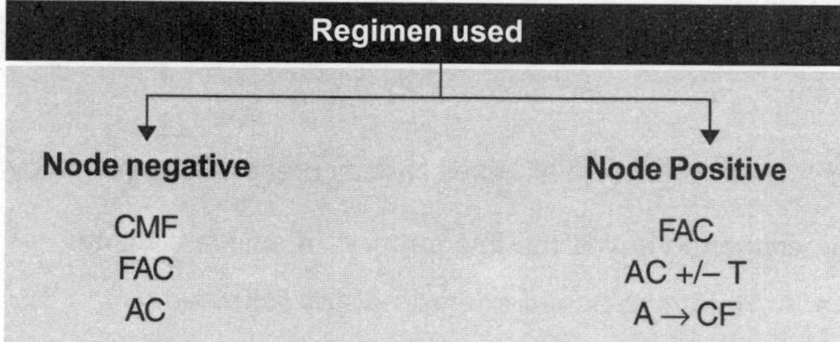

12. Ans. is d i.e. Clinical examination, mammogram and FNAC

Ref. Bailey 25/e, p 829; Harrison 17/e, p 564

In any patient who present with breast lump or other symptoms suspicious of carcinoma, ***the diagnosis should be made by a combination of clinical assessment, radiological imaging (mammography) and tissue sampling*** for either cytological or histological examination.

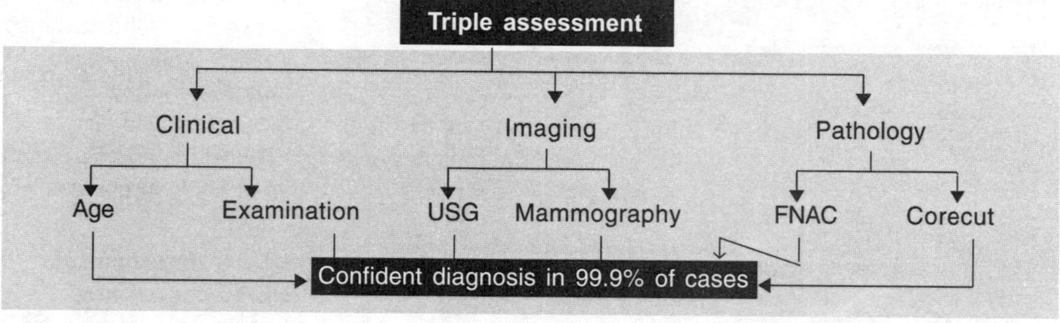

Remember:
- In premenopausal women, lesions that are either equivocal or non suspicious on physical examination, should be reexamined in 2-4 weeks during the follicular phase of menstrual cycle
- Days 5-7 of the cycle are the best time for breast examination

13. Ans. is b i.e. Atypical hyperplasia

Ref. Robbin's 7/e, p 1130, 8/e, p 1074; Schwartz 8/e, p 464

Breast Lesion	Relative risk of breast cancer
• *Non proliferative breast changes* – Duct ectasia – Apocrine change – Mild hyperplasia – Adenosis – Fibroadenoma without complex feature – Cysts	*1.0*
• *Proliferative breast disease without atypia* – Moderate or florid hyperplasia – Sclerosing adenosis – Papilloma – Complex sclerosing lesion (radial scar) – Fibroadenoma with complex features	*1.5 – 2.0 (Low)*
• *Proliferative disease with atypia* – Atypical lductal hyperplasia – Atypical lobular hyperplasia	*4.0 – 5.0 (Moderate)*
• *Carcinoma in situ* – Lobular Ca *in situ* – Ductal Ca *in situ*	*8.0 – 10.0 (High)*
• *Cancer in one breast—risk of Ca inother breast*	

14. Ans. is a i.e. Mammography *Ref. Grainger 5/e, p 1190, 1188*

I, think confusion is between mammography and MRI.

Now see, Grainger.

Screening with MRI is superior to mammography in detecting invasive breast cancer ***in younger women where the sensitivity of mammography is low due to presence of dense breast parenchyma.***

Although ***mammography remains more sensitive for detecting Ductal carcinoma in sits [DCIS].***

Sensitivity of ultrasound for detecting breast mass is significantly low, that's why ultrasound is not a useful screening test for breast cancer.

Indications for breast MRI

- Suspicion of lobular carcinoma
- Staging of primary breast cancer
- For screening in younger women
- Assessing the integrity of breast implant
- To detect site of occult primary tumor, in cases with malignant axillary lymphodenopathy with normal mammogram and breast USG.

Role of PET

- PET may plat a role in imaging atypical lesions but is less sensitive for early breast cancer than is MRI or mammography.

15. **Ans. is d, e i.e. Old age; Surgery is the treatment of choice**

Ref. Harrison 17/e, p 569; Devita 8/e, p 1643

Male Breast Cancer

- 1/150th in incidence compared to female breast Ca
- **Risk Factors** – Any condition with increased estrogen or reduced androgen
  - Cirrhosis
  - Undescended testes
  - Testicular injury
  - Mumps orchitis
  - Klinefelter's syndrome
  - Gynecomastia is seen preceding or accompanying in 20% of cases
- *Infiltrating ductal ca is most common type*
- Average age of presentation is ***60 year***
- Present with asymmetric, unilateral lump
- Majority of male breast Ca are ER positive
- **Staging and prognostic factor** are same as that for female breast Ca

Treatment

- Modified radical mastectomy followed by postoperative radiation therapy in cases with increased chance of local recurrence.
- Though none of the trial has compared systemic chemotherapy in male, it is advocated with similar guidelines as for females
- Breast conserving therapy is not feasible due to small account breast tissue present in males

Remember Gynecomastia alone does not appear to be a risk factor

... Devita 8/e, p 1643

16. **Ans. is a, b, c i.e. Letrozole; Anastrozole; Exemestene** *Ref. Devita 8/e, p 1636-1638*

Already explained See Answer No. 7

17. **Ans. is d i.e. Ataxia telangiectasia** *Ref. Robbins 8/e, p 1077; Harrison 17/e, p 563*

All of the given options increase risk of breast carcinoma. But the least incidence is with ataxia telaniectasia, hence answer.

Incidence of Sporadic, Familial, and Hereditary Breast cancer	
Sporadic breast cancer	65 – 75%
Familial breast cancer	20 – 30%
Hereditary breast cancer	5 – 10%
BRCA - 1a	45%
BRCA - 2	35%
p53 (Li-Fraumeni syndrome)	1%
STK11/LKB1 (Peutz-Jeghers syndrome)	< 1%
PTEN (Cowden disease)	< 1%
MSH2 / MLH1 (Muir-Torre syndrome)	< 1%
ATM (Ataxia - telangiectasia)	< 1%
Unknown	20%

Remember :
- Not more than 10% of human breast cancer can be directly linked to germline mutation.
- Ataxia telangiectasis is an autosomal recessive disorder characterized by ataxic-dyskinetic syndrome begining in early childhood, caused by neuronal degeneration predominantly in the cerebellum. There is defect in ATM gene which is associated with DNA repair. These patient also have an increased frequency of breast Ca in addition to lymphomas, leukemias (T-cell type).

18. Ans. is c i.e. Areas of spiculated microcalcifications

Ref. Chapman 3/e, p 350; CSDT 13/e, p 285, 289

Mammography

- *Most useful technique for detection of early breast cancer.*
- **Indications :**
  - *Screening* of Ca breast.
  - *Evaluation* of ill defined breast mass.
  - *Fibroadenosis.*
  - Search for *occult Ca* breast in women with metastatic disease.
  - *Follow up* of breast Ca.
  - Prior to *cosmetic operation and biopsy.*
- **Procedure :**
  - Breast is exposed to ***low voltage and high ampere X-ray*** with lateral oblique projection.
  - Film screen mammography deliver 0.1 CGy per view and ***replaced*** the ***older xero mammo-graphic technique.***
- **Sensitivity :**
  - 60 - 90%
- **Specificity :**
  - 30 - 40% for non palpable
  - 85 - 90% for clinically evident

- **Advantage :** – 40% reduction in stage II disease in screened population with 30% increased in survival rate, due to early detection.
- **Disadvantage :** It may not reveal carcinoma in :
  - *Very dense breast*
  - Medullary Ca
  - Cancer in *young women* with fibrocystic change
  - Repeated mammography i*ncrease risk of carcinoma* due to radiation exposure.

Differences in Benign and Malignant lesions seen in Mammography

	Benign	Malignant
1. Opacity	Smooth margin Low density Homogenous *Thin* 'halo'	• Ill defined margin-stellate, spiculated • High density • In homogenous • *Wide* 'halo'
2. Calcification	Smooth, widely separated/ linear thick rod like 'Popcorn' – Fibroadenoma 'Floating' – 'Milk of calcium' Widespread – all one/both	• Microcalcification segmented, cluster distribution mixture of size and shape • Eccentrically located
3. Surrounding parenchyma	Normal	Disrupted
4. Nipple/areola	± Retracted	± Retracted
5. Skin	Normal	Thickened
6. Cooper's ligaments	Normal	Thickened
7. Ducts	Normal	Focal dilatation
8. Subcutaneous/ retromammary space	Normal	Obliterated

19. Ans. is a i.e. Tumor necrosis *Ref. Robbin's 8/e, p 1089; Anderson 10/e, p 2373*

- The most commonly used grading system for breast ca is ***Scarf bloom Richardson.***
- Grading is done by *evaluating* :
  - **T**ubule formation
  - **M**itotic rate
  - **N**uclear polymorphism

Mnemonic **-TNM**

- Grading is directly related to survival.
- 80% of patient with ***grade I tumor***, 60% of women with ***grade II tumor***, 15% of patient with ***grade III tumor*** *survive for 10 years.*

HISTOLOGIC GRADING	
Feature	**Score**
Percent tubule formation	
> 75	1
10 – 75	2
< 10	3
Nuclear polymorphism	
Mild (Small and uniform)	1
Intermediate	2
Severe	3
Mitotic counts	
<9	1
10 – 19	2
>20	3
Total Score	**3** – 5 **Well differentiated**
	6 – 7 Moderate differentiated
	8 – 9 Poorly differentiated

20. **Ans. is b i.e. Pectoralis major** *Ref. Harrison 17/e, p 566*

Extension to chest wall is included in Stage 4a.

Extension to chest wall does not include pectoralis muscle.

For details, see theory portion

21. **Ans. is a i.e. P53** *Ref. Robbin's 8/e, p 1078; Harrison 16/e, p 516 - 517*

Genetic mutation associated with breast cancer are of two types :

Germline mutations/Inherited mutation	Somatic mutation or acquired mutation
• Cause familial breast cancer (less common) • Involves : BRCA - 1 ***(MC)*** BRCA - 2 p53 • BRCA - 1 is involved in 3% of all breast cancer & 60 - 70% of familial breast cancer	• Cause sporadic or primary breast cancer ***(MC)*** • Involves p53 and *not involved BRCA-1* • p53 is involved in 40% of breast cancer

Since P53 is involved in both types of mutation and ***sporadic breast cancer is more common*** so, p53 is involved commonly than BRCA-1. ***Hence answer -***

Remember :

– Most common mutation in ***familial breast cancer***	:	BRCA 1
– Most common mutation in ***sporadic breast cancer***	:	p53
– Most common mutation in ***breast cancer***	:	p53

22. Ans. is c i.e. Duct papilloma *Ref. Bailey 25/e, p 831*

Already explained in Ans. No. 6

23. Ans. is c i.e. Pectoralis major myocutaneous flap *Ref. Devita 8/e, p 1629*

Breast reconstruction

1. **Prosthetic reconstruction**
   - A ***tissue expander implant is placed*** in subpectoral plane *between pectoralis major and pectoralis minor.*
   - Two types of implant are used :
     - ***Silicone gel prosthesis*** : Chances of silicone induced autoimmune disorders.
     - ***Saline filled prosthesis*** : Less chance of post prosthetic autoimmune disorders.
2. **Autologus tissue reconstruction**
   - It includes ***placement of local and distant flaps*** for breast reconstruction.
   - ***Local flaps** include* :
     - *Latissimus dorsi myocutaneus flap :* Easy to harvest with minimal donor site morbidity but provide limited volume of tissue, so suitable only for small breast or when concomitant implant is placed.
     - *Transverse rectus abdominous myocutoneous flap* **(TRAM) :** Most common method of *autologus breast reconstruction* because of large volume and texture which closely resemble breast.
     - *Depending* on volume, the TRAM flap is transferred on a single pedicle, double pedicle or as a free flap
     - *Main disadvantage* is loss of abdominal wall strength (10% in unilateral and loss of 40% strength in double pedicle graft), hernia formation.
   - **Distant flaps :** Most recent technique in breast reconstruction and *involves use of perforator flaps.*
     - **It include :**
       - Deep inferior epigastric artery perforator (DIEP) flap
       - Superficial inferior epigastric artery perforator
       - Inferior gluteal flap
       - Superior gluteal flap
       - Rubens flap.
     - *Main disadvantage* of these flaps are more operating time, venous congestion, fat necrosis & flap loss.

24. Ans. is a, c and d i.e. Distant metatasis; Axillary LN involvement; and Supraclavicular LN involvement *Ref. See below*

Guy's question is very simple as.

MRM or Surgery is indicated for stage I, stage II and early stage III tumour or late stage III, stage IV are contraindication to MRM.

Now see :

• Distant metastasis	M_1	– Minimum stage would be stage IV
• Fixity to chest wall	T_4	– Minimum stage would be stage IIIb
• Axillary LN involvement	N_1	– Minimum stage would be stage Ia
• Supraclamicular LN	N_3	– Minimum stage would be stage IIIc

25. Ans. is a i.e. Lobular Ca *Ref. Robbin's 8/e, p 1083*

Already explained, kindly see answer no. 5

26. Ans. is a and b i.e. ER +ve (receptor); and Progesterone (receptors) +ve

Already explained

27. Ans. is c i.e. Multicentricity *Ref. Devita 8/e, p 1620-1624*

Breast conservation therapy (BCT)

Indication :
- Early stage T_1 - T_2 tumor
- Solitary lesion
- Enough size of breast

Contraindication	
Absolute	**Relative**
– Persistent positive margin after reasonable surgical attempts – *Two or more* primary tumor in separate areas of breast – *Diffuse* malignant appearing microcalcification – *History* of prior therapeutic irradiation – *Pregnancy*	– Large tumor relative to breast size – Bilateral tumor – Women with very large pendulous breast – Active collagen vascular disease *(SLE)* *... Devita 7/e, p 1437*

Breast conservation therapy sequence

↓

Core needle biopsy

Lumpectomy and sentinel lymph node (SLN) biopsy and *axillary dissection if SLN positive*

Adjuvant systemic chemotherapy + breast irradiation

Adjuvant hormone therapy if receptor positive.

Note : Subareolar primary tumor, positive axillary lymphnodes and extremes of age were ***previously considered as contraindication*** for BCT but now not.

Remember : Inspite of giving chemotherapy after surgery ***trend is now moving towards chemotherapy prior to surgery*** i.e. neoadjuvant chemotherapy, which results in decrease in size of tumor and makes surgery more feasable.

28. Ans. is a, b, c, d i.e. Axillary nodes are most commonly involved; Internal mammary nodes are also involved; If supraclavicular LN is involved then it is N_3; and Axillary nodes are surgically resected in treatment *Ref. Robbin's 7/e, p 1146*

Spread of Breast Ca

Local :	To involve remaining portion of breast, skin, pectoral muscle and even chest wall.
Lymphatic :	Axillary LN (Most common), internal mammary lymph node. Supraclavicular and any contralateral LN represent advanced disease.
Hematogenous route :	Bone (Most common) > liver > lung. Most common ***bones involved*** are lumbar vertebrae.

29. Ans. is a, b and c i.e. Indicated in 50-70 years of age; Mortality reduced by 30%; and Radiation due to mammography can cause carcinoma

Ref. CMDT 10, p 655; Grainger 5/e p 1190

MRI is definitively better than mammography but it can't be used for screening.
- MRI has got high sensitivity but low specificity, this results in multiple unnecessary biopsies if lesion is suspicious on MRI.
- Thus for normal population it is not used as screening modality.

Role of MRI in Breast masses :
- ***MRI*** is gold standard for imaging the breasts of women with implants.
- Useful to ***differentiate*** between scar ***from*** recurrence in women who had previous breast conservation therapy.

Role of Ultrasound in Breast masses :
- It is particularly ***useful in young women*** with ***dense breast*** in whom mammograms are difficult to interpret.
- In ***distinguishing*** cysts from solid lesion.
- It is not useful as screening tool.

30. Ans. is c i.e. Carcinoma in contralateral breast

Ref. KDT 6/e p 304; Goodman 10/e p 1141

Tamoxifen decreases the risk of developing cancer in contralateral breast.

Adverse effects of tamoxifen

- *Endometrial hyperplasia and endometrial cancer:* Tamoxifen blocks estrogen receptors on the breast (antagonistic action), while it stimulates these receptors in the uterus bone, liver, pituitary (partial agonistic action). This stimulation increase the risk of endometrial hyperplasia and cancer.

- *Cataract:* Tamoxifen causes retinal deposits, decreased visual aqcuity and cataract in occasional patients.
- *Thromboembolism*.
- *Other side effects include:* Hot flushes, vomiting, vaginal bleeding, vaginal discharge, menstrual irregularities. Dermatitis, anorexia, depression, mild leucopenia can also be seen rarely.

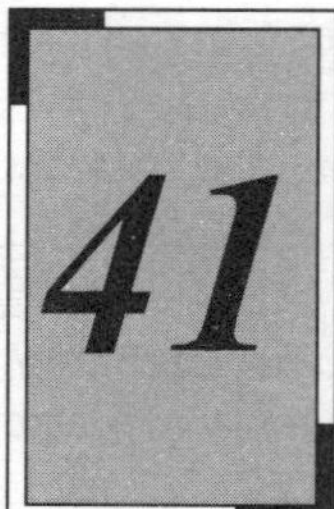

Pediatric Tumour

What's Important ?

- **Cytogenetics and Treatment of Wilm's Tumour**
- **Prognostic Factor of Every Tumour**

- ***Cancer is the fourth leading cause of death*** in pediatric age group
- Pediatric cancers have good prognosis; and the overall 5 year survival rate of pediatric malignancy is now greater than 75%
- For treatment planning and recommendition the apex society is children oncology group (COG), it is the amalgamation of four prior pediatric cooperative group (children cancer group, pediatric oncology group, rhabdosarcoma study group, and National Wilm's tumor study group)
- ALL (Acute lymphoblastic leukemia) is the most common malignancy of childhood. Peak age of onset is 4 years ... *CPDT 19/e, p 853*
- Brain tumor are the most common solid tumor of childhood ... *CPDT 19/e, p 860*
- Neuroblastoma is the most common neoplasm of Infancy
- Neuroblastoma is the most common solid intraabdominal pediatric tumor
- Osteosarcoma is the most common pediatric bone tumor
- Retinoblastoma is the most common intraocular tumor in pediatric patients

In this chapter we are going to cover, those pediatric tumor which are not discussed in other chapters.

WILM'S TUMOUR / NEPHROBLASTOMA

- Arise from kidney and is usually composed of ***three elements*** - blastema, epithelium and stroma.
- ***Majority*** of Wilms tumour are of sporadic type.
- Most commonly ***left kidney*** involved (in 50% cases). > Rt Kidney (45%) > bilateral (5%)

Genetics

Wilms tumor can be the manifestation of some genetic disorders. These are:

Disorder	Features	Defect
WAGR syndrome	Wilm's tumor, Aniridia genital anomalies, Mental retardation	11 p 13 deletion
Denys-Drash syndrome	Genitourinary defects, renal mesangial sclerosis, intersex disorder, Wilm's tumor	11 p 13 WT_1 point mutation
Frasier syndrome	Genitourinary defects, focal glomerulosclerosis, intersex disorder. Wilm's tumor (low incidence)	Point mutation in WT-1 gene
Beckwith Weidemann syndrome	Organomegaly, macroglossia, hemihyper-trophy, umbilical hernia, hypoglycemia, increased risk of Wilm's tumor, hepato-blastoma, adrenocortical carcinoma	11 p 15.5 (WT-2 locus) deletion Duplication 11 p 15.5

Other rare syndrome which increase risk of WT are Pearlman syndrome, Solos syndrome, Neurofibromatosis, von Willebrand disease, sporadic aniridia

- Genitourinary anomalies most commonly associated with WT are hypoplasia, fusion and ectopia of kidney, duplication of collecting system, hypospadia, cryptoorchidism
- Patient with these disease and genetic disorder have higher incidence of bilateral disease

Clinical Features

- Seen commonly between ages 2 and 5 years, unusual after 6 years.
- Most common presenting feature is asymptomatic ***abdominal mass or swelling.***
- Fever, hematuria, hypertension might be seen.

Diagnosis

- **USG** (most important investgation) or CT of abdomen.
- Plain X ray chest to detect lung metastasis CT chest is not recommended as lung metastasis of WT can be seen on plain X-ray ... *Nelson 18/e, p 2142*
- ***Calcification*** tends to be more *crescent shaped, discrete,* and **peripheral** in comparison of **finely stippled** calcification of *neuroblastoma.*

  It can form tumor thrombus that extends through renal vein to IVC. IVC thrombus must be ruled out prior to surger

Staging

Two staging are currently used:

a. Prechemotherapy staging system developed by National Wilms tumor study group
b. Postchemotherapy based system developed by International Society of Pediatric Oncology

Treatment

***Surgical excision* is treatment of choice. :** The aim of surgery is to completely remove the tumour (nephrectomy) and ureter with out spill age via transabdominal transperitoneal approach and to determine the tumor stage by virtue of its extent and the presence of lymphnode involvement.

Preoperative treatment with or chemotherapy is indicated in :

- Wilms tumor in solitary kidney.
- Bilateral tumors.
- Tumor in horeshoe kidney.
- Extensive pulmonary metastases.
- In child with bilateral disease primary goal of treatment is removal of tumor with a secondary goal to preserve maximum normal renal tissue.

After excision further treatment depends upon histology.

Post surgical treatment of Wilms tumor		
Histological type	**Stage**	**Treatment**
Favourable (common) characterized by blastema, epithelia, and stroma devoid of ectopia or anaplasia	I, II	18 weeks (dactinomycin and vin cristine
	III and IV	24 weeks (dactinomycin, vincristine, and doxorubicin with radiation
Unfavourable Marked enlargement of nuclei, hyperchromatism of the enlarged nuclei, and multipolar mitotic figure	I	
	I III IV	24 weeks (vincristine, doxorubin, etoposide, and cyclophosphamide) with radiation

- Chemotherapy should optimally begin within 5 days after surgery where as radiation therapy should be started within 10 days

Prognostic factors:
- Histologic grade
- Pathology
- Staging
- Ploidy (diploid tumor have better prognosis)

NEUROBLASTOMA

- Neuroblastoma is an embryonal cancer of peripheral sympathetic nervous system. It include spectrum of tumor with variable degree of neuronal differentiation, ranging from undifferentiated small, round cells ***(typical neuroblastoma)*** to tumor containing mature ganglion cells (ganglioneuroblastoma or ganglioneuroma)
- ***Most common*** site is (adrenal) > paravertebral retroperitoneum > posterior mediastinum.
- It is the MC tumour diagnosed in infants ***less than 1 year of age.***
- It is the MC ***intraabdominal neoplasm*** of child.
- Majority of tumours are ***sporadic*** in origin.
- Predisposing conditions include neurofibromatosis, Hirschsprung's disease, Turner syndrome, Beckwith-Weidmann syndrome
- It comes under differential diagnosis of small round blue cell tumours (SRBCTs) which includes:
  - Neuroblastoma
  - Rhabdomyosarcoma
  - Peripheral neuroepithelioma
  - Lymphoma
  - Ewing sarcoma
  - Non hodgkin lympoma and occasionally wilm's tumour.
- *Spontaneous regression in stage 4-S disease* (small primary with metastasis confined to liver, skin or bone marrow) and spontaneous or induced *differentiation to benign neoplasm (ganglioneuromas)* are ***unique behaviour*** of this tumour.
- In characteristic lesions, ***homer-wright pseudorosettes*** can be found.

- Germline mutation in the anaplastic lymphoma kinase gene (ALK) has been identified as major cause of familial predisposition to neuroblastoma ... *Robbins 8/e, p 475*

Clinical features

- 90% of patients present before 6 years.
- Most common symptom is ***pain*** (from primary or metastatic disease).
- Usually firm nodular mass is palpable in flank or midline.
- ***Orbital metastases*** commonly present with peri-orbital ecchymoses and proptosis called as Raccoon eyes.
- Infants with stage ***IV-s disease*** may display cutaneous metastases called as blueberry muffin lesions.
- ***Chronic watery diarrhea*** due to secretion of VIP and opsoclonus- myoclonus are unusual paraneoplastic manifestation called as dancing eyes-dancing feet syndrome.
- Most common site of metastases in ***unfavourable histology are bones***, characteristically to the long bones, facial bones, skull (in particular sphenoid bone); bone marrow and lymph nodes.
- ***In favourable histology*** metastases is confined to liver or subcutaneous tissue.

Diagnosis

- Anemia, thrombocytopenia/***thrombocytosis*** (more common).
- ↑ LDH, ferritin, ***urinary catecholamines*** (vanillyl mandelic and homovanllic acid), neuron specific enolase.
- Plain X-ray or CT show ***stippled calcification.*** It is the MC *abdominal tumour to demonstrate calcification prior to chemotherapy.*
- It displaces ***kidney inferolaterally*** which helps to *differentiate if from wilms tumour.*
- ***Ultrasound is the initial radiologic study for evaluating pediatric abdominal mass.*** On USG neuroblastoma appear as solid mass with cystic lesion
- MRI is superior to CT in assessing vessel encasement, vessel patency, spinal cord compression and BM involvement in selected cases.
- MIBG (meta iodo benzyl guanidine) or somatostatin receptor scintigraphy is ***very sensitive*** in detecting tumours which concentrate catecholamines, so used in the diagnosis of primary, residual and metastic disease in neuroblastoma.
- Bone scan with Tc 99m for osseous metastasis.
- Appearance of neuroblastoma in bone marrow may simulate appearance of ALL, differentiation can be done by monoclonal antibody phenotyping.

Prognostic factors in Neuroblastomas		
Variable	**Favourable**	**Unfavourable**
Stage	Stage 1, 2A, 2B, 4S	Stage 3, 4
Age (Single most important)	< 18 months	> 18 months
Histology (Shimada index)		
Evidence of Schwannian stroma and gangliocytic differentiation	Present	Absent
Mitosis-karyorrhexis index*	<200/5000 cells	>200/5000 cells

Contd...

Contd...

Variable	Favourable	Unfavourable
DNA ploidy	Hyperdiploid or near-triploid	Near-diploid
N-MYC (Most important molecular event)	Not amplified	Amplified
Chromosome 17q gain	Absent	Present
Chromosome 1p loss	Absent	Present
Chromosome 11q loss	Absent	Present
TRKA expression	Present	Absent
TRKB expression	Absent	Present
Telomerase expression	Low or absent	Highly expressed

* ***Mitotic karyorrhexis index*** (MKI) is defined as the number of mitotic or karyorrhectic cells per 5000 tumor cells in random foci

Treatment

- Low risk tumor (Stage I or II with favourable features) are treated are surgery alone. Stage 4S shows high rate of spontaneous regression and these patients require only observation. However 4S tumor in infants younger than 2 months or with unfavourable histologic features require chemotherapy
- Intermediate risk tumor (Stage II unfavourable, Stage III favourable) tumour are treated by surgery, chemotherapy and in some case radiotherapy. Preoperative chemotherapy can shrink the tumor and make surgery more feasable
- High risk tumor is treated by induction chemotherapy followed by surgery followed by focal irradiation to residual tumor
- Effective chemotherapeutic agents include cisplatin, cyclophosphamide, etoposide and doxorubicin

RHABDO MYOSARCOMA

- Arise from embryonic mesenchyme with potential to differentiate into skeletal muscle.
- It is the MC *pediatric soft tissue sarcoma.*
- ***Associated*** with *neurofibromatosis, Beckwith wiedemann syndrome,* Li-fraumenii cancer family syndrome, fetal alcohol syndrome.
- Most common ***nonocular orbital*** *tumour in young children.*

Pathology

- Histological type : ***Embryonal rhabdomyosarcoma (60%) > Alveolar > Pleomorphic***
- Diagnostic cell : ***Rhabdomyoblast.***
- May also contain tadpole or strap cells.
- ***Embryonal type*** consist of spindle cell variant and sarcoma botryoides (tumour cells resemble tennis racket and tumour cells form submucosal zone of hypercellularity known as cambium layer).
- ***Genetic markers*** : t (2;13), t (1;13) → alveolar type.
  Ilp deletion → embryonal type

Clinical features

- Most common presenting ***feature*** is mass that may or may not be painful.
- Most common *site* is ***head and neck > Genitourinary tract > extremities> trunk.***

... Nelson 18/e, p 2144

- Most common site of primary head and neck rhabdomyosarcoma in children is orbit and nasopharynx > paranasal sinuses and middle ear.
- ***Age :*** Bi-modal. First peak between 2-5 and second peak between 15-19 years.
- Extremity rhabdomyosarcoma are more common in older children (upper limb > lower limb)
- Vaginal rhabdomyosarcoma may present as a grape like mass or tumor tissue bulging through the vaginal orifice, known as sarcoma botryoides and can produce urinary tract or large bowel symptoms
- Most common site for ***metastasis*** : lung.

Diagnosis

- **Definitive diagnosis** is established by biopsy, microscopic appearance and immunohistochemical stain.
- Plain X ray, CT (especially lung CT to rule out lung metastasis) and MRI (preferred for extent of disease).

Treatment

– ***Surgical management*** is ***site specific*** and includes complete wide excision of primary tumour and surrounding involved tissue while preserving cosmetic appearance and function.
– Tumours ***not amenable to primary excision*** should be amply biopsied and then treated with ***neoadjuvant agent, secondary excision*** is then performed.
– ***Radiation therapy*** is generally administered to ***all patients,*** the only exception being those with group I non-alveolar rhabdomyosarcoma.
– ***Chemotherapy*** is administered to ***all patients*** even when tumour is fully resected at diagnosis.
– If intracranial extension is detected than, additional radiotherapy is given to base of brain with whole brain irradiation as well as intrathecal chemotherapy.

Prognosis

Best prognosis is of botryoid followed by embryonal, pleomorphic, alveolar.

- ***Diploid tumors have better prognosis*** than hyperdiploid tumours.
- Prognosis is related to site also.

Favourable primary sites	***Unfavorable primary site***
– Orbit (best prognosis) – Vagina – Parameningeal	– Extremity – Paratesticular

Other soft tissue sarcoma

Non-rhabdomyosarcoma soft tissue sarcoma's (NRSIS) accounts for 3% of all childhood tumor. The most common histological types are synovial sarcoma > fibrosarcoma > malignant fibrous histrocytoma. Surgery is main stay of treatment

LANGERHAN'S CELL HISTOCYTOSIS (LCH) / HISTIOCYTOSIS X

- It comes under ***class I of childhood histicytoses.***
- The hallmark of LCH is proliferation of cells of the monocyte lineage containing the characteristic electron microscopic finding of Langerhan's cell

Pathology

- ***Tumour cells*** are *dendritic and antigen presenting with* coffee bean *shaped nuclei and express HLA-DR.*
- ***Diagnostic characteristic :***
  - Presence of HX bodies / Birbeck granules having tennis racket appearance.
  - Positive immuno staining for S-100 protein.
  - CD-1a positivity.

Clinical features

- Most common involvement is of ***skeleton.***
- Most common site are ***skull bones***, long bones, spinal vertebrae, mastoid and mandible.
- **It present as three clinicopathologic entities :**
  i. ***Acute disseminated LCH (Letterer-siwe disease)***
  Typically present at under 2 years with seborrheic skin rash in scalp and back; fever; weight loss; lymphadenopathy; hepatosplenomegaly; pulmonary lesions; osteolytic bone lesions; extensive infitration of bone marrow leading to anemia, thrombocytopenia and recurrent infections such as otitis media, mastoiditis.
  ii. ***Unifocal and multifocal LCH (unifocal and multifocal eosinophilic granuloma)*** are characterized by expanding, erosive accumulation of Langerhan's cell within medullary cavities of bones admixed with eosinophils, lymphocytes, plasma cells and neutrophils. It may be confined to lungs.
  iii. ***Hand-Schuller-Christian triad*** consist of CDE i.e., calvarial defects, diabetes insipidus and exophthalmos.

Diagnosis

- Tissue ***biopsy*** on skin / bone lesion is diagnostic.

Treatment

- Usually resolves ***spontaneously.***
- ***Intralesional corticosteroid***, curettage or low dose radiation are useful *local* treatment for symptomatic lesions.
- *Multifocal* disease is treated with ***systemic chemotherapy*** (best is vinblastine and etoposide, prednisolone).
- *Unresponsive disease :* ***Immunosuppressive therapy*** with cyclosporine/antithymocyte globulin and 2 chloro deoxyadenoside and stem cell transplant.

Remember : Age and degree of organ involvement are the most important prognostic factors.

HEPATOBLASTOMA

Hepatoblastoma is the ***MC*** hepatic malignancies, in children under 5 years

- Median age at diagnosis is 16 months. M > F
- Risk factors include low birth weight, FAD, Gardner's syndrome, Beckwith Weidmann syndrome, hemihypertrophy, trisomy 18

Clinical Presentation

- ***Most frequently*** present as *abdominal mass or abdominal distention.*
- Children diagnosed with hepatoblastoma have ***additional anomalies*** including *hemihypertrophy, Meckel's diverticulum, congenital absence of the kidney, congenital absence of the adrenal gland and umbilical hernia.*
- Child with Beckwith-Wiedemann syndrome have an increased risk of developing hepatoblastoma.

Pathology

- Hepatoblastoma may be divided into two broad histologic subsets :
  - Pure epithelial type consits of either fetal or embryonal elements.
  - Combination of both cell types.

Diagnosis

- The serum level of ***AFP is increased*** in approximately 90% of patients with hepatoblastoma.
- Abdominal ***ultrasonography*** demonstrates the presence and extent of a solid mass.
- Abdominal radiographic examination should include ***CT and MRI*** imaging.

Staging

- ***Two staging system are used***
  a. COG (Children oncology group) staging is surgical staging and is determined by surgical resectability
  b. SIOPEL (European International Society of Pediatric Oncology) staging uses a pretreatment extent of disease (Pretext). This scheme identifies four pretext categories depending upon the number of liver sections free of tumor
- Pretext scoring more accurately predict outcome

Treatment

- ***Surgery resection*** is the cornerstone of treatment for hepatoblastoma.
- ***Radiation therapy*** has a *limited role* in the treatment of hepatoblastoma or HCC.
- ***Chemotherapy :*** Both neoadjuvant and post surgical chemotherapy are used. Cisplatin and doxorubicin are most effective agent.

Prognosis : For Hepatoblastoma, ***resectability*** of the primary tumor and ***disease extent*** at diagnosis remain the strongest predictors of survival.

QUESTIONS

1. **Commonest childhood malignancy is :**
   a. Leukemia [AI 07]
   b. Lymphoma
   c. Neuroblastoma
   d. Brain tumour

2. **The prognosis of rhabdomyosarcoma is likely to be poor if the site of tumour is :**
   a. Orbit [AI 06]
   b. Paratesticular
   c. Extremity
   d. Urinary bladder

3. **A malignant tumour of childhood, that metastasizes to bones most often is :**
   a. Wilm's tumour [AI 06]
   b. Neuroblastoma
   c. Adrenal gland tumours
   d. Granulosa cell tumour of ovary

4. **The ideal timing of radiotherapy for Wilm's tumour after surgery is :** [AI 06]
   a. Within 10 days
   b. Within 2 weeks
   c. Within 3 weeks
   d. Any time after surgery

5. **The most important determinant of prognosis in Wilim's tumour is ?** [AI 06]
   a. Stage of disease
   b. Loss of heterozygosity of chromosome 1p
   c. Histology
   d. Age less than one year at presentation

6. **The most common malignant neoplasm of infancy is :** [AI 05]
   a. Malignant teratoma
   b. Neuroblastoma
   c. Wilm's tumour
   d. Hepatoblastoma

7. **The most common presentation of a child with Wilms' tumour is :** [AI 05]
   a. An asymptomatic abdominal mass
   b. Hematuria
   c. Hypertension
   d. Hemoptysis due to pulmonary secondaries

8. **Aniridia is associated with :**
   a. Nephroblastoma
   b. Medulloblastoma [AIIMS Nov 09]
   c. Hepatoblastoma
   d. Neuroblastoma

9. **A child with partial nephrectomy for Wilms tumor shows nephroblastosis on histopathology. What does it indicates :**
   a. Risk to contralateral kidney
   b. Increase risk of LM involvement
   c. Increased susceptibility to chemotherapy [AIIMS Nov 09]
   d. Chances of Denys drash syndrome

10. **Abdominal Ultra-sonography in a 3 year old boy shows a solid well circumscribed hypo-echoic renal mass. Most likely diagnosis is :** [AI 06]
    a. Wilm's tumour
    b. Renal cell carcinoma
    c. Mesoblastic nephroma
    d. Oncocytoma

11. **Which of the following is the post-chemotherapy based staging system in Wilm's tumor :** [AI 09]
    a. National Wilm's tumor staging system (NWTSG)
    b. International society of pediatric oncology (SIOP)
    c. AJCC TNM
    d. Chadwick

12. **A 7 year old boy with left renal mass had bone pain and was detected to have bone metastatic deposits. The most likely renal tumour is :** [AIIMS 08]
    a. Favourable histology Wilm's tumour
    b. Renal cell carcinoma
    c. Clear cell sarcoma
    d. Rhabdoid tumour

13. Which of the following statement about neuroblastoma is not true : [AIIMS 09]
a. Most common extracranial solid tumor in childhood
b. >50% present with metastasis at the time of diagnosis
c. Lung metastasis are common
d. Often encase aorta and its branches at the time of diagnosis

14. All are true about Langerhans' histiocytosis except: [AIIMS 09]
a. Common before 3 years of age
b. Letterer Siwe disease is systemic manifestation
c. Radio sensitive
d. Testis is commonly involved

15. α Fetoprotein is increased in:
a. Hepatoblastoma **[AIIMS 09]**
b. Neuroblastoma
c. RCC
d. Seminoma

16. Wilm's tumor can be associated with all of the following, except:
a. Hemihypertrophy **[AIIMS 10]**
b. Aniridia
c. Hypertension
d. Bilateral polycystic kidney

17. Common tumors of childhood are:
a. Nephroblastoma **[PGI Dec, June 08]**
b. Leukemias
c. Retinoblastoma
d. Brain tumors
e. Osteosarcoma

18. Embryonal rhabdomyosarcoma can be seen in:
a. Face **[PGI 08]**
b. Neck
c. Nasal cavity
d. Vagina
e. Prostate

19. Wilms tumor and neuroblastoma differentiating features with respect to Wilm's tumor are:
a. Less calcification **[PGI 08]**
b. Intraspinal extension
c. Aorta and IVC invasion
d. Crossing midline

20. Neuroblastoma originates from:
a. Adrenals **[PGI 08]**
b. Mediastinum
c. Chest wall
d. Peripheral nerves
e. Neck

ANSWERS, REFERENCES, EXPLANATIONS WITH INFORMATIVE ILLUSTRATIONS

1. **Ans. is a i.e. Leukemia** *Ref. Ghai 6/e, p 561; Nelson 18/e, p 2097*

Childhood malignancies (in decreasing order)

- Leukemia (Most common is ALL).
- Brain tumors : Infratentorial (medulloblastoma) > supratentorial tumour but within Ist year of life supratentorial *(MC is choroid plexus tumour)* is common than infratentorial.
- Lymphoma
- Neuroblastoma : MC ***intra-abdominal*** solid tumour in childhood.
- Wilms tumour : MC ***malignant tumour of kidney*** in childhood.
- Soft tissue sarcoma: MC soft tissue sarcoma in children under 15 year is rhabdomyosarcoma.
- Bone tumour - Osteosarcoma is MC primary malignant bone tumour in children and adolescents followed by Ewing (but in children < 10 years Ewing's sarcoma > osteosarcoma).
- Retinoblastoma : MC primary ocular tumour of childhood.

Note : In India, sequence is leukemia > Brain tumour > Retinoblastoma > Lymphoma > Neuroblastoma > Soft tissue sarcoma > Wilm's = Bone tumour.

2. **Ans. is c i.e. Extremity** *Ref. Devita 8/e, p 2069*

On the basis of **sites,** *rhabdomyosarcoma is divided into :*

Favourable primary sites	Unfavorable primary site
(Low risk)	*(High risk)*
– Orbit	– Extremity
– Vagina	– Parameningeal
– Paratesticular	

Other bad prognostic factor for rhabdomyosarcoma :
- – Alveolar histology
- – Children > 10 years
- – Tumour size > 5 cm
- – Hyperdiploidy

3. **Ans. is b i.e. Neuroblastoma** *Ref. Nelson 18/e, p 2138*

- Most common site of metastases in neuroblastoma are ***long bones,*** skull, bone marrow, liver, lymph nodes and skin. Metastasis to facial bones is characteristic.
- Most common site of metastases in *Wilm's tumour* : ***Lung***
- Most common site of metastases in *Rhabdomyosarcoma* : ***Lung***
- Most common tumour of adrenal gland is pheochromocytoma which is uncommon in children.
- Most common site of metastases of *Granulosa cell tumour of ovary* : ***Opposite ovary***

4. **Ans. is a i.e. Within 10 days** *Ref. CPDT 19/e, p 871; Devita 7/e, p 1904*

Treatment of Wilm's tumour

- *Chemotherapy is started within* **5 days** *after surgery. Vincristine, doxorubicin, Actinomycin are most frequently used drugs*
- *Radiotherapy is started within* **10 days** *after surgery.*

5. **Ans. is c i.e. Histology** *Ref. Devita 7/e, p 1904; Robbins 8/e, p 481*

"The histology of Wilm's tumour is identified as the most important determinant of prognosis." *... Devita 7/e, p 1904*

- **On the basis of histology Wilm's tumour is classified into :**
  1. ***Unfavorable histology type (UH) :*** Marked enlargement of nuclei, hyperchromatism, multipolar mitotic figure, clear cell sarcoma.
  2. ***Favorable histology type :*** Blastoma, epithelia and stroma devoid ectopia or anaplasia.

  Anaplasia can be focal or diffuse. Only diffuse anaplasia comes under UH category

- **Prognostic factor of Wilm's Tumour :**
  - Histology
  - Tumor size
  - Ploidy
  - Staging
  - Age of patient
  - Lymphnode metastases
  - Local features of tumour such as capsular or vascular invasion.

6. **Ans. is b i.e. Neuroblastoma** *Ref. Nelson 18/e, p 2137*

"Neuroblastoma is the most frequently diagnosed neoplasm in infants."

Accounting 28-39% of neonatal malignancy.

- It is MC ***intraabdominal*** neoplasm of child.

Remember : Most common tumour of child is Leukemia > Brain tumour > Lymphoma.

7. **Ans. is a i.e. An asymptomatic abdominal mass** *Ref. Nelson 18/e, p 2141*

Clinical features of Wilms tumour :

- Painless abdominal mass (MC)
- Abdominal pain
- Hematuria
- Hypertension (25%)
- Fever
- Malaise, weakness, anorexia, weight loss.

Associated Anomalies	Associated Syndromes
Cryptorchidism	WAGR syndrome : IIpl3
Macroglossia and organomegaly	Beckwith-Weidman syndrome
Hemihypertrophy	Dennys-Drash syndrome
Hypospadias	Sotos syndrome
Aniridia	Perlmann syndrome
Neurofibromatosis	Gonadal dysgenesis
Pseudohermaphroditism	Neurofibromatosis
Horse shoe kidney	
Gonadoblastoma	

- Most common genitourinary anomalies associated with Wilm's tumour are *hypoplasia, fusion and ectopia of kidney, duplication of collecting system, hypospadias and cryptorchidism.*

8. **Ans. is a i.e. Nephroblastoma** *Ref. Nelson 18/e, p 2140*

Already explained

9. **Ans. is a i.e. Risk to contralateral kidney** *Ref. Robbins 8/e, p 480; Devita 8/e, p 205*

'Presence of neprogenic rests in resected specimen, suggest increase risk of developing Wilm's tumor in contralateral kidney and these patient require regular and frequent surveillance'

Nephrogenic rest
- Putative precurser lesion of WT, seen in renal parenchyma adjacent to WT in 25-40% of unilateral tumors and in nearly 100% cases of bilateral WT
- Appearance varies from expansile mass (that resemble wt) to sclerotic rest consisting predominantly of fibrous tissue
- Nephroblastomatosis refers kidney with multifocal or diffuse nephrogenic rest patient with nephroblastomatosis have increased chance of recurrence and development of contralateral tumor

10. **Ans. is a i.e. Wilm's tumour** *Ref. Rumack Ultrasonography 3/e, p 361, 1926 - 1927*

Most important point in the question is age of patient i.e. 3 year
- Wilm's tumour is MC primary renal tumour in childhood.
- On sonography tumours shows a large solid mass ***distorting the sinus***, pyramids, cortex and contour of kidney.
- Echogenicity is usually quiet ***hyperechoic*** and homogenous, although there may be ***hypoechoic*** areas that represent hemorrhage and necrosis.

Remember :
- ***Mesoblastic nephroma or fetal renal hamartoma (congenital Wilm's tumour)*** is the MC neonatal renal neoplasm to occur within the first few months of life.
- ***Oncocytomas*** occur in parathyroid, thyroid, adrenal, salivary glands and kidneys. It occur mostly in men with peak incidence in 6th and 7th decade.
- **Renal oncocytoma produce typical *spoke wheel pattern* on angiography.**
- Peak age of renal cell carcinoma is ***50-70 years;*** it is rare in childhood.

11. Ans. is b i.e. International Society of Pediatric Oncology *Ref. Devita 8/e, p 2051*

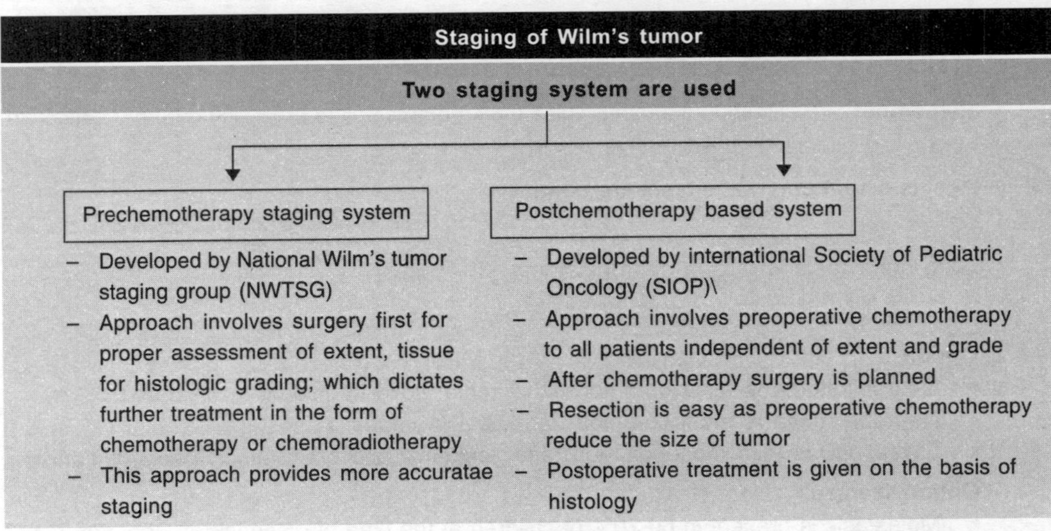

Staging System Developed by the Third National Wilms Tumor Study

Stage	Description
Stage I	Tumor is limited to kidney and is completely excised Capsular surface intact; no tumor rupture; no residual tumor apparent beyond margins of excision
Stage II	Tumor extends beyond kidney but is completely excised. No residual tumor apparent at or beyond margins of excision
Stage III	Residual non-hematogenous tumor confined to the abdomen. Lymph node involvement of hilus, periaortic chains, or beyond; diffuse peritoneal contamination by tumor spillage; peritoneal implants of tumor, tumor extends beyond surgical margins microscopically or macroscopically; tumor not completely removable because of local infiltration into vital structures
Stage IV	Deposits beond stage III (e.g., lung, liver, bone, brain)
Stage V	Bilateral renal involvement at diagnosis

Modified from National Wilms' Tumor Study Committee: Wilms tumor status report, 1990. J Clin Oncol 1991;9:877-887

12. Ans. is c i.e. Clear cell sarcoma *Ref. Nelson 18/e, p 2140*

Clear cell sarcoma is the subtype of Wilm's tumour which usually metastasize to bone.

Histologically Wilm's tumour is of two types :

Favourable type	Unfavourable type
Conventional type of Wilm's.	Clear cell sarcoma is its subtype.
Characterized by blastema, epithelia, and stromal elements.	Marked enlargment of nuclei, hyperchromatism and multipolar mitotic figures.
Devoid of ectopia or anaplasia.	Focal or diffuse areas of anaplasia.
Age 2-5 year	Occur in older children.
Most common site of metastases lung	Usually metastases to bone.

Remember : Rhabdoid tumour which may metastasize to brain, is no longer classified as subtype of Wilm's tumour.

13. Ans. is c i.e. Lung metastasis are common

Ref. Nelson 18/e, p 2138; Devita 8/e, p 2047

Lung metastasis is rare in neuroblastoma (3% cases)

Other options

Option 'a'

- Neuroblastoma is most common extracranial solid neoplasm in children
- Neuroblastoma is most common neoplasm in infant
- Overall NB is third most common (after leukemia and brain tumor) pediatric cancer

Option 'b and c'

- Metastasis is present in 60-70% of children at the time of diagnosis ...*Ghai 8/e, p 573*
- Most common site of metastasis are: Long bones, facial bones, bone marrow, lymphnode, liver, skin
- Metastasis to facial bones (sphenoid) is characteristic

Option 'd'

- Adrenal and retroperitoneal neuroblastoma characterstically involve and displace or encase the major vessels
- Exact frequency is not known, but at the time of evaluation, it is essential to rule out the major vessel (aorta and IVC) involvement or displacement by MRI or CT

Remember:

Feature	Neuroblastoma	Wilm's tumor
Incidence	Most common intraabdominal solid tumor in children	Most common renal tumor in children
Stage	Already metastatic in greater than 50% of patients	Generally confined to the kidney
Lung metastasis	Rare	Common
Encashment of aorta	Characteristic	Uncommon
Calcification	Common	Rare
Crossing midline	Common	Rare

14. Ans. is d i.e. Testis is commonly involved

Ref. Robbins 8/e, p 631; Nelson 18/e; p 2159-2162

Most common site of LCH are bones skull bones, long bones, vertebra, mastoid and mandible); skin, liver

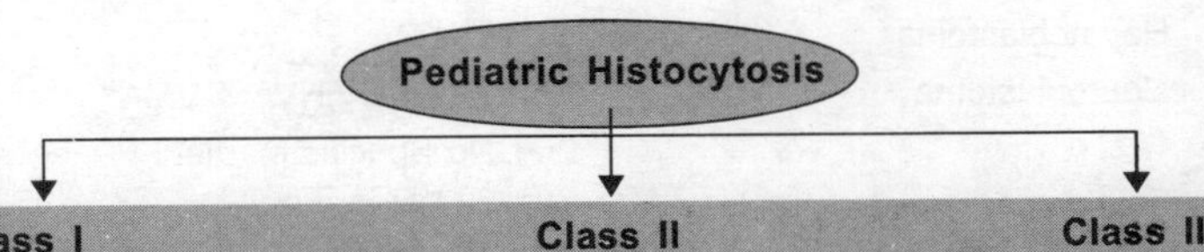

Class I	Class II	Class III
Langerhan's cell histiocytosis • Proliferation of abnormal histiocytes (Langerhan's cell) • ***Include:*** – Hand-Schuller Christian syndrome – Letterer Siewe disease – Eosinophilic granuloma • Birbeck granules in cytoplast and CD 1a positivity is diagnostic • Single system disease is treated by radiotherapy • Multisystem disease is treated by systemic chemotherapy	Hemophagocytic lymphohistiocytosis • Proliferation of macrophages ***Include:*** – Familial hemophagocytic lymphohistiocytosis (FHLH) – Infection associated hemophagocytic syndrome (secondary HLH) - Tissue infiltration by activated CD8 T lymphocytes, and activated macrophages in presence of hypercytokinemia is characteristic • FHLH is treated by etoposide, corticosteroids and intrathecal steroids. Allogenic stem cell transplantation can cure 60% of cases • Secondary HLH usually responds spontaneously when etiologic infection get cured	True malignant histiocytosis – Malignancy of cell of monocyte macrophage lineage ***Include:*** – Acute monocytic leukemia – True malignant histiocytosis

Langerhan's cell histiocytosis

Letterer Siewe disease	Eosinophillic granuloma	Hand-Schuller Christian
• Age <2 years disease • Multifocal multisystem LCH characterized by involvement of skin seborrhic eruptions. Bone (osteolytic lesion) with concurrent hepato-splenomegaly, lymphadenopathy	• Age 5-15 years • Usually involve bones, most commonly the calvarium. Other sites are skin, lung or stomach	• Age 2-10 years • Multifocal unisystem disease characterized by triad of calvarial bone defect diabetes insipidus, exophthalmos

15. **Ans. is a i.e. Hepatoblastoma (see below)**

Serum level of α Fetoprotein are elevated in 90% of patients with hepatoblastoma

Malignancy	Tumor Marker
Hepatoblastoma	↑ AFP
Neuroblastoma	↑ Urinary HVA & VMA
RCC	No Specific marker
Seminoma	↑ LDH; PLAP

16. **Ans. is d i.e. Bilateral polycystic kidney**

Ref. Nelson 18/e, p 2141; CPDT 19/e, p 870

There is confusion between option c and d as Ghai 5/e, p 574 has mentioned cystic kidney disease to be associated with Wilm's tumor. CPDT and Nelson have not mentioned such association and above all hypertension is seen in 25% of patients with WT at the time of presentation. *So, the answer would be bilateral polycystic kidney disease.*

Refer Ans. No. 7 for details

17. **Ans. is a, b, c, d and e i.e. All options are correct** *Ref. Ghai 5/e, p 561*

Relative frequency of cancer in pediatric patients (decreasing order)

1	Leukemia	(1)*
2	Brain tumor	(2)*
3	Lymphoma	(4)*
4	Neuroblastoma	(5)*
5	Wilm's tumor	(8)*
6	Soft tissue sarcoma	(6)*
7	Osteosarcoma	(7)*
8	Retinoblastoma	(3)*

* Indicates rank in India

18. **Ans. is a, c, d and e i.e. Face, Nasal cavity, Vagina and Prostate**

Ref. CPDT 19/e, p 874; Devita 8/e, p 2068

Embryonal rhabdomyosarcoma commonly arise in the head, neck and genitourinary regions. In contrast alveolar tumor affect older patients and arise in trunk and extremity

Characteristics of rhabdomyosarcoma

Site	Frequency (%)	Symptoms and signs	Predominant pathologic subtype
Head and neck	**35**		Embryonal
Orbit		Proptosis	
Parameningeal		Cranial nerve palsies; aural or sinus obstruction with or without drainage	

Contd...

Contd...

Site	Frequency (%)	Symptoms and signs	Predominant pathologic subtype
Other		Painless, progressively enlarging mass	
Genitourinary	**22**		Embryonal (botryyoid variant in bladder and vagina)
Bladder and prostate		Hematuria, urinary obstruction	
Vagina and uterus		Pelvic mass, vaginal discharge	
Paratesticular		Painless mass	
Extremities	**18**	Adolescents, swelling of affected body part	Alveolar (50%), undifferentiated
Other	**25**	Mass	Alveolar, undifferentiated

19. Ans. is a i.e. Less calcification *Ref. Nelson 18/e, p 2140-43*

Already explained, see Answer No. 13.

20. Ans. is a, b and e i.e. Adrenals, Mediastinum, Neck *Ref. OP Ghai, 6/e, p 573*

Site of origin of Neuroblastoma

- Adrenal gland (30%)
- Paraverebral retroperitoneum (28%)
- Posterior mediastinum (15%)
- Pelvis (5%)
- Cervical area

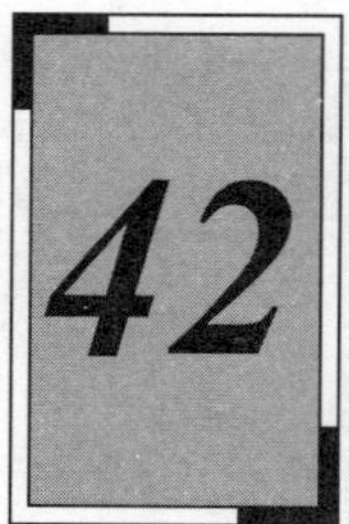

Ophthalmic Tumour

What's Important ?

- Treatement of Retinoblastoma
- Optic Nerve Glioma

MALIGNANT MELANOMA OF CHOROID

- Most common primary intraocular malignant tumour of adults.
- Arise from ***neural crest*** derived pigment cells of uvea (outer layers of choroid).

Pathology

- Grossly it is of two types :
  - Circumscribed (pedunculated) tumour (***collar stud tumour***) MC
  - Diffuse (flat) malignant melanoma
- Histopathology (***Callender's classification***)
  - ***Mixed cell melanoma :*** MC
  - ***Spindle A melanoma :*** Best prognosis
  - Spindle B melanoma
  - ***Epitheloid cell melanoma :*** Worst prognosis
  - Necrotic melanoma

Clinical features

- It can be divided into ***four*** stages :

Quiescent stage

- If tumour at *periphery* : No symptom
- If tumour at *posterior* pole : Early visual loss
- *Small tumour :* Earliest pathognomic sign is appearance of orange patches in pigment epithelium due to accumulation of lipofuscin.
- *Large tumour :* Exudative Retinal detachment ***(marked vision loss).***

Glaucomatous stage

- Caused by forward movment of lens and iris; infiltration of trabecular meshwork and pressure upon vortex veins.
- If RD is accompanied by raised IOP, growth may be diagnosed with certainity.

Stage of extraocular extension

- Occur through sclera usually at limbus and usually accompanied by marked proptosis.

- Tumours usually fill the globe before perforating the sclera but perforation may occur relatively early along the perivascular space of vortex veins.

Stage of metastasis

- Most common in liver and is MC cause of death.

Differential diagnosis :
- Choroidal naevus
- Cavernous hemangioma
- Posterior scleritis.

Diagnosis

- ***USG :*** *Classic mushroom shape* of melanoma can be seen with acoustic hollowing within the mass.
- ***Radioactive tracers :*** P^{32} and $Gallium^{67}$ (more sensitive).
- ***Fluorescein angiography :*** Double circulation with increased fluorescence in the mass is characteristic of malignant melanoma.

Treatment

- Tumour **< *10mm*** across and upto 2mm thick : Brachytherapy.
- Medium sized tumours ***10-15 mm*** in diameter and 3-5 mm in height : Plaque or external proton beam radiation.
- Orbital spread require, exenteration but metastasis elsewhere can be treated by enucleation and radiation.

RETINOBLASTOMA / GLIOMA RETINAE

- Most common intraocular tumour of childhood (M = F), usually seen between ***1-2 years.***
- Arise from ***primitive retinal cell*** which is capable of differentiation into both glial and neuronal cells.

Genetics : Marker is ***13q 14 (RB)*** deletion/mutation.

- It arise in two ways :
  - ***Sporadic / Non hereditary cases*** (MC) : Usually unilateral
  - ***Hereditary / Familial cases :*** Autosomal dominant inheritance. They are usually bilateral, can be associated with pinealoblastoma (so called *trilateral retinoblastoma*). They also have increase the risk of osteosarcoma.

Pathology

- Two pattern are seen:
  - ***Glioma exophytum*** (MC) : Causing exudative retinal detachment
  - ***Glioma endophytum :*** Causing vitreous or anterior chamber seeding giving ***"cottage cheese appearance".***
- Microscopically consist of :
  - ***Flexner - Winter steiner rosettes (highly specific)*** and fleurettes resembling photoreceptor differentiation. Also contains *Homer-wright and pseudorosette.*
  - Focal zones of *dystrophic calcification are characteristic* of retinoblastoma.

Spread

- Metastasis first occurs in the pre-auricular and neighbouring lymph nodes. Direct extension to the optic nerve and brain is more common than metastasis to liver.

Clinical features

- Most common presentation is ***leucocaria*** on amaurotic cat's eye. Other features include squint, cataract buphthalmous. Globe may burst at limbus resulting in marked proptosis.

Differential diagnosis

Conditions causing leukocoria other than retinoblastoma (pseudoglioma) are:

It includes :

- Inflammatory deposit in vitreous with or without
- Congenital cataract
  detachment of retina following cyclitis or choroiditis
- Coloboma of choroid
- Retrolental fibroplasia (retinopathy of prematurity)
- Persistent hyperplastic primary vitreous
- Toxocara endophthalmitis
- Exudative retinopathy of coats
- Noirre disease
- Retinal dysplasia
- Retinocytoma
- Retinal astrocytoma
- Incontinentia pigmenti (Bloch Sulz boiger's syndrome)

Diagnosis

- ***Examination under anaesthesia :*** *Intraocular pressure* (IOP) *is raised more often in retinoblastoma whereas lowered* IOP *is common in pseudoglioma.*
- ***X-ray :*** Shows calcification within tumour which is pathognomonic of retinoblastoma.
- ***USG :*** *B-scan* shows cauliflower like mass arising from retina while *A-scan* shows *characteristic V-Y* pattern.
- ***LDH :*** Activity is raised.
- ***CT or MRI :*** For extraocular and optic nerve involvement.

Treatment

– ***Tumour < 10 mm and optic nerve is not involved i.e early stage I :*** conservative treatment by radiotherapy, photocoagulation (for posterior lesions), cryotherapy (for anterior lesions).

– ***Tumour > 10 mm or when optic nerve involved i.e. late stage I and stage II :*** Enucleation and optic nerve is cut as far as possible followed by radiochemotherapy.

– ***Stage III and IV :*** Debulking of orbit followed by radiochemotherapy.

Remember :
– Routine ophthalmologic examination should continue until **6 year** of age to detect new lesions.
– Rarely spontaneous regression may occur.
– Most common orbital tumor in children : Rhabdomyosarcoma

... Nelson 17/e, p 1722

Prognosis

- ***Poor prognostic factors :*** Optic nerve involvement, undifferentiated tumour cells, massive choroidal invasion, extraocular extension.
- It has the ***best prognosis of all childhood tumours*** with over 80% survival.

TUMOURS OF OPTIC NERVE AND ITS SHEATHS

1. ***Optic nerve glioma / Juvenile pilocytic astrocytoma***
   - It is MC tumour of optic nerve in childhood.
   - Arise from any part of optic nerve.
   - It is benign tumour derived from ***astrocytes and oligodendroglial cells*** of optic nerve.
   - Can be seen as a component of ***Von - Recklinghausen neurofibromatosis (NF1).***
   - Usually congenital with peak age 2-5 years.
   - Present with unilateral visual loss with gradual painless proptosis.
   - ***Signs :***
     - Relative afferent pupillary defect
     - Optic atrophy
     - Disc edema
     - Enlarged optic canal (always present).
   - It grows centripetally and may involve chiasma (poor prognosis).
   - **Diagnosis** : MRI is better than CT.
   - **Treatment** :
     - Best managment is usually periodic observation.
     - Surgical removal is advised for tumor arising from intraorbital, intracanalicular or prechiasmal portion of nerve if patient has nearly complete loss of vision of affected eye.
     - For tumour of chiasma, resection with chemoradiation is advised.

2. ***Meningioma***

   It is of two types :

Primary intra-orbital meningioma (optic nerve sheath meningioma)	Secondarily orbital meningioma
– Arise from the cap cells of arachnoid around the intra-orbital portion of optic nerve – Clinically present with early visual loss with small degree of proptosis – Occur predominantly in middle aged women – Presence of ***opticociliary shunt is pathognomonic*** of nerve sheath meningioma – CT confirms the origin of tumour	– Include intracranial meningioma which secondarily involves orbit – Produce greater proptosis due to hyperostosis and lesser visual impairment. – Typically occur in middle aged women – Orbital invasion may occur through floor of anterior cranial fossa, superior orbital fissure and optic canal

QUESTIONS

1. **Which one of the following statement is incorrect about optic glioma ? [AI 06]**
   a. Has a peak incidence in first decade
   b. Arises from oligodendrocytes
   c. Causes meningeal hyperplasia
   d. Is associated with type I neurofibromatosis
2. **The most common retrobulbar orbital mass in adults is : [AI 06]**
   a. Neurofibroma
   b. Cavernous hemangioma
   c. Meningioma
   d. Schwannoma
3. **The most common second malignancy in survivors of retinoblastoma is :[AI 06]**
   a. Thyroid cancer
   b. Nasopharyngeal carcinoma
   c. Optic glioma
   d. Osteosarcoma
4. **The mother of a one and a half year old child gives history of a white reflex from one eye for the past 1 month. On computed tomography scan of the orbit there is clacification seen within the globe. The most likely diagnosis is : [AI 05]**
   a. Congenital cataract
   b. Retinoblastoma
   c. Endophthalmitis
   d. Coats disease
5. **Most common malignancy in eye lid is:**
   a. Basal cell carcinoma [AIIMS 09]
   b. Squamous cell carcinoma
   c. Malignant melanoma
   d. Sebaceous carcinoma
6. **As regards to intraocular retinoblastoma, which one of the following statements is false : [AIIMS 06]**
   a. 94% of cases are sporadic
   b. Patients with sporadic retinoblastoma do not pass their genes to their offsprings
   c. Calcification in the tumour can be detected on ultrasound scan
   d. Reese-Ellsworth classification is useful in predicting visual prognosis following radiotherapy.
7. **Which of the following is not of prognostic significance in chorodial melanoma ?**
   a. Presence of retinal detachment
   b. Size of the tumour [AIIMS 06]
   c. Cytology of the tumour cells
   d. Presence of extraocular extension
8. **The inheritance pattern of familial retinoblastoma: [AIIMS 05]**
   a. Autosomal recessive
   b. Autosomal dominant
   c. X-linked dominant
   d. X-linked recessive
9. **Childhood malignancy producing proptosis is/are: [PGI 05]**
   a. Neuroblastoma
   b. Hepatoma
   c. Retinoblastoma
   d. Germ cell tumor
   e. Nephroblastoma
10. **Retinoblastoma can be associated with:**
    a. Osteosarcoma [AI 10]
    b. Renal cell carcinoma
    c. Pinealoblastoma
    d. None of the above
11. **True about retinoblastoma: [PGI 09]**
    a. Leukocoria seen
    b. Visual loss is the earliest presentation
    c. Squint seen
    d. Nystagmus common

ANSWERS, REFERENCES, EXPLANATIONS WITH INFORMATIVE ILLUSTRATIONS

1. **Ans. is c i.e. Causes meningeal hyperplasia**

Ref. Parson 20/e, p 463; Nelson 17/e, p 2121

Meningeal hyperplasia is not seen in optic nerve glioma.

Important features of Optic nerve gliomas (Juvenile pilocytic astrocytoma)

- Cytologic benign hamartoma which is generally stationary or grow only slowly.
- Arise from astrocytes and oligodendroglial cells of optic nerve.
- Usually congenital, with peak age 2 - 5 years (1st decade).
- ***Clinical presentation :***
  - **If involves intraorbital portion of nerve :**
    - U/L loss of vision
    - Proptosis
    - Deviation of eye
    - Optic atrophy
    - Congestion of optic nerve head.
  - **If involves chiasma :**
    - Defects of vision
    - Visual field defect (often bitemporal hemianopia)
    - Increase ICT
    - Papilledema / Optic atrophy
    - Hypothalmic / Pituitary dysfunction.
- It occur with increased frequency in Neurofibromatosis I.
- Best management is usually periodic observation.

Features	Optic nerve glioma	Meningioma
Age	Usually < 5 year	Usually middle aged women
Margin	Well defined	More infiltrative
Calcification	Rare	More common
Orbital hyperostosis	Absent	Present
Widened optic canal	In 90% cases	In 10% cases
Associated with NF - 1	More	Less
Optic Nerve	Kinkling and buckling	Straight
Enhancement	Heterogenous	Diffuse homogenous

2. **Ans. is b i.e. Cavernous hemangioma** *Ref. Parson 20/e, p 461*

Orbital space occupying lesion (Causes of Proptosis)

Children	Adults
Dermoid cyst	Cavernous haemangioma
Teratoma	Haemangiopericytoma
Capillary haemangioma	Optic nerve meningioma
Lymphangioma	Schwannoma, Neurofibroma
Optic nerve glioma	Fibrous histiocytoma
Plexiform neurofibroma	Lymphomas
Rhabdomyosarcoma	
Acute myeloid leukaemia	
Histiocytosis	
Neuroblastoma	Metastasis from breast, lung, prostate carcinoma
Wilm's tumour	
Ewing sarcoma	

Important points about Cavernous hemangioma

- Most common benign orbital tumour of adults
- Well encapsulated
- 2nd – 3rd decade
- Usually located in retrobulbar muscle cone
- Presents with slowly progressing unilateral proptosis
- **Treatment** : Surgical through lateral orbitotomy.

3. **Ans. is d i.e. Osteosarcoma**

Ref. Robbin's 7/e, p 300; Devita 8/e, p 2054, 8/e, p 2054; Nelson's 17/e, p 1717, 1723

"Patients with hereditary retinoblastoma have significantly increased risk of osteosarcoma." *... Nelson 17/e, p 1717*

Important points of Retinoblastoma

- Most common intraocular tumour of childhood.
- Caused by defective RB1 gene, which is located on 13q 14.
- It occur in ***two*** forms :

Sporadic / Nonhereditary	Familial / Hereditary
– More common	– Less common
– Usually U/L, unifocal	– Usually B/L, multifocal
– There is increased risk of of second malignancies	– ***Autosomal dominant***
	– Patient have significant risk for development of ***second malignancies*** primarily osteosarcoma ***(MC),*** soft tissue sarcoma, melanoma, brain tumour

- It is ***small round blue cell tumour*** with Flexner-Winter steiner rosette (highly specific), Homer-Wright and pseudorosette.
- Can arise from any ***nucleated layers*** of retina.
- Only about *10%* of tumour are detected by *routine ophthalmologic screening* in context of positive family history.
- ***Calcification within the tumor*** on X-ray / CT is pathognomonic.
- ***Clasically presents*** with leukocoria (white pupillary reflex).
- Radiation given for treatment increase risk of osteosarcoma, cataract, orbital growth deformities, lacrimal dysfunction, late retinal vascular injury.

4. **Ans. is b i.e. Retinoblastoma** *Ref. Nelson 17/e, p 1722*

Already explained, kindly see answer no. 3

5. **Ans. is a i.e. Basal cell carcinoma** *Ref. Khurana Ophthalmology 4/e, p 360*

Basal cell carcinoma is the commonest malignant tumor of lid (90%)

Tumors of the Lid	
Benign	**Malignant**
• Papilloma (MC) • Hemangioma • Neurofibroma	• Basal cell carcinoma (MC) • Squamous cell carcinoma • Malignant melanoma • Sebaceous gland adenocarcinoma

Malignant tumors of lid

Features	BCC	SCC	SGC	MM
Incidence	Most common (90%)	5%	1-2%	1-2%
Site	Lower lid > medial Canthus > upper lid	Lid margin	Meibomian gland	
Clinical features	• Small nodule which undergoes ulceration (with rolled margin) to form rodent ulcer	• Ulcerated growth with elevated and indurated margin • May present as polypoid verrucous lesion also	• Nodule which grows to form big growth • Initially mistaken as chalazion	• Flat or slightly elevated naevus with irregular border and variegated pigmentation
Treatment	• Surgical excision with 3 mm circumferential margin • Radiotherapy and cryotherapy for inoperable cases	• Same as BCC	• Surgical excision with reconstruction of lid	• As tumor is radio-resistant surgical excision with reconstruction is treatment of choice

BCC—Basal cell Ca; SCC—Squamous cell Ca; MM—Malignant melanoma, SGC—Sebacious gland Ca

6. **Ans. is b i.e. Patients with sporadic retinoblastoma do not pass their genes to their offsprings**

See below

Lets consider all options.

Option 'a' and Option 'b'

Genetics of Retinoblastoma *... Devita 8/e, p 2054*

- Retinoblastoma results from loss or inactivation of the both alleles of retinoblastoma gene *(located on chromosome 13q14 which is a tumor suppressor gene).*
- The timing of the loss or inactivation determines whether the disease is heritable (germinal) or nonheritable (somatic).
- *In germinal or heritable case,* at least one normal allele must be lost or incactivated prior to the first mitoic division of embryogenesis. This occurs if the sperm or the egg contains defective DNA from affected or carrier parent or if the defect develops by means of spontaneous mutation prior to fertilisation.
- *In sporadic or nonheritable cases,* both alleles are present and active beyond the stage of the fertilized egg, but one or more subsequent spontaneous mutation occur to delete or inactivate both alleles in at least one immature retinal cell.
- An analysis of the offspring of patients with sporadic b/l retinoblastoma demonstrated that 49% offsprings developed the disease. This suggest that essentially all patient with sporadic retinoblastoma have a germ line mutation that is transmitted in a manner identical to hereditary retinoblastoma.
- The individuals with germinal or heritable form of disease have one altered allele in every cell of the body. They develop the malignancy only if the other allele in an immature retinal cell is deleted or inactivated by spontaneous mutation *(90% of heritable cases develop retinoblastoma).*
- Heritable cases tend to be bilateral and multifocal and develop earlier in childhood.
- Non-heritable cases tend to be unilateral and unifocal and generally appear later.
- Heritable cases also have a strong tendency to develop non-retinoblastoma malignancies *(i.e. pineoblastoma, osteosarcoma, soft tissue sarcoma).*

Option 'c' *... Ultrasound of Eye by Sandra 2/e, p 180*

Sonographic features of Retinoblastoma

- B scan show cauliflower like mass arise from retina while A scan shows characteristic v-y pattern. Calcification when detected is highly suggestive.

  Note : CT scan and X-ray orbit are best investigation for detection of calcification.

Option 'd'

Reis and Ellsworth developed a classification to predict which eyes were likely to survive local therapy and keep useful vision after local therapy such as radiation therapy and cryotherapy.

Remember : *Esson prognosis classification* was also used for assessing prognosis of retinoblastoma.

7. **Ans. is a i.e. Presence of retinal detachment** *Ref. Devita 7/e, p 1815*

Prognostic factor for Choroidal and Ciliary body melanoma are :

- Age of the patient
- Location of its anterior border
- Height of tumour
- Cell type
- Scleral infiltration by tumour cells
- Location of tumour
- Largest tumour diameter in contact with sclera
- Integrity of Bruch's membrane
- Pigmentation

Remember : *Size is the most useful prognostic factor.*

8. **Ans. is b i.e. Autosomal dominant** *Ref. Robbin's 7/e, p 300*

Already explained

9. **Ans. is a, c, d and e i.e. Neuroblastoma; Retinoblastoma; Germ cell tumour; and Nephroblastoma** *Ref. Parson 20/e, p 461*

Already explained

10. **Ans. is c i.e. Pineoblastoma** *Ref. Robbins 8/e, p 1365*

Retinoblastoma arising in the context of germline mutations not only may be bilateral but also may be associated with pinealoblastoma (trilateral retinoblastoma) which is associated with a poor outcome.

Note: Patients with familial retinoblastoma are also at greatly increased risk ***(not associated)*** of developing osteosarcoma and other soft tissue sarcoma. These tumors are usually developed later and thus association is very rare.

11. **Ans. is a, c i.e. Leukocoria seen, Squint seen** *Ref. Parson 20/e, p 358*

Clinical features of Retinoblastoma

- Earliest feature is peculiar yellow reflex from the pupil called leucocoria or amaurotic cats eye

Other modes include:

- Divergent squint
- Cataract
- Bupthalmos
- Hypopyon

If left untreated retinoblastoma runs through the same stage as melanoma of choroid:

1. Questent stage : Six month to year
2. Glaucomatous stage : Proptosis (Real or apparent), severe pain
3. Extraoccular extension : When tumor bursts through sclera (usually at limbus)
4. Metastasis : First occurs in the preauricular and neighbouring lymph nodes, later in cranial or other bones

43 Miscellaneous

QUESTIONS

1. **Fine needle aspiration cytology is not suitable for diagnosing : [AI 06]**
   a. Tubercular lymphadenitis
   b. Papillary carcinoma of thyroid
   c. Plasmacytoma
   d. Aneurysmal bone cyst

2. **AIDS associated malignancies are :**
   a. Kaposi sarcoma [PGI 10, 09]
   b. Bronchgenic carcinoma
   c. Breast carcinoma
   d. Non-Hodgkin's lymphoma
   e. Invasive cervical carcinoma

3. **A 45 years old man present with progressive cervical lymph nodes enlargement, since 3 months; most diagnostic investigation is : [AIIMS 05]**
   a. X-ray soft tissue
   b. FNAc
   c. Lymph node biopsy
   d. None of the above

4. **Smoking is a causative factor for all the carcinomas except : [AIIMS 10, AI 10]**
   a. Esophageal carcinoma
   b. Laryngeal carcinoma
   c. Nasopharyngeal carcinoma
   d. Urinary bladder carcinoma

5. **Psammoma bodies may be seen in all of the following, except : [AI 09; AIIMS 10]**
   a. Follicular carcinoma of Thyroid
   b. Papillary carcinoma of Thyroid
   c. Meningioma
   d. Serous cystadenocarcinoma of ovary

6. **Which of the following is not a true malignant tumor : [AI 08]**
   a. Plasmacytoma
   b. Askins tumor
   c. Fibromatosis
   d. Chloroma

7. **Concomitant chemoradiotherapy is indicated in all of the following, except :**
   a. Stage III B Ca Cervix [AI 09]
   b. T2 N0 M0 Anal Cancer
   c. T2 N0 M0 Glottic Cancer
   d. T1 N2 M0 Nasopharyngeal Cancer

8. **Which of the following tumour may regress spontaneously: [PGI 10]**
   a. Retinoblastoma
   b. Malignant melanoma
   c. Osteosarcoma
   d. Choriocarcinoma

9. **A 35 year old premenopausal patient has recently developed a 1.5 cm sized pigmented lesion on her back. Which of the following forms of tissue diagnosis will you recommend for her ? [AIIMS 06]**
   a. Needle biopsy
   b. Trucut biopsy
   c. Excision biopsy
   d. Incisional biopsy

10. **Which is the most common site of metastatic disease : [AIIMS 05]**
    a. Lung b. Bone
    c. Liver d. Kidney

11. **All of the following are examples of a round cell tumor, except : [AIIMS 05]**
    a. Neuroblastoma
    b. Ewing's sarcoma
    c. Non Hodgkin's lymphoma
    d. Osteosarcoma

12. **WHO ladder is for rational titration of :**
    a. Oral analgesia [AIIMS 05]
    b. Chemotherapy
    c. Radiotherapy
    d. Antideprassant

13. **A 40 year old patient is suffering from carotid body tumor. Which of the following is the best choice of treatment for him : [PGI 08]**
    a. Excision of tumor
    b. Radiotherapy
    c. Chemotherapy
    d. Carotid artery ligation both proximal and distal to the tumor

14. **Which of the following malignancy can be seen in anorectal fistula : [PGI 05]**
    a. Squamous cell carcinoma
    b. Transitional carcinoma
    c. Adeno carcinoma
    d. Columnar carcinoma
    e. Lymphoma

ANSWERS, REFERENCES, EXPLANATIONS WITH INFORMATIVE ILLUSTRATIONS

1. **Ans. is d i.e. Aneurysmal bone cyst** *Ref. Anderson 10/e, p 75 - 77, 1115*

Aneurysmal bone cyst can not be diagnosed by FNAC.

- ***FNAC*** is the *first investigation done* in ***thyroid, parotid, breast*** and ***lymphnode enlargement.***
  But it can't differentiate follicular adenoma from follicular carcinoma of thyroid.
- It is ***contraindicated*** in testicular cancer, RCC, Pheochromocytoma.
- ***CT or MRI guided FNAC*** help in confirming solitary plasmacytoma.

... Devita 7/e, p 2170

Aneurysmal bone cyst is diagnosed by :

- **X-ray** – Eccentric – Radiolucent
  – Expansile – Metaphyseal swelling.
- **CT** – *Diagnostic.*

Remember :

Excisional biopsy –	Entire tumours mass is removed with a small margin of normal tissue surrounding it.
–	*Best and most diagnostic.*
Incisional biopsy –	A wedge of tissue is removed and an effort is made to include the majority of cross- sectional diameter of the tumours.
Core needle biopsy –	When diagnosis is being made through endoscopy or fluoroscopy guided.
–	Considerably less tissue is obtained and the has less diagnostic capacity.
FNAC –	Least diagnostic, as obtains only a suspension of cells.

2. **Ans. is a, d and e i.e. Kaposi sarcoma; Non-Hodgkin's lymphoma; and Invasive cervical carcinoma** *Ref. Devita 7/e, p 2248*

Kaposi sarcoma, Non Hodgkin lymphoma, Invasive cervical cancer are AIDS defining neoplasm. *... Devita 7/e, p 2248*

Cancers associated with AIDS (in ↓ order of frequency)

1. Kaposi sarcoma
2. Non hodgkin's lymphoma (Primary CNS Lymphoma)
3. Invasive cervical cancer
4. Anal cancer
5. Angiosarcoma
6. Hodgkin's disease
7. Leukemia
8. Multiple myeloma
9. Melanoma
10. Seminoma or germinoma
11. Lung adenocarcinoma

Remember : CNS lymphoma is most common CNS neoplasm in AIDS patient.

3. **Ans. is c i.e. Lymph node biopsy** *Ref. Harrison 17/e, p 370*

"Prompt biopsy of lymph node is required if the patient history and physical finding suggest a malignancy. Examples include a solitary, hard, non tender cervical node, supraclavicular adenopathy; and solitary or generalized adenopathy that is firm, movable and suggestive of lymphoma."

But, If there is any mucosal lesion than it should be biopsed first. If no mucosal lesion is detected, an excisional biopsy of the largest node should be perfomed. **Fine needle aspiration** should *not be performed as the first diagnostic procedure.*

Cause of Supraclavicular adenopathy	
Neoplastic	***Non neoplastic***
– Gastrointestinal malignancy	– Tuberculosis
– Carcinoma lung	– Sarcoidosis
– Carcinoma breast	– Toxoplasmosis
– Carcinoma testes	– Ovarian carcinoma

4. **Ans. is c i.e. Nasopharyngeal Ca** *Ref. Harrison 17/e, p 2736; Devita 7/e, p 194*

Causal association between smoking and cancer		
Highly associated	***Probable***	***No association***
Pancreatic cancer	Acute myeloid leukemia	Acute lymphocytic leukemia
Renal cell cancer	Cervical cancer	Breast cancer
Oropharyngeal cancer	Colorectal cancer	Childhood cancers
Bladder cancer	Liver cancer	Ovarian cancer
Esophageal cancer	Prostate cancer	Skin cancer
Stomach cancer		Testicular cancer
Lung cancer		Lymphoma
Laryngeal cancer		

Mnemonic = **PROBE SLL**

Remember : – Smoking ↓ risk of Ca endometrium.
– Smoking is much more harmfull than tobacoo chewing.

So, Guys please don't adopt smoking habit as your life is valuable for others too.

5. **Ans. is a i.e. Follicular carcinoma of thyroid** *Ref. Robbins 8/e, p 1122*

Psammoma bodies are never found in follicular and medullary variant of thyroid carcinomas.

Psammoma bodies is a type of dystrophic calcification in which a necrotic cells is surrounded by layers of calcification in lamellar form.

Psammoma bodies are found in :
- **M**eningioma
- Papillary carcinoma of **T**hyroid
- **S**erous cystadenoma of ovary
- **R**enal cell carcinoma (papillary type)

Mnemonic **: M**ujhe **T**ere **S**ang **R**ehna hai

- Breast Ca
- Lung Ca
- Mesothelionas

} Rare

6. **Ans. is c i.e. Fibromatosis** *Ref. Robbins 8/e, p 1252*

Fibromatosis is a benign condition

Fibromatosis

- Fibromatosis represent a group of fibrous ***benign tumors or tumor like conditions*** and are classified into superficial and deep fibromatosis.

Superficial Fibromatosis (Palmar, Plantar and Penile Fibromatoses

- These are ***tumor like lesions*** (not true tumors) which include a group of fibrous tissue lesions that are more bothersome than serious :
  - Palmar fibromatoses (Depuytren contracture)
  - Plantar fibromatoses
  - Penile fibromatoses (Peyronie's disease)

Deep Fibromatosis (Desmoid tumors)

- Deep fibromatoses represent a ***group of benign*** but locally aggressive ***fibrous tumors***.
- *They do not metastasize and hence are not considered malignant despite their locally aggressive nature*
- They may however recur after surgical excision (due to their locally infiltrative nature).

Other options

Plasmacytoma : Malignant tumor of plasma cells

Askin tumor :
- Rare malignant neoplasm arising from chest wall of children and young adults
- It originates from primitive neuroectodermal rest and is associated with very high mortality rate

Chloromas : (Extramedullary leukaemia) are seen in AML

7. **Ans. is c i.e. T_2 N0 M0 Glottic cancer** *Ref. Harrison 17/e, p 550*

I think there is confusion between option 'c' and option 'd'

Now see

T_2 N0 M0 Glottic cancer represent Stage II disease for which treatment of choice is surgery

T_1 N_2 N0 nasopharyngeal cancer represent Stage III disease in which surgery is not possible

Concomitant chemotherapy and radiotherapy appears to be the most effective approach for locally and regionally advanced nasopharyngeal Ca *... Harrison*

8. **Ans. is a, b, d i.e. Retinoblastoma, Malignant melanoma, Choriocarcinoma**

See below

Spontaneous regression is seen in :

- **R**enal cell Carcinoma
- **R**etinoblastoma
- **C**horiocarcinoma
- **N**euroblastoma
- Malignant **M**elanoma

Mnemonic : Rahal **R**oy '**Ci** **N**ai' **M**ovei

9. **Ans. is c i.e. Excision biopsy** *Ref. Schwartz 9/e, p 415; Sabiston, 17/e, p 783 - 784*

- The pigmented lesion in this patient should be evaluated for possibility of *malignant melanoma* and hence biopsied.
- The choice of biopsy depends on the *size of the lesion* and *anatomic location.*
- Method of choice is excisional biopsy.
- In circumstances when complete excisional biopsy could not be performed, **punch biopsy** or **incisional biopsy** should be done. These conditions are :

- Large lesion whose removal would create too large defect.
- Proximity of lesion to important structures such as the eye, nose or ear.

Remember : The frequency of melanoma is rapidly increasing. Infact the rise in the rate of melanoma is highest of any cancer

10. **Ans. is a i.e. Lung** *Ref. Robbins 8/e, p 730*

"Lung is the most common site of metastasis."

Both carcinomas and sarcomas arising anywhere in the body may spread to lungs via the blood or lymphatics or by direct continuity

11. **Ans. is d i.e. Osteosarcoma** *Ref. Anderson 10/e, p 2514 - 2515*

Small round cell tumours are group of sarcomas that usually occur in children and consist of *small round 'blue' cells.* **They include :**

- Rhabdomyosarcoma
- Ewing's sarcoma
- Neuroblastoma
- Non Hodgkin lymphoma
- Occasionally wilm's tumour
- Other Primitive neuroepthelial tumours (PNET)
- Intraabdominal Desmoplastic small round cell tumours (DSRCT)
- Lymphomas (lymphoblastic lymphoma)
- Carcinoma (small cell carcinoma)
- Askins tumours (small cell tumours of thoracopulmonary region)

12. **Ans. is a i.e. Oral analgesia** *Ref. Devita 8/e, p 2771*

The WHO has devised a simple and effective method for rational titration of oral analgesia in cancer patients called the *WHO ladder.*

The ladder has follow the Three steps :

1. ***For mild to moderate pain***, one begins with acetaminophen aspirin or a nosteroidal anti-inflammatory agent (NSAID; eg. ketoprofen), with or without an adjuvant such as a glucocorticoid (dexmethasone) or antidepressant (amitriptyline).
2. When ***pain persists for or increases***, an opioid such as codeine or hydrocodone should be added (not substituted).
3. Pain that is persistent or that is ***moderate to severe*** at the outset should be abandoned. ***Adjuvants*** may be used at all steps.

The critical features of this approach are :

- Treatment is ***oral***, should be given around the clock with supplemental doses as needed to control pain, and is tailored to the individual patient.
- Transmucosal fentanyl (in lolliopop form) may aid in control of breakthrough pain.
- Records of pain control should be a prominent component of the medical record.
- When opoids are used, the patient should be placed on a prophylactic regimen to prevent constipation.

13. Ans. is a i.e. Excision of tumour *Ref. Bailey & Love 25/e, p 732*

CAROTID BODY TUMOR = CHEMODECTOMA = POTATO TUMOR

- ***Carotid body tumor is a non chromaffin paraganglioma arising from chemoreceptor on medial side of carotid body.***
- Common in people living in high *altitude* (probably due to hypoxic stimulation of carotid body); 10-15% have family history.
- Most common in 5th decade, ***M = F***
- Associated with *pheochromocytoma.*
- ***Benign*** tumor, but *metastases* is ***seen in some cases.***

Clinical feature

- Main symptom is slowly growing painless swelling at the bifurcation of common carotid artery.
- Swelling is firm, pulsatile, nontender with sidewise mobility, bruit may be present.

Diagnosis

- *Carotid angiogram* - ***Diagnostic***
- *MRI* - To know exact extent
- *Open biopsy* - ***Most specific*** but contraindicated due to risk of uncontrollable bleeding.

Treatment

- ***Surgical*** exicision is only treatment available.
- In older individual with long history the tumour may be left as such.
- In younger individuals and if growth rate is high tumour should be removed.
- Tumor is radioresistant.

Remember :

Other sites of nonchromaffin paraganglioma or chomedectomas.

- Aortic body
- Glomus jugulare (located in the adventia of jugular bulb)
- Glomus intravagale (located in the ganglion nodosum of vagus nerve)
- Paraganglion tympanicum (distributed along the tympanic branch of glosso-pharyngeal nerve).

14. Ans. is a and c i.e. Squamous cell carcinoma; and Adeno carcinoma

Ref. Bailey & Love 24/e, p 1267

Carcinoma arising from Perianal fistulae

- Colloid carcinoma.
- Adenocarcinoma *(develop from anal granular tissue).*
- Squamous cell ca *(from squamous epithelium lining the fistula).*

Index

A

B

C

D

E

F

G

H

I

J

K

L

M

U

V

W

Y